PRINCIPLES OF OSTEOARTHRITIS – ITS DEFINITION, CHARACTER, DERIVATION AND MODALITY-RELATED RECOGNITION

Edited by **Bruce M. Rothschild**

Principles of Osteoarthritis – Its Definition, Character, Derivation and Modality-Related Recognition
Edited by Bruce M. Rothschild

Published by InTech
Janeza Trdine 9, 51000 Rijeka, Croatia

Publishing Process Manager Vana Persen

Technical Editor Teodora Smiljanic

Cover Designer InTech Design Team

Additional hard copies can be obtained from orders@intechopen.com

Principles of Osteoarthritis – Its Definition, Character,
Derivation and Modality-Related Recognition, Edited by Bruce M. Rothschild
p. cm.
978-953-51-0063-8

For EU product safety concerns:
IN TECH d.o.o., Prolaz Marije Krucifikse Kozulić 3, 51000 Rijeka, Croatia,
info@intechopen.com or visit our website at intechopen.com.

Meet the editor

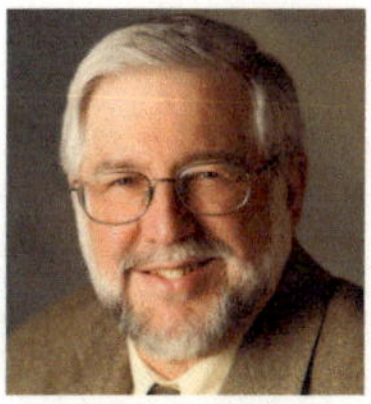

Dr. Bruce M. Rothschild is a Fellow of the American College of Physicians, American College of Rheumatology and Society of Skeletal Radiology, and was elected to the International Skeletal Society. He is recognized for his work in Rheumatology and Skeletal Pathology, where his special interests focus on clinical-anatomic-radiologic correlation and evolution, and management of arthritis. He is widely recognized for contributions to understanding radiologic manifestations of rheumatologic disease. He has published over 700 papers and abstracts, including authoritative papers on the character of bone changes with disease, and is the author of five books. Dr. Rothschild is Professor of Medicine at Northeast Ohio Medical University in Rootstown, Ohio, and Adjuvant Professor of Anthropology at the University of Kansas. He holds Research Associateships at the Carnegie Museum and the Biodiversity Institute at the University of Kansas. He was first director of the Rheumatology Division at The Chicago Medical School, and a prime force behind the resurgence of data-based paleorheumatology and comparative osseous pathology.

Contents

Preface

The inevitability of a disease sounds a clarion for its prevention, or at least its control. Understanding its pathophysiology is essential to that process. For osteoarthritis, preconceived notions and mythology must be transcended to allow identification of its essentials. The first step was to establish a scientific basis for its recognition. Sorting associated phenomenon allowed identification of those which are non-diagnostic, and one major finding which is pathognomonic: the joint osteophyte. Once that was distinguished from the asymptomatic vertebral body, osteophytes identifying spondylosis deformans, a major impediment to disease understanding, was eliminated. While animal models have been sought or manufactured to address the question, this new understanding afforded a new perspective. There is a major dichotomy between the frequency of osteoarthritis in wild-caught and captive animals. The former were seldom afflicted, while the latter commonly develop osteoarthritis. The commonality with the human condition is the artificiality of the environments that we share to varying degrees. Transformation from an arboreal to a terrestrial habitat, alteration of ground conditions, alteration of gait, and design of footwear are a few of the factors to consider.

This work is divided into sections on the basis of epidemiology, biomechanics, altered morphology and its imaging, biochemistry, immunology, genetic contributions, environmental and sports-related trauma, and quality of life. The question of primacy of cartilage or bone in the induction of osteoarthritis is reviewed, examining also the role of synovial and other extra-osseous, extra-cartilaginous tissues. Recognizing osteoarthritis and alteration in joint morphology and kinesiology and their interactions is explored.

Osteoarthritis has variably been referred to as a non-inflammatory and as an inflammatory form of arthritis. The latter perspective seems to derive from the apparent role of inflammation and immune response in wound healing. Therefore, the role of mediators of healing, inflammation, and modulators of immune response are reviewed. The role of the nervous system in development and progression of osteoarthritis is explored. Absence of certain nerve functions (e.g. position sense) leads to accelerated joint damage (a neuropathic joint), while cholinergic effectors may also contribute to joint damage.

Epidemiological studies afford the opportunity to identify possible factors which mitigate the occurrence or severity of osteoarthritis. Genetic analyses suggest possible vectors and genetic models allow the resultant hypotheses to be tested. Their use obviates the need to create artificial surgical models of disease. The inherent role of joint instability can be directly evaluated, rather than artificially produced instability. The latter perhaps directly models osteoarthritis related to trauma.

Trauma modifies tissue relationships, creating an artificial state which may itself be a major factor in development of osteoarthritis. So, too, it is with sports. Inherent in many sports activities is joint trauma, and training often includes efforts to allow the body to accept more punishment. "Work hardening" may predispose to osteoarthritis, as may injudicious training programs. Optimizing training to increase the rate and level of preparation for sports must be individed. Nonetheless, it carries risk of injury and precipitation of osteoarthritis. The resultant quality of life often reflects the care taken during those life events.

Osteoarthritis is the most common disease affecting humans. It has been suggested that the only reason the entire human population is not afflicted is because we die too soon. As life expectancy is extended, the prevalence of osteoarthritis can be expected to increase. Osteoarthritis appears to be the inevitable result of the human condition, or at least as it exists today. Understanding its nature and contributing factors may allow prevention. Redesign of walking surfaces and initiation of exercise programs oriented to maintenance of joint stability have seen reasonable recommendations to start that process. Understanding the nature and character of osteoarthritis should facilitate its control and perhaps prevention. This book specifically examines opportunities for intervention in the process. Medicinal applications are a subject for a second volume.

Dr. Bruce Rothschild
Professor of Medicine, The Northeastern Ohio Universities, College of Medicine,
Director, Arthritis Center NEO,
USA

Part 1

Overview of Osteoarthritis

1

Epidemiology and Biomechanics of Osteoarthritis

Bruce M. Rothschild and Robert J. Woods
Northeast Ohio Medical University
USA

1. Introduction

Defending the term osteoarthritis may appear unusual to many who study skeletal anatomy. Often referred to as degenerative joint disease in early studies, recognition of the hyperactive nature of the involved tissues led to discarding that designation (Moskowitz et al, 1984). In keeping with contemporary usage, our terminology will designate the condition, osteoarthritis. While the suffix "itis" is used, this is not meant to designate the presence of inflammation. While a controversy has raged whether the term osteoarthrosis is a better designation (and it probably is), contemporary usage supports use of the term osteoarthritis (Rothschild & Martin, 2006). Arthritis implies inflammation of a diarthrodial (synovial membrane-lined) joint, yet in osteoarthritis (as in the majority of the 100+ varieties of arthritis) there is negligible inflammation (Rothschild, 1982; Resnick, 2002). Any associated inflammation actually appears to be related to complications (of osteoarthritis) (Altman & Gray, 1985; Dieppe & Watt, 1985; Gibilisco et al., 1985; Lally et al., 1989; Schumacher et al., 1977). Such complications are usually crystalline in nature: Hydroxyapatite, calcium pyrophosphate, or urate (gout) crystals.

The primary sites of tissue injury in osteoarthritis are the cartilage of the joint and the subchondral bone, directly underlying and supporting it (Resnick, 2002). This gives rise to microfractures (Acheson et al., 1976; Layton et al., 1988) and proliferation of new bone at the periphery of the cartilage, forming a spur. The microfractures are accompanied by a healing process that increases the density of the bone just under the cartilage surface, resulting in subchondral sclerosis. Subchondral, in this usage, refers to that component of cortical bone located just under the articular cartilage of the metaphysis. In osteoarthritis, overgrowth of bone occurs, but not bone resorption. Those overgrowths are called osteophytes.

Although osteoarthritis was though to be common in prehistory, its identification in a 150 million years old (Jurassic) pliosaur (Jurmain, 1977) actually represents a different disorder sharing only characteristics determined by semantics (Rothschild, 1989; Rothschild & Martin, 2006). Spinal involvement with osteophyte formation, so common in dinosaurs and marine reptiles (e.g., pliosaurs) actually represents a very different phenomena (spondylosis deformans). The presence of osteophytes in osteoarthritis and spondylosis deformans defines overgrowth of joint and disc marginal bone, respectively. Although the term osteophyte is used for both, they appear to represent quite different pathophysiologies. Osteoarthritis represents a disease of diarthrodial joints (those articulating bones at which movement takes place and which are lined by a synovial membranes) (Resnick, 2002;

Rothschild, 1982; Rothschild & Martin, 2006). Spondylosis deformans involves a disc space, not a "joint." (Without a joint, it is difficult to diagnose arthritis). Spinal osteophytes are essentially an asymptomatic phenomena (Rothschild, 1989). Osteoarthritis, on the other hand, clearly is a disorder of joints characterized by morbidity (Moskowitz et al, 1984). Diarthrodial joint osteophytes, though diagnostic for osteoarthritis (Altman et al., 1986, 1990, 1991) must be distinguished from enthesiophytes. The latter represent calcification of sites of tendon, ligament or joint capsule insertion (Resnick, 2002; Rothschild & Martin, 2006). Calcific tendonitis can result from trauma, genetic, or metabolic phenomenon (Holt & Keats, 1993). While related bone divots have been considered erosions, they actually appear to represent tendon avulsions (Shaibani et al., 1993). Neither avulsions nor enthesiophytes are related to osteoarthritis.

Full loss of the cartilaginous joint surface in severe osteoarthritis allows bone to rub on bone. The articular surface becomes polished and sometimes even grooved, a process called eburnation. That process occurs whenever cartilage loss in an area is at least focally complete, independent of etiology. It is not diagnostic of osteoarthritis. Eburnation occurring in the course of another disease sometimes is referred to as secondary osteoarthritis, but that represents semantics. The disease, not osteoarthritis, caused the damage (in secondary osteoarthritis). Referring to eburnation simply as a sign of severe osteoarthritis would therefore appear misleading. Eburnation is simply evidence that cartilage destruction was so severe as to allow bone to rub on bone.

1.1 Pathophysiology of osteoarthritis

The congruence of articular surfaces is essential in reducing the frictional component of joint movement. It allows the formation of a boundary layer of surface lubrication, which is quite efficient not only in facilitating motion, but also in generating the fluid waves necessary to provide nutrition to the avascular cartilage. Impaired cartilage nutrition, secondary to loss of congruence or exposure to toxins, results in impairment of chondrocyte metabolism, which in turn leads to inefficient production of mucopolysaccharide ground substance. The ground substance is highly hygroscopic and allows the turgor necessary to maintain resilience and congruence. Because the ground substance is contained by the meshwork of collagen fibrils, any disruption of the fibrils, by trauma, inflammation, intrinsic metabolic defects, or toxic agents, will deleteriously affect the turgor and congruence of the cartilage and contribute to its destructive process. Elasticity of bone is essential in protecting cartilage. Trauma may also produce microfractures and/or remodeling resulting in less bone elasticity (Acheson et al., 1976; Layton et al., 1988). The bone is then less able to distribute the stresses of daily microtrauma, increasing their transmission to the cartilage. As the cartilage serves more for congruence and the bone for shock absorption, stiffening of the bone transfers stresses to the cartilage component, which is not designed to withstand it.

Excessive weight (obesity) has been suggested as a factor in the development of osteoarthritis in humans (Goldin et al., 1976; Leach et al., 1973; Silberberg & Silberberg, 1960; Sokoloff et al., 1960; Saville & Dickson, 1968), but the opposite was found in birds (Rothschild & Panza, 2006a,b). Mechanical disadvantage (e.g., joint instability) appears to be the more important variable influencing the development of osteoarthritis (Jurmain, 1977; Rothschild & Martin, 2006). The role of joint stability is emphasized by the occurrence of osteoarthritis in 80% of humans with severe instability, versus only 30% with slight or moderate (O'Donoghue et al., 1971). The construction of the joint appears to be a major factor. Highly stabilized joints appear to be protected (Harrison et al., 1953; Puranen et al., 1975). For example, the human ankle, when ligamentous structures are intact and joint congruity is maintained, is rarely affected by osteoarthritis, even with overuse (Cassou et al., 1981; Funk, 1976). On the other hand, the human knee, the most complicated and least constrained joint (Radin, 1978), is the most susceptible to the development of osteoarthritis.

There apparently has been selection against development of osteoarthritis, probably when the vertebrate skeleton was first developing. This selection can be observed in the properties of the anatomical and morphological features adapted to maintain the joint (e.g., articular cartilage, subchondral bone, synovial fluid, specific mechanical design). Osteoarthritis provides important (otherwise often inaccessible) clues to structure-function relationships (Jurmain, 1977; Silberberg & Silberberg, 1960; Woods, 1986, 1995). Therefore, a logical method of assessing the factors which can contribute to osteoarthritis development is to analyze the basic joint features, and to use the maintenance properties of the features as indicators of the factors of joint damage.

1.2 Biomechanics of osteoarthritis

Synovial joints are much more complex than the mechanical bearings (i.e., ball-and-socket, hinge, and cochlear joints) which are often used as explanatory analogies. As physical mechanisms, they are, however, subject to the same basic principles of static and dynamic force distribution and transmission. In order to further understand the role of these basic mechanical influences in the development of osteoarthritis, several factors must be investigated:

1. The contribution of the functional anatomy of the joint to the magnitude, rate, and duration of joint forces.
2. The effects of contact area on the distribution and transmission of those forces.
3. The resulting patterns of osteoarthritis which can develop from the interaction of functional forces and the biomechanical design of specific joints.

Although the anatomy of a quadrupedal and bipedal locomotor system is nearly identical, the morphological differences have produced a transition of mechanical function of certain muscle groups (Jenkins, 1972; Kummer, 1975; Lovejoy, 1975; Sigmon, 1975). The reorientation of the line of action of muscles (through skeletal morphology changes) suggests alterations in the concentrated areas of force transmission and the joint reaction force magnitudes between the two systems. A priori, a different topographic pattern of osteoarthritis would be anticipated among the species. Human and ape patterns are discussed below.

1.2.1 Biomechanics of the hip

In order to understand the resultant forces acting on the hip joint during the normal walking cycle, it is necessary to review the action of the musculature which produces the forces (Seedhom & Wright, 1981). The bipedal walking cycle consists of the heel-strike, foot-flat position, toe-off, and subsequent heel strike of the other foot (Fig. 1). During this cycle the limb completes a stance phase and a swing phase. The stance phase includes 60% of the walking cycle. During the stance phase (the period when the foot is in contact with the ground surface), the foot goes from heel-strike, to foot-flat, to toe-off. The swing phase includes 40% of the walking cycle. During the swing phase (the period when the limb is swinging forward), the foot goes from toe-off to heel-strike. At the end of the stance phase is a period of double support, when both feet are in contact with the ground surface. As the rate of walking increases, this period becomes shorter in duration. As a walk changes to a run, there is no longer a period of double support (Lovejoy, 1973).

Muscular load sharing during the walking cycle, can alternatively be derived through the study of muscle groups, correlated with mathematical models of torque about the hip joint (Seireg & Arvikar, 1975; Sorbie & Zalter, 1965). The action of the musculoskeletal system in producing bipedal locomotion should, if it is to be understood thoroughly, be studied as an interacting system involving the entire postcranial organism. In view of the specific interest in joint reaction force, discussion of the action of various muscle groups will be focused on the associated joints.

During normal level walking, the forces on the hip joint have been described as quasi-static, and thus have mainly been treated as the resultants of a progression of static postures at successive intervals (Seireg & Arvikar, 1975). At faster rates of walking, other factors of dynamics (e.g., inertia forces/moments) can be calculated from the linear and angular accelerations identified for each body segment.

The hip joint reaction force has two significant peaks of magnitude. The larger peak, with a magnitude of about seven times body weight, occurs at about 55% of the cycle, just prior to toe-off. While the rate of application of this force is rapid, its actual time of application represents a period extending from 45% to 70% of the cycle. Associated with this peak force is the firing of the hip flexors, the adductors, and to a lesser extent, the gluteus maximus and hamstring group. The hip flexors, mainly the ilio-psoas and rectus femoris, fire concentrically (about 45% to 70% of the cycle), initiating swing-through and raising the thigh. The adductors, primarily the posterior group, also act as hip flexors, firing concentrically from 45% to about 75% of the cycle. The gluteus maximus fires concentrically at a low magnitude from 45% to about 70% of the cycle, and serves to prevent horizontal rotation (due to the force of toe-off by the opposite limb) of the pelvis about the stance hip. The hamstring group (which also crosses the hip joint and contributes to the hip joint reaction force) fires concentrically at low magnitude from 45% to about 70% of the cycle, also facilitating knee flexion.

The other peak hip joint reaction force, with a magnitude of about four times body weight, occurs at about 10% of the cycle, just after heel-strike. The rate of application is very rapid, with duration from 0% (heel-strike), to about 25% of the cycle. Associated with this peak force is the firing of the hamstring group, the gluteus maximus, the ilio-psoas, the abductors and the adductors. The hamstring group fires eccentrically from 90% to about 20% of the cycle (from just before heel-strike to just afterward). This action decelerates the forward swinging limb and counteracts the forward and downward momentum of the trunk and pelvis, as the body weight shifts to the other limb. In conjunction with the hamstring group, the gluteus maximus fires eccentrically, controlling the forward rotation of the trunk and pelvis about the hip joint at heel-strike. The ilio-psoas fires eccentrically at low magnitude, from 95% to about 10% of the cycle. It produces stability at the hip joint, counterbalancing the hip effect of the hamstrings (while decelerating the thigh just before heel-strike).

The abductor group, a major contributor to hip joint reaction force, fires concentrically from 90% to 40% of the cycle (just before heel-strike and well into stance phase). This action counteracts the downward gravitational list of the trunk about the hip joint, limiting it to about 4 degrees (Lovejoy, 1973). The adductors fire from 90% to 20% of the cycle, and act as stabilizers of the forces of heel-strike. The anteriorly arising muscles fire eccentrically, while the posteriorly arising muscles fire concentrically during this period. Three-dimensional representation, of the magnitude and direction of the resultant hip joint force throughout the walking cycle (Seireg & Arvikar, 1975), reveals that the force vectors transmit through the joint at a relatively concentrated area on the most superior portion of the femoral head.

1.2.1.1 Hip joint contact areas

During the walking cycle, the entire available cartilage surface on the acetabulum (with the exception of the dome) comes into contact with the femoral head (Greenwald & Haynes, 1972; Greenwald & O'Connor, 1971). However, femoral head cartilage does not share the same fate. The peripheral inferior and peri-foveal regions of femoral head cartilage come into contact with the acetabulum only during the extremes of the walking cycle. As the range of motion during walking is small (about 35-40 degrees) (Nordin & Frankel, 1980a), this area is infrequently compressed. An alternative approach to assessment of contact areas is supported by analysis of femoral trabecularization patterns. X-ray examination reveals that these trabecular "rays" pass through the femoral neck toward the anteriosuperior and posterosuperior regions of the femoral head (identifying the areas of contact) (Harrison et al, 1953; Trueta, 1968).

Although the acetabulum and femoral head appear to be spherical in outline with congruent surfaces, cross-sectional examination of hip joints reveals subtle incongruencies (Day et al., 1975; Greenwald & O'Connor, 1971; Kempson et al., 1971). The acetabulum has its thickest cartilage at the periphery, becoming progressively thinner in the area of the superior dome. The femoral head has its thickest cartilage at the center, just superior to the fovea capitus, becoming progressively thinner towards the periphery (Kempson et al., 1971; Day et al., 1975). The area in the superior dome of the acetabulum has been identified as only coming into contact under extreme joint loads (Day et al., 1975; Greenwald & Haynes, 1972; Greenwald & O'Connor, 1971), a phenomena which requires (according to load-deflection curves) a load of three to four times body weight.

An advantage to this incongruity has been suggested by Bullough and associates (1973). If the methods of cartilage lubrication are contemplated, it is apparent that an area of high stress, such as the dome, is much in need of adequate amounts of synovial fluid. Suggesting that the cartilage is wetted through a sump action, they propose that a joint of perfect congruity would restrict circulation of synovial fluid within the dome area, producing malnourished cartilage.

Analyzing the hip joint reaction force, clarifies that the concentrated area of force transmission [found by Seireg & Arvikar (1975)] corresponds to the incongruent superior dome of the acetabulum. In the walking cycle, the supporting leg is in full extension at the time of the major force peak. Given that the reaction force is transmitted through a concentrated area on the most superior aspect of the femoral head, the corresponding area of force transmission on the acetabulum would be the anterior portion of the dome. The smaller peak reaction force would likewise be transmitted through the posterior portion of the dome when the leg is in flexion.

1.2.1.2 Anatomical distribution of osteoarthritis in the human hip

The highest concentration of osteoarthritis in the human femoral head is just superior to the fovea capitus (Wood, 1986), in the area of the acetabular notch (an area of habitual non-contact of articular surfaces during gait). Areas of habitual non-contact develop malnourished cartilage (with depleted mechanical properties, similar to cartilage of older individuals) rendering such an area more susceptible to damage (Sokoloff, 1969). The area superior to the fovea is under high magnitude stress during contact, thus the resulting quantitative increase in osteoarthritis sequelae. The area of least quantifiable osteoarthritis (the upper half of the femoral head) is the area which is in constant contact with another articulating surface during gait. This supports the contention that regular, but variable pressure application maintains healthy articular cartilage in the presence of normal joint motion.

1.2.1.3 Anatomical distribution of osteoarthritis in the great ape hip

The pattern of osteoarthritis in the gorilla hip, are mild and distributed over most of the articulation, although more concentrated in the distinctly larger anterior horn area (Woods, 1986). The gorilla manifests a concentration around the periphery of the notch, which is not as pronounced in the chimpanzee. The femoral heads display a striking difference, compared to the acetabulae. Osteoarthritis in the gorilla femoral head presents as a highly concentrated band, lacking in the chimpanzee. Disregarding the dense band in the gorilla, the femoral heads of both gorillas and chimpanzees are practically void of disease. Trueta (1968) suggests that, theoretically, osteoarthritis of the hip should not be the problem for quadrupeds that it is for humans. This is based on the contention that the weight-bearing area, unlike that of humans, is continuously moved over the entire surface of the hip articulation during locomotion due to the larger range of motion.

The femoral head of a quadrapedal animal probably has more of its total surface involved as a regular contact area, and unlike that of humans, possesses healthy articular cartilage. The band of osteoarthritis in the gorilla femoral head is so common and severe, yet unseen in the chimpanzee, that a fundamental difference in anatomy and/or behavior is suggested. When the gorilla hip joint is rotated and articulated to simulate hip flexion (the common quadrupedal posture) the band lies over the acetabular notch. Two factors may be responsible. The gorilla is much less active than the chimpanzee, spending most of its time in a position of hip flexion. It is possible that the band of osteoarthritis is in a relatively malnourished cartilage area (due to lack of contact), which is therefore less able to tolerate the high stresses generated when the animal does move. The design of the acetabulum in both the gorilla and chimpanzee hip provides a distinctly larger anterior surface area, which better accommodates high magnitude joint forces. The force of forward propulsion is directed anteriorly into this enlarged dome of the acetabulum (Kummer, 1975). Secondly, the ligamentum teres of the chimpanzee runs from the fovea capitus femoris and divides in two, where it combines with the transverse acetabular ligament and inserts into the acetabular notch, just as in humans (Sonntag, 1923). However, the ligamentum teres of the gorilla runs from the fovea capitus femoris, into the acetabular notch and posteriorly along the joint capsule at the posterior horn of the acetabulum. It passes through the gemellus inferior and quadratus femoris, where it branches out and finally inserts into the innominate (Gregory, 1950). It is possible that this larger type of ligamentum teres applies pressure (i.e. mechanical force) to the joint capsule area which is not a factor in the anatomy of humans or chimpanzees. Action of the gemellus inferior and quadratus femoris could possibly aggravate condition.

1.2.2 Biomechanics of the knee

The knee is a two-joint structure consisting of the distal femur, patella and proximal tibia. The tibiofemoral articulation provides the primary motion of the joint, while the patellofemoral articulation serves to increase the contact area and give mechanical advantage to the quadriceps femoris muscle group. Motion in the knee joint is mainly in the sagittal plane, allowing approximately 140 degrees of flexion. However, only 67 degrees of flexion are actually utilized in the normal walking cycle (Nordin & Frankel, 1980b). The knee is actually quite a complex joint. While often thought of as a hinge joint, its motion actually encompasses a significant rotary or geocentric component. Transverse or rotary motion of up to 45 degrees of external rotation and 30 degrees of internal rotation is found in the knee. Motion in the coronal plane is restrained by ligaments and soft tissue.

The impetus of forward progression begins approximately 45% into the walking cycle (Fig. 1), just prior to toe-off, when the quadriceps group fires concentrically (producing knee extension at toe-off). Facilitation of knee extension by the tensor fascia lata lasts until just after toe-off. Gastrocnemius firing initiates just prior to quadriceps concentric firing and lasts until toe-off. Concentric muscle contraction from 30% to 60% into the cycle produces plantar flexion of the ankle joint. As it is a two-joint muscle, it also produces knee flexion. Conjoined action of the gastrocnemius and quadriceps produces stability of the knee during the high stress periods. The action of these muscles is associated with a peak joint reaction force magnitude equivalent to three (Morrison, 1970) to seven times body weight (Seireg & Arvikar, 1975). The rate of application is moderate and the duration is from about 30% to 60% of the cycle.

A second period of peak muscular action at the knee relates to heel strike. The quadriceps femoris fires eccentrically, from approximately 95% to 20% of the cycle (just prior until just after heel-strike). At heel-strike the knee "lock" is broken. Eccentric quadriceps firing then absorbs the vertical forces attempting to buckle the knee. During this same interval (90% to 20% of the cycle), the hamstring group fires eccentrically (thus decelerating the forward moving thigh. These actions are associated with peak joint reaction force magnitude of three (Morrison, 1970) to six times body weight (Seireg & Arvikar, 1975). The rate of application is rapid, representing 90% to 20% of the cycle.

1.2.2.1 Knee joint contact areas

During bipedal progression, the knee is habitually in a more extended position, due to the narrow range of flexion and extension necessary for walking. Static analysis of the knee joint reaction force has shown that it is transmitted through the tibiofemoral articulation approximately centered up the axis of the tibial shaft (Nordin & Frankel, 1980b). The distal femoral condyles must transmit up to seven times body weight (Seireg & Arvikar, 1975), and the knee has adapted to give maximum cartilage contact to this area by flattening the condyles (Heiple & Lovejoy, 1971; Kettlekamp & Jacobs, 1972; Maquet et al., 1975; Walker & Hajek, 1972). When viewed laterally, the long axis of the condyle is about 90 degrees to the vertical shaft, indicating that the largest true contact takes place during full extension, when the contact surface is perpendicular to the stresses passing through the joint (Heiple & Lovejoy, 1971; Lovejoy, 1973).

Studies to determine actual weight bearing areas and stress distribution at different degrees of flexion have focused mainly on the role of the menisci in force transmission. The menisci are two C-shaped fibrocartilages overlying the tibial condyles and anchored firmly in the intercondylar area. Their inferior surface is flat and flush with the tibial articular surface, while their superior surface is thick at the periphery and gets increasingly thinner toward the center, exposing the more central articular cartilage. The articular cartilage of the tibial condyles is thickest at this exposed area (McLeod et al., 1977; Simon, 1970).

Poisson's principle appears directly applicable to the menisci: When an object undergoes vertical strain, it also undergoes a proportionate horizontal expansion (Shrive et al., 1978). As the spherical condyles compress the menisci, they impart vertical and horizontal components of force. Since the base of the menisci is flat, it can only resist the vertical component, leaving the horizontal component to displace the menisci outwards. The fibers of the menisci course circumferentially around the periphery. Their tensile strength limits the amount of displacement possible, under an applied load (Shrive et al., 1978). The displacement on the medial side is also restricted by the peripheral attachment to the meniscofemoral and meniscotibial ligaments (Fukubayashi & Kurosawa, 1980). This allows a simple mechanism for increased contact area. As the menisci displace in different directions, contact is maximized throughout flexion, in spite of changes in geometry of the articulating portions of the femoral condyles. This changing condylar geometry results in a contact area during full extension distributed anterio-posteriorly, compared to medio-laterally during full flexion (Shrive et al., 1978).

Throughout increasing flexion, the contact area gets increasingly smaller, and the stress therefore becomes increasingly concentrated and moves posteriorly. External and internal rotation cause the contact area to move laterally, relative to the direction of rotation (Ahmed & Burke, 1983).

During the two peak periods of joint reaction force, the knee joint is in full extension or just slightly flexed. These positions correspond with the periods when contact area is the greatest. The result is a minimization of load per unit area. Activities which place the knee into a much higher degree of flexion (e.g., climbing stairs or stooping to lift an object) produce much higher joint reaction forces (Nordin & Frankel, 1980b). The result of such activity is a very high load per unit area, transmitted at the very posterior aspect of the articulating surfaces.

During dynamic activities it has been shown that the patellofemoral joint reaction force is a consequence of the magnitude of the quadriceps muscle, which has been shown to increase as flexion increases (Nordin & Frankel, 1980b). The patellofemoral joint reaction force is only one-half body weight (Nordin & Frankel, 1980b) at the middle of stance phase.

The retropatellar articular surface has three facets. Corresponding to the lateral and medial walls of the femoral surface are lateral and medial facets on the patella. The third facet runs adjacent to the most inferior aspect of the medial facet. Rarely described and difficult to observe outside of cadaveric material (although quite distinct on the macerated patellae of robust individuals), the third facet is referred to as the "odd medial facet" (Goodfellow et al., 1976). This facet does not come into contact until extreme degrees of flexion.

Patellofemoral contact areas have been identified on the basis of dye methodology (Goodfellow et al., 1976), radiographic techniques (Matthews et al., 1977), and from pressure transducer measurements in cadaveric specimens (Ahmed et al., 1983). Pressure distribution is transmitted through the vertical ridge separating the lateral and medial facets (Ahmed et al., 1983) during low degrees of flexion (from 0 to 10 degrees). From 20 to 40 degrees of flexion, the contact area was found to change to a horizontally oriented band along the inferior portion of the articulation. From 45 to 75 degrees of flexion, the contact area was a horizontal band in the central area of the articulation. From 75 to 90 degrees, the contact area was found to be a horizontal band across the superior portion of the articulation. The bands of contact area do not extend into the odd medial facet until 110 degrees of flexion is achieved (Goodfellow et al., 1976; Ahmed et al., 1983). Beyond 110 degrees of flexion, the band begins to divide into two areas of contact: Lateral and slightly superior and on the odd medial facet. It should be noted that the knee comes into this high of a degree of flexion only during extreme activities. When the knee is in extreme flexion, the patella rotates slightly. The odd medial facet then comes into contact with the medial femoral condyle. During extreme flexion, the majority of the patella has recessed into the intercondylar notch. The quadriceps tendon then lies over the synovial membrane and joint capsule at the superior portion of the patellar surface of the femur.

1.2.2.2 Anatomical distribution of osteoarthritis in the human knee

The distal femoral concentrations conform very well to the relative joint reaction force magnitudes established for the joint. The femoral condyles show a marked osteoarthritis, compared with the patellofemoral area, in accordance with the relative joint reaction forces transmitted by each area (Woods, 1986). The posterior most portion of the femoral condyles experience the highest load per unit area and have the highest concentrations of osteoarthritis. Osteoarthritis was prominent in the areas found to transmit the highest load per unit area (the most posterior portions of each side, underlying the menisci).

The patella displays greater osteoarthritis than the opposing surface on the femur, especially on the odd medial facet, in accordance with the contention that this is a site of habitual non-contact and cartilage malnutrition. Damage apparently occurs during periods of extreme flexion and high joint reaction force, when this area does come into contact.

1.2.2.3 Anatomical distribution of osteoarthritis in the great ape knee

The distal femur of gorillas and chimpanzees presents the converse concentration pattern from that noted in human knees. The patellofemoral area, especially in the chimpanzee, displays greater osteoarthritis than the tibiofemoral area (Woods, 1986). The quadriceps femoris subjects the quadrupedal patellofemoral articulation to high joint reaction forces, in spite of existing morphological differences exist between bipedal and quadrupedal knee joints. The patellofemoral joint reaction force of the gorilla and chimpanzee increases with the degree of flexion, as occurs in the human knee. During the locomotory cycle, and in common postural positions, the gorilla and chimpanzee knees are habitually flexed. Relative to the bipedal knee, the quadrupedal knee is therefore subjected to more frequent applications of a high patellofemoral joint reaction force.

Gorilla and chimpanzee femoral condyles, viewed laterally, have a distinctly rounded contour (Heiple & Lovejoy, 1971; Lovejoy, 1975; Lovejoy & Heiple, 1970). The human distal femur has an elliptical contour, providing maximum contact and minimizing loads during full extension, whereas quadrupedal tibiofemoral articulation loading occurs throughout a larger range of motion. The rounded contour in gorillas and chimpanzees results in a loading condition where high magnitude forces are not concentrated on any specific area. This may explain the contrasting reduction of tibiofemoral osteoarthritis in the gorilla and chimpanzee (relative to the human distal femur, which has a distinctly higher concentration in the tibiofemoral area than the patellofemoral area).

The gorilla distal femur does not display quite the contrast seen in chimpanzees. This may be related to the gorilla's massive size, resulting in extreme tibiofemoral articulation applied forces/surface area. The gorilla species may be nearing the size limit for this type of knee design to be effective. Considering the degree of flexion and extension involved in gorilla locomotion, they may be reaching the limits of the design capabilities of their joints for their body size. (The larger the animal, the lesser the amount of joint excursion).

The chimpanzee distal femur has a quite highly concentrated band of osteoarthritis across the most superior portion of the patellar surface. The high concentration and position of this band suggests that malnourished cartilage may also be involved. The patella retreats toward the intercondylar notch as the joint reaction force increases (when the knee is in a high degree of flexion). The superior portion of the articulation is probably only in contact during extension, predisposing to a malnourished state. The lateral condyle of the chimpanzee also has a high concentration on the most posterior portion. This is probably due to the amount of time spent in a flexed posture, when forces would be concentrated on this area.

Unlike the proximal tibia of humans, the gorilla and chimpanzee proximal tibiae do not display the posterior osteoarthritis associated with high magnitude stress application. The distribution is more generalized, as would be expected from a more distributed load application.

1.2.3 Biomechanics of the ankle joint

The ankle is actually composed of two joints, the tibiotalar and subtalar joints. Motion in the tibiotalar joint is primarily in the saggital plane. Inversion and eversion occur at the subtalar joint (Alexander et al., 1982). The latter is important for ambulation on uneven ground. The total range of saggital motion, estimated at about 45 degrees, varies greatly with age (Alexander et al., 1982). Estimates of the range of plantar flexion (20 degrees) and dorsiflexion (25 degrees) of the tibiotalar joint (Barnett & Napier, 1952; Close, 1956; Stauffer et al., 1977) have been compromised by the arbitrary division between the two, resulting in a relatively large standard deviation (Sammarco et al., 1973; Stauffer et al., 1977).

1.2.3.1 Ankle joint contact areas

The weight-bearing contact area of the ankle joint is primarily tibiotalar. Ramsey and Hamilton (1976) studied the contact area of the ankle joint and found that the primary contact and weight bearing area is along the lateral side of the main talar surface, with a band of contact extending medially across the apex of the talar articulation. Damage to the ankle ligaments results in deviation of the primary contact area to the medial side of the main talar surface. A role of the fibulotalar joint in weight-bearing has been suggested (Lambert, 1971) but awaits clarification. The notably large contact area of the ankle joint makes it particularly tolerable of compressive forces (Stauffer et al., 1977). Studies of the instant centers of joint rotation (Sammarco et al., 1973) indicate that shear forces are highest during stance phase, but are not of a significant magnitude.

Plantar flexion during the stance phase of the walking cycle is the resultant of post-tibial group muscle concentric firing, representing 10% to 60% of the cycle (early foot-flat to toe-off). Maximum muscle force magnitude (five times body weight) occurs at approximately 45% into the cycle. This major peak of joint reaction force is moderate in rate of application, lasting from about 20% to 60% of the cycle.

1.2.3.2 Anatomical distribution of osteoarthritis in the ankle of humans

The talus shows prominent osteoarthritis at areas where contact is irregular (Woods, 1986). The corners of the main weight-bearing portion of the articulation and the malleolar articulations are opposed by areas of the distal tibia, which are frequently irregular in shape and without a complete articular surface. The distal tibia is notably void of high concentrations of osteoarthritis, except at the anterior and posterior edges (perhaps related to ligamentous damage).

1.2.3.3 Anatomical distribution of osteoarthritis in the great ape ankle

Almost negligible osteoarthritis was found in the ankle joints of the gorilla and chimpanzee (Woods, 1986). Greater range of motion during locomotion in the apes (distributing load application over a larger area) probably explains this lesser involvement.

2. Epidemiology of osteoarthritis

2.1 Understanding the anthropologic record

The critical studies by Altman et al (1986, 1990, 1991) clearly established the importance of the osteophyte for identification of osteoarthritis. Much of the anthropology literature has lumped a variety of forms of joint pathology as osteoarthritis (Bridges, 1991; Waldron, 1991), predicating their diagnoses on presumptive criteria, such as eburnation (discussed above), porosity and other joint surface disruption and any new bone formation in the vicinity of a joint. Pitting (porosity) has no correlation in clinical practice (Resnick 2002). It is not visualized on x-ray. When critically examined in knees (Rothschild, 1997), there was no correlation of porosity (pitting) with the documented unequivocal sign of osteoarthritis (diarthrodial joint osteophytes).

Comparing frequencies of osteoarthritis must be based on age and gender-based cohorts, as osteoarthritis is a phenomenon of aging (Rothschild, 1982; Resnick, 2002). It is more common in men than in women prior to age 45 and in women than in men after age 55 (Moskowitz et al., 1984). As the relateionship of osteoarthritis to age appears independent of socioeconomic status, at least in the United States and Great Britain (Davis, 1988), such cohorts should be comparable. Bremner et al. (1968) suggested that osteoarthritis is found less frequently as one travels farther from the equator. Blumberg et al. (1961) reported lower frequencies in Inuit and Lawrence et al. (1963) in Finland (versus Netherlands).

However, the frequency of osteoarthritis is equal in Jamaica and Great Britain (Bremner et al., 1968). Variations in race, culture, and environment, however, limit such comparisons. Prevalence and distribution of osteoarthritis vary with ethnicity and geography [Table 1 (Davis, 1988)]. Southern Chinese, South African Blacks and East Indians have a lower incidence of hip osteoarthritis than European or American Caucasians (Felson, 1988; Hoaglund et al., 1973; Mukhopadhaya & Barooah, 1967; Solomon et al., 1975). Amerindians had earlier onset and higher frequencies of osteoarthritis than other United States populations, in contrast to Inuit, in whom the frequency was lower.

Osteoarthritis should also be divided into primary and secondary. Secondary includes that due to an injury, another form of arthritis or a congenital predisposition. When osteoarthritis of the hip is common in a population, its occurrence is often considered secondary to acetabular dysplasia (Felson, 1988; Gofton, 1971; Murray, 1965; Solomon, 1976).

The genetics of osteoarthritis is beyond the scope of this discussion. Familial occurrence of distal and proximal interphalangeal joint osteoarthritis (Stecher, 1961) and role of gene polymorphism (e.g., Type III procollagen gene COL2A1) (Knowlton, et al., 1990) exemplify the challenge. COL2A1 mutation results in spondyloepiphyseal dysplasia congenital. Thus suggesting that the resultant osteoarthritis is actually not primary, but caused by the change in joint shape. How much apparent geographic variation is genetic in origin? The genetics of osteoarthritis is delegated to articles specifically addressing this developing knowledge.

Joint Affected-Gender	Locale /Percent affected by age	30	40	50	60	70	80
1st carpal-metacarpal-M	Goteborg, Sweden					27	52
	Zoetermeer Holland	1	3	5	18	18-22	30-42
	Leigh/Wensleydale, England	1	3	5	12	35	
	Kamitonda, Japan	1	1	5	5	18	30
	Twswana, South Africa	1	3	5	8		
	Tsikundamalema, South Africa	1	3	2	15		
1st carpal-metacarpal-F	Goteborg, Sweden					28	54
	Zoetermeer, Holland	1	3	14	22	29-45	48-55
	Leigh/Wensleydale, England	1	3	8	20	50	
	Kamitonda, Japan	1	1	4	12	12	20
	Tswana, South Africa	1	3	4	1	10	
	Tsikundamalema, South Africa	1	3	2	1	1	
Interphalangeal (hands) M	Goteborg, Sweden					75	77
	Zoetermeer, Holland		8	15	50	47-55	65-71
	Sofia, Bulgaria		3	7	10	14	
	Leigh/Wensleydale, England		10	25	30	55	60
	Tswana, South Africa		3	12	20	55	
	Tsikundamalema, South Africa		25		75	80	
	Hong Kong				24		
	Kamitonda, Japan		10	15	50	72	75
	United States – Caucasian/Black		7	18	32-57	71-78	79
	-- Blackfeet/Pima Amerindians		45	80-90		98-100	
Interphalangeal (hands) F	Goteborg, Sweden					86	86
	Zoetermeer Holland		10	40	75	66-72	72-76
	Sofia, Bulgaria		5	12	14	21	
	Leigh/Wensleydale, England		8	20	50	77	
	Tswana, South Africa		5	7	40	65	
	Tsikundamalema, South Africa		40	55	65	75	
	Hong Kong				35		
	Kamitonda, Japan		8	20	50	75	85
	United States – Caucasian/Black		6		25-65	49-69	88
	-- Blackfeet/Pima Amerindians		45	55	80	92-97	
Knee - M	Goteborg, Sweden						33
	Malmo, Sweden		0	3	5	5	5
	Zoetermeer, Holland			9	17	21	22
	Sofia, Bulgaria	3	4	7	10	10	

Joint Affected-Gender	Locale /Percent affected by age	30	40	50	60	70	80
	Northern England		7	12	29	42	
	South Africa/Greenland		40/34				
	Hong Kong				5		
	Framingham, Massachussetts, United States					31	31
	NHANES, United States	0	2	2	4	8	
Knee - F	Goteborg, Sweden						45
	Malmo, Sweden		7	4	11	27	36
	Zoetermeer, Holland			14	19	35	44
	Sofia, Bulgaria	2	5	10	11	10	
	Northern England		6	17	49	56	
	South Africa/Greenland		28/26				
	Hong Kong				13		
	Framingham, Massachussetts, United States					31	42
	NHANES, United States	0	2	4	7	18	

Table 1. Frequency of osteoarthritis as a function of joint affected, locale, age and gender, from Bagge et al (1992), Butler (1988), Felso (1988), Hoaglund (1973), van Saase (1989).

2.2 Joint distribution of human osteoarthritis

Hip osteoarthritis is more common in farmers than in other vocations (Peyron, 1984). Van Saase et al. (1989) suggested 2.5-4.8% of Zoetermeer men aged 45-74 had osteoarthritis of the shoulder and 10% after age 80. This contrasts with 1.4-7.7% of women in the former age group and 11.1% in the latter.

The shoulders, hips, and knees are especially affected in miners, contrasted with fingers, elbows, and knees in dockworkers (Partridge, 1968), and fingers in cotton workers (Lawrence, 1961). Hand involvement was greater in craftsmen, miners, and construction workers (Davis, 1988), and osteoarthritis of the knee in individuals involved in occupations demanding knee flexion (Anderson & Felson, 1986), but also had geographic variation, more common in Japanese and Korean than Caucasian women (Bang et al., 2011; Toba et al., 2006).

The wrist is uncommonly affected in osteoarthritis. Much of what has been called osteoarthritis of the wrist may actually be another disorder, calcium pyrophosphate deposition disease (Rothschild & Martin, 2006; Rothschild et al., 1992). Butler (1988) recorded frequencies of wrist osteoarthritis of less than 0.6% of men prior to age 60 and 1.6% after age 60 in the United States. Frequencies in women were 0.1% and 0.8%, respectively. Van Saase (1989) suggested 1% under age 44, 5% age 45-59, 10-15% in the sixties, 15-20% in the seventies, and 20-25% in the eighties, the higher frequencies representing men. However, his data fit more the age curve of wrist calcium pyrophosphate deposition disease (Rothschild et al., 1992). Kellgren & Lawrence (1958) found that 16%-27% of knee osteoarthritis was related to previous injury (Davis, 1987).

2.3 Severity of osteoarthritis in the anatomic record

The severity of osteoarthritis is determined by the amount of cartilage loss (recognized on the basis of joint space narrowing). This measurement can only when cartilage is preserved, not in "bare" bones. End stage osteoarthritis often, but not invariably, results in bone rubbing on bone. This rubbing, which represents the end stage of many forms of arthritis, produces eburnation. It is one marker for severity, but does not always occur, even with end stage disease. Its sensitivity has never been established for determining the frequency of end stage of disease and its specificity for osteoarthritis has been falsified. Radiologic evidence of joint space narrowing remains the best measure of severity.

Any discussion of severity must carry a caveat. Only a fraction of osteoarthritis is symptomatic. Peyron (1984) reported that 2.3% of working British men and 1.3% of women retired because of it and that in precluded working for only 3 months in 5% of individuals aged 55-64. Additionally, there is no linear relationship between structural changes and functional limitations (Mankin & Radin, 1993).

2.4 Osteoarthritis in the zoologic/paleontologic record

It may seem paradoxical to start with the paleontologic record, but that forms the basis for the hypothesis that osteoarthritis is actually a phenomenon of artificial environments or mechanical disadvantage. It proved to be extremely rare in dinosaurs (Rothschild, 1990b). It was not present in any sauropod [e.g., *Camarasaurus*, *Apatosaurus* (formally called *Brontosaur*), *Diplodocus*], and actually has been documented in weight-bearing bones only in the ankles of 2 of 39 *Iguanodon* found in a coal mine under Brussels (Rothschild, 1991). Given phylogenetic classification of dinosaurs, it is perhaps not surprising that osteoarthritis is extremely rare in both fossil and extant reptiles (Rothschild, 2008, 2010) Osteoarthritis was present in the ankles of 27% of fossil *Diprotodon*, the marsupial cow with a ball and socket ankle joint (Rothschild & Molnar, 1988.

Fox (1939) found no osteoarthritis in 173 rodent genera, while Sokoloff (1959) described it in the knees of laboratory mice and guinea pigs, and in the shoulders of guinea pigs. However, comparison of captive and wild-caught guinea pigs revealed almost invariable occurrence in the former and absence in the latter (Rothschild, 2003). Analogous to the observation in guinea pigs, osteoarthritis is frequently reported in domestic mammals. Bovine osteoarthritis was noted in 20% of Holstein-Friesian bulls more than 9 yrs old (Neher & Tietz, 1959) and horses, but as only isolated occurrences in non-domestics (Rothschild & Martin, 2006). Ten percent of large captive cats had osteoarthritis affecting shoulders, elbows and stiffles (Rothschild et al., 1998).

Examination of non-human primates revealed the same pattern, with a similar increase in frequency with age noted in rhesus macaques in captive environments (Rothschild & Woods, 1992a,b; Rothschild et al, 1999). As the distribution of arthritis in captive animals [predominant shoulder (33%) and elbow (47%)] was quite different from that [predominant knee (80%)] of free-ranging individuals, this cannot be simply written off as age/survival variation.

Birds present a totally different picture. Frequency of osteoarthritis is independent of captive or wild-caught status (Rothschild & Panza, 2004, 2005, 2006a,b). Previous reports analyzed domestic chickens and turkeys (Poulos, 1978; Rejno & Stromberg, 1978; Sokoloff, 1959), attributing pathology to nutritional factors (e.g., selection for weight production) and dysplasia. However systematic examination of birds revealed species-dependent variation in frequency, with more than 25% of some species affected (Rothschild & Panza, 2004,2005, 2006a,b).

3. Conclusions

Osteoarthritis is clearly a disease of artificial environments in mammals, the group in which humans are categorized. Comparison of wild and zoo animals show this disparity, which is not relieved by other "unnatural environments." The conditions on Cayo Santiago are probably among the best that can be offered. Rhesus macaques have the run of an island, where the only human intervention includes observation and some provisioning. However, the hurricanes that afflict that locale reduce the canope to one level, with greater resultant ground activity than would be found in the wild. Absence of predators on the island also minimize ground risk. Behavior changes. Conversely, birds represent a natural model for understanding the underlying causes of osteoarthritis. With frequency variation in birds being species, rather than genus-determined, perhaps greater understanding of bird behavior will provide insights to osteoarthritis that will have clinical benefit.

4. References

Acheson, R., Chan, Y. & Clemett, R. (1976). New Haven survey of joint diseases. XII. Distribution and symptoms of osteoarthritis in the hands with reference to handedness. *Annals of the Rheumatic Diseases*, Vol. 35, pp. 274-278.

Ahmed A.; & Burke, D. (1983). In-vitro measurements of static pressure distribution in synovial joints. Part I: Tibial surface of the knee. *Journal of Biomechanical Engineering*, Vol.105, pp. 216-225.

Ahmed A.; Burke D., & Yu, A. (1983). In vitro measurements of static pressure distribution in synovial joints. Part II: Retropatellar surface. *Journal of Biomechanical Engineering* Vol.105, pp. 226-235.

Alexander R.; Battye, C., Goodwill, C. & Walsh, J. (1982). The ankle and subtalar joints. *Clinics of Rheumatic Disease*, Vol.8, pp,. 703-711.

Altman, R. & Gray, R. (1985). Inflammation in osteoarthritis. *Clinics in the Rheumatic Diseases*, Vol.ll, pp. 353-365.

Altman, R.; Asch, E., Bloch, D., Bole, G., Borenstein, D., Brandt, K., Cooke, T., Christy, W., Greenwald, R., Hochberg, M., Howell, D., Kaplan, D., Koopman, W., Longley, S., McShane, D., Mankin, G., Medsger, T., Medsger, R., Mikkelsen, S., Moskowitz, R., Murphy, W., Rothschild, B., Segal, M., Sokoloff, L. & Wolfe F. (1986). Development of criteria for the classification and reporting of osteoarthritis: Classification of osteoarthritis of the knee. *Arthritis & Rheumatism*, Vol.29, pp. 1039-1049.

Altman, R.; Alarcon, G., Appelrouth, D., Bloch, D., Borenstein, D., Brandt, K., Brown, C., Cooke, T., Daniels, W., Feldman, D., Gray, R., Greenwald, R., Hochberg, M., Howell, D., Ike, R., Kapila, P., Kaplan, D., Koopman, W., Longley, S., McShane, D., Medsger, T., Michel, B., Murphy, W., Osial, T., Ramsey-Goldman, R., Rothschild, B. & Wolfe F. (1990). Criteria for classification and reporting of osteoarthritis of the hand. *Arthritis & Rheumatism*, Vol.33, pp. 1601-1610.

Altman, R.; Alarcon, G., Appelrouth, D., Bloch, D., Borenstein, D., Brandt, K., Brown, C., Cooke, T., Daniels, W., Feldman, D., Gray, R., Greenwald, R., Hochberg, M., Howell, D., Ike, R., Kapila, P., Kaplan, D., Koopman, W., Longley, S., McShane, D., Medsger, T., Michel, B., Murphy, W., Osial, T., Ramsey-Goldman, R., Rothschild, B.

& Wolfe F.(1991). Criteria for classification and reporting of osteoarthritis of the hip. *Arthritis & Rheumatism*, Vol.34, pp. 505-514.

Anderson, J. & Felson, D. (1986). Factors associated with knee osteoarthritis (OA) in a national survey. *Arthritis & Rheumatism*, Vol.29 (Suppl), p. 16.

Bagge. E/, Bjelle. A. & Svanborg, A. (1992) Radiographic osteoarthritis in the elderly. A cohort comparison and a longitudinal study of the "70-year old people in Göteborg." *Clinical Rheumatology*, Vol.11, pp.486–491.

Bang, S.-Y.; Son, C.-N., Sung, Y.-K., Choi, B., Joo, K.-B. & Yun, J.-B. (2011) Joint-specific prevalence and radiographic pattern of hand arthritis in Korena. *Rheumatology International*,Vol.31, pp. 361-364.

Barnett, C.; & Napier, J. (1952). The axis of rotation at the ankle joint in man. Its influence upon the form of the talus and the mobility of the fibula. *Journal of Anatomy*, Vol.86, pp. 1-9.

Blumberg, B., Bloch, K. & Black, R. (1961). A study of the prevalence of arthritis in Alaskan Eskimos. *Arthritis & Rheumatism*, Vol.4, pp. 325-341.

Bremner, J., Lawrence, J. & Miall, W. (1968). Degenerative joint disease in a Jamaican rural population. *Annals of the Rheumatic Diseases*, Vol.27, pp. 326-332.

Bridges, P. (1991). Degenerative joint disease in hunter-gatherers and agriculturalists from the southeastern United States. *American Journal of Physical Anthropology*, Vol.85, pp. 379-391.

Bullough, P.; Goodfellow, J. & O'Connor, J. (1973). The relationship between degenerative changes and load-bearing in the human hip. *Journal of Bone and Joint Surgery* Vol. 55B, pp. 746-758.

Butler, W., Hawthorne, V., Mikkelsen, W., Carman, W., Bouthillier, D., Lamphiear D. & Kazi, I. (1988). Prevalence of radiologically defined osteoarthritis in the finger and wrist joints of adult residents of Tecumseh, Michigan, 1962-65. *Journal of Clinical Epidemiology*, Vol.41, pp. 467-473.

Cassou, B., Camus, J. & Peyron J.(1981). Recherche d`une arthrose primitive de la cheville chez les sujets de plus de 70 ans. In: *Epidemiologie de l'Arthrose*, J.G. Peyron (Ed.), pp. 180-184, Geigy,Paris.

Close, J. (1956). Some applications of the functional anatomy of the ankle joint. *Journal of Bone and Joint Surgery*, Vol.38A, pp. 761-781.

Davis, M., Ettinger, W. & Neuhaus, J. (1987). Knee injury and obesity as risk factors for unilateral and bilateral osteoarthritis of the knee (OAK). *Arthritis & Rheumatism*, Vol.30 (Suppl), p. 130.

Davis, M. (1988). Epidemiology of osteoarthritis. *Clinical Geriatric Medicine*, Vol.4, pp. 241-255.

Day, W.; Swanson, S. & Freeman M. (1975). Contact pressures in the loaded human cadaver hip. *Journal of Bone and Joint Surgery*,Vol.57B, pp. 302-313.

Dieppe, P. & Watt, I. (1985). Crystal deposition in osteoarthritis: An opportunistic event? *Clinics in the Rheumatic Diseases*, Vol. 11, pp. 367-392.

Felson, D. (1988). Epidemiology of hip and knee osteoarthritis. *Epidemiologic Review*, Vol.10, pp. 1-28.

Fox, H. (1939). Chronic Arthritis in Wild Mammals. *Transactions of the American Philosophical Society* (New Series), Vol. 31(Part II), pp. 73-149.

Fukubayashi, T. & Kurosawa, H. (1980). The contact area and pressure distribution pattern of the knee. *Acta Orthopaedica Scandinavica,*Vol.51, pp. 871-879.

Funk, F. Jr. (1976). Osteoarthritis of the foot and ankle. In: *Symposium on Osteoarthritis*, American Academy of Orthopedic Surgeons (Ed.), pp. 287-301, C.V. Mosby, St. Louis.

Gibilisco, P., Schumacher, H. Jr., Hollander, J. & Soper, K. (1985). Synovial fluid crystals in osteoarthritis. *Arthritis & Rheumatism*, Vol.28, pp. 511-515.

Gofton, J. (1971). Studies in osteoarthritis of the hip. III. Congenital subluxation and osteoarthritis of the hip. *Canadian Medical Association Journal*, Vol.104, pp. 911-915.

Goldin, R., McAdam, L. & Louie, J. (1976). Clinical and radiological survey of the incidence of osteoarthrosis among obese patients. *Annals of the Rheumatic Diseases*, Vol.35, pp. 349-353.

Goodfellow, J.; Hungerford, D. & Zindel M. (1976). Patellofemoral joint mechanics and pathology. 1. Functional anatomy of the patellofemoral joint. *Journal of Bone and Joint Surgery,*Vol.58B, pp. 287-290.

Greenwald, A. & Haynes, D. (1972). Weight-bearing areas in the human hip joint. *Journal of Bone and Joint Surgery*, Vol. 54B, pp. 157-163.

Greenwald, A. & O'Connor, J. (1971). The transmission of load through the human hip joint. *Journal of Biomechanics*, Vol.4, pp. 507-528.

Gregory, K. (1950). *The anatomy of the gorilla*, Columbia University Press, New York, pp. 161.

Harrison, M.; Schajowicz, F. & Trueta J. (1953). Osteoarthritis of the hip: A study of the nature and evolution of the disease. *Journal of Bone and Joint Surgery*, Vol.35B, pp. 598-626.

Heiple, K. & Lovejoy, C. (1971). The distal femoral anatomy of Australopithecus. *American Journal of Physical Anthropology*, Vol.35, pp. 75-84.

Hoaglund, F., Yau, A. & Wong W. (1973). Osteoarthritis of the hip and other joints in southern Chinese in Hong Kong: Incidence and related factors. *Journal of Bone and Joint Surgery*, Vol.55A, pp. 645-657.

Holt, P. & Keats, T. (1993). Calcific tendinitis: A review of the usual and unusual. *Skeletal Radiology*, Vol.22, pp. 1-9.

Jenkins, F. (1972). Chimpanzee bipedalism: Cineradiographic analysis and implications for the evolution of gait. *Science*, Vol.178, pp. 877-879.

Jurmain, R. (1977). Stress and the etiology of osteoarthritis. *American Journal of Physical Anthropology*, Vol.46, pp. 353-366.

Kellgren, J. & Lawrence J. (1958). Osteo-arthrosis and disk degeneration in an urban population. Annals *of the Rheumatic Diseases*, Vol. 17, pp. 388-396.

Kempson, G.; Spivey, C., Swanson, A. & Freeman, M. (1971). Patterns of cartilage stiffness on normal and degenerate human femoral Heads. *Journal of Biomechanics*, Vol.4, pp. 597-609.

Kettlekamp, D. & Jacobs, A. (1972). Tibiofemoral contact area. Determination and implications. *Journal of Bone and Joint Surgery,* Vol.54A, pp. 349-356.

Kummer, B. (1975). Functional adaptation to posture in the pelvis of man and other primates, In: Primate *Functional Morphology and Evolution,* R.H. Tuttle (Ed.), 281-290, Mouton, Paris, France.

Lally, E., Zimmermann, B., Ho, G. Jr. & Kaplan, S. (1989). Urate-mediated inflammation in nodal osteoarthritis: Clinical and roentgenographic correlations. *Arthritis & Rheumatism,* Vol.32, pp. 86-90.

Lambert, K. (1971). The weight-bearing function of the fibula. *Journal of Bone and Joint Surgery,* Vol.53A, pp. 507-513.

Lawrence, J. (1961). Rheumatism in cotton operatives. *British Journal of Industrial Medicine,* Vol.18, pp. 270-276.

Lawrence, J., DeGraff, R. & Laine, V. (1963). Degenerative joint disease in random samples and occupational groups. In: *The Epidemiology of Chronic Rheumatism,* J.H. Kellgren, M.R. Jeffrey & J. Ball (Eds.), Blackwell, Oxford, England.

Layton, M., Goldstein, S., Goulet, R., Feldkamp, L., Kubinski, D. & Bole, G. (1988). Examination of subchondral bone architecture in experimental osteoarthritis by microscopic computed axial tomography. *Arthritis & Rheumatism,* Vol.31, pp.1400-1405.

Leach, R., Baumgard, S. & Broom, J. (1973). Obesity: Its relationship to osteoarthritis of the knee. *Clinical Orthopaedics and Related Research,* Vol.93, pp. 271-273.

Lovejoy, C. (1973). The gait of Australopithecines. *Yearbook of Physical Anthropology,* Vol.17, pp. 147-161.

Lovejoy, C. (1975). Biomechanical perspectives on the lower limb of early Hominids, In: Primate *Functional Morphology and Evolution,* R.H. Tuttle (Ed.), 291-326, Mouton, Paris, France.

Lovejoy, C. & Heiple, K. (1970). A reconstruction of the femur of *Australopithecus africanus. American Journal of Physical Anthropology,* Vol.32, pp. 33-40.

Mankin, H. & Radin, E. (1993). Structure and function of joints. In: *Arthritis and Allied Conditions,* D.J. McCarty & W.J. Koopman (Eds.), 12th edition, pp. 181-193, Lea and Febiger, Philadelphia.

Maquet, P.; Van De Berg, A. & Simonet, J. (1975). Femorotibial weight-bearing areas. *Journal of Bone and Joint Surgery,* Vol.57A, pp. 766-771.

Matthews, L.; Sonstegard, D. & Henke, J. (1977). Load bearing characteristics of the patellofemoral joint. *Acta Orthopaedica Scandinavica,* Vol.48, pp. 511-516.

McLeod, W.; Moschi, A., Andrews, J. & Hughston, J. (1977). Tibial plateau topography. *American Journal of Sports Medicine,* Vol.5, pp. 13-18.

Morrison, R. (1970). The mechanics of the knee joint in relation to normal walking. *Journal of Biomechanics,* Vol.3, pp. 51-61.

Moskowitz, R.; Howell, D., Goldberg, V. & Mankin, H. (1984).*Osteoarthritis: Diagnosis and Management.* Saunders, Philadelphia.

Mukhopadhaya, B. & Barooah, B. (1967). Osteoarthritis of hip in Indians: An anatomical and clinical study. *Indian Journal of Orthopaedics,* Vol.1, pp. 55-62.

Murray, R. (1965). The aetiology of primary osteoarthritis of the hip. British Journal of Radiology, Vol.38, pp. 810-824.

Neher, G. & Tietz, W. Jr. (1959). Observations on the clinical signs and gross pathology of degenerative joint disease in aged bulls. *Laboratory Investigation,* Vol.8, pp. 1218-1222.

Nordin, M. & Frankel, V. (1980a). Biomechanics of the knee, In: *Basic Biomechanics of the Skeletal System,* V.H. Frankel & M. Nordin (Eds.), 113-148, Lea and Febiger, Philadelphia.

Nordin, M. & Frankel, V. (1980b). Biomechanics of the hip. In: *Basic Biomechanics of the Skeletal System,* V.H. Frankel & M. Nordin (Eds.), 149-177, Lea and Febiger, Philadelphia.

O'Donoghue, D., Frank, G. & Jeter, G. (1971). Repair and reconstruction of the anterior cruciate ligament in dogs - factors influencing long-term results. *Journal of Bone and Joint Surgery,* Vol.53A, pp. 710-718.

Partridge, R. & Duthie, J. (1968). Rheumatism in dockers and civil servants: A comparison of heavy manual and sedentary workers. *Annals of the Rheumatic Diseases,* Vol.27, pp. 559-568.

Peyron, J. (1984). The epidemiology of osteoarthritis. In: *Osteoarthritis: Diagnosis and Management,* R.W. Moskowitz, D.S. Howell, V.M. Goldberg & H.J. Mankin (Eds.), pp. 9-27, Saunders, Philadelphia.

Poulos, P. (1978). Tibial dyschondroplasia (osteochondrosis) in the turkey. *Acta Radiologica,* Vol.Suppl 358, pp. 197-203.

Puranen, J., Ala-Ketola, L. & Peltokallio, P. (1975). Running and primary osteoarthritis of the hip. *British Medical Journal,* Vol.2, pp. 424-425.

Radin, E. (1978). Our current understanding of normal knee mechanics and its implications for successful knee surgery. In: *American Association of Orthopedic Surgeons Symposium on Reconstructive Surgery* Ramsey, P. & Hamilton, W. (1976). hanges in tibiotalar area of contact caused by lateral talar shift. *Journal of Bone and Joint Surgery,* Vol.58A, pp. 356-357.

Rejno, S. & Stromberg B. (1978). Osteochondrosis in the horse. *Acta Radiologica,* Vol.Suppl 358, pp. 153-178.

Resnick, D. (2002). *Diagnosis of Bone and Joint Disorders,* Saunders, Philadelphia.

Rothschild, B. (1990). Radiologic assessment of osteoarthritis in dinosaurs. *Annals of the Carnegie Museum,* Vol.59, pp. 295-301.

Rothschild, B. (1991). Skeletal paleopathology of Rheumatic Diseases: The sub-Homo connection. In: *Arthritis and Allied Conditions,* D.J. McCarty (Ed.), 12th edition, pp. 3-7, Lea& Febiger, Philadelphia.

Rothschild, B. (1982). *Rheumatology: A Primary Care Approach.* Yorke Medical Press, New York.

Rothschild, B. (1989). Skeletal paleopathology of rheumatic diseases: The subprimate connection. In: *Arthritis and Allied Conditions,* D. McCarty (ed.), 3-7, 11th ed., Lea and Febiger, Philadelphia.

Rothschild, B. (1997). Porosity: A curiosity without diagnostic significance. *American Journal of Physical Anthropology,* Vol.104, pp. 529-533.

Rothschild, M. (2003). Osteoarthritis as a complication of artificial environment: The Cavia (guinea pig) story. *Annals of the Rheumatic Diseases*, Vol.62, pp. 1022-1023.

Rothschild, B. (2008). Scientifically rigorous reptile and amphibian, osseous pathology: Lessons for forensic herpetology from comparative and paleo-pathology. *Applied Herpetology*, Vol.10, pp. 39-116.

Rothschild, B. (2010). Macroscopic recognition of non-traumatic osseous pathology in the post-cranial skeletons of crocodilians and lizards. *Journal of Herpetology*, Vol.44, pp. 13-20.

Rothschild, B. & Molnar RE. (1988). Osteoarthritis in fossil marsupial populations of Australia. *Annals of the Carnegie Museum*, Vol.57, pp.

Rothschild B. & Panza, R. (2005). Epidemiologic assessment of trauma-independent skeletal pathology in non-passerine birds from museum collections. *Avian Pathology*, Vol.34, pp. 212-219.

Rothschild B. & Panza, R. (2006a). Osteoarthritis is for the birds. *Clinical Rheumatology*, Vol.25, pp. 645-647.

Rothschild B. & Panza, R. (2006b) Inverse relationship of osteoarthritis to weight: The bird lesson. *Clinical and Experimental Rheumatology*, vol. 24, p. 218.

Rothschild, B. & Woods, R. (1992a). Osteoarthritis, calcium pyrophosphate deposition disease, and osseous infection in Old World monkeys and prosimians. *American Journal of Physical Anthropology*, Vol.87, pp. 341-347.

Rothschild, B. & Woods, R. (1992b). Arthritis in New World Monkeys: Osteoarthritis, Calcium Pyrophosphate Deposition Disease and Spondyloarthropathy. *International Journal of Primatology*,

Rothschild, B., Woods R. & Rothschild, C. (1992). Calcium pyrophosphate deposition disease: Description in defleshed skeletons. *Clinical and Experimental Rheumatology*, Vol.10, pp. 557-564.

Rothschild, B., Hong, N. & Turnquist, J. (1999). Skeletal survey of Cayo Santiago rhesus macaques: Osteoarthritis and apical plate excrescences. *Seminars in Arthritis and Rheumatism*, Vol. 29, pp. 100-111.

Sammarco, G.; Burstein, A. & Frankel, V. (1973). Biomechanics of the ankle. *Orthopedic Clinics of North America*, Vol.4, pp. 75-96.

Saville, P. & Dickson, J. (1968). Age and weight in osteoarthritis of the hip. *Arthritis & Rheumatism*, Vol.11, pp. 635-644.

Schumacher, H., Smolyo, A., Tse, R. & Maurer, K. (1977). Arthritis associated with apatite crystals. *Annals of Internal Medicine*, Vol.87, pp. 411-416.

Seedhom, B. & Wright, V. (1981). Biomechanics. *Clinics of the Rheumatic Diseases*, Vol.7, pp. 259-281.

Seireg, A. & Arvikar, F. (1975). The prediction of muscular load sharing and joint forces in the lower extremities during walking. *Journal of Biomechanics*, Vol.8, pp. 89-102.

Shaibani, A.; Workman, R. & Rothschild, B. (1993). The significance of enthesitis as a skeletal phenomenon. *Clinical and Experimental Rheumatology*, Vol.11, pp. 399-403.

Shrive, N,; O'Connor, J. & Goodfellow, J. (1978). Load-bearing in the knee joint. *Clinical Orthopaedics and Related Research*, Vol.131, pp. 279-287.

Sigmon, B. (1975). Functions and evolution of Hominid hip and thigh musculature. In: *Primate Functional Morphology and Evolution*, R.H. Tuttle (Ed.), 235-252, Mouton, Paris, France.

Silberberg, M. & Silberberg, R. (1960). Osteoarthritis in mice fed diets enriched with animal or vegetable fat. *Archives of Pathology*, Vol.70, pp. 385-390.

Simon, W. (1970). Scale effects in animal joints I. Articular cartilage thickness and compressive stress. *Arthritis & Rheumatism*, Vol.13, pp. 244-255.

Sokoloff, L. (1959). Osteoarthritis in laboratory animals. *Laboratory Investigation*, Vol.8, pp. 1209-1217.

Sokoloff, L. (1969). *The Biology of Degenerative Joint Disease*, University of Chicago Press, Chicago, Illinois.

Sokoloff, L., Mickelsen, O., Silverstein, E., Jay, G. Jr. & Yamamoto, R. (1960). Experiment obesity and osteoarthritis. *American Journal of Physiology*, Vol.198, pp. 765-770.

Solomon, L. (1976). Patterns of osteoarthritis of the hip. *Journal of Bone and Joint Surgery*, Vol.58B, pp. 176-183.

Solomon, L., Beighton P. & Lawrence, J. (1975). Rheumatic disorders in the South African Negro. Part II. Osteoarthrosis. *South African Medical Journal*, Vol.49, pp. 1737-1740.

Sonntag, C. (1923). On the anatomy, physiology, and pathology of the chimpanzee. *Proceedings of the Zoological Society (London)*, Vol.1923 , pp. 323-426.

Sorbie, C. & Zalter, R. (1965). Bio-engineering studies of the forces transmitted by joints. I: The phasic relationship of the hip muscles in walking. In: *Biomechanics and Related Bio-Engineering Topics*, 359-367, R.M. Kenedi (Ed.), Pergamon Press, Glasgow.

Stauffer, R.; Chao, E. & Brewster, R. (1977). Force and motion analysis of the normal, diseased, and prosthetic ankle joint. *Clinical Orthopaedics and Related Research*, Vol.127, pp. 189-196.

Toba, N.; Sakai, A., Aoyagi, K., Yoshida, S., Honda, S. & Nakamura. T. (2006). Prevalence and involvement patterns of radiographic hand osteoarthritis in Japanese women: The Hizen-Oshima study. *Journal of Bone & Mineral Metabolism*, Vol.24, pp. 344-348.

Trueta, J. (1968). Studies of the development and decay of the human frame. *Journal of Bone and Joint Surgery*, Vol. 43B, pp. 376-386.

Van Saase, J., van Romunde. L., Cats, A., Vandenbroucke, J. & Valkenburg, H. (1989). Epidemiology of osteoarthritis: Zoetermeer survey. Comparison of radiological osteoarthritis in a Dutch population with that in 10 other populations. *Annals of the Rheumatic Diseases*, Vol.48, pp. 271-280.

Waldron, H. (1991). Prevalence and distribution of osteoarthritis in a population from Georgian and early Victorian London. *Annals of the Rheumatic Diseases*, Vol.50, pp. 301-307.

Walker, P. & Hajek, J. (1972). The Load-bearing area in the knee joint. *Journal of Biomechanics*, Vol.5, pp. 581-589.

Woods, R. (1986). Biomechanics and Degenerative Joint Disease in Humans, Gorillas, and Chimpanzees. Masters Thesis, Kent State University, Kent, Ohio.

Woods, R. (1995) . Biomechanics and Osteoarthritis of the Knee. Ph.D. Thesis, Ohio State University, Columbus, Ohio.

2

Symptoms, Signs and Quality of Life (QoL) in Osteoarthritis (OA)

Keith K.W. Chan and Ricky W.K. Wu
The Hong Kong Institute of Musculoskeletal Medicine (HKIMM), Hong Kong SAR, China

1. Introduction

Osteoarthritis is a syndrome with heterogeneous clinical presentations. Joint pain is the cardinal symptom accompanied by varying degrees of functional alterations like joint stiffness and instability. Clinical presentations are diversified, depending on which joint is affected, how severely it is affected, and the number of joints involved. The disease onset is usually subtle and unrecognized, but at the later stages, symptoms can be overt and debilitating. In between the onset and the late stages, the symptoms progress at variable rate and the patterns can be stepwise, continual, or static. The implications of osteoarthritis towards individual's quality of life (QoL) are different among different individuals and may not be directly proportional to the severity of structural abnormalities of the joints. Biopsychosocial factors come into play, and associated co-morbidities may further complicate the situation.

2. Symptoms in osteoarthritis

2.1 Joint pain

It is usually the chief complaint of symptomatic osteoarthritis which leads patients to seek medical attention. There are 2 types of pain in joint osteoarthritis, the mechanical and inflammatory pain. Typical mechanical OA pain is often described as deep and dull ache, localized to one or a few joints. The pain is aggravated by prolonged use or after extreme-ranged movements of the involved joint(s), by the end of the day, or after an increased mechanical load (O'Reilly & Doherty, 1998). Usually, the mechanical pain is relieved by rest or by gentle massage. Early in the disease, the pain is only episodic; its precipitants are usually known and predictable and the pain episodes are self-limiting. With the progression of the disease, the pain may become constant; occur at rest or even at night. At late stages, this mechanical joint pain may turn into unanticipated episodes of sharp pain superimposed on the pain at baseline (Hawker et al., 2008). This sharp pain is stabbing in character, more severe and stressful, occurring more frequently during movements after a period of resting (Chan, K.K.W. & Chan, L.W.Y., 2011). In contrast, the onset and frequency of inflammatory pain was less predictable. It could be triggered by weather changes, prolonged walking, a minor sprain, or from misplacement of the feet during walking. Sometimes, inflammatory pain occurred as flares in the form of exaggerated pain on the background of mechanical pain. According to a qualitative study on knee OA, most patients (80%) could distinguish between mechanical and inflammatory pain, describing the character of each very differently. Inflammatory pain was described as a burning pain that could persist for days without treatment. Patients found resting and ice packing helpful, but most help came from taking analgesics, especially the non-steroidal anti-inflammatory drugs (NSAIDs). The frequency of inflammatory pain was highly unpredictable, varying from once every few weeks to once every few months. Sometimes the inflammatory pain might have a relapsing pattern, with the pain regressing gradually and relapsing again a few days later. This pattern could persist for 3 to 4 months of a year. Irrespective of whether pain was mechanical or inflammatory in nature, patients would avoid events that would trigger or aggravate the pain or take analgesics before the event as a preventive measure (Chan, K.K.W. & Chan, L.W.Y., 2011).

Although joint pain from osteoarthritis is typically local, in some patients the pain may be referred. For example, pain from OA hip may refer to the knee; and pain from OA cervical facet joints may refer to shoulder, arm, forearm and hand. In case of OA involving cervical or lumber facet joints, the pain may involve radicular components with features of sharp shooting pain different from the typical OA pain which are dull and achy. Most patients with symptomatic OA had symptoms in more than one joint. In a study of 500 patients with limb joints OA, only 6% had symptoms confined to a single joint (Cushnaghan & Dieppe, 1991). The most frequently affected joints were knees (41%), hands (30%) and the hips (19%).

The cause of joint pain in osteoarthritis is not well understood. It has been suggested that different mechanisms may produce pain characteristics by different joint structures (Kellgren, 1983):

- As cartilage is aneural, joint pain should arise from adjacent structures.
- Subchondral bone microfracture and osteophytes which stretch nerve endings in the periosteum may cause consistent joint pain on use.
- Bone angina caused by distortion of medullary blood flow and by thickened subchondral trabeculae, leading to intraosseous hypertension and intraosseous stasis. This may contribute to nocturnal joint pain (Arnoldi et. al., 1972).
- Joint inflammation involving the enthesis, joint capsules and synovium may cause pain at rest.
- Structural alteration, muscle weakness and altered usage of the joint with osteoarthritis would lead to stretching of the joint capsule, muscle spasm, enthesopathy and bursitis which in turn lead to the typical mechanical or activity-induced joint pain.

The degree of joint pain does not always correlate with the degree of structural changes of osteoarthritis which is usually defined by abnormal change in appearance of the joints on radiographs (Hannan et al., 2000), e.g. pain can be absent in spite of severe joint damage in some cases. Nevertheless, those with significant radiographic changes are more likely to have joint pain than those with mild changes (Duncan et al., 2007), and the concordance between symptoms and radiographic osteoarthritis are greater with more advanced structural damage (Peat et al., 2006).

2.2 Joint stiffness

Joint osteoarthritis may present with joint stiffness especially in the morning. It is a tight and "gelling" sensation of the joints, periarticular soft tissues and musculature, rendering the joint difficult and slow to move. Unlike diffuse stiffness in rheumatoid arthritis, stiffness of OA is confined to the region around the affected joint. Typical OA joint stiffness occurs after prolonged period of immobilization, not restricted to the time in the morning, and usually lasts less than 30 minutes. As the disease progresses, prolonged stiffness would be evident. It is attributable to joint incongruity and capsular fibrosis as a result of the process of osteoarthritis.

2.3 Joint instability

Patients with osteoarthritis of joints in lower limbs frequently experience a sensation of instability or buckling, i.e. shifting without actually falling or giving way. It tends to be more common in patients who have OA in multiple joints of lower limbs. Such buckling can be the results of:

- Weakness of periarticular musculature from joint disuse
- Muscle fatigue because the peri-articular musculature have to work harder to move the joint as the coefficient of friction increases due to the cartilage surface fissures or loses integrity
- Laxity of ligaments as a result of narrowing of joint spaces from the loss of the supporting cartilage or from other joint deformities

3. Signs in osteoarthritis

3.1 Crepitus

It is an audible and palpable cracking or crunching over a joint during its active or passive movement. It is presumably caused by irregular articular surface attributable to the degenerative process rubbing against each other during motion. The degree of crepitus may be correlated with the degree of degenerative process (Ike & O'Rourke, 1995). However, many people have significant crepitus at their joints in the absence of any joint pain.

3.2 Restricted joint motion

The restricted movement over the degenerated joint can be caused by pain, effusion, capsular contractures, muscle spasm or weakness, intra-articular loose bodies, mechanical constraints by loss of joint cartilage and joint misalignment. Such feature may or may not associate with stress pain at extreme range. In order to make a differentiation, both active and passive ranges of joint motion are tested. The active movements give a rough idea of range of motions available in the joint, the pain experienced by the patient and the power in the peri-articular muscle groups. Passive joint movement particularly gives information on pain, range and the end-feel, i.e. the specific sensation imparted from the joint onto the examiner's hands at the extreme of passive movement (Cyriax J & Cyriax P, 1993). The quality of the end-feel is dependent upon the nature of tissue that is compromising full motion of the joint. For example:

- Elastic end-feel may be attributable to joint effusion.
- A springy end-feel is appreciated when the joint is springing or bouncing back at the end range by an intra-articular loose body.
- An abnormal hard end-feel may be attributable to involuntary muscle spasm or capsular contracture
- A bony-hard end-feel could be due to bony restraints by loss of joint cartilage, osteophytes impingement and joint misalignment.

For better interpretation of abnormal end-feel of a joint, one can compare the sensation with the joint on the contralateral side.

3.3 Bony changes and joint deformity

Bony enlargement in OA is attributable to the formation of osteophytes and the remodeling process leading to peri-articular bony hypertrophy and subchondral cyst formation. Incongruent degeneration of the joints will also contribute to joint angulations and misalignment. The classical example is the deformities in the nodal OA of hand (Figure 1) which causes bony enlargement at the distal and proximal interphalangeal joints known respectively as *Heberden's nodes* and *Bouchard's nodes*; and the angular deformity of the carpometacarpal and metacarpophalangeal joint of the thumb giving rise to the *squared hand*.

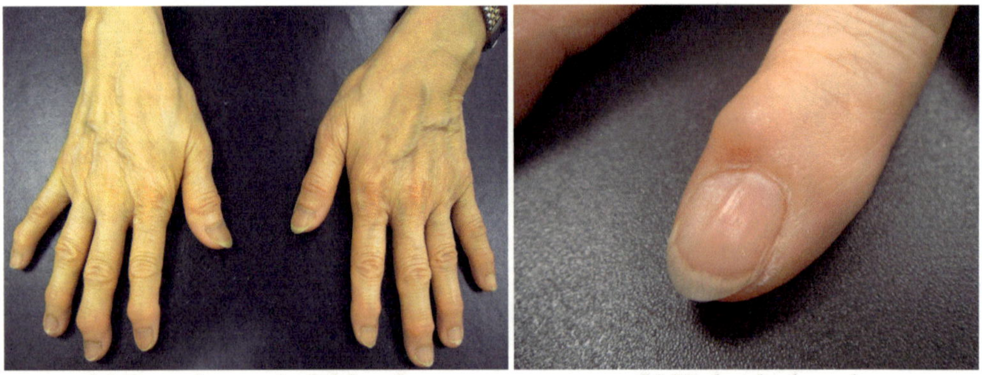

(a) Bony changes in OA hand (b) Herberden's node

Fig. 1. Nodal OA of hand

3.4 Joint tenderness

Tenderness with pressure along the joint margin is typical for OA. However, peri-articular structures may also be tender contributing to the joint pain, e.g. myofascial trigger points, adjacent bursitis or tendonitis, and ligament enthesopathy. Point tenderness should be sought away from the joint line to find out concomitant painful structures to guide management.

3.5 Variable levels of inflammation

Variable degree of synovitis may be found in the joints with osteoarthritis, giving rise to local palpable warmth, effusion and synovial thickening (Figure 2). This could also be one of the sources of joint tenderness. These features are usually intermittent and appear with the flare-ups in the osteoarthritic joint.

3.6 Muscle atrophy

Peri-articular muscular wasting may be apparent as a result of OA of the corresponding joint due to disuse muscle atrophy. The associated muscle weakness would compromise joint stability and muscle tones around the joint which further jeopardize the integrity of the joint (Hurley, 1999). For assessment of muscle strength and size, examiner can perform resisted movement of the joint and by direct measurement of the diameter of the muscle bulk compared to that on contralateral limb.

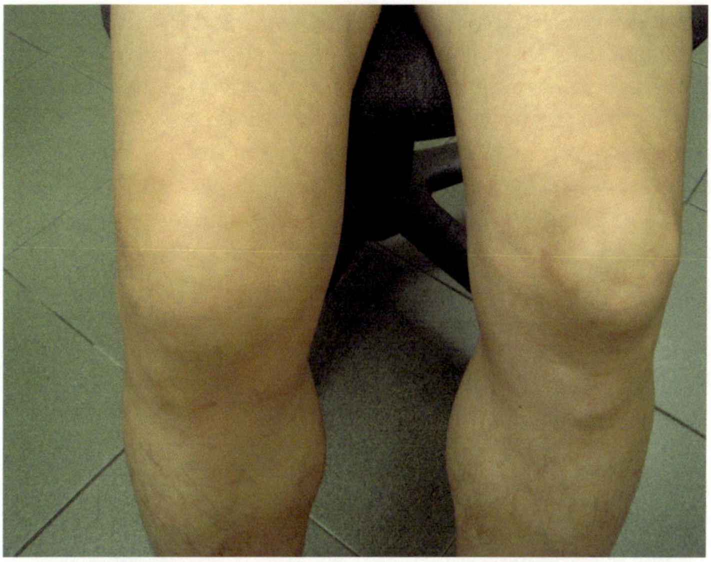

Fig. 2. Warm right knee effusion caused by synovitis in knee OA.

3.7 Absence of systemic manifestation

Symptoms of osteoarthritis are usually localized to the affected joint and systemic manifestations like fever, weight loss, anemia, fatigue and malaise are not features of primary OA. The presence of such features should alert the physician to consider other differential diagnoses like rheumatoid arthritis, although some subsets of OA occasionally give rise to systemic manifestation such as those crystal associated OA.

4. Clinical patterns and subsets

Osteoarthritis affects many joints, with heterogeneous clinical patterns, and may be triggered by diverse constitutional and environmental factors. The causes and clinical presentations among individuals with osteoarthritis could be quite different from each other. The trend in recent years is to separate osteoarthritis into more homogeneous grouping as subsets in order to better define respective etiological factors and to determine corresponding natural history and prognosis. The grouping of subsets was made according to the following clinical characteristics (Altman, 1991):

- Identifiable causes of osteoarthritis
- Joint sites involved
- The number of joints involved
- The pattern of joints involvement
- The presence of associated crystal deposition
- The presence of marked inflammation
- The radiographic bone response

It is important to note that the subset grouping of osteoarthritis is arbitrary and sharp distinction between subsets does not exist. It is possible that different subsets appear in one individual and evolution from one subset to another could occur with time and at different sites.

4.1 Nodal generalized OA (NGOA) or primary generalized OA (PGOA)

It is the best recognized OA subset. It has a female preponderance, marked familial predisposition, peaked onset in the middle age. Joints involved are symmetrically affected. Characteristically, it affects the distal interphalangeal joints (DIPJ) of the fingers with gelatinous cyst and bony outgrowth at the dorsal surface of the involved joints known as Heberden's nodes (Figure 1). In addition to DIPJ of the fingers, similar lesions may affect the proximal interphalangeal joints (Bouchard's nodes) of the fingers. Other frequently involved joints are carpometacarpal, metacarpophalangeal and interphalangeal joints of the thumbs, the acromioclavicular joint, the spinal facet joints, the hips, the knees and the first metatarsophalangeal joint. The disease typically goes through an episodic symptomatic phase (over one to three years) with considerable inflammation. In most cases, symptoms then subside resulting in a good deal of deformity but seldom give rise to serious disability (Pattrick et al., 1989).

4.2 Erosive OA (Punzi, 2004)

This is a rare condition and is considered as a more aggressive form of PGOA primarily affecting small joints of the hands. It has been documented to actually be a manifestation of calcium pyrophosphate deposition disease (Rothschild, 2006; Rothschild and Bruno, 2011; Rothschild and Yakubov, 1997; Rothschild et al., 1992). Women between 45 and 55 years are most typically affected and it has a strong familial predisposition. Joints are symmetrically affected and both the distal and proximal interphalangeal joints are equally affected with the typical Heberden's nodes and Bouchard nodes. The inflammatory features of the disease are florid with overt pain, synovial swelling and erythema. The hallmarks of the condition are the presence of destructive crumbling erosion demonstrated radiographically, with occasional joint instability at the interphalangeal joints. As a result, the functional outcome of the hand is much less favorable.

4.3 Local large joint OA

4.3.1 Hip

The classical symptom of hip OA is groin pain on weight bearing. The patients typically have difficulty in flexing and internally rotating their hips, so they may feel pain when getting in or out of the car, or when bowing forward to reach the ground or their feet. In rare cases, the patients may only present with referred knee pain from the hip. The condition is more common among white Caucasians, but is significantly less common among Chinese (Nevitt et al., 2002) and black African populations. There are two major subgroups of hip OAs defined by radiological patterns: the superior pole OA and the medial pole OA.

4.3.1.1 Superior pole OA

It is the common form of hip OA where degenerative process affects the weight bearing superior surface of the femoral head and the adjacent acetabulum. It has a male preponderance and associated with obesity or local structural abnormality. The disease is usually unilateral at presentation but likely to progress and may involve another hip as the disease evolves. The hallmark is superolateral femoral head migration with osteophytes at lateral acetabulum and medial femoral margins combined with typical buttressing of medial femoral neck cortex on hip radiographs (Figure 3).

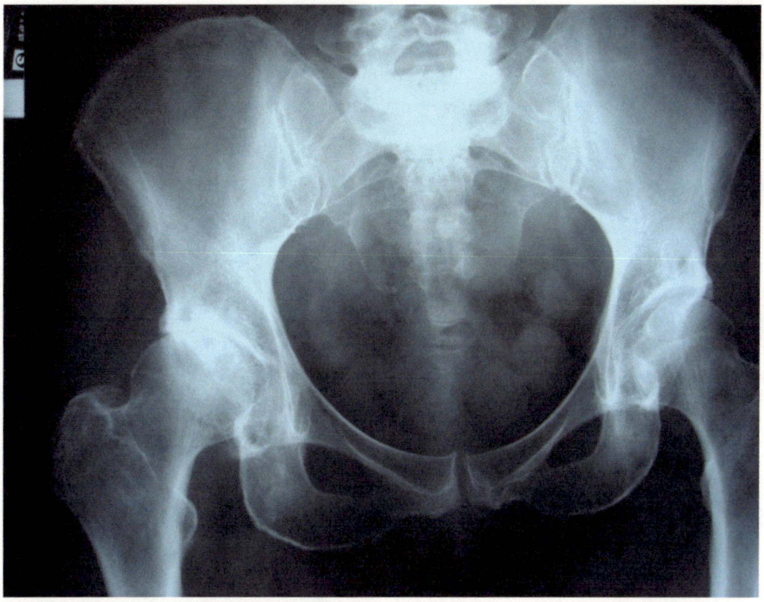

Fig. 3. Radiograph of Superior pole OA hip.

4.3.1.2 Medial pole OA

It is less commonly seen where more widespread, central cartilage loss are present at the hip. It has a female preponderance and usually associated with hand OA as part of the PGOA syndrome. The disease is more likely bilateral at presentation but less likely to progress.

Signs involve reproduction of the groin pain, typically on internal rotation and flexion of the hip. Trendelenburg sign may be present. When the patient stands on the unaffected side, the pelvis as viewed from the back remains level; while the patient stands on the painful side as a result of hip OA, the unsupported side of the pelvis will drop as a result of weak gluteus medius muscle on the side of painful hip. In moderate to severe diseases, hip flexion contracture may be demonstrated.

4.3.2 Knee

The knee is the commonly involved joint of osteoarthritis. The condition is primarily affecting elderly people with female preponderance and associated with obesity. There are three compartments of the knee that can be affected by OA: the medial tibiofemoral compartment is more commonly affected than the lateral tibiofemoral compartments; but there is a lack of data addressing prevalence of patellofemoral OA (chondromalacia patellae) and its correlation to tibiofemoral disease (McAlindon et al., 1992). The classical symptom of knee OA is knee pain on weight bearing. The pain is particularly aggravated when walking downstairs and raising up from chair after prolonged sitting if patellofemoral disease (chondromalacia patellae) is involved. Stiffness and gelling of the joint are frequent complaints of knee OA. Signs involve bony enlargement, joint tenderness, crepitus on movement and occasional joint effusion. Popliteal (Baker's) cysts are the bursae that communicate with the knee joint space which may become quite large and tense leading to posterior knee pain (Figure 4). Sometimes, patients with knee OA may have their Baker's cysts ruptured and present to the clinician with signs and symptoms mimic that of deep vein thrombosis. In moderate to severe knee OA, there may be joint deformity (varus for medial compartment disease and valgus for lateral compartment disease).

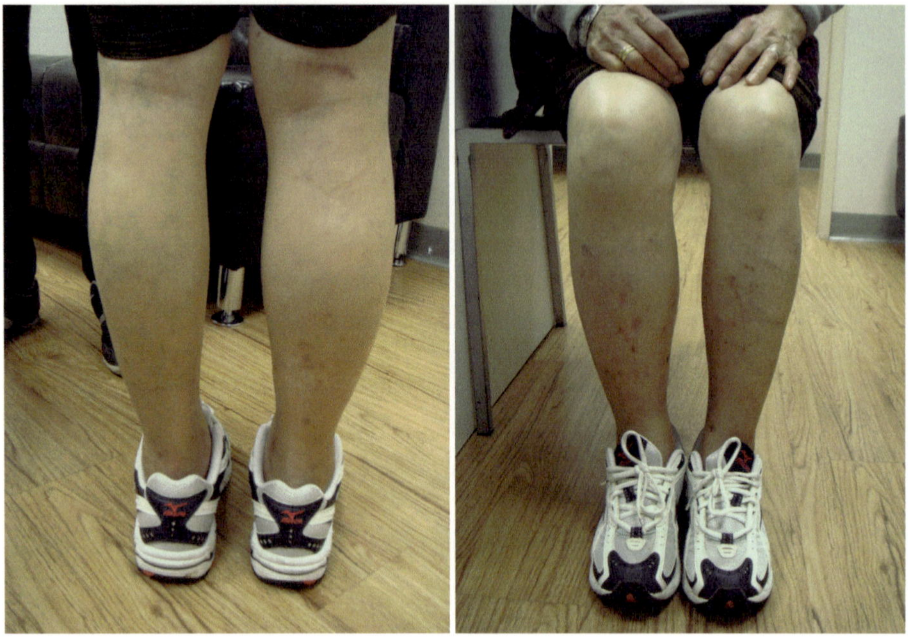

Fig. 4. Ruptured Baker's cyst of right knee with OA

	PGOA	Erosive OA	Superior pole hip OA	Medial pole hip OA	Knee OA
Preponderance	Female	Female	No	Female	Female
Familial predisposition	Marked	Marked	Sporadic	Marked	Mostly sporadic
Age	Middle age	45-55	↑ with age	Middle age	↑ with age
Symmetry	Yes	Yes	No	Yes	No
Joints involved	Multiple, DIPJ, PIPJ commonly involved	Mainly PIPJ & DIPJ	Superior pole of hip	Medial pole of hip	Medial > Lateral knee compartments
Inflammation*	Episodic	Florid	Episodic	Episodic	Episodic
Systemic manifestation	No	Yes	No	No	No
Progression	Slow	Aggressive	Variable	Less likely	Variable
Outcome disability	Low	High	Variable	Low	Variable
Hallmark	Herberden's/ Bouchard's nodes	Subchondral erosion on radiographs	Superolateral femoral head migration + osteophytes at lateral joint margin	Radiograhs: widespread central joint space narrowing	Bowed leg, Baker's cyst

* Any inflammation can be caused by the co-existing crystal arthritis

Table 1. Comparison between different OA clinical subsets

5. Natural history of osteoarthritis

Few studies assessed the natural history of knee OA (Dieppe et al., 1997; Ledingham et al., 1995; Massardo et al., 1989; Schouten et al., 1992); and the conclusions are that the natural history of osteoarthritis is highly variable (Hochberg, 1996). In a large scale prospective observational study of 188 participants with OA knees follow-up over 1-5 years, approximately 50% of the patients described worsening of their symptoms with time. However, a significant portion reported improvement (Schouten et al., 1992). In another smaller scale retrospective study on 72 patients with symptomatic knee OA even found that more than 50% of clinical phenomena improved within 6 months (Berkhout et al., 1985). Factors that may associate with the progression of disease especially pain remain speculative. But it is observed that the disease progression is the result of a complex interplay between structural changes of the joint(s) and related psychosocial factors of the affected patients which highlights the importance of study of morbidity associated with OA.

6. Morbidity with different degrees of quality of life (QoL) impairments

In 1947, the World Health Organization (WHO) defined health not just by the absence of disease or infermity, but as a state of complete physical, mental and social well-being (World Health Organization, 1980). The departure from such a state is morbidity. The health related QoL is used to describe different domains within such a broader term of health or as a measure of morbidity associated with any health conditions. The specific dimensions found in most health related QoL definitions include: degrees of physical symptoms, functional limitations, emotional well-being, social functioning, role activities, life satisfaction and health perception (Fioravanti et al., 2005; Rejeski & Shumaker, 1994). Osteoarthritis, being a highly diversified clinical condition, would lead to morbidity with different degrees of QoL impairments among affected individuals (Woo et al., 2004).

6.1 Physical symptoms: Pain

Pain is usually the predominant symptom in patients with symptomatic OA. Pain in OA affects different domains of one's QoL: sleep interruption (Leigh et al., 1998; Wilcox et al., 2000), psychological stress (Downe-Wamboldt, 1991), reduced independence (Gignac et al., 2000), poorer perceived health (Loborde & Powers, 1985) and increased healthcare utilization (Badley & Wang, 1996). The likelihood of mobility problems increases as pain increases (Wilkie et al., 2007).

Yet, some patients experience significant pain and with subsequent QoL compromise even before OA has progressed enough to produce radiographic abnormalities. The reverse is also common; some patients feel little or no discomfort with low morbidity even though their radiographs show advanced OA. Why is there such a great discrepancy? Several observations suggest that pain in OA is not simply attributable to the structural changes in the affected joint, but the result of interplay between structural change, peripheral and central pain processing mechanism (Creamer & Hochberg, 1997) which can be explained by multi-dimensional concept of pain via Loeser's onion ring pain model (Figure 5): although pain is a nociceptive event (cognition of pain sensation from nociceptors), whether pain may lead to suffering (negative affection) and subsequent pain behaviors e.g. absence from work or healthcare utilization is mainly shaped by external psychosocial and other environmental factors (Loeser & Cousins, 1990).

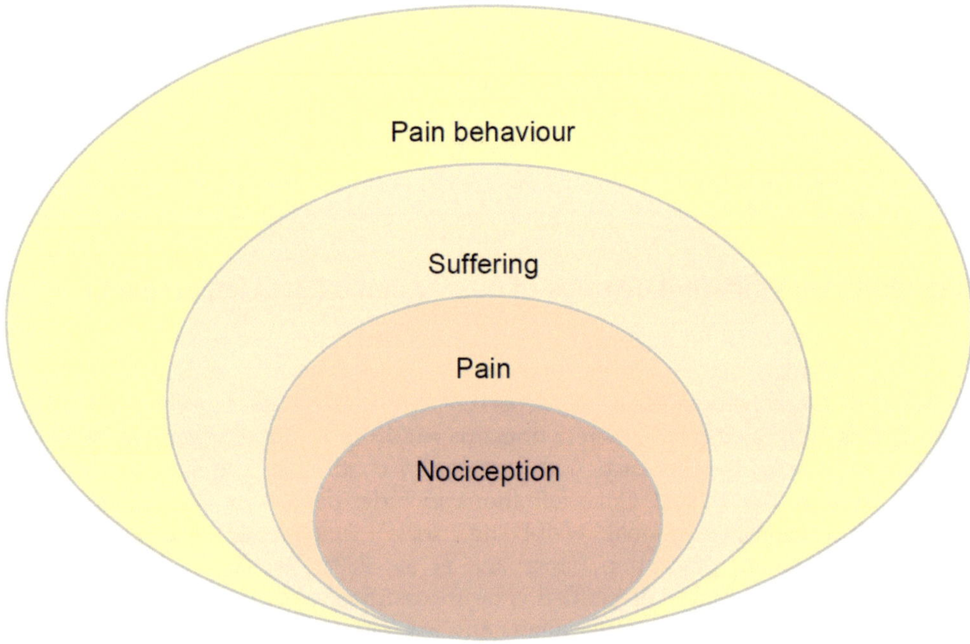

Fig. 5. Loeser's pain model

6.2 Biopsychosocial impairments

Similar concept which explains the impact of diseases upon individuals is the biopsychosocial (BPS) model (Engel, 1977). In such a model, OA is a *disease* which involves objective disorder at molecular, cellular, physiological, mechanical and structural levels confined to the affected individual. The affected individual will have a psychological awareness and perception of dysfunction at the personal level; such subjective state is known as the *illness*. The physical and/or psychological dysfunction as a result of the disease or illness at the personal level e.g. difficulty in climbing stairs is the *disability*. The compromised social role assumed by the affected individual as a result of the disease, associated illness and disability is termed as *handicap*. All the biological, psychological and social parameters are important determinants in the final outcomes, impairment of which would greatly compromise individuals' overall QoL in the context of the disease.

In the context of osteoarthritis, studies showed that pessimism was associated with poor physical outcomes (Brenes et al., 2002; Ferreira & Sherman, 2007). Observational studies found negative mood was correlated with more joints involvement and disability by OA and vice versa (Van Baar et al., 1998). Qualitative studies noticed patients with OA expressed declined life satisfaction and that depression and anxiety were their major mood problems (Tak & Laffrey et al., 2003). Patients felt distressed with not being able to participate in activities that they used to be able to do. The most frequently quoted activities are leisure activities such as travel, social activities, close relationships, community mobility, employment and heavy housework (Gignac et al., 2006). Some patients with advanced OA even perceived the disease threatened their self identities and felt lack of power to change their situation. However, studies also showed that a main bulk of OA patients would ignore their disease and tried to carry on their normal life regardless of symptoms exacerbation (Cook et al., 2007). From these studies, we can have a glimpse of the highly diversified OA morbidity as a result of inter-relationship between biopsychosocial factors among different OA patients.

6.3 Co-morbidities

Co-morbidity is defined as the co-existence of two or more health problems in a person. As OA is an age-related condition, patients with OA are also likely to suffer from a number of other disabling and chronic health conditions (Kadam et al., 2004). In a cross-sectional study of 455 patients suffering from knee OA, 78% of patients had at least one musculoskeletal co-morbidity and 82% had at least one non-musculoskeletal co-morbidity, on average they had 3.2 co-morbidities (Chan et al., 2009). The presence of co-morbidities would further complicate the clinical outcomes and impair patients' QoL in the following ways:

- Co-morbidities can interact with each other to produce high levels of disability. For example, there are increased pain and decreased mobility in patients with musculoskeletal co-morbidities (Croft et al., 2005); decreased ambulation and general health in patients with concomitant angina, chronic obstructive pulmonary disease, previous stroke or obesity.
- Polypharmacy issues may intervene. For examples, drug safety issues of COX-2 inhibitors among patients with cardiovascular co-morbidity; risk of gastro-intestinal upset or bleeding from the use of non-steroidal anti-inflammatory drugs (NSAIDs) among patients with gastro-intestinal co-morbidity.
- Depression can accompany any chronic condition like OA and lead to significant morbidity according to biopsychosocial model of disease. Treatment of the depressed individual with OA with antidepressants can improve pain, function, and quality of life scores (Lin et al., 2003).
- The presence of severe co-morbid conditions may influence the choice of treatment for OA, for example exercise, and joint replacement surgery.

7. Conclusions (Figure 6)

Osteoarthritis (OA) is not just a degenerative disease, but a clinical syndrome of joint pain with highly diversified clinical presentations. It is accompanied by varying degrees of functional limitation and reduction in quality of life. Discordance between osteoarthritis pathology, symptoms and disability is frequently encountered; hence structural pathology is not the absolute determinant to the clinical outcome. Psychosocial factors and co-morbidities are crucial issues which amalgamate the final health status of the affected individuals.

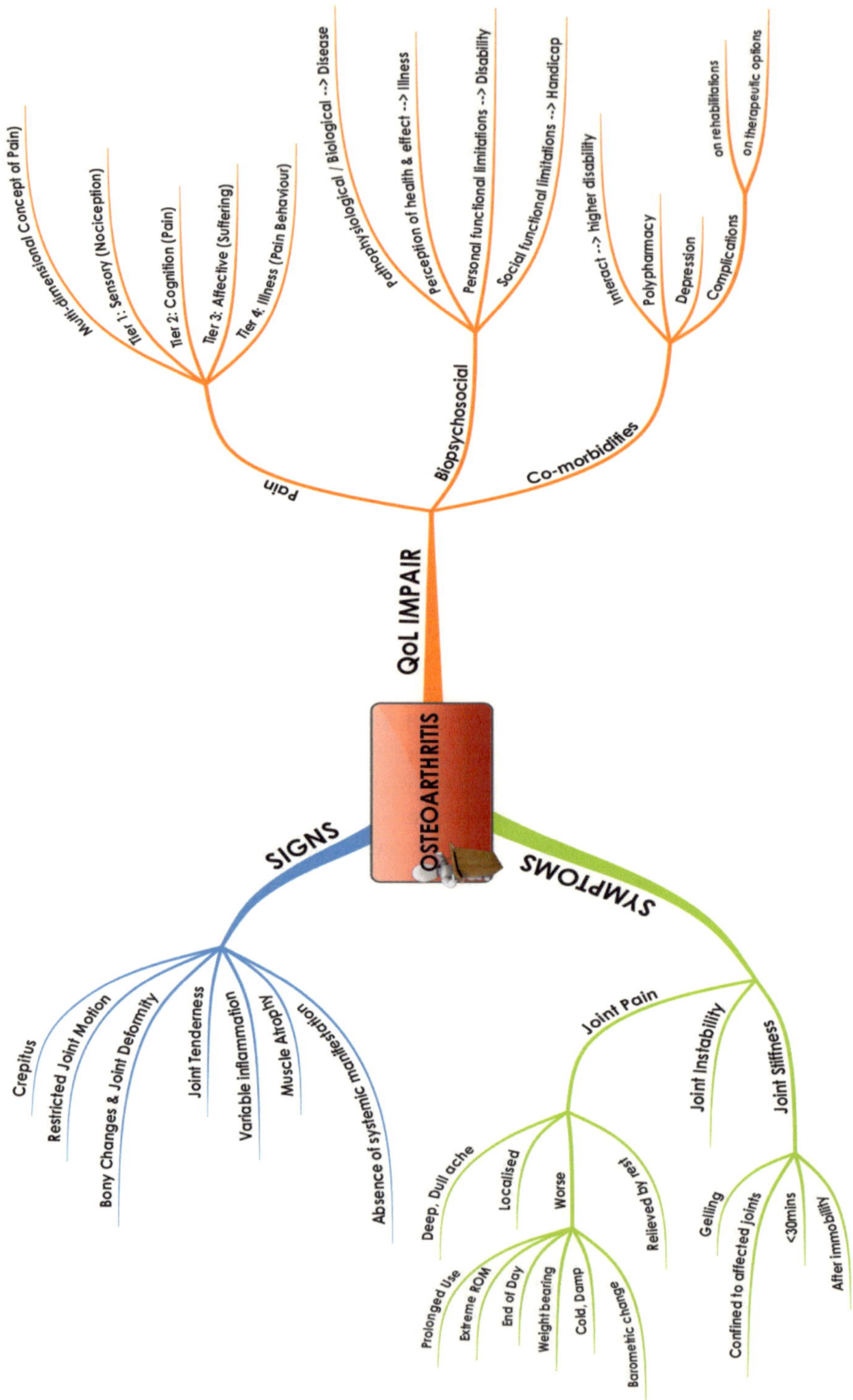

Fig. 6. Summary of symptoms, signs and QoL in OA.

8. References

Altman, R.D. (1991) Criteria for classification of clinical osteoarthritis. *J Rheumatol.*, 18(Suppl.27): pp.10-12.

Arnoldi CC, Linderholm H, Mussbichler H. (1972). Venous engorgement and intraosseous hypertension in osteoarthritis of the hip. *J Bone Joint Surg.* 54B: 409-421.

Badley, E.M. & Wang, P. (1996). Determinants of consultation with health professionals for musculoskeletal disorders in a population with universal health insurance. *Arthritis Rheum.*, 39: pp.S263.

Berkhout, B., MacFarlane, J.D. & Cats, A. (1985). Symptomatic osteoarthritis of the knee: A follow up study. *Br J Rheumatol.* 24: pp.40-45.

Brenes, G.A., Rapp, S.R. & Rejeski, W.J. (2002). Do optimism and pessimism predict physical functioning? *Journal of Behavioral Medicine.* 25(3): pp.219-231.

Chan, K.K.W. & Chan, L.W.Y. (2011). A qualitative study on patients with knee osteoarthritis to evaluate the influence of different pain patterns on patient's quality of life and to find out patients' interpretation and coping strategies for the disease. *Rheumatology Reports.* Volume 3:*e3*

Chan, K.K.W., Ngai, A.H.Y., Ip, A.K.K., Lam, S.K.H., Lai, M.W.W. (2009). Co-morbidities of patients with knee osteoarthritis. *HKMJ.* 15(3): pp.31-37.

Cook, C., Pietrobon, R. & Hegedus, E. (2007). Osteoarthritis and the impact on quality of life health indicators. *Rheumatology International.* 27(4): pp.315-321.

Creamer, P. & Hochberg, M.C. (1997). Why does osteoarthritis of the knee hurt sometimes? *Br J Rheumatol.* 37: pp.726-728.

Croft, P., Jordan, K. & Jinks, C. (2005). "Pain elsewhere" and the impact of knee pain in older people. *Arthritis Rheum* 52: pp.2350–2354.

Cyriax, J.H. & Cyriax, P.J. (1993). *Cyriax's illustrated Manual of Orthopaedic Medicine.* Butterworth Heinemann, ISBN 07506 3274 7, Oxford.

Cushnaghan J, Dieppe P. (1991). Study of 500 patients with limb joint osteoarthritis, part I: analysis by age, sex, and distribution of symptomatic joint sites. *Ann Rheum Dis.* 50: 8-13.

Dieppe, P.A., Cushnaghan, J. & Shepstone, L. (1997). The Bristol "OA500" study: progression of osteoarthritis (OA) over 3 years and the relationship between clinical and radiographic features at the knee joint. *Osteoarthritis Cartilage.* 5: pp.87-97.

Downe-Wamboldt, B. (1991). Coping and life satisfaction in elderly women with osteoarthritis. *J Adv Nurs* 16: pp.1328-1335.

Duncan, R., Peat, G. & Thomas, E. (2007). Symptoms and radiographic osteoarthritis: not as discordant as they are made out to be? *Annals of the Rheumatic Diseases.* 66(1): pp.86-91.

Engel, G.L. (1977). The need for a new medical model: A challenge for biomedicine. *Science.* 196: pp.129–136.

Ferreira, V.M. & Sherman, A.M. (2007). The relationship of optimism, pain and social support to well-being in older adults with osteoarthritis. *Aging & Mental Health.* 11(1): pp.89-98.

Fioravanti, A., Cantarini, L., Fabbroni, M., Righeschi, K. & Marcolongo, R. (2005). Methods used to assess clinical outcome and quality of life in osteoarthritis. *Semin Arthritis Rheum.* 34(6 Suppl 2): pp.70-72.

Gignac, M.A., Cott, C., Badley, E.M. (2000). Adaptation to chronic illness and disability and its relationship to perceptions of independence and dependence. *J Geronto B Psychol Sci Soc Sci.* 55: pp.362-372.

Gignac, M.A., Davis, A.M. & Hawker, G. (2006) "What do you expect? You're just getting older": a comparison of perceived osteoarthritis-related and aging –related health experience in middle- and older-age adults. *Arthritis & Rheumatism* 55(6): pp.905-912.

Hannan, M.T., Felson, D.T. & Pincus, T. (2000). Analysis of the discordance between radiographic changes and knee pain in osteoarthritis of the knee. *J Rheumatol.* 27: pp.1513.

Hawker, G.A., Stewart, L., French, M.R., Cibere, J., Jordan, J.M., March, L., Suarez-Almazor, M. & Gooberman-Hill, R. (2008) Understanding the pain experience in hip and knee osteoarthritis – an OARSI/OMERACT initiative. *Osteoarthritis Cartilage.* 16: pp.415-422.

Hochberg, M.C. (1996). Prognosis of osteoarthritis. *Ann Rheum Dis.* 55: pp.685-88.

Hurley, M.V. (1999) The role of muscle weakness in the pathogenesis of osteoarthritis. *Rheum Dis Clin North Am.* 25: pp.283-298.

Ike, R.W. & O'Rourke K.S. (1995). Compartment-directed physical examination of the knee can predict articular cartilage abnormalities disclosed by needle arthroscopy. *Arthritis Rheum.* 38: pp.917-925.

Jaovisidha, K., Rosenthal, A.K. (2002). Calcium crystals in osteoarthritis. *Current Opinion in Rheumatology.* 14: pp.298–302

Kadam, U.T., Jordan, K., Croft, P.R. (2004). Clinical comorbidity in patients with osteoarthritis: a case-control study of general practice consulters in England and Wales. *Ann Rheum Dis.* 63: pp.408-414.

Kellgren, J.H. (1983). Pain in osteoarthritis. *J Rheumatol.* 10(suppl 9): pp.108-9.

Ledingham, J., Regan, M., Jones, A. & Doherty, M. (1995). Factors affecting radiographic progression of knee osteoarthritis. *Ann Rheum Dis.* 54: pp.53-58.

Leigh, T.J., Hindmarch, I., Bird, H.A. & Wright, V. (1988). Comparison of sleep in osteoarthritic patients and age and sex matched healthy controls. *Ann Rheum Dis.* 47: pp.40-42.

Lin, E.H.B., Katon, W. & Von-Korff, M. (2003) Effect of improving depression care on pain and functional outcomes among older adults with arthritis. A randomized controlled trial. *JAMA* 290: pp.2428-2434.

Loborde, J.M., Powers, M.J. (1985). Life satisfaction, health control orientation, and illness-related factors in persons with osteoarthritis. *Res Nurs Health.* 8: pp.183-190.

Loeser, J.D., Cousins, M.J. (1990). Contemporary pain management. *Med J Aust.* 153: pp.208-212.

Massardo, L., Watt, I., Cushnaghan, J. & Dieppe, P. Osteoarthritis of the knee joint: an eight year prospective study. *Ann Rheum Dis.* 48: pp.893-7.

McAlindon, T.E., Snow, S., Cooper, C., & Dieppe, P.A. (1992). Radiographic patterns of osteoarthritis of the knee joint in the community: the importance of the patellofemoral joint. *Ann. Rheum. Dis.* 51: pp.844-849.

Nevitt, M.C., Xu, L. & Zhang, Y. (2002). Very low prevalence of hip osteoarthritis among Chinese elderly in Beijing, China, compared with Whites in the United States. *Arthritis and Rheumatism.* 46: pp.1773–1779.

O'Reilly, S. & Doherty, M. (1998) Clinical featuers of osteoarthritis and standard approaches to the diagnosis. In: Brandt, K.B., Doherty, M., Lohmander, L.S., eds. *Osteoarthritis.* Oxford, UK: Oxford University Press. pp.197-217.

Pattrick, M., Aldridge, S., Hamilton, E., Manhire, A. & Doherty, M. (1989) A controlled study of hand function in nodal and erosive osteoarthritis. *Ann. Rheum. Dissease.* 48: pp.978-982.

Peat, G., Thomas, E. & Duncan, R. (2006). Clinical classification criteria for knee osteoarthritis: performance in the general population and primary care. *Annals of the Rheumatic Diseases.* 65: pp.1363-1367.

Punzi, L., Ramonda, R. & Sfriso, P. (2004). Erosive osteoarthritis. *Best Practice & Research Clinical Rheumatology.* 18(5): pp.739-758.

Rejeski, W.J., Shumaker, S. (1994). Knee osteoarthritis and health-related quality of life. *Med Sci Sports Exerc.* 26(12): pp.1441-1445.

Rothschild BM. (2006). Pathologic acromioclavicular and sternoclavicular manifestations in rheumatoid arthritis, spondyloarthropathy and calcium pyrophosphate deposition disease. *Skeletal Radiol.* 35:367.

Rothschild BM, Bruno MA. (2011). Calcium pyrophosphate deposition disease. *eMedicine Radiology.* http://www.emedicine.com/radioTOPIC125.HTM

Rothschild BM, Woods RJ, Rothschild C. (1992). Calcium pyrophosphate deposition disease: Description in defleshed skeletons. *Clin Exp Rheumatol* 10:557-564.

Rothschild BM, Yakubov LE. (1997). Prospective six month, double-blind trial of hydroxychloroquine treatment of calcium pyrophosphate deposition disease. *Contemp Ther* 23:327-331.

Schouten J.S.A.G., Van denOuweland F.A. & Valkenburg H.A. (1992). A 12 year follow-up study in the general population on prognostic factors of cartilage loss in osteoarthritis of the knee. *Ann Rheum Dis.* 51: pp.932-937.

Tak, S.H. & Laffrey, S.C. (2003). Life satisfaction and its correlates in older women with osteoarthritis. *Orthopaedic Nursing* 22(3): pp.182-189.

Van Baar, M.E., Dekker, J. & Lemmers, J.A. (1998). Pain and disability in patients with osteoarthritis of hip or knee. *J Rheumatol.* 25: pp.125-133.

Wilcox, S., Brenes, G.A. & Levine, D. (2000). Factors related to sleep disturbance in older adults experiencing knee pain or knee pain with radiographic evidence of knee osteoarthritis. *J Am Geriatr Soc.* 48: pp.1241-1251.

Wilkie, R., Peat, G. & Thomas, E. (2007). Factors associated with restricted mobility outside the home in community-dwelling adults aged 50 years and older with knee pain: an example of use of an international classification of functioning to investigate participation restriction. *Arthritis Care & Research.* 57(8): pp.1381-9.

Woo, J., Lau, E. & Lee, P. (2004). Impact of osteoarthritis on quality of life in a Hong Kong Chinese population. *J Rheumatol* 31: pp.2433-2438.

World Health Organization. (1980). International classification of impairments, disabilities and handicap (ICIDH): a manual of classification relating to the consequences of disease. Geneva WHO 1980.

Part 2

Imaging

3

An Atlas-Based Approach to Study Morphological Differences in Human Femoral Cartilage Between Subjects from Incidence and Progression Cohorts: MRI Data from Osteoarthritis Initiative

Hussain Tameem and Usha Sinha
San Diego State University
USA

1. Introduction

Recent advances in magnetic resonance (MR) imaging have made it the modality of choice for assessment of cartilage status for osteoarthritis (OA) (Roemer et al., 2009; Eckstein, 2007). MRI allows assessment of morphological changes using high resolution 3D imaging as well as evaluation of changes at the biochemical/molecular level using MR relaxometry techniques (T2: spin-spin relaxation and T1ρ: spin-lattice relaxation with spin locking) and delayed Gadolinium enhanced MRI of cartilage (dGEMRIC) (Blumenkrantz & Majumdar, 2007). Research on the potential application of MRI to detect and classify osteoarthritis and monitor progression is an area of intense research (Hunter et al., 2009).

A number of review articles detail the technical limits, accuracy and precision of MRI including the choice of pulse sequences and image analysis methods for morphological assessment in osteoarthritis (Raynauld, 2003; Eckstein et al., 2009; Xing, 2011). Cartilage morphology metrics from MRI are now being actively explored as imaging biomarkers of disease status and progression. The sequences that provide the best contrast of cartilage to adjacent tissue as well as the best resolution are the fat-suppressed spoiled gradient echo and fast double echo and steady state (DESS) with water excitation (Blumenkrantz & Majumdar, 2007; Roemer et al., 2010). Segmentation of the cartilage is a challenging task and few completely automated segmentation algorithms have been proposed. A fully automated segmentation algorithm based on Active Shape Modeling (Fripp et al., 2007) has been implemented and evaluated for normal cartilage. A more recent automated algorithm that is extensible to osteoarthritic cartilage first segments the bone-cartilage interface and then classifies cartilage voxels based on texture analysis. However, the large-scale applicability of these algorithms to normal and diseased cartilage is not yet demonstrated. Semi-automated algorithms using region growing, edge detection, and spline fitting have been used successfully in large-scale projects (Raynauld, 2003; Duryea et al., 2007). Morphological indices used to classify disease status and progression, include global and regional measures of total cartilage volume (raw and normalized), cartilage surface area, cartilage thickness (global and regional), and denuded area (Pelletier et al., 2007; Eckstein et al., 2009; Hunter et al., 2009). However, several research groups are still trying to determine which cartilage morphometric measure is most responsive or valid in predicting progression (Eckstein et al., 2006; Hunter et al., 2009). Several studies have also established the superiority of using MR at 3.0T for measuring cartilage thickness and volume in an accurate way (Kshirsagar et al., 1998; Raynauld, 2003; Eckstein et al., 2006; Dam et al., 2007; Guermazi et al., 2008). Eckstein et al. performed a study to measure thickness, volume, and surface area of the femorotibial cartilage. These measurements were obtained from MR images that were acquired at 1.5T and 3.0T field strength at same slice thickness. The authors show that the precision for quantitative cartilage morphology measurements at 3.0T was significantly higher when compared to those at 1.5T demonstrating importance of MR imaging at 3.0T for cartilage in determining OA progression (Eckstein et al., 2005).

Early longitudinal studies showed that MR morphometric data was highly sensitive to cartilage loss (cartilage volume or thickness changes of the order of -4 to -6%); however more recent studies report cartilage volume/thickness changes lower at -1 to 3% per year (Hunter et al., 2009). Phan et al. in their study calculated the rate of cartilage loss using MR images at 1.5T in subjects with knee OA in a longitudinal study. They also compared and correlated this value along with other parameters to the clinical Western Ontario and McMaster University Osteoarthritis (WOMAC) score. Their results showed the suitability of using MR for tracking OA in longitudinal studies. They were able to visualize cartilage degradation not seen through regular radiographs. However, they did not find any correlation with the WOMAC score which was attributed to patients getting used to their pain (Phan et al., 2006). Several studies have utilized the longitudinal MR image data available from the Osteoarthritis Initiative (OAI) to study cartilage in OA (Eckstein et al., 2001; Duryea et al., 2010; Thompson, et al., 2010; Guermazi et al., 2011; Iranpour-Boroujeni et al., 2011; Wirth et al., 2011a, 2011b). Eckstein et al. performed a study where they investigated the rate at which cartilage deterioration occurs when looking at OAI participants grouped in three categories described as healthy, with no radiographic evidence or risk and knees with radiographic evidence of OA (Kellgren/Lawrence score of 2-4). Sub-regional thickness calculated from coronal MR images showed that there was no significant difference seen between the healthy group and group with no radiographic evidence of OA in the weight bearing sub-regions of the femorotibial cartilage. However, significant difference in cartilage thickness (loss) was seen in knees from the group with radiographic evidence of OA (higher K&L scores) when compared to knee for participants in the healthy group (Eckstein et al., 2001). Wirth et al. demonstrated that standardized response mean (SRM) calculated from the femorotibial cartilage thickness values were modestly higher when the observation are made for a period of 2 years as compared to 1 year for knees with radiographic evidence of OA (Wirth et al., 2011). A study by Duryea et al. proposes measuring the joint space width (JSW) as an improved alternative to the current MR methodology for cartilage morphology. The study demonstrates that the SRM values for radiographic JSW are very much comparable to those obtained from the MRI measures and hence can be a more cost effective alternative (Duryea et al., 2010). Increasingly, studies indicate that sub regional assessment of cartilage volume/thickness is more sensitive than global assessment of longitudinal changes.

As the preceding discussion summarizes, morphological changes detected by imaging techniques provide an important tool for diagnosis and assessment of osteoarthritis. However biochemical changes precede these morphological changes and thus the ability to detect biochemical changes will be essential to the early diagnosis and treatment of pathologies. MRI affords this ability through measurement of MR indices that are sensitive to local biochemical changes. The MR indices that have been established as sensitive markers of osteoarthritis are: T2, T1ρ and dGEMRIC (Blumenkrantz et al., 2007). Findings from these studies have shown these parameters to correlate with clinical findings and a potential to uses these parameters in a clinical environment to detect and monitor OA. These techniques have the power of detecting cartilage loss at an early stage when the damage is still reversible (David-Vaudey et al., 2004; Li et al., 2005; Phan et al., 2006; Regatte et al., 2006; Koff et al., 2007; Li et al., 2007; Link et al., 2007).

T2 relaxation time (spin-spin relaxation) is a noninvasive marker of cartilage integrity as it is sensitive to tissue hydration and the collagen-proteoglycan matrix (Blumenkrantz et al., 2007; Taylor et al., 2009; Link et al., 2010). In normal cartilage, T2 is low due to the immobilization of the water protons in the collagen-proteoglycan matrix. Depletion of collagen and proteoglycan in osteoarthritis renders protons more mobile which is reflected as longer T2 relaxation times. Another factor that contributes to the increased T2 is due to an increase in water content in diseased cartilage. However, the link between T2 and biochemical changes is complex; T2 changes have been correlated with changes in collagen content but not with proteoglycan loss (Regatte et al., 2002). An interesting feature of cartilage T2 is the spatial distribution within the cartilage with a steep gradient from the subchondral bone to the cartilage surface. Prior studies have explored the relationship between T2 and cartilage morphometry: T2 has been found to be inversely correlated with cartilage volume and thickness (Dunn et al., 2004). Studies analyzing MRI T2 relaxation time have also been performed on the data from OAI (Carballido-Gamio et al., 2011; Pan et al., 2011). Carballido-Gamio et al. propose a new improved technique that involves flattening of the cartilage and application of texture analysis to create T2 maps. The texture analysis performed using gray-level co-occurrence matrix in direction parallel and perpendicular to the cartilage layers. The longitudinal analysis is performed on data at baseline, 1-year follow-up, and 2-year follow-up. The results show several textures features showing higher values perpendicular to the cartilage layers where other texture feature exhibiting higher values parallel to the cartilage layers. These finding provide initial results to an alternative approach to study cartilage in OA (Carballido-Gamio et al., 2011). Another study investigates the correlation between T2 values obtained from MR images at 3.0T and the vastus lateralis/vastus medialis cross-sectional area (VL/VM CSA) in a group of middle aged subjects from the incidence cohort (non-symptomatic). The authors used axial T1W images to calculate the CSA values of the thigh muscles. The results showed that higher values of T2 correlated with greater loss of cartilage in OA. Regression values indicated that the VL/VM CSA values are inversely proportional to the T2 values (Pan et al., 2011).

T1ρ refers to measurement of T1 in the rotating frame and probes very low frequency interactions such as between water and large macromolecules (like proteoglycan) that are present in the extracellular matrix of the cartilage (Blumenkrantz et al., 2007; Taylor et al., 2009). T1ρ has been shown to be correlated with proteoglycan disruption and shows regional variations similar to T2. Studies have shown that cartilage T1ρ values in OA subjects to be increased compared to controls that is in accordance with the model of proteoglycan disruption with disease. Comparing T2 and T1ρ, Majumdar et al. found T1ρ to be more sensitive than T2 in distinguishing OA cartilage from healthy cartilage (Majumdar 2006).

In dGEMRIC studies, the charged contrast agent $GdDTPA^{2-}$ is injected intravenously into a patient and allowed to diffuse into articular cartilage and imaging is performed 2-3 hours after contrast administration (Blumenkrantz et al., 2007; Taylor et al., 2009). The proteoglycan molecule consists of a central protein core to which a large number of negatively charged side chains called glycosaminoglycan (GAG) are attached. The GAG side chains repel the negatively charged contrast agent so that regions of low GAG concentration (as in diseased cartilage) show greater contrast uptake than normal cartilage. The distribution of the contrast agent (and GAG) is calculated from a T1 map of the cartilage. Like T2 maps, the T1 maps are heterogeneous indicating that the spatial distribution of GAG is heterogeneous. The dGEMRIC has been used to evaluate osteoarthritis in knee cartilage and T1 values correlate to the KL grading scale (Williams et al., 2005). dGEMRIC has shown potential in early detection of osteoarthritis as it provides direct information on the distribution and content of GAG in cartilage.

From the discussion so far, it is clear that regional quantitative assessment of morphological/biochemical cartilage is more sensitive than global changes, and the analysis requires one to account for spatial heterogeneity in the indices as well as the variability of these indices in a normal population. To address these factors, studies have used T and Z scores successfully to study cartilage loss, T2, $T1\rho$ and dGEMRIC changes in OA (Blumenkrantz et al., 2007). T and Z scores provide an estimation of the difference between patients and healthy young subjects and the difference between patients and their age matched healthy subjects respectively. Burgkart et al. showed in their study that the cartilage volume measurements when normalized on joint surface area before diseased state increase the accuracy and applicability of T and Z scores by reducing inter-subject variability (Burgkart et al., 2003). However, the T or Z score are still based on the mean value for normal subjects in a cartilage compartment. Thus, it averages the spatial distribution of the index over the compartment and given the spatial variation of the MR indices, this approach may mask subtle changes.

Morphological quantification of osteoarthritis currently includes measurement of sub-regional cartilage loss. Detailed studies have revealed a small loss of 1-2% in cartilage thickness annually and a high degree of spatial heterogeneity for cartilage thickness changes in femorotibial sub-regions between subjects (Eckstein et al., 2010; Frobell et al., 2010; Wirth et al., 2010). Most quantitative studies divide the cartilage into a few compartments and report cartilage thickness (mean and standard deviation) for each compartment. Wirth et al. reported a technique for regional analysis of femorotibial cartilage thickness based on quantitative MRI (Wirth et al., 2008). The latter paper uses an elegant algorithm driven identification of sub-regions with user-controlled parameters to define the sub-regions. Wirth et al proposed that these parameters could be tuned according to the regional cartilage progression with OA. This technique represents a significant advancement in the automated and quantitative assessment of cartilage thickness. However, localized changes smaller than the size of the sub-regions may escape detection even with this technique. Eckstein et al explored the magnitude and regional distribution of differences in cartilage thickness and subchondral bone area associated with specific Osteoarthritis Research Society International (OARSI) JSN grades. Their regional analysis provided quantitative estimates of JSN related cartilage loss and revealed that the central part of the weight-bearing femoral condyle as the most strongly affected (Eckstein et al., 2010). In a recent paper, Wirth et al extended their regional analysis to identify spatial patterns of cartilage loss in the medial femoral condyle. They localized the posterior aspect of the central, weight-bearing medial femoral condyle as showing the greatest sensitivity to change in disease status (Wirth et al., 2010).

These regional analyses clearly indicate that cartilage loss occurs in a spatially heterogeneous manner and sometimes, in very localized regions. Stammberger et al. proposed elastic registration of 3D cartilage surfaces to detect local changes in cartilage thickness; in both synthetic and volunteer data, thickness differences recovered from the registration method were similar to that from using Euclidean distance transformations (Stammberger et al., 2000). Cohen et al. generated templates of cartilage of the patellofemoral joint and demonstrated the potential of using the standard thickness maps by comparing it with thickness maps generated for individual patients to identify regions with maximum loss of cartilage in patients with Osteoarthritis (Cohen et al., 2003). Recently, Carballido-Gamio et al. performed inter-subject comparison of knee cartilage thickness after registration to a common reference space (Carballido-Gamio et al., 2008). They measured the thickness at each point on the bone-cartilage interface and used affine and elastic registration techniques for point-wise comparison of cartilage thickness. They established the reproducibility of this method for intra- and inter- subject cartilage thickness comparisons and concluded that the techniques could be used to build mean femoral shapes and cartilage thickness maps. They showed that the proposed technique was an accurate and robust way to analyze inter-subject thickness point wise. However, there are no reports to date on the construction of a cartilage atlas to automatically characterize cartilage morphology in a population group (i.e., a cartilage atlas), which can be used to assess localized morphological or parametric differences between cohorts.

Our approach extends prior work on creation of standard maps of cartilage thickness to an atlas-based approach. The atlas-based approach allows automatic detection of voxel based differences between cohorts (e.g., segregated by age, gender, ethnicity, disease status) as well as enables tracking of longitudinal changes. The approach is general and differences are not restricted to morphological differences at the voxel level but extend to parametric maps of T2, T1ρ, and dGEMRIC. The approach has the potential to allow automatic and accurate detection of subtle changes as it leverages the statistical power of the cohort size. Thus, it is possible to model variability within the cohort and identify significant differences between the cohorts at the voxel level. This unique approach allows measuring localized changes in cartilage morphometry without any previous knowledge of probable regions of changes. The approach is also not restricted to detecting differences/changes in cartilage; it can also be extended to other anatomical structures that are impacted by osteoarthritis (e.g., bone). In this chapter, we outline the atlas based method and apply it (i) to detecting disease-based differences in cartilage morphometry, and (ii) to creating a bone atlas from knee MRI of normal healthy young adults.

2. Methodology

2.1 Data selection criteria and MRI

Data for the current project was obtained from the Osteoarthritis Initiative. Realizing the importance of OA and its impact on millions of patients (socially and economically) National Institute of Health (NIH) started a four-year observational study called the Osteoarthritis Initiative (OAI). This initiative was lead by the National Institute of Health (NIH) in collaboration with an academic and industrial consortium to obtain clinical, biochemical and imaging data on a large cohort of subjects to follow the onset and progression of osteoarthritis. The OAI provides an extremely rich database of high resolutions MR images of human knees and is made publicly available to the research community (www.ucsf.edu). OAI provides MR images for 4,796 participants (ver. 0.E.1) at baseline and the follow-up data for these participants at periodic intervals through other data release versions. Availability of this rich dataset, have resulted in several promising research methodologies and significant findings.

This study uses sagittal knee magnetic resonance images made available in OAI data release version 0.A.1. A water-excitation double echo steady state (DESS) imaging sequence was used to generate the MR images on a Magnetom Trio, Siemens acquisition machine at 3.0T. The imaging parameters used in the acquisition protocol are repetition time (TR)/echo time (TE): 16.3/4.7ms, x and y resolution: 0.365, slice thickness: 0.7 mm and field of view (FOV): 140 mm.

The OAI data version 0.A.1 for images (MRI and X-ray) refers to the baseline line data and represents its first public release. This release contains 200 incidence and progression cohort participants. The participants in this group were further stratified based on gender and clinic (four recruitment centers). OAI adopts the following criteria to classify subjects as belonging to the progression or incidence sub-cohort. The progression cohort consists of participants that have symptomatic OA at the onset of the study. The incidence cohort contains participants with no prior symptomatic OA at the start of the study, but is at a higher risk of knee OA. OAI defines symptomatic knee OA in participants if they meet both of following criteria: 1. Knee symptoms defined by "pain, aching, or stiffness in or around the knee on most days" for at least a month in the past year and 2. Radiographic evidence of tibiofemoral osteophytes that is comparable to Kellgren and Lawrence grade $\geq$ 2. Participants with no symptomatic knee OA (as defined above) in either knee at baseline, but exhibit characteristics such as frequent knee symptoms with no radiographic OA or meeting two or more eligibility factors, are classified in the incidence sub cohort.

The cartilage atlas was created from 30 participants chosen from the available set of 200 incidence and progression cohorts. All atlas subjects belong to the incidence cohort and are Caucasian males. Further, subjects in the incidence group with KLG scores in the range of 0-2 ('absent' to 'mild' OA) were used to create the atlas. Sagittal knee MR images of the selected 30 male participants were used to create the femoral cartilage image atlas. The demographics of the participants are as follows: mean $\pm$ standard deviation of the age 66.5 $\pm$ 8.2 years and mean $\pm$ standard deviation of the KLG grade 1.56 $\pm$ 1.1 (more details can be obtained from our previous publication (Tameem et al., 2011). In addition to the 30 participants chosen to create the cartilage atlas, 10 male participants were chosen from the incidence and progression group each to compare localized changes in femoral cartilage with disease condition. It should be noted that the ten incidence cohort subjects chosen for the comparison were not part of the atlas cohort. The mean $\pm$ standard deviation of age for participants chosen from the incidence and progression cohort was 64 $\pm$ 8.87 and 67.5 $\pm$ 8.78 respectively. The average knee osteophyte (KOST) grade, average knee joint space-medial (KJSM) grade, average knee joint space-lateral (KJSL), and Kellgren and Lawrence (K&L) grade for the incidence cohort is 1, 0, 0, and 1 respectively. The average KOST, KJSM, KJSL, and K&L grade for participants from the progression cohort is 1.8, 0.5, 0.1, and 2.3 respectively. Table 1 provides the detailed demographics of all participants.

	Incidence					Progression				
Subject	Age	KOST	KJSM	KJSL	K&L	Age	KOST	KJSM	KJSL	K&L
Pat01	50	1	0	0	1	58	2	0	0	2
Pat02	69	0	0	0	0	68	2	0	0	2
Pat03	60	0	0	0	0	69	2	1	0	3
Pat04	65	2	0	0	2	53	1	0	0	1
Pat05	55	2	0	0	2	75	2	0	0	2
Pat06	66	0	0	0	0	61	2	0	1	3
Pat07	75	2	0	0	2	78	1	1	0	1
Pat08	54	2	0	0	2	72	2	1	0	3
Pat09	72	1	0	0	1	79	2	1	0	3
Pat10	74	0	0	0	0	62	2	1	0	3

Table 1. Demographics of participants from incidence and progression sub-cohort

2.2 Overview of the femoral atlas creation process

The femoral cartilage atlas was generated from the MR images of the right knee of the 30 chosen participants from the incidence cohort using the following steps.

2.2.1 Delineation of the cartilage from the MR knee images

The image on the left top corner in figure 1 shows a slice from the MR images of the knee. Automatic identification of the cartilage from the knee image is a challenging endeavor because of low contrast in some areas and is an area of intense research activity. A robust completely automated algorithm has not yet been validated on a large number of image volumes. However, for this study our focus was to develop the cartilage atlas and a manual segmentation was used. It was critical to be precise in accurately segmenting the cartilage from the entire knee image. For this purpose, two operators (graduate students) in consultation with and verified by an experienced musculo-skeletal radiologist manually segmented the femoral cartilage from the knee images. An iterative approach was taken where the operators consulted the radiologist before and after performing segmentation for small sets of images. Consultations after segmenting each small set ensured high accuracy and reduced fatigue for the operators; this was critical considering the large number of slices for each participant because of the high resolution MR scans (0.365×0.365×0.70) and 30 datasets for creating the atlas (Tameem et al., 2007, 2011).

2.2.2 Image pre-processing steps

As a first step, a cubic interpolation scheme was applied to the segmented images to achieve an isotropic resolution of 0.365×0.365×0.365 mm^3 for datasets of all 30 participants. A reference subject was selected with age and KL grade close to the average of the cohort as the initial representative of the cohort. All subjects were than aligned to the reference subject. This initial alignment was achieved using a mutual information based affine transform technique available through the FMRIB Software Library (FSL) (Jenkinson & Smith, 2001). The affine transformation corrects for global size and positional differences between a subject and the chosen reference. The affine transformed subject data is then mapped to the reference using an elastic registration technique that is based on the Demons algorithm (Thirion 1998). This mapping results in a 3-dimensional deformation field that spatially maps each voxel in a subject dataset to the coordinate system of the reference. This process is iterative and is computed using the equation 1 (Ardekani & Sinha, 2006).

$$u_{n+1} = G_\sigma \otimes \left(u_n + G_\sigma \otimes \frac{1}{2} \left[\frac{C(T-S)\|\nabla S\|\|\nabla T\|}{(\|\nabla T\|^2 + \|\nabla S\|^2)(\|\nabla S\|^2 + \|\nabla T\|^2 + 2(T-S)^2)} \nabla S \right] \right) \quad (1)$$

In equation 1, u_{n+1} denotes the correction vector field at iteration $n+1$, G_σ is a Gaussian filter with variance σ, $\otimes$ represents the convolution, scaling factor denoted by C, and T and S denote the reference and transformed image intensities respectively. The displacement $u(q)$ is estimated by the algorithm such that for every voxel location (q) in the reference image (T) it maps the corresponding location in the subject's transformed images (S). To preserve the morphology, the algorithm computes deformation fields through both forward and backward transformations. The Gaussian filter was optimized to a 3x3x3 kernel to make sure the deformation is smooth and registration is more accurate. A mean intensity image is created when the transformed images of the entire group are averaged. Similarly, averaging the deformation fields of all images in the group yields a mean deformation field. Combining this mean deformation field with the mean intensity image creates an image template for the group. In the next iteration the image template produced replaces the reference image and the whole process of affine and elastic transformation for all 30 image set is repeated again. This process continues until there is no substantial change in the deformation field between two consecutive computations. This was observed after 4-5 iterations when creating the cartilage atlas. The final image created is the average shape atlas that converges to the centroid of the population data set (Kochunov et al., 2001, 2005). The entire process is visualized in figure 1.

2.3 Active shape models

Active shape models (ASM) developed in the past (Cootes et al., 1994) have been used extensively to determine the patterns of variability within a group of subjects. Using principal component analysis, ASMs can be created from the deformation fields that are available after the last step in the atlas creation process. We define the deformation field as a 3-dimensional matrix that stores the amount of displacement needed to move a voxel on the atlas to its corresponding voxel location in the subject (this is achieved with the freeform transformation). The analysis was performed in the following steps also discussed in detail in our recent publication (Tameem et al., 2011). The mean deformation value over N subjects is calculated by averaging the deformation field for all subjects over every voxel as shown in equation 2.

$$d_{mean} = (\Sigma di / N) \quad (2)$$

Using equation 3 we can calculate the deviation of each subject from the mean value calculated in equation 2.

$$\Delta di = di - dmean \quad (3)$$

A covariance matrix of dimension n×n is calculated as show in equation 4. This covariance matrix enables calculating the basis as shown in equation 4.

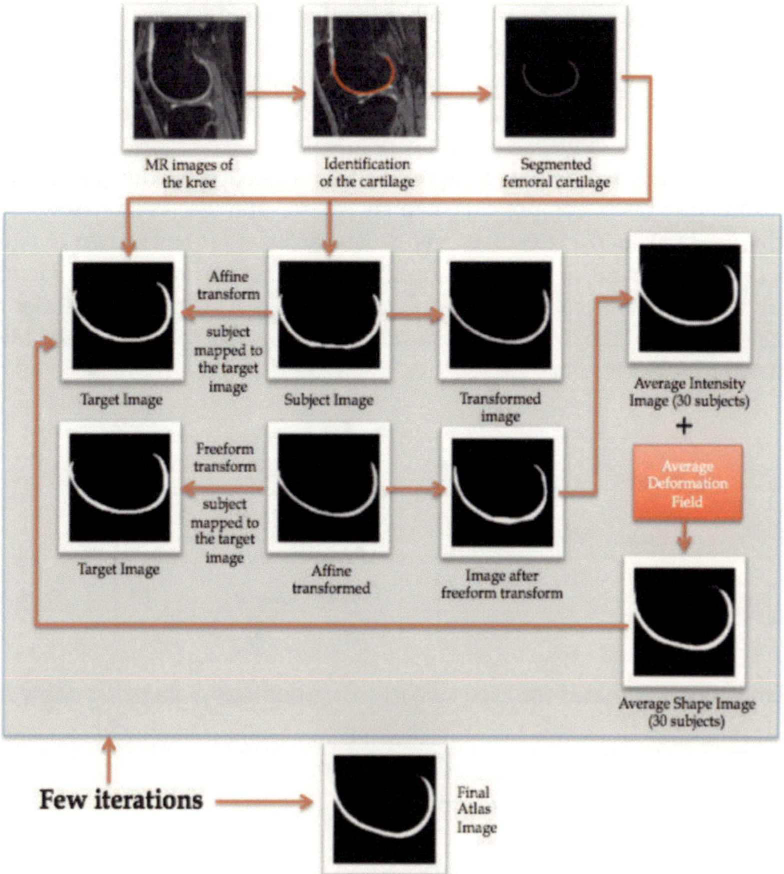

Fig. 1. An illustration of various steps involved in the atlas creation process: starting from the initial data selection, manual segmentation, affine registration, and freeform registration. Iterating the freeform registration and updating the template results in convergence to the centroid of the cohort.

$$d_{mean} = (\sum \Delta d_i \Delta d_i^T / N) \quad (4)$$

Finally, the eigenvectors and eigenvalues are calculated by diagonalizing the covariance matrix. Using equation 5 a linear model is created which is our shape model.

$$d = d_{mean} + \nu W_s \quad (5)$$

In equation 5, υ = (υ1, υ2... υk) is a matrix of the first eigenvectors, and Ws is a vector of weights called the shape coefficient. The principal component analysis on the deformation fields of all 30 participants results in the lead modes of shape variation. Shape variations are calculated along the two leading modes of variations at ±2SD and ±3D from the mean image. The shape variance for the femoral cartilage within the group of participants used to create the atlas can be visually represented through the images synthesized using ASMs.

2.4 Tensor morphometric analysis to detect local shape changes

Local variations in shape between populations can be estimated using the jacobian values of the deformation fields available from the non-linear warping algorithm. The deformation fields obtained from the last step of atlas creation process provide for a voxel (q) in the atlas reference frame, a three dimensional map of displacement values. For every voxel (q) mapped from the reference image (atlas) to the subject image (i), the displacement values can be broken into three components namely u_i, v_i, and w_i. Each voxel itself can be expressed by its three coordinates x, y, and z. The jacobian $J_i(q)$ as shown in equation 6, is defined as the determinant of the gradient mapping function and I is the identity matrix. The jacobian values that are calculated are always positive. A value of 1 indicates no volume change, values greater than 1 represent positive volume change, and values lower than 1 represent a negative volume change.

$$J_i(\boldsymbol{q}) = \left|\nabla(\boldsymbol{q}+\boldsymbol{u}_i(\boldsymbol{q}))\right| = \left| I + \begin{pmatrix} \frac{\partial u_i(\boldsymbol{q})}{\partial x} & \frac{\partial u_i(\boldsymbol{q})}{\partial y} & \frac{\partial u_i(\boldsymbol{q})}{\partial z} \\ \frac{\partial v_i(\boldsymbol{q})}{\partial x} & \frac{\partial v_i(\boldsymbol{q})}{\partial y} & \frac{\partial v_i(\boldsymbol{q})}{\partial z} \\ \frac{\partial w_i(\boldsymbol{q})}{\partial x} & \frac{\partial w_i(\boldsymbol{q})}{\partial y} & \frac{\partial w_i(\boldsymbol{q})}{\partial z} \end{pmatrix} \right| \qquad (6)$$

The jacobian values calculated for each subject in a group are averaged as show in equation 7.

$$J_P(x,y,z) = \frac{1}{N}\sum_{i=1}^{N} J_i(x,y,z) \qquad (7)$$

J_p denotes to the mean of the jacobian values over all subject in the cohort under consideration. N represents the number of subjects in each population group, and J_i (x, y, z) denotes the jacobian value at each voxel location for subject i. When images are warped the calculated jacobian values provide information on the localized volume changes between two populations. Using statistical techniques regions with significant differences between the two populations (the incidence and progression cohort) can be identified on a voxel level. Jacobian maps provide a powerful visual description that highlights these changes.

2.5 Statistical analysis

The jacobian values were obtained after aligning each subject in the incidence and progression cohort to the atlas as described in the previous step. Some processing steps such as smoothing the deformation fields using a 4mm full-width-half-maximum Gaussian kernel were performed. Smoothing takes care of any inaccuracies in the registration and ensures a normal distribution. The statistical analysis is performed using the Statistical Parametric Mapping (SPM) application (version 5) in MATLAB (Ashburner, 2009). A two-sample t-test voxel based analysis was performed on the dataset between the incidence and progression cohort to determine the local variations in the cartilage morphology between the populations. A false discovery rate (FDR) correction was used to control for multiple comparisons (Benjamini & Hochberg, 1995). FDR is an established method to correct for multiple comparisons in brain voxel-based morphometry. Statistical analysis yields some regions with higher "t" values that indicate areas of larger morphological differences in the femoral cartilage between the incidence and progression group.

3. Results

3.1 Registration and atlas

Accuracy in segmentation and registration are critical components in the atlas creation process. The initial affine transformation correct for positional and size differences. The freeform transformation applied after affine transformation measures true morphological differences. Figure 2 shows the alignment results of one of the slices of a 3D image volume. The contour shown on the reference image is transferred to the subject image before and after affine and non-linear transformation to confirm accuracy achieved in the registration process. It is fairly evident from the results that the affine transform does a very good job of correcting the positional shape changes, whereas, the non-non-linear transform corrects the local changes.

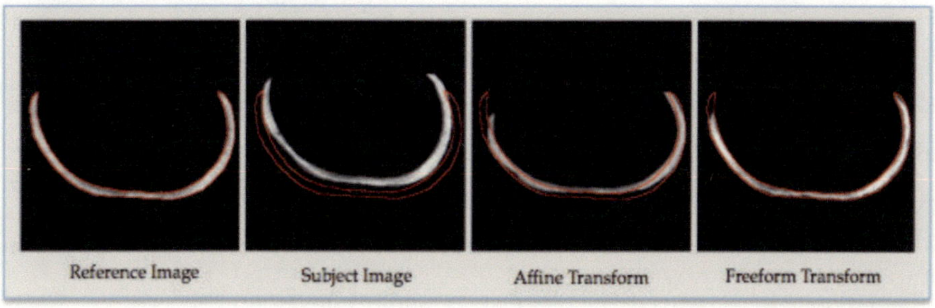

Fig. 2. Image showing registration accuracy achieved during the atlas creation process. (From left to right): The contour traced on the reference image is overlaid on the subject image, subject image after affine transform, and subject image after freeform transformation.

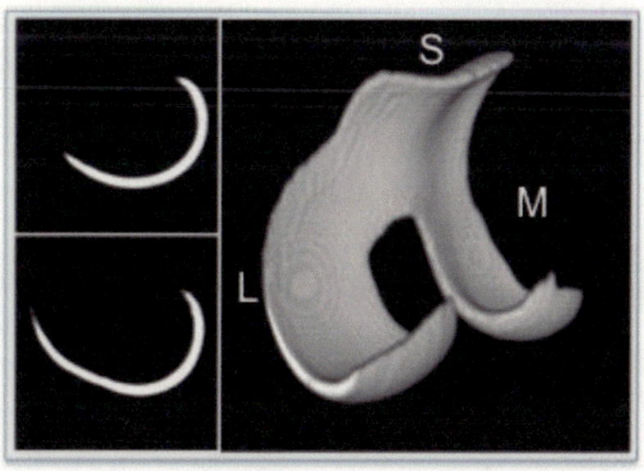

Fig. 3. Figure illustrates the 2D slices of the atlas image in the left column and a 3D image in the right column. The sharp edges displayed on the atlas image are evidence of high registration precision (S-superior, L-lateral, and M-medial).

After 3 iterations, no significant change in the deformation field values was observed in successive iterations. The atlas converged to the population centroid after three iterations and the sharp edges seen in the atlas (figure 3) confirm the accuracy of the free form registration.

3.2 Visualizing deformation maps

The mean and standard deviation of the femoral cartilage calculated from the magnitude of the 3D deformation fields across 30 subjects are visualized in figure 4 (2D display) and figure 5 (3D display).

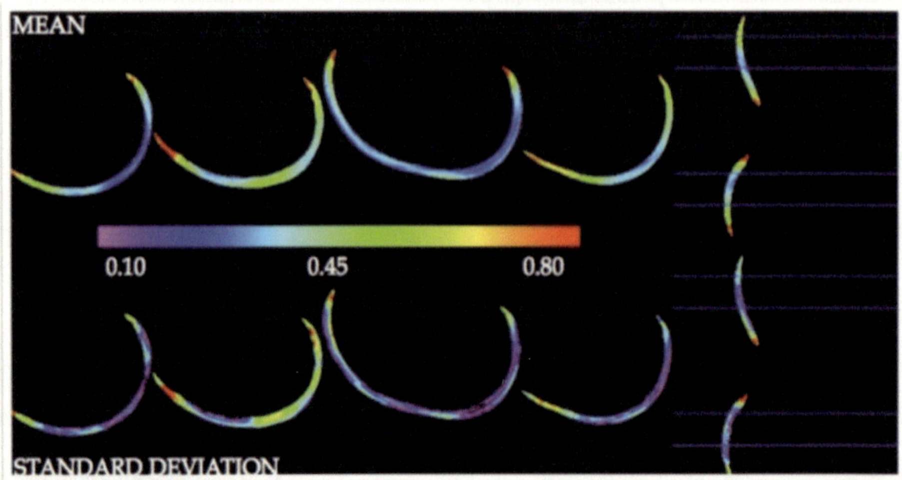

Fig. 4. Two-dimensional maps of the mean and standard deviation values of the magnitude of the 3D deformation vector fields of the 30 subjects used to create the atlas. The values are displayed over several cross-sectional slices in the entire atlas volume.

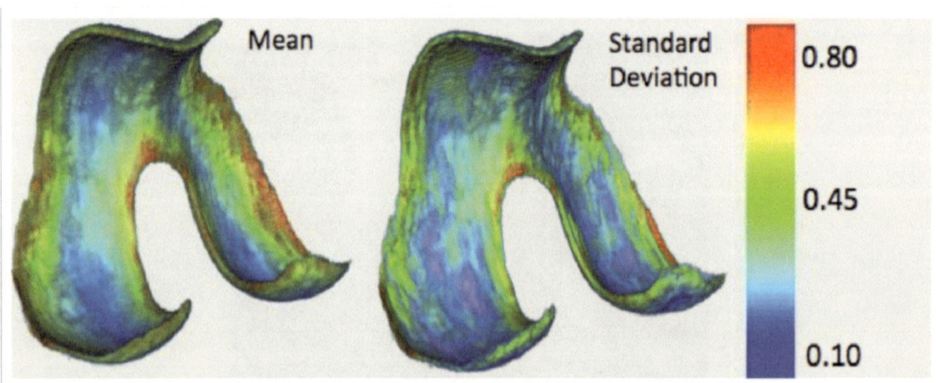

Fig. 5. Three-dimensional map of the mean and standard deviation of the magnitude of the 3D deformation vector fields across the 30 subjects used to create the atlas.

The regions of large deformations and standard deviation values are seen along the edges (Figure 5). A possible explanation resulting to this finding is the inaccuracies in the manual segmentation process. The trochlea region near the intercondylar notch and in the medial aspect shows higher deformation and standard deviation values (Figure 5). Between the medial and lateral aspects of the cartilage, the medial condyle regions show slightly higher deformation than the lateral regions.

3.3 Active shape models from atlas cohort

Synthesized images using principal component analysis based active shape models were created. Using the first 2 dominant eigenvectors the images generated at ±2SD and ±3SD and the 3D maps are visualized in figure 6.

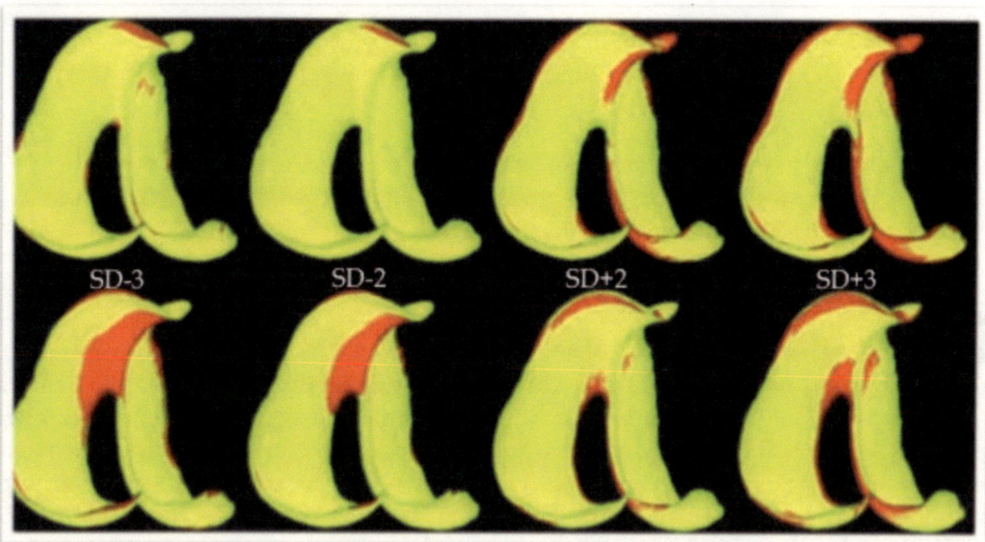

Fig. 6. Synthesized images along ±2SD and ±3SD overlaid on the atlas. The first and second row corresponds to images generated along the 1st and 2nd eigenmodes respectively.

The synthesized images (along 1st and 2nd eigenvectors and different standard deviations) are overlaid on the atlas. Regions where the atlas and the synthesized images completely overlap are shown in yellow. Regions where either the atlas or the synthesized images extended beyond each other are shown in red and green respectively. It should be noted that the shape of the atlas remains the same and the extension of synthesized images beyond the atlas changes for different standard deviations. Looking closely at the synthesized shape images at the positive and the corresponding negative SD it is observed that the areas visualized in red (and green) in one image are visualized as green (and red) in the corresponding image. Also, the magnitude of shape difference is evidently higher in at $|\pm 3SD|$ than at $|\pm 2SD|$.

3.4 Statistical analysis

Statistical analysis performed in SPM results in 't' values that are obtained after comparing the jacobian values for incidence and progression cohorts. The regions with significant differences are overlaid on the atlas and can be clearly visualized in the 3D map shown in figure 7. Regions such as the medial weight-bearing region and the lateral posterior condyle exhibit significant differences between the incidence and progression cohorts.

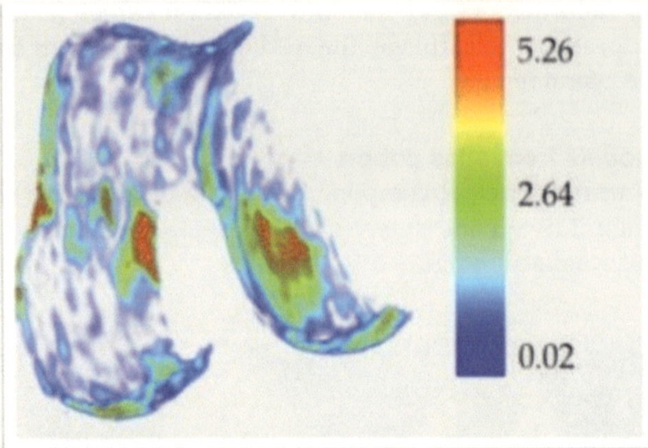

Fig. 7. Results from the statistical analysis overlaid on the atlas. Regions with most difference between the incidence and progression cohort is shown on the 3D map. The regions in white indicate no change.

4. Discussion

Extending the previous work of Cohen et al. and Carballido-Gamio et al. (Cohen et al., 2003; Carballido-Gamio et al., 2008), the focus of this study was to create a femoral cartilage atlas from high-resolution 3D MR images made available by the OAI through version 0.A.1. The atlas-based approach to study localized morphological changes has been well established for brain and we extend this to study localized changes in cartilage morphology in osteoarthritis. Figure 2 confirms the accuracy of the registration steps involved in the atlas creation process (affine and freeform) by overlaying the contour traced on the atlas over the subject image obtained before and after the two registration steps. In addition to this visual confirmation, 3D residual distance maps have confirmed that the nonlinear algorithm used here provides registration accuracy within 1-2 pixels. Figure 3 shows the 2D slices and 3D volume of the femoral cartilage atlas that was created from 30 Caucasian male subjects from the incidence group. The accuracy of the registration techniques (both affine and freeform) can be confirmed by the sharp edges observed in the 3D image. Several non-linear deformation algorithms are available to warp an image volume to a target volume. The accuracy of the algorithm is usually verified by the accuracy of the registration. However, this still does not guarantee that the jacobian values calculated from the deformation fields reflect the actual local volume changes. Rohlfing et al. has confirmed, using synthetic image volumes and deformations, that the demons algorithm used in the current work does provide accurate estimates of local volume changes (Rohlfing, 2006).

The deformation values obtained for the 30 subjects used to create the atlas are averaged and the voxel-wise mean and standard deviation values are visualized in figure 4 and 5. It is observed that the overall deformation values are quite small (in the order of ~0.4 mm) and hence exhibit very less variation within the population used to create the atlas. However, higher values are observed around the edges and that can be attributed to registration errors. The low variability seen in the current atlas can be credited to the fact that the participants selected to create the atlas had to meet strict selection criteria of age, gender, race and low K&L score. Past studies found the inter-subjects variability across morphological parameters such as cartilage thickness and volume to be significantly higher (Eckstein et al., 2001). In our study the inter-subject variability was minimized by using the affine transformation as the first step in the atlas creation process and accounts for global size changes. In figure 5, higher mean and standard deviation of the deformation values are realized on the patellofemoral compartment of the trochlear (femoral) side. Previous distal femoral bone studies have indicated that shape changes in the intercondylar notch when comparing normal against diseased subjects as a discriminant of OA (Shepstone et al., 2001) and hence has there is a possibility of a potential link between the findings of this study to what has been observed in the past. The active shape models generated using principal component analysis along first two eigenmodes and ±2SD and ±3SD are shown in figure 6. These models display small morphological variability that is in agreement with the findings using the deformation magnitude values. Integrating active shape models with segmentation algorithms can provide a-prior information about cartilage shape variability (Duchesne et al., 2002). Also, active shape indices derived can be used to discriminate between cohorts or classify single subjects.

Results from the voxel based statistical analysis performed using SPM in Matlab as shown in in figure 7 display specific weight bearing regions such as the lateral side of the intercondylar notch and medial posterior femoral regions displaying significant morphological differences between the incidence group and the progression group. These findings are consistent with other studies. Eckstein et al. showed that cartilage degradation is significantly higher in knees with radiographic evidence of OA in comparison to healthy knees and knees with no radiographic evidence of OA. Subjects were grouped as non-exposed controls (n = 112), calculated K&L grade 2 (n = 310), calculated K&L grade 3 (n = 300), and calculated K&L grade 4 (n = 109). Regional and sub-regional thickness values calculated from coronal MR images showed that there was significant difference seen in the weight bearing sub-regions of the femorotibial cartilage in subjects with K&L grade of 4 (Eckstein et al., 2010). Bredbenner et al. recently investigated the potential of using statistical shape modeling as a tool to detect onset of OA. The authors use SSM to effectively characterize the variability in the subchondral bone region in femur and tibia. They also show the potential of combining SSM with rigid body transformation to distinguish subjects at risk and no risk of developing OA (Bredbenner et al., 2010).

As an extension to our current work, we have created statistical atlases of the femur and tibia bone. We aim to use these atlases to characterize morphological variations in the bone in a well-defined group and use it as a predictor for osteoarthritis and osteoporosis. For this study MR images of the knee were acquired on 10 normal subjects and the femur and tibia were segmented from the sagittal MR images. The atlas of the femur and tibia are created as outlined in section 2.2. The accuracy of registration is shown in figure 10 where the contour traced on the atlas is overlaid on the test subject and the remaining images.

The atlas for femur and tibia are visualized in figure 9. The sharp edges and the thin growth plate seen in the cross-sectional images is a visual confirmation of extremely accurate alignment during the atlas creation process. We present some initial results and in future hope to utilize the rich data set available from OAI and conduct a detail study to investigate morphological variation in the bone using the atlas based approach.

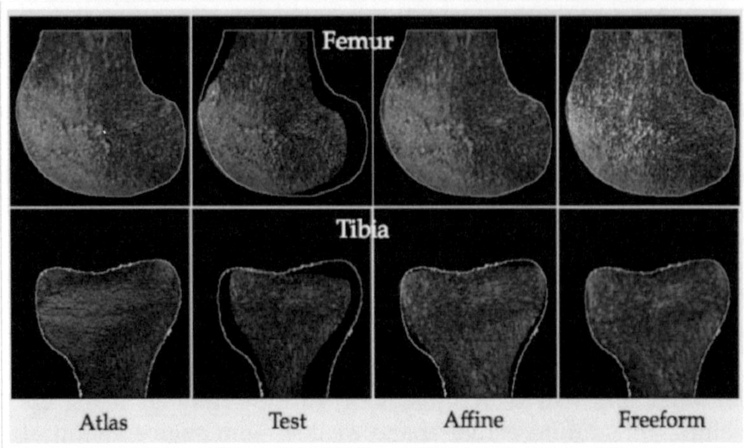

Fig. 8. Selection on the reference image is overlaid on the subject before and after affine and freeform registration. For Row 1: Femur and Row 2: Tibia

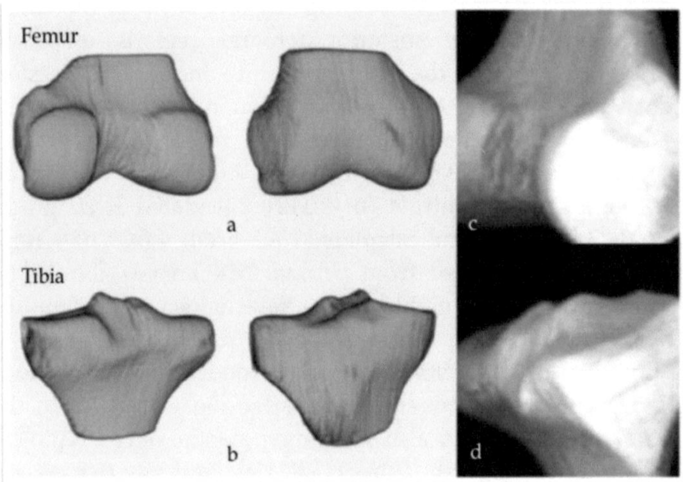

Fig. 9. 3D images of the femur and tibia atlas

5. Conclusion

This chapter is focused on the atlas-based approach for automated image analysis for cartilage and bone. The primary area of application is to characterize and monitor progression of osteoarthritis. In this chapter, the atlas approach is applied to the study of morphological differences between population cohorts at different stages of osteoarthritis. The second area of application is a preliminary study of femoral and tibial bone atlas with the aim of identifying morphological differences in bone in matched cohorts with osteoarthritis. The atlas approach is not limited to identification of morphological differences (between cohorts) or changes (in longitudinal studies). It is readily extendable to the analysis of parametric image datasets such as T2, T1rho and dGEMRIC.

6. Acknowledgment

The OAI is a public-private partnership comprised of five contracts (N01-AR-2-2258; N01-AR-2-2259; N01-AR-2-2260; N01-AR-2-2261; N01-AR-2-2262) funded by the National Institutes of Health, a branch of the Department of Health and Human Services, and conducted by the OAI Study Investigators. Private funding partners include Merck Research Laboratories; Novartis Pharmaceuticals Corporation, GlaxoSmithKline; and Pfizer, Inc. Private sector funding for the OAI is managed by the Foundation for the National Institutes of Health. This manuscript was prepared using an OAI public use data set and does not necessarily reflect the opinions or views of the OAI investigators, the NIH, or the private funding partners.

7. References

Ardekani, S. & Sinha U. (2006). Statistical representation of mean diffusivity and fractional anisotropy brain maps of normal subjects. *Journal of magnetic resonance imaging : JMRI,* Vol.24, No.6, (November 2006), pp. 1243-1251, DOI 10.1002/jmri.20745

Ashburner, J. (2009). Computational anatomy with the SPM software. *Magnetic resonance imaging,* Vol.27, No. 8, (October 2009), pp. 1163-1174, DOI 10.1016/j.mri.2009.01.006

Benjamini, Y. & Hochberg, Y. (1995). Controlling the False Discovery Rate: a Practical and Powerful Approach to Multiple Testing. *Journal of the Royal Statistical Society,* Vol. 57, No.1, (1995), pp. 289-300

Blumenkrantz, G. & Majumdar, S. (2007). Quantitative Magnetic Resonance Imaging of Articular Cartilage in Osteoarthritis. *European Cells and Materials,* Vol.13, (2007), pp. 75- 86

Bredbenner, T. L.; Eliason, T.D.; Potter R.S.; Mason R.L.; Havill, L.M. & Nicolella, D.P. (2010). Statistical shape modeling describes variation in tibia and femur surface geometry between Control and Incidence groups from the osteoarthritis initiative database. *Journal of biomechanics,* Vol.43, No.9, (March 2010), pp. 1780-1786, DOI 10.1016/j.jbiomech.2010.02.015

Burgkart, R.; Glaser, C.; Hinterwimmer, S.; Hudelmaier, M.; Englmeier, M.R.; Reiser, M. & Eckstein, F. (2003). Feasibility of T and Z scores from magnetic resonance imaging data for quantification of cartilage loss in osteoarthritis. *Arthritis and rheumatism,* Vol.48, No.10, (October 2003), pp. 2829-2835, DOI 10.1002/art.11259

Carballido-Gamio, J.; Bauer, J.S.; Stahl, R.; Lee, K.Y.; Krause, S.; Link, T.M. & Majumdar, S. (2008). Inter-subject comparison of MRI knee cartilage thickness. *Medical image analysis,* Vol.12, No.2, (April 2008), pp. 120-135, DOI 10.1016/j.media.2007.08.002

Carballido-Gamio, J.; Joseph, G.B.; Lynch, J.A.; Link, T.M. & Majumdar, S.(2011). Longitudinal analysis of MRI T2 knee cartilage laminar organization in a subset of patients from the osteoarthritis initiative: a texture approach. *Magnetic resonance in medicine : official journal of the Society of Magnetic Resonance in Medicine / Society of Magnetic Resonance in Medicine,* Vol.65, No.4, (April 2011), pp. 1184-1194, DOI 10.1002/mrm.22693

Cohen, Z.; Mow, V.C.; Henry, J.H.; Levine, W.N. & Ateshian, G.A. (2003). Templates of the cartilage layers of the patellofemoral joint and their use in the assessment of osteoarthritic cartilage damage. *Osteoarthritis and Cartilage,* Vol.11, No.8, (August 2003), pp. 569-579, DOI 10.1016/S1063-4584(03)00091-8

Cootes, T.F.; Taylor, C.J. & Cooper, D.H. (1994). Active Shape Models - Their Training and Application. *Computer Vision and Image Understanding,* Vol.61, No.1, (January 1995), pp. 38-59, DOI 1077-3142195

Dam, E.B.; Folkesson, J.; Pettersen, P.C. & Christiansen, M.D. (2007). Automatic morphometric cartilage quantification in the medial tibial plateau from MRI for osteoarthritis grading. *Osteoarthritis and cartilage / OARS, Osteoarthritis Research Society,* Vol.15, No.7, (July 2007), pp. 808-818, DOI 10.1016/j.joca.2007.01.013

David-Vaudey, E.; Ghosh, S.; Ries, M. & Majumdar, S. (2004). T2 relaxation time measurements in osteoarthritis. *Magnetic resonance imaging,* Vol.22, No.5, (June 2004), pp. 673-682, DOI 10.1016/j.mri.2004.01.071

Duchesne, S.; Pruessner, J.C. & Collins, D.L. (2002). Appearance-Based Segmentation of Medial Temporal Lobe Structures. *NeuroImage,* Vol.17, No.2, (October 2002), pp. 515-531, DOI 10.1006/nimg.2002.1188

Dunn, T. C.; Lu, Y.; Ries, M.D. & Majumdar, S. (2004). T2 relaxation time of cartilage at MR imaging: comparison with severity of knee osteoarthritis. *Radiology,* Vol.232, No. 2, (June 2004), pp. 592-598

Duryea, J.; Neumann, G.; Brem, M.H.; Koh, W.; Noorbakhsh, F.; Jackson, R.D.; Yu, J.; Eaton, C.B. & Lang, P. (2007). Novel fast semi-automated software to segment cartilage for knee MR acquisitions. *Osteoarthritis and cartilage/OARS, Osteoarthritis Research Society,* Vol.15, No.5, (December 2006)), pp. 487-492.

Duryea, J.; Neumann, G.; Niu, J.; Totterman, S.; Tamez, J.; Dabrowski, C.; Le Graverand, M.P.; Luchi, M.; Beals, C.R. & Hunter, D.J. (2010). Comparison of radiographic joint space width with magnetic resonance imaging cartilage morphometry: analysis of longitudinal data from the Osteoarthritis Initiative. *Arthritis care & research,* Vol.62, No.7, (July 2010), pp. 932-937, DOI 10.1002/acr.20148

Eckstein, F.; Charles, H.C.; Buck, R.J.; Kraus, V.B.; Remmers, A.E.; Hudelmaier, M.; Wirth, W. & Evelhoch, J.L. (2005). Accuracy and precision of quantitative assessment of cartilage morphology by magnetic resonance imaging at 3.0T. *Arthritis and rheumatism,* Vol.52, No.10, (October 2005), pp. 3132-3136, DOI 10.1002/art.21348

Eckstein, F.; Cicuttini, F.; Raynauld, J.P.; Waterton, J.C. & Peterfly, C. (2006). Magnetic resonance imaging (MRI) of articular cartilage in knee osteoarthritis (OA): morphological assessment. *Osteoarthritis and cartilage / OARS, Osteoarthritis Research Society,* Vol.14, No. Suppl A, (May 2006), pp. 46-75, DOI 10.1016/j.joca.2006.02.026

Eckstein, F.; Guermazi, A. & Roemer, F.W. (2009). Quantitative MR imaging of cartilage and trabecular bone in osteoarthritis. *Radiologic clinics of North America,* Vol.47, No.4, (July 2009), pp. 655-673

Eckstein, F.; Nevitt, M.; Gimona, A.; Picha, K.; Lee, J.H.; Davies, R.Y.; Dreher, D.; Benichou, O.; Hellio Le Graverand, M.; Hudelmaier, M.; Mascheck, S. & Wirth, W. (2010). Rates of change and sensitivity to change in cartilage morphology in healthy knees and in knees with mild, moderate, and end stage radiographic osteoarthritis. *Arthritis care & research,* Vol.63, No. 3, (March 2011), pp. 311-319, DOI 10.1002/acr.20370

Eckstein, F.; Winzheimer, M.; Hohe, J.; Englmeier, K.H. & Reiser, M. (2001). Interindividual variability and correlation among morphological parameters of knee joint cartilage plates: analysis with three-dimensional MR imaging. *Osteoarthritis and cartilage / OARS, Osteoarthritis Research Society,* Vol.9, No.2, (February 2001), pp. 101-111, DOI 10.1053/joca.2000.0365

Eckstein, F.; Wirth, W.; Hudelmaier, M.L.; Mascheck, S.; Hitzi, W.; Wyman, B.T.; Nevitt, M.; Hellio LeGravererand, M.P. & Hunter, D. (2009). Relationship of compartment-specific structural knee status at baseline with change in cartilage morphology: a prospective observational study using data from the osteoarthritis initiative. *Arthritis research & therapy*, Vol.11, No.3, (June 2009), pp. R90

Eckstein, F.; Wirth, W.; Hunter, D.J.; Guermazi, A.; Hwoh, C.K.; Nelson, D.R. & Benichou, O. (2010). Magnitude and regional distribution of cartilage loss associated with grades of joint space narrowing in radiographic osteoarthritis-data from the Osteoarthritis Initiative (OAI). *Osteoarthritis and Cartilage/OARS, Osteoarthritis Research Society*, Vol.18, No.6, (February 2010), pp. 760-768

Eckstein, F.; Mosher, T. & Hunter, D. (2007). Imaging of knee osteoarthritis: data beyond the beauty. *Current opinion in rheumatology*, Vol.19, No.5, (September 2007), pp. 435-443

Fripp, J.; Crozier, S.; Warfield, S. & Ourselin, S. (2007). Automatic segmentation of articular cartilage in magnetic resonance images of the knee. *Medical Image Computing And Computer-Assisted Intervention*, Vol.4792, (2007), pp. 186-194

Frobell, R.B.; Nevitt, M.C.; Hudelmaier, M.; Wirth, W.; Wyman, B.T.; Benichou, O.; Dreher, D.; Davies, R.; Lee, J.H.; Baribaud, F.; Gimona, A. & Eckstein, F. (2010). Femorotibial subchondral bone area and regional cartilage thickness: a cross-sectional description in healthy reference cases and various radiographic stages of osteoarthritis in 1,003 knees from the Osteoarthritis Initiative. *Arthritis care & research*, Vol.62, No.11, (May 2010), pp. 1612-1623

Guermazi, A.; Burstein, D.; Conaghan, P.; Eckstein, F.; Hellio Le Graverand, M.; Keen, H. & Poemer, F. (2008). Imaging in osteoarthritis. *Rheumatic diseases clinics of North America*, Vol.34, No.3, (August 2008), pp. 645-687, DOI 10.1016/j.rdc.2008.04.006

Guermazi, A.; Hunter, D.J.; Li, L.; Benichou, O.; Eckstein, F.; Kwoh, C.K.; Nevitt, M. & Hayashi, D. (2011). Different thresholds for detecting osteophytes and joint space narrowing exist between the site investigators and the centralized reader in a multicenter knee osteoarthritis study-data from the Osteoarthritis Initiative. *Skeletal radiology*, (April 2011), (Epub ahead of print), DOI 10.1007/s00256-011-1142-2

Hunter, D.J.; Le Graverand, M.P. & Eckstein, F. (2009). Radiologic markers of osteoarthritis progression. *Current opinion in rheumatology*, Vol.21, No. 2, (April 2009), pp. 110-117

Hunter, D.J.; Niu, J.; Zhang, Y.; Totterman, S.; Tamez, J.; Dabrowski, C.; Davies, R.; Le Graverand, M.P.; Luchi, M.; Tymofyeyev, Y. & Beals, C.R. (2009). Change in cartilage morphometry: a sample of the progression cohort of the Osteoarthritis Initiative. *Annals of the Rheumatic Diseases*, Vol.68, No.3, (April 2008), pp. 349-356

Iranpour-Boroujeni, T.; Watanabe, A.; Bashtar, R. Yoshioka, H. & Duryea, J. (2011). Quantification of cartilage loss in local regions of knee joints using semi-automated segmentation software: analysis of longitudinal data from the Osteoarthritis Initiative (OAI). *Osteoarthritis and cartilage / OARS, Osteoarthritis Research Society*, Vol.19, No.3, (March 2011), pp. 309-314, DOI 10.1016/j.joca.2010.12.002

Jenkinson, M. & Smith, S. (2001). A global optimisation method for robust affine registration of brain images. *Medical image analysis*, Vol.5, No.2, (June 2001), pp. 143-156, DOI 10.1016/S1361-8415(01)00036-6

Kochunov, P.; Lancaster, J.; Hardies, J.; Thompson, P.M.; Woods, R.P.; Cody, j.D.; Hale, D.E.; Laird, A. & Fox, P.T. (2005). Mapping structural differences of the corpus callosum in individuals with 18q deletions using targetless regional spatial normalization.

Human brain mapping, Vol.24, No.4, (April 2005), pp. 325-331, DOI 10.1002/hbm.20090

Kochunov, P.; Lancaster, J.; Thompson, P.; Woods, R.; Mazziotta, J.; Hardies, J. & Fox, P. (2001). Regional Spatial Normalization: Toward an Optimal Target. *Journal of Computer Assisted Tomography*, Vol.25, No.5, (September-October 2001), pp. 805-816, ISSN 0363-8715

Koff, M.F.; Amrami, K.K. & Kaufman, K.R. (2007). Clinical evaluation of T2 values of patellar cartilage in patients with osteoarthritis. *Osteoarthritis and cartilage / OARS, Osteoarthritis Research Society*, Vol.15, No.2, (February 2007), pp. 198-204, DOI 10.1016/j.joca.2006.07.007

Kshirsagar, A.; Watson, P.; Tyler, J.A. & Hall, L.D. (1998). Measurement of Localized Cartilage Volume and Thickness of Human Knee Joints by Computer Analysis of Three-Dimensional Magnetic Resonance Images. *Investigative Radiology*, Vol.33, No.5, (May 1998), pp. 289-299, ISSN 0020-9996

Li, X.; Benjamin Ma, C.; Link, T.M.; Castillo, D.D.; Blumenkrantz, G.; Lazano, J.; Carballido-Gamio, J.; Ries, M. & Majumdar, S. (2007). In vivo T(1rho) and T(2) mapping of articular cartilage in osteoarthritis of the knee using 3 T MRI. *Osteoarthritis and cartilage / OARS, Osteoarthritis Research Society*, Vol.15, No.7, (July 2007), pp. 789-797, DOI 10.1016/j.joca.2007.01.011

Li, X.; Han, E.T.; Ma, C.B.; Link, T.M. & Majumdar, S. (2005). In vivo 3T spiral imaging based multi-slice T(1rho) mapping of knee cartilage in osteoarthritis. *Magnetic resonance in medicine : official journal of the Society of Magnetic Resonance in Medicine / Society of Magnetic Resonance in Medicine*, Vol.54, No.4, (October 2005), pp. 929-936, DOI 10.1002/mrm.20609

Link, T.M. (2010). The Founder's Lecture 2009: advances in imaging of osteoporosis and osteoarthritis. *Skeletal radiology*, Vol.39, No.10, (June 2010), pp. 943-955

Link, T.; M., Stahl, R. & Woertler, K. (2007). Cartilage imaging: motivation, techniques, current and future significance. *European radiology*, Vol.17, No.5, (November 2006), pp. 1135-1146, DOI 10.1007/s00330-006-0453-5

Majumdar, S.; Li, X.; Blumenkrantz, G.; Saldanha, K.; Ma, CB.; Kim, H.; Lozano, J. & Link, T. (2006). MR imaging and early cartilage degeneration and strategies for monitoring regeneration. *Journal of Musculoskelet Neuronal Interact*, Vol.6, No.4, (December 2006), pp. 382-384

Pan, J.; Stehling, C.; Muller-Hocker, C.; Schwaiger, B.J.; Lynch, J.; McCulloch, C.E.; Nevitt, M.C. & Link, T.M. (2011). Vastus lateralis/vastus medialis cross-sectional area ratio impacts presence and degree of knee joint abnormalities and cartilage T2 determined with 3T MRI - an analysis from the incidence cohort of the Osteoarthritis Initiative. *Osteoarthritis and cartilage / OARS, Osteoarthritis Research Society*, Vol.19, No.1, (January 2011), pp. 65-73, DOI 10.1016/j.joca.2010.10.023

Pelletier, J.P.; Raynauld, J.P.; Berthiaume, M.J.; Abram, F.; Choquette, D.; Haraoui, B.; Beary, J.F.; Cline, G.A.; Meyer, J.M. & Martel-Pelletier, J. (2007). Risk factors associated with the loss of cartilage volume on weight-bearing areas in knee osteoarthritis patients assessed by quantitative magnetic resonance imaging: a longitudinal study. *Arthritis research & therapy*, Vol.9, No. 4, (August 2007), pp. R74

Phan, C.M.; Link, T.M.;Blumenkrantz, G.; Dunn, T.C.; Ries, M.D.; Steinbach, L.S. & Mujumdar, S. (2006). MR imaging findings in the follow-up of patients with different stages of knee osteoarthritis and the correlation with clinical symptoms.

European Radiology, Vol.16, No.3, (March 2006), pp. 608-618, DOI 10.1007/s00330-005-0004-5

Raynauld, J. (2003). Quantitative magnetic resonance imaging of articular cartilage in knee osteoarthritis. *Current opinion in rheumatology*, Vol.15, No.5, (September 2003), pp. 647-650

Raynauld, J.P.; Kauffmann, C.; Beaudoin, G.; Berthiaume, M.J.; de Guise, J.A.; Bloch, D.A.; Camacho, F.; Godbout, B.; Altman, R.D.; Hochberg, M.; Meyer, J.M.; Cline, G.; Pelletier, J.P. & Martel-Pelletier, J. (2003). Reliability of a quantification imaging system using magnetic resonance images to measure cartilage thickness and volume in human normal and osteoarthritic knees. *Osteoarthritis and Cartilage*, Vol.11, No.5, (May 2003), pp. 351-360, DOI 10.1016/S1063-4584(03)00029-3

Regatte, R.; Akella, S.; Borthakur, A.; Kneeland, J. & Reddy, R. (2002). Proteoglycan Depletion–Induced Changes in Transverse Relaxation Maps of Cartilage☆Comparison of T2 and T1ρ. *Academic Radiology*, Vol.9, No.12, (2002), pp. 1388-1394.

Regatte, R.R.; Akella, S.V.; Lonner, J.H.; Kneeland, J.B. & Reddy, R. (2006). T1rho relaxation mapping in human osteoarthritis (OA) cartilage: comparison of T1rho with T2. *Journal of magnetic resonance imaging : JMRI*, Vol.23, No.4, (April 2006), pp. 547-553, DOI 10.1002/jmri.20536

Roemer, F.W.; Eckstein, F. & Guermazi, A. (2009). Magnetic resonance imaging-based semiquantitative and quantitative assessment in osteoarthritis. *Rheumatic diseases clinics of North America*, Vol.35, No.3, (November 2009), pp. 521-555

Roemer, F.W.; Kwoh, C.K.; Hannon, M.J.; Crema, M.D.; Moore, C.E.; Jakicic, J.M.; Green, S.M. & Guermazi, A. (2010). Semiquantitative assessment of focal cartilage damage at 3 T MRI: A comparative study of dual echo at steady state (DESS) and intermediate-weighted (IW) fat suppressed fast spin echo sequences. *European Journal of Radiology*, doi 10.1016/j.ejrad.2010.07.025

Rohlfing, T. (2006). Transformation Model and Constraints Cause Bias in Statistics on Deformation Fields. *Medical Image Computing And Computer-Assisted Intervention – MICCAI 2006*, pp. 207-214, DOI 10.1007/11866565, Copenhagen, Denmark, October 1-6, 2006

Shepstone, L.; Rogers, J.; Kirwan, J. & Silverman, B. (2001). Shape of the intercondylar notch of the human femur: a comparison of osteoarthritic and non-osteoarthritic bones from a skeletal sample. *Annals of the Rheumatic Diseases*, Vol.60, No.10, (October 2001), pp. 968-973, DOI 10.1136/ard.60.10.968

Stammberger, T.; Hohe, J.; Englmeier, K.H.; Reiser, M. & Eckstein, F. (2000). Elastic Registration of 3D Cartilage Surfaces From MR Image Data for Detecting Local Changes in Cartilage Thickness. *Magnetic Resonance in Medicine*, Vol.44, No.4, (October 2000), pp. 592-601, DOI 10.1002/1522-2594(200010)44:4

Tameem, H.Z.; Ardekani, S.; Seeger, L.; Thompson, P. & Sinha, U.S. (2011). Initial results on development and application of statistical atlas of femoral cartilage in osteoarthritis to determine sex differences in structure: Data from the osteoarthritis initiative. *Journal of magnetic resonance imaging : JMRI*, (June 2011) DOI 10.1002/jmri.22643 (Epub ahead of print)

Tameem, H.Z., Selva, L.E. & Sinha, U.S. (2007). Morphological Atlases of Knee Cartilage: Shape Indices to Analyze Cartilage Degradation in Osteoarthritic and Non-Osteoarthritic Population. *Engineering in Medicine and Biology Society (EMBS) 2007.*

29th Annual International Conference of the IEEE, pp. 1310-1313, ISBN 978-1-4244-0787-3, Lyon, France, August 23-26, 2007

Taylor, C.; Carballido-Gamio, J.; Majumdar, S. & Li, X. (2009). Comparison of quantitative imaging of cartilage for osteoarthritis: T2, T1rho, dGEMRIC and contrast-enhanced computed tomography. *Magnetic resonance imaging,* Vol.27, No.6, (March 2009), pp. 779-784

Thirion, J.P. (1998). Image matching as a diffusion process: an analogy with Maxwell's demons. *Medical image analysis,* Vol.2, No.3, (September 1998), pp. 243-260, DOI 10.1016/S1361-8415(98)80022-4

Thompson, L.R.; Boudreau, R.; Newman, A.B.; Hannon, M.J.; Chu, C.R.; Nevitt, M.C. & Kent Kwoh, C. (2010). The association of osteoarthritis risk factors with localized, regional and diffuse knee pain. *Osteoarthritis and cartilage / OARS, Osteoarthritis Research Society,* Vol.18, No.10, (October 2010), pp. 1244-1249, DOI 10.1016/j.joca.2010.05.014

Williams, A.; Sharma, L.; McKenzie, C.A.; Prasad, P.V. & Burstein, D. (2005). Delayed gadolinium-enhanced magnetic resonance imaging of cartilage in knee osteoarthritis: findings at different radiographic stages of disease and relationship to malalignment. *Arthritis and rheumatism,* Vol.52, No.11, (November 2005), pp. 3528-3535

Wirth, W.; Benichou, O.; Kwoh, C.K.; Guermazi, A.; Hunter, D. Putz, R. & Eckstein, F. (2010). Spatial patterns of cartilage loss in the medial femoral condyle in osteoarthritic knees: data from the Osteoarthritis Initiative. *Magnetic resonance in medicine : official journal of the Society of Magnetic Resonance in Medicine / Society of Magnetic Resonance in Medicine,* Vol.63, No.3, (Feburary 2010), pp. 574-581

Wirth, W.; Buck, R.; Nevit, M.; Le Graverand, M.P.; Benichou, O.; Dreher, D.; Davies, R.Y.; Lee, J.H.; Picha, K.; Gimona, A.; Maschek, S.; Hudelmaier, M. & Eckstein, F. (2011). MRI-based extended ordered values more efficiently differentiate cartilage loss in knees with and without joint space narrowing than region-specific approaches using MRI or radiography - data from the OA initiative. *Osteoarthritis and cartilage / OARS, Osteoarthritis Research Society,* Vol.19, No.6, (June 2011), pp. 689-699, DOI 10.1016/j.joca.2011.02.011

Wirth, W.; Larroque, S.; Davies, R.Y.; Nevitt, M.; Gimona, A.; Baribaud, F.; Lee, J.H.; Benichou, O.; Wyman, B.T.; Hudelmaier, M.; Maschek, S. & Eckstein, F. (2011). Comparison of 1-year vs 2-year change in regional cartilage thickness in osteoarthritis results from 346 participants from the Osteoarthritis Initiative. *Osteoarthritis and cartilage / OARS, Osteoarthritis Research Society,* Vol19, No.1, (January 2011), pp. 74-83, DOI 10.1016/j.joca.2010.10.022

Wirth, W. & Eckstein, F. (2008). A Technique for Regional Analysis of Femorotibial Cartilage Thickness Based on Quantitative Magnetic Resonance Imaging. *IEEE Transactions on Medical Imaging,* Vol.27, (June 2008), pp. 737-744

Xing, W.; Sheng, J.; Chen, W.H.; Tian, J.M.; Zhang, L.R. & Wang, D.Q. (2011). Reproducibility and accuracy of quantitative assessment of articular cartilage volume measurements with 3.0 Tesla magnetic resonance imaging. *Chinese Medical Journal,* Vol.124, No.8, (April 2011), pp. 1251-1257

4

The Application of Imaging in Osteoarthritis

Caroline B. Hing, Mark A. Harris, Vivian Ejindu and Nidhi Sofat
St George's Hospital NHS Trust, London, UK

1. Introduction

Osteoarthritis (OA) is the most common articular disorder worldwide and affects multiple tissues of a joint in response to biomechanical factors. Novel developments in radiographic techniques allow imaging at a macroscopic and microscopic level, quantifying this dynamic process allowing the application of metrics to both disease progression and response to different treatment modalities. This chapter aims to outline how both invasive and non-invasive radiographic modalities can be implemented to allow quantification of the structure of osteoarthritic joints.

Plain-film radiography remains the most common imaging modality for initial assessment and grading of osteoarthritis. Newer techniques such as magnetic resonance imaging (MRI), ultrasound (US) and computed tomography (CT) allow a multimodal approach to the assessment of architectural change within the articular and peri-articular tissues.

We performed a literature search to identify pertinent review articles investigating advances in imaging techniques in humans using the MesH terms and Boolean operators 'osteoarthritis' AND 'ultrasound' OR 'magnetic resonance imaging' OR 'computed tomography'. We identified 24165 relevant articles and limited our search to review articles on humans in English. The structure of the chapter is divided into subheadings covering the different imaging modalities: conventional radiography (CR), MRI , US, CT and bone scintigraphy. Within each subheading, further sections address the use of imaging to quantify disease progression with grading techniques and also cover the use of radiopharmaceuticals such as SPECT (single positron emission computed tomography) and dGEMRIC (delayed gadolinium enhanced MRI of cartilage). A further section outlining the use of imaging as a measure of the molecular composition and structure of osteoarthritic joints is included prior to the final section outlining future advances.

2. Conventional radiography

Conventional radiography (CR) is the primary investigative tool for the diagnosis and follow-up assessment of osteoarthritis (OA). Radiographs are typically obtained in two standardised orthogonal planes. Their acquisition is relatively inexpensive, technically simple, non-invasive and readily available. Differing attenuation of X-ray signal within soft tissues compared to bone allows excellent visualisation of the pathological changes of the osseous structures of a joint. Recognised pathological features include marginal osteophytosis, subchondral sclerosis with joint space narrowing, subchondral cysts and deformation of the bone ends (Figure 1).

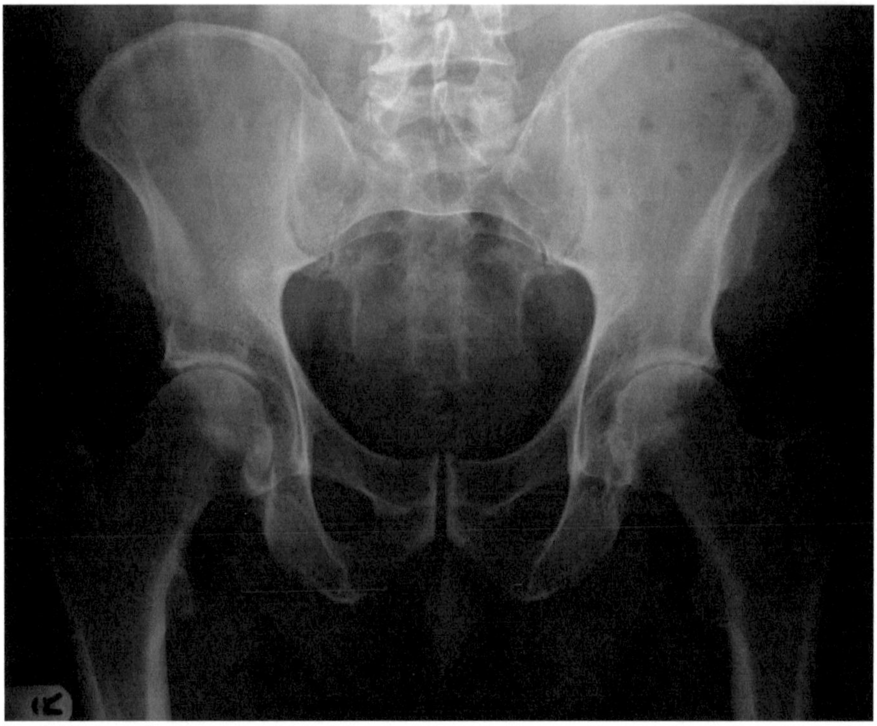

a. Bilateral hip involvement in OA with superior joint space loss and subchondral sclerosis

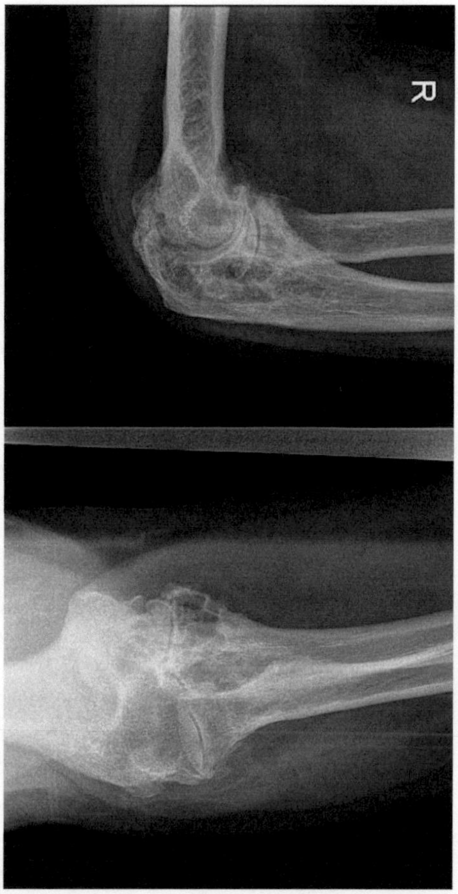

b. Severe joint space narrowing, osteophyte formation and cysts in the elbow joint

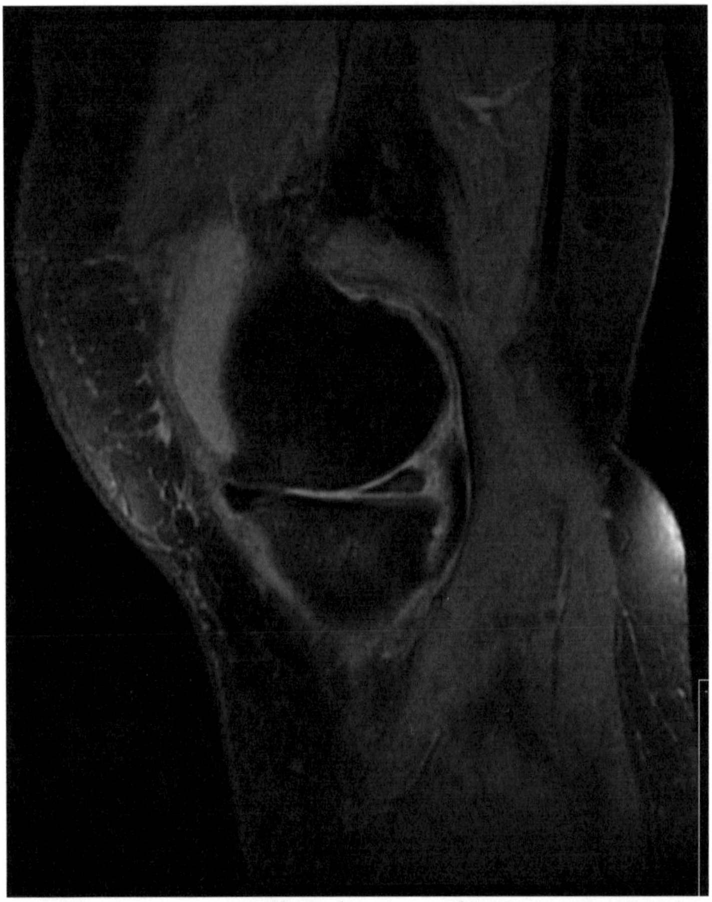

c. Knee MRI demonstrating severe cartilage damage and joint space narrowing

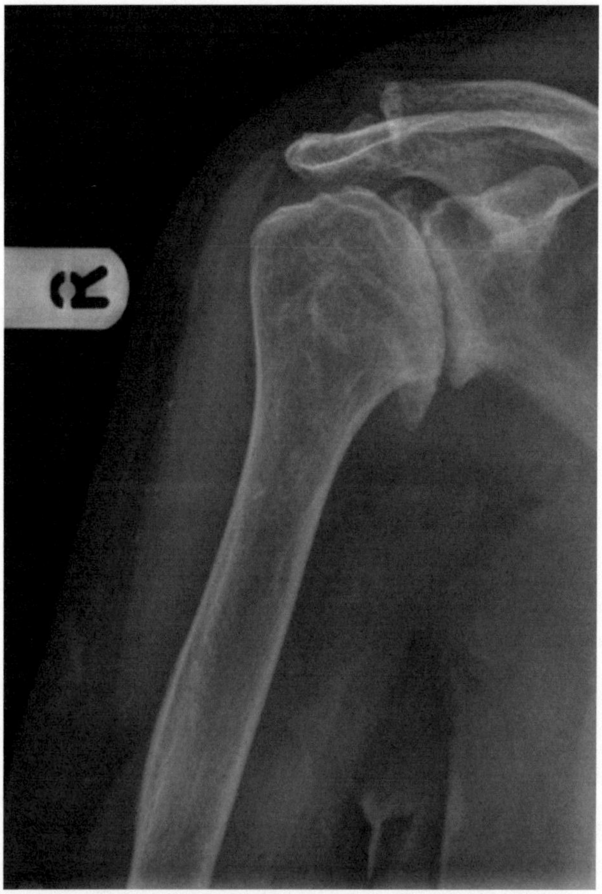

d. Osteoarthritis of the glenohumeral joint

Fig. 1. X rays and MRI demonstrating range of joints involved in OA

In 1957 Kellgren and Lawrence incorporated the common features of OA into a grading system (Kellgren and Lawrence 1957) that was subsequently adopted by the world health organisation in 1961. They produced an atlas of standard radiographs demonstrating increasing grades of OA. Grades 0 and 1 were normal and doubtful respectively. Grades 2, 3 and 4 showed definite OA divided into mild, moderate and severe (Figure 2). Similar grading system atlases have been produced as variations on the same theme. Of these the most notable is the Osteoarthritis Research Society International (OARSI) score published by Altman et al. (Altman and Gold 2007). These grading systems are used to monitor the progression of OA. The primary variable used for the assessment of progression of OA is the joint space width (JSW) which is a surrogate for cartilage thickness and demonstrates cartilage loss with decreased JSW. There are a number of pitfalls in the acquisition and subsequent measurement of JSW with CR that increase error and subsequently increase the number of participants needed in a study to achieve adequate power. Changes in the position of the joint relative to the x-ray source and film will alter the JSW through magnification, parallax or superimposition of normal bone.

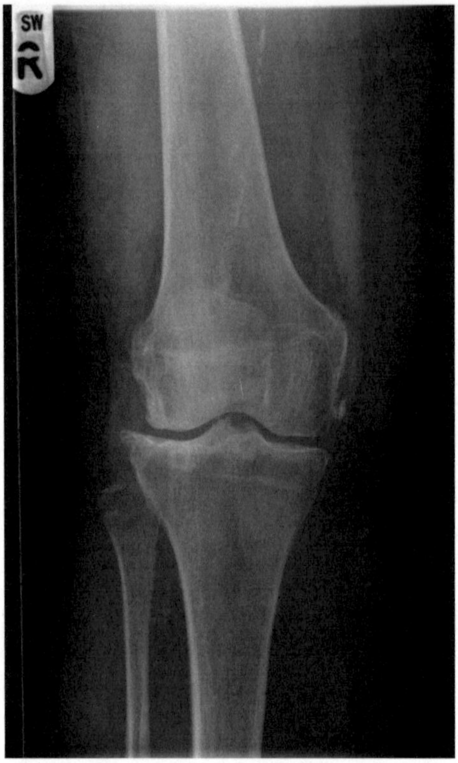

a. Kellgren-Lawrence grade 2, showing minimal joint space narrowing and osteophyte formation

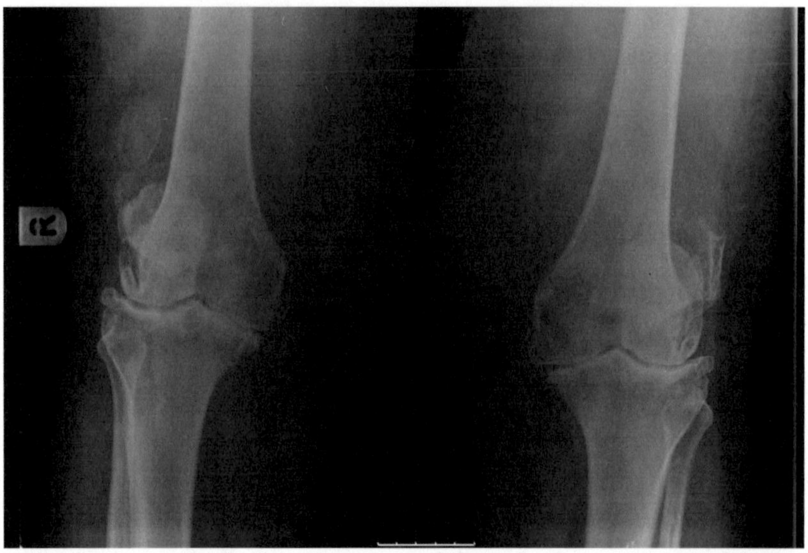

b. Kellgren-Lawrence grade 4, showing severe bilateral tricompartmental knee OA with multiple ossific loose bodies

Fig. 2. Kellgren Lawrence grading

Typically the knee is used in assessment of JSW in disease modifying OA drugs (DMOAD) trials. Standardised protocols have evolved to improve the reliability of the JSW measurement. The JSW is most accurate when measured perpendicular to the x-ray beam and joint, and parallel to the film (Buckland-Wright 2006). Non-weight bearing films are inaccurate and their use is historical. Partial flexion of the knee or tilting of the x-ray beam is required to achieve the perpendicular alignment of beam to joint. The degree of flexion or tilt can be ascertained with fluoroscopic assistance or using standardised positioning. The semi-flexed anteroposterior view described by Buckland-Wright (Buckland-Wright, Marfarlane et al. 1995) and the Lyon Schuss view use fluoroscopy to ensure that the joint line is parallel to the x-ray beam before taking the radiograph. The fixed flexion and metatarso-phalangeal views (Buckland-Wright, Ward et al. 2004) are simpler in that they don't require fluoroscopy to obtain radio-anatomic alignment (Figure 3).

Although CR is the primary investigation in osteoarthritis, it has significant limitations. The earliest histological changes in the development of OA occur within the cartilage and precede radiographically detectable changes. Such changes are unable to distinguish primary from secondary OA. In the former, there is no other underlying cause identified; in the latter, OA changes may be secondary to other underlying joint pathology such as haemochromatosis or other inflammatory arthropathies. There is little difference in the x-ray absorption between varying soft tissues such as cartilage, ligaments, tendons and synovium. As a result the "whole organ" of the synovial joint cannot be assessed directly. Progression of the early stages of OA, which are a target for (DMOADs), is therefore not adequately characterised.

Bagge *et al.* conducted a study of 79 to 85 year-olds and found that more than half of patients with advanced radiographic signs of disease have no significant self-reported complaints (Bagge, Bjelle et al. 1991). Another disadvantage of these CR grading systems is their lack of sensitivity to change. Amin *et al.* conducted a longitudinal study (Amin, LaValley et al. 2005) of participants with knee OA, showing radiographic progression of joint space narrowing (JSN) was predictive of cartilage loss on MRI. However, 42% had cartilage loss visible on MRI with no radiographic progression of JSN. Radiographic progression appeared specific (91%) but not sensitive (23%) for cartilage loss. Conventional radiographs are a 2 dimensional (2D) representation of a 3 dimensional (3D) structure. The pathological changes of OA can also be obscured by superimposed normal bone. Chan *et al.* demonstrated a 60% detection rate of osteophytes in conventional knee radiographs versus 100% on MR imaging (Chan, Stevens et al. 1991).

Microfocal radiography utilises a micron sized x-ray source which emits divergent x-rays. The joint to be imaged is close to the source, but the film is approximately 2 meters away. The resultant image is of high resolution and magnified four to twenty times (Buckland-Wright, MacFarlane et al. 1995). These magnified images can yield a more accurate quantitative assessment of JSW measurements and also allow computerised Fractal Signature Analysis to quantify the changes in the trabeculae of subchondral bone seen in OA (Messent, Ward et al. 2007). The authors hypothesise that these changes in the subchondral and subarticular bone will correspond to the severity of knee OA defined by the reduction in JSW (Messent, Ward et al. 2007).

Conventional radiography still remains the primary imaging modality in the diagnosis and follow up of OA. However, the inability of CR to visualise the "whole organ" of the joint and differentiate early pathological changes is a major weakness that other modalities, particularly MRI, do not share.

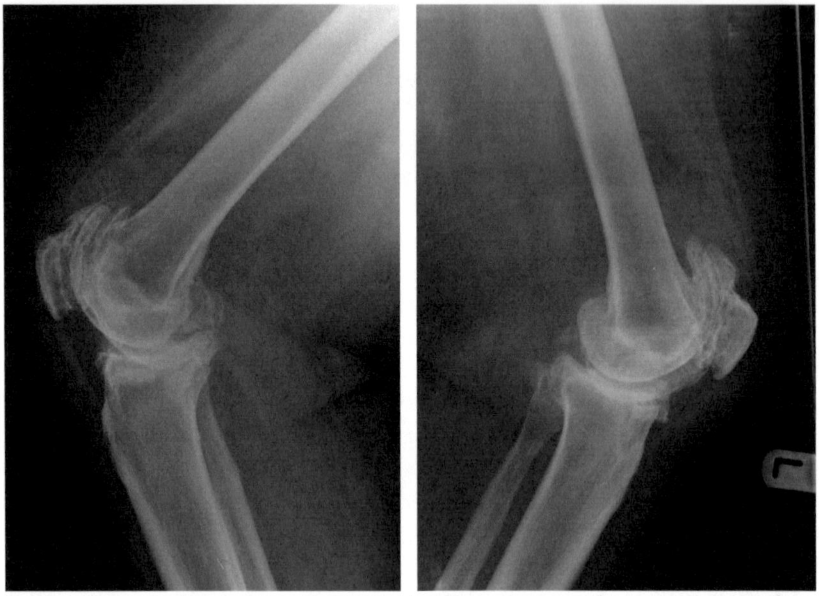

a. Fixed flexion knee radiographs stressing the importance of correct views for assessing changes on plain X ray

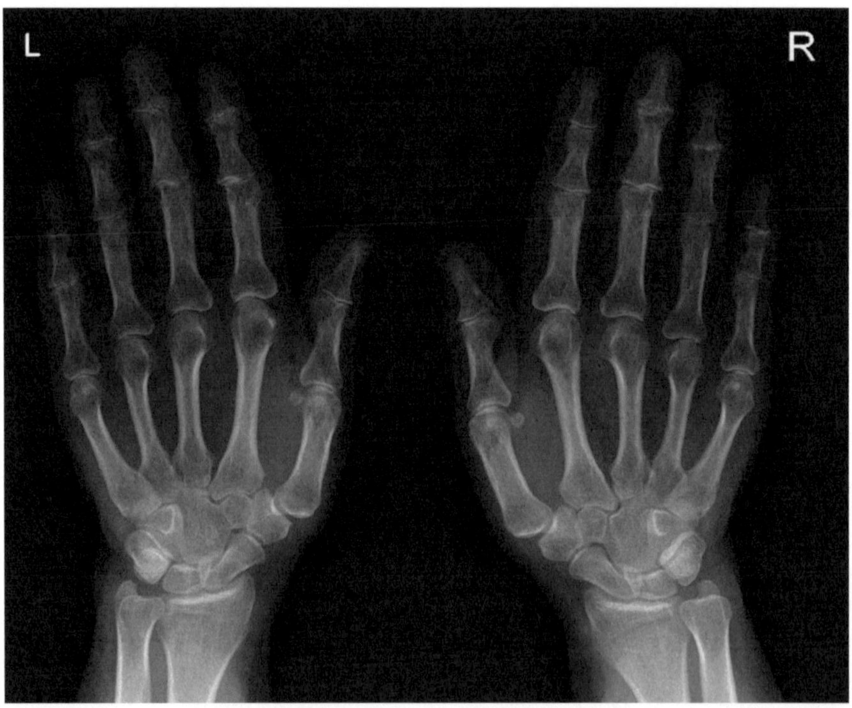

b. Bilateral hand OA demonstrating predominantly proximal and distal interphalangeal joint involvement

Fig. 3. Optimal views for assessing degree of change

3. The contribution of MRI and CT to our understanding of OA pathophysiology

Radiographic imaging advances over recent years have led to a better understanding of the hierarchical structure of cartilage allowing delineation of early OA change at a molecular level. Articular cartilage is primarily hyaline cartilage which exhibits 3D anisotropic characteristics (physical and biological properties are direction dependent). The matrix composition and organization vary according to the depth from the articular surface including a superficial zone, a transitional zone, a radial zone and a zone of calcified cartilage (Potter, Black et al. 2009).

Cartilage can be conceptualized as a biphasic model consisting of a solid phase (glycoproteins, collagen, proteoglycans and chondrocytes) and a fluid phase (water and ions) that comprises 75% of cartilage by weight (Peterfy and Genant 1996). Proteoglycans (PG) consist of a protein core and glycosaminoglycans (GAG) side chains (Xia, Zheng et al. 2008). An osmotic pressure is generated by the heavily sulphated GAG molecules that carry a high concentration of negative charge. Counter ions such as Na^+ draw water into cartilage osmotically with the osmotic pressure contributing to the stiffness of cartilage thereby defining its load bearing properties both in healthy and disease states (Xia, Zheng et al. 2008). The collagen fibrils are thus maintained under pressure by the 'swelling pressure' that maintains the articular cartilage in an 'inflated' form (Peterfy and Genant 1996). Equilibrium exists between the swelling pressure that is resisted by the collagen framework which in turn determines the degree of compression of the PG molecules and the ensuing number of negative charges exposed (Peterfy and Genant 1996).

Disease states that disrupt the collagen framework allow PGs to expand resulting in exposure of more negatively charged moieties and a resultant increase in water content typically found to varying degrees in osteoarthritis, rheumatoid arthritis and traumatic cartilage damage (Peterfy and Genant 1996). Reduction of GAG concentration is also the biomarker of early disease and can be exploited by newer imaging modalities which provide a nondestructive high resolution image of hierarchical structure.

Newer imaging techniques primarily involving MRI (magnetic resonance imaging) have evolved to allow quantitative assessment of zonal changes in cartilage architecture in OA. Semi-quantitative scoring methods include WORMS (whole organ MR imaging score), BLOKS (Boston-Leeds osteoarthritis knee score and KOSS (knee osteoarthritis scoring system) (Peterfy, Guermazi et al. 2004; Kornaat, Ceulmans et al. 2005; Hunter, Lo et al. 2008). Conventional MRI techniques that can be exploited include spin-echo (SE) and spoiled gradient-recalled echo (SPGR) sequences, fast SE sequences and 3D sequences (Crema, Roemer et al. 2011). Fast SE sequences can be performed in 2D and 3D.

Two dimensional fast SE has been tested in clinical trials and provides excellent contrast between fluid and cartilage as well as allowing assessment of bone marrow oedema, synovial thickening, menisci and ligaments (Crema, Roemer et al. 2011) (Figure 4). However 2D fast SE has the disadvantage of producing 2D images in all planes with gaps between images, meaning that detail can be lost when assessing thin 3D structures such as cartilage. 3D fast SE obtains information from the entire volume of the scanned joint which therefore allows manipulation of images in all planes and construction of volumetric images for quantitative assessment of cartilage morphology. It also permits assessment of bone marrow lesions (BMLs), menisci and ligaments but as yet has not been tested in clinical trials (Crema, Roemer et al. 2011).

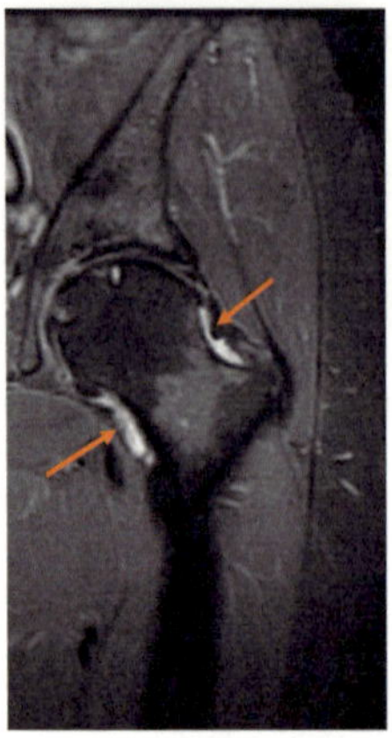

a. MRI hip demonstrating synovial thickening (orange arrows)

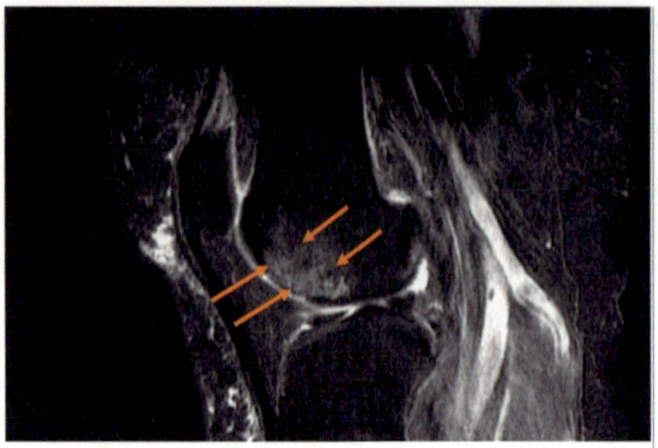

b. MRI knee demonstrating bone marrow lesions (orange arrows)

Fig. 4. Magnetic Resonance Imaging in Osteoarthritis

Spoiled gradient-recalled echo sequences (SPGR) also obtain 3D information, allowing multi-planar reformatting and have the advantage of higher sensitivity when compared to 2D fast SE (Crema, Roemer et al. 2011). However they are susceptible to artifacts due to a long acquisition time making them less reliable for assessment of bone marrow oedema when compared to fast SE.

Other imaging techniques include sampling perfection with application-optimized contrast using different flip-angle evolutions (SPACE), dual-echo steady state (DESS), balanced steady state free precession (bSSFP) and driven equilibrium Fourier transform (DEFT) but these techniques have not been well validated as yet in clinical studies (Crema, Roemer et al. 2011).

Compositional assessment techniques include T2 mapping, delayed gadolinium-enhanced MR imaging of cartilage (dGEMRIC), T1rho (T1ρ) imaging, sodium (Na) imaging and diffusion-weighted imaging (Crema, Roemer et al. 2011). These imaging modalities aim to quantify changes in water content, collagen content and GAGs.

T2 mapping utilizes the interaction between water and surrounding macromolecules with increased interactions resulting in decreased T2 dependent changes in hydration and indirectly collagen concentration that can be objectively assessed in 2D either on colour or grey-scale maps using full thickness mean values, Z-score maps, laminar approaches, texture analysis and flattened cartilage relaxation time maps analysed with grey-level co-occurrence matrices (Burstein, Gray et al. 2009; Carballido-Gamio, Joseph et al. 2011; Crema, Roemer et al. 2011). The relaxation times of T1 and T2 are thus dependent on water content and indirectly the associated collagen network allowing imaging without contrast.

T2 mapping is essentially the pixel by pixel solving of the T2 relaxation curve and can be used to delineate collagen composition of cartilage as well as menisci, ligaments and tendons by utilizing special pulsed sequences (ultrashort echo time techniques) (Potter, Black et al. 2009). Early OA generates a more heterogenous T2 map than normal cartilage but should be interpreted with caution since T2 maps are affected by physical activity and there is no direct correlation between OA grade and T2 changes (Crema, Roemer et al. 2011). Additionally T2 artefacts are generated by the 'magic angle effect' whereby there is an artefactual increase in T2 signal when the ordered structure of collagen is orientated at 55 degrees to the magnetic field resulting in zero dipole-dipole interactions and a prolongation of T2 relaxation time. T2 also exhibits a non-monoexponential behaviour of T2 in cartilage which can make quantification of proton density difficult and has a long acquisition time (Burstein, Gray et al. 2009; Crema, Roemer et al. 2011). Further preventable errors can result from variations in voxel size, parameter selection, signal-to-noise ratio and receiver coil between institutions (Potter, Black et al. 2009).

T1ρ measures the spin-lattice relaxation time in the rotating frame and is similar to T2 relaxation except that an additional radiofrequency pulse is applied after the magnetization is tipped into the transverse plane with an exponential relationship of signal decay to the time constant T1ρ (Burstein, Gray et al. 2009). Experimental studies have shown that T1ρ may be more sensitive than T2 weighted MRI to proteoglycan depletion which is characteristically seen in early OA (Crema, Roemer et al. 2011). However T1ρ requires special pulsed sequences, multiple data sets and has low spatial resolution (Crema, Roemer et al. 2011). Comparison of T1ρ, T2 and dGEMRIC images with histological studies of proteoglycan distribution have shown no correlation, suggesting that other factors such as collagen fibre orientation and concentration as well as the presence of other macromolecules may contribute to variations in T1ρ (Burstein, Gray et al. 2009; Crema, Roemer et al. 2011). However its nonspecific sensitivity may provide a future tool for quantification of molecular changes in early OA.

The diffusion coefficient of water in cartilage correlates to the degree of hydration (Burstein, Gray et al. 2009). Since hydration increases with cartilage degeneration in early OA this is potentially an exploitable biomarker of both the collagen network and GAGs (Xia, Farquhar et al. 1995; Crema, Roemer et al. 2011). The movement of water molecules can be measured in a noninvasive manner without the use of contrast material using pulsed-gradient spin-echo (PGSE) by utilizing a pair of gradient pulses separated by a time interval to detect an irreversible loss of signal due to Brownian motion (Xia, Farquhar et al. 1995). Spatial resolution can be used to localize cartilage degradation in disease but monitors microscopic tissue damage rather than PG content and is more difficult in thin cartilage layers (Xia, Farquhar et al. 1995; Crema, Roemer et al. 2011).

Collagen structure changes in early OA but its concentration does not. Increased levels of degraded collagen have been observed in the superficial and middle zones (Burstein, Bashir et al. 2000). Measurement of collagen using experimental techniques include T2 relaxation times, magnetization transfer (MT) and quantum studies (Burstein, Bashir et al. 2000). T2 techniques are susceptible to the 'magic angle effect' (an artefact signal produced when tissues with an ordered collagen structure are placed at a certain angle to the magnetic field). Magnetization transfer delineates the interaction of water molecules and more slowly rotating molecules with collagen contributing to the majority of the effect and GAG to a lesser extent in cartilage (Burstein, Bashir et al. 2000).

The magnetization transfer in cartilage depends on both collagen structure and concentration with experimental pilot studies showing a variation in MT images in the form of saturation over full magnetization that corresponds to variations in collagen without changes to water or proteoglycan content (Bageac, Gray et al. 1999). However techniques are still experimental and subject to variation according to the parameters of the saturation and correlation to other imaging modalitics (Burstein, Bashir et al. 2000). Multiple quantum studies again offer a potential technique for visualizing changes in macromolecules in early OA that result in a change in the protons or sodium associated with the proteoglycans (Morris and Freemont 1992).

MRI imaging techniques such as dGEMRIC and Na imaging specifically quantify changes in GAG concentration by exploiting the correlation of change in ionic concentration with GAG concentration since proteoglycans have substantial negative fixed charge (Burstein, Bashir et al. 2000; Xia, Zheng et al. 2008; Potter, Black et al. 2009; Crema, Roemer et al. 2011).

The dGEMRIC technique uses T1 mapping of an intravenously administered anionic contrast agent gadopentate dimeglumine (Gd-DTPA^{2-}) which allows quantitative assessment of GAG content. Time is needed to allow penetration of Gd-DTPA^{2-} through the full cartilage thickness. Hence it is called 'delayed' gadolinium enhanced MRI and can require a delay of an hour and a half from injection to the start of image acquisition (Crema, Roemer et al. 2011). The distribution of Gd-DTPA^{2-} will be high in areas where GAG content is low with resultant decreased T1. Since the concentration of Gd-DTPA^{2-} in the blood is time dependent, a state of equilibrium between GAG content and Gd-DTPA^{2-} is never reached and the T1 measurement after penetration of Gd-DTPA^{2-} is referred to as the dGEMRIC index which varies directly with GAG content (Crema, Roemer et al. 2011). There is a correlation between areas of low dGEMRIC index and cartilage lesions which also directly correlates to an increasing Kellgren/Lawrence radiographic severity grade (Williams, Sharma et al. 2005).

A low dGEMRIC index is associated with an increased risk of developing radiographic OA within 6 years (Owman, C.J et al. 2008). Potentially a reduced GAG content in cartilage may increase susceptibility to an increased loading stress on the collagen network resulting in increased mechanical shearing with subsequent fibrillation of the cartilage and resultant OA change (Owman, C.J et al. 2008). Furthermore dGEMRIC has also been applied to imaging of the meniscus and the dGEMRIC index has been shown to correlate with cartilage variations indicating that both may undergo a parallel degradative process (Krishnan, Shetty et al. 2007). The dGEMRIC index of the meniscus was not found to vary consistently with different zones of the meniscus and may be affected by vascular supply or steric hindrance (the size of atoms within collagen prevent certain chemical reactions) by the collagen matrix (Krishnan, Shetty et al. 2007).

The extracellular matrix has a negative fixed charge density due to the sulfate and carboxyl groups in the GAG molecule. Positive charged ions of sodium are therefore present in higher concentrations in cartilaginous interstitial fluid than in synovial fluid or bone (Felson, McLaughlin et al. 2003). Areas of cartilage where GAG depletion has occurred will therefore have a lower sodium ion concentration. Sodium MRI imaging measures the resonance frequency produced by Na's nuclear spin momentum and has the advantage in cartilage that sodium is naturally present with a higher concentration than the surrounding tissues (Felson, McLaughlin et al. 2003). Disadvantages of sodium imaging include the low spatial resolution compared to proton MR imaging with some spatial variation present in normal cartilage and the need for special hardware (Zanetti, Bruder et al. 2000).

Bone marrow lesions (BML) have been cited as a potential biomarker of structural deterioration in knee OA using sagittal short inversion time inversion-recovery (STIR), T1- and T2- weighted turbo spin-echo MR imaging (Zanetti, Bruder et al. 2000; Felson, McLaughlin et al. 2003; Link, Steinbach et al. 2003; Kijowski, Stanton et al. 2006). A natural history study by Felson et al. using a 1.5T MRI system showed that in the knee the presence of BML was a powerful risk factor for further structural deterioration (Felson, McLaughlin et al. 2003). In the medial compartment the presence of BMLs was found to correlate with an increased progression of medial compartment OA by a factor of six (Felson, McLaughlin et al. 2003). Furthermore there was an association between frontal plane malalignment and BML. However other studies have shown that whilst BMLs are associated with OA they may not directly correlate with severity of Kellgren-Lawrence grading. Bone marrow lesions may instead correlate with a number of non-characteristic histological abnormalities including bone marrow necrosis, bone marrow fibrosis and trabecular abnormalities (Zanetti, Bruder et al. 2000; Link, Steinbach et al. 2003; Hayashi, Guermazi et al. 2011). Further MRI studies of the relation of BMLs to pain in OA have been more encouraging. Pain incidence and severity correlate to the presence and size of BMLs (Felson, Chaisson et al. 2001; Felson, Niu et al. 2007). Felson et al found that BMLs were present in 77.5% of patients with painful knees compared to 30% of patients with no knee pain (Felson, Chaisson et al. 2001; Felson, Niu et al. 2007).

Recently microCT has also been used, predominantly in animal models to define the nature of osteophytes and change in bone marrow volume in OA (Hayashi, Guermazi et al. 2011; Sampson, Beck et al. 2011). Such studies have reported that osteophyte size and localization may be better visualized using microCT. Increased bone volume is also observed in OA lesions (Sampson, Beck et al. 2011).

4. Ultrasound assessment in OA

Ultrasound (US) provides a cost-effective, real time, non-invasive multi-planar imaging modality in the assessment of OA and also to guide therapeutic injections (Moller, Bong et al. 2008). Ultrasound has the advantage over MRI and bone scintigraphy in that it is more readily available and non-invasive. However its main disadvantage is that it is operator dependent with a long learning curve (Iagnocco 2010). It is portable and therefore allows repeated assessment of subtle progression of joint pathology in both static and dynamic modes (Moller, Bong et al. 2008). Whilst CR changes such as JSN, subchondral sclerosis, marginal osteophytes and cysts are used to assess OA progression, in the hand these may be late findings. Thus US may provide a useful adjunct to the early assessment of subclinical manifestations of OA (Iagnocco 2010).

The recent development of high resolution high frequency transducers, multi-frequency probes, matrix probes and volumetric probes has expanded the application of US in the assessment of cartilage thickness, menisci, tendons, ligaments, joint capsule, synovial membrane, synovial fluid and bursae as well as to a lesser extent subchondral bone. Recent studies have indicated an association between synovial proliferation and BML with pain in OA making their assessment with US particularly attractive (Moller, Bong et al. 2008; Kortekaas, Kwok et al. 2010).

Anatomic sites most frequently assessed with US include the hand, the foot, the knee and hip joints both in terms of primary evaluation of early disease, therapeutic interventions and response to treatment (Walther, Harms et al. 2002; Kuroki, Nakagawa et al. 2008; Mancarella, Magnani et al. 2010). The anatomical site and type of tissue under investigation will determine the US technique used (Moller, Bong et al. 2008). Scanning protocols are tailored to specific joints with established guidelines ensuring standardization of images in two planes (Keen, Wakefield et al. 2009; Iagnocco 2010). For example, in the small joints of the hand, longitudinal and transverse scans in flexion for the dorsal aspects and in neutral to visualize the volar aspects are performed with a high frequency (more than 12 MHz) probe (Moller, Bong et al. 2008; Iagnocco 2010; Mancarella, Magnani et al. 2010; Wittoek, Carron et al. 2010). In order to visualize the weight bearing surfaces of the femoral condyles in the knee, the scan is performed with the knee flexed in the supine position (Moller, Bong et al. 2008; Yoon, Kim et al. 2008). In the hip the leg is extended and externally rotated to allow visualization of the anterior surface of the femoral head using a lower frequency (8-12 MHz) probe (Backhaus, Burmester et al. 2001; Moller, Bong et al. 2008; Iagnocco 2010). Studies in the literature vary as to how the joint is positioned and which planes are scanned (Naredo, Acebes et al. 2008).

The shape and size of the probe also has a role in image acquisition with smaller hockey stick probes being more appropriate for the small joints of the hand and larger footprint probes more suited for knee and hip joints (Iagnocco 2010). Both grey-scale and Doppler scans provide complementary modalities for the thorough assessment of osteoarthritic joints (Iagnocco 2010). Using an initial grey-scale setting and by altering the probe frequency both superficial and deeper structures can be viewed in small joints such as in the hand and larger joints such as the hip (Iagnocco 2010; Mancarella, Magnani et al. 2010). Power Doppler settings allow the assessment of active inflammation, or at least to vascular hyperaemia in the synovium thus defining both disease state and response to therapy modalities (Iagnocco 2010; Mancarella, Magnani et al. 2010; Arrestier, Rosenberg et al. 2011).

The application of US in the assessment of OA includes definition of the extent of changes in the cartilaginous matrix, changes in intra-articular and peri-articular soft tissues as well as assessment of changes to the bony cortex (Moller, Bong et al. 2008). Early disease progression is reflected in loss of sharpness of the superficial cartilaginous margin corresponding to micro-cleft formation and later loss of echogenicity (Moller, Bong et al. 2008; Iagnocco 2010). Diffuse thinning eventually progresses to cartilage loss and asymmetric JSN with good reproducibility and agreement between ultrasonographers and histological findings (Moller, Bong et al. 2008; Iagnocco 2010).

Bone changes in early OA include the presence of a hyperechoic signal in the area of joint capsule attachment (Moller, Bong et al. 2008). Later disease changes include the formation of osteophytes as cortical protrusions at the corresponding joint margin (Iagnocco 2010). In the hand osteophytes can be accompanied by cartilage erosions visualized as a step-down contour defect (Iagnocco 2010; Wittoek, Carron et al. 2010). Recent evidence has shown that US is more sensitive than CR for the detection of osteophytes and JSN in hand OA (Wakefield, Balint et al. 2005; Iagnocco 2010).

With reference to OA changes affecting intra-articular soft tissues, synovial thickening, joint effusion and increased vascularity can be detected using both grey-scale and Doppler modalities (Moller, Bong et al. 2008; Iagnocco 2010). Furthermore, increased synovial flow detected with Doppler modalities is also a sign of increased synovial vascularity which correlates well with corresponding histological changes (Backhaus, Burmester et al. 2001). The Outcome Measures in Rheumatoid Arthritis Clinical Trials (OMERACT) definitions of synovial fluid and synovial hypertrophy applied in rheumatoid arthritis are also applicable to OA (Moller, Bong et al. 2008; Koutroumpas, Alexiou et al. 2010). Synovial thickening is defined as abnormal hypoechoic intra-articular material that is non-displaceable, poorly compressible and may exhibit power Doppler signal (PDS). Effusion is defined as abnormal intra-articular material that is hypoechoic or anechoic, displaceable and does not exhibit PDS (Koutroumpas, Alexiou et al. 2010). Synovial thickening is frequently found in inflamed OA joints and synovial fluid can be defined by its quantity and content with respect to US imaging in OA (Iagnocco 2010). It is unclear if any inflammation perceived is from OA or from complicating crystalline arthritis.

Specific US findings related to anatomical location of the joint under investigation have also been defined in the literature, with the majority of studies involving the joints of the hand (Walther, Harms et al. 2002; Kuroki, Nakagawa et al. 2008; Wittoek, Carron et al. 2010; Wittoek, Jans et al. 2010; Arrestier, Rosenberg et al. 2011). Several studies have also investigated the diagnostic accuracy of US compared to CR, CT and MRI in the hand (Keen, Wakefield et al. 2008; Moller, Bonel et al. 2009; Mancarella, Magnani et al. 2010).

Ultrasound is more sensitive than CR in detecting cartilage erosions in the hand which may provide a tool for allowing earlier identification of cartilage loss in joints (Wittoek, Carron et al. 2010). However longitudinal studies are required to validate the development of US detected cartilage erosions into CR detected erosions. Osteophytes are also detected with a higher sensitivity using US compared to CR due to its ability to assess the joint under investigation in multiple planes (Wakefield, Balint et al. 2005; Wittoek, Carron et al. 2010). By contrast, estimating JSN with US is dependent on the acoustic window since osteophytes can block adequate visualization and the central portion of the joint cannot be visualized with US (Wakefield, Balint et al. 2005). Evaluation of JSN is subjective with no validated criteria defined in the literature. Cartilage thickness may provide a surrogate marker of JSW since reduced cartilage thickness in the hand has been shown to correlate with JSN (McNally 2007). In order to improve near field resolution, increased sensitivity for detection of blood flow and minimize compression / obliteration of small quantities of effusion or synovial thickening, a lightly held probe with a generous amount of contact jelly reduces contact pressure (Koski, Saarakkala et al. 2006).

Effusion and PDS do not appear to be specific for cartlage erosion with effusion also found in 'normal' joints and conflicting results found in current studies (Chao, Wu et al. 2010; Kortekaas, Kwok et al. 2010; Mancarella, Magnani et al. 2010; Wittoek, Carron et al. 2010; Wittoek, Jans et al. 2010; Arrestier, Rosenberg et al. 2011). Subclinical inflammation has been reported in some studies with no correlation found with PDS or patients' reported pain levels but may indicate future disease progression (Kuroki, Nakagawa et al. 2008; Kortekaas, Kwok et al. 2010; Wittoek, Jans et al. 2010). Scanning of the sagittal (longitudinal) extensor and flexor sides is performed in relaxed finger extension with axial imaging used to view the metacarpophalangeal joints and coronal imaging used to view the interphalangeal joints (Koski, Saarakkala et al. 2006). Gentle flexion of the joints allows detection of intra-articular changes such as osteophytes and synovial thickening (Koski, Saarakkala et al. 2006) (Figure 5). Ultrasound shows good agreement with MRI for the assessment of cartilage erosion and grey-scale synovial thickening (Moller, Bonel et al. 2009). Osteophytes can produce a signal void on MRI due to the presence of densely packed calcium, making US more sensitive than CR and MRI (Moller, Bonel et al. 2009).

Similar techniques can be employed to image the small joints of the forefoot (Koski, Saarakkala et al. 2006). The extensor approach is used to probe the interphalangeal joints as well as the meta-tarsophalangeal joints to detect joint erosions and synovial thickening.

In the knee US probes can also be used arthroscopically to assess cartilage morphology as well as conventional scanning protocols to assess cartilage thickness in the weight bearing areas of the femoral condyles, protrusion of the medial meniscus in the knee and the presence of Baker's cysts (Kuroki, Nakagawa et al. 2008; Yoon, Kim et al. 2008; Iagnocco 2010). Alternative imaging protocols such as the longitudinal sagittal US scan may also provide visualization of a larger area of femoral condyle than the suprapatellar transverse axial scan (Yoon, Kim et al. 2008). Synovial thickening can also be detected but may not correspond to clinical response to intra-articular corticosteroid injections (Hattori, Takakura et al. 2005).

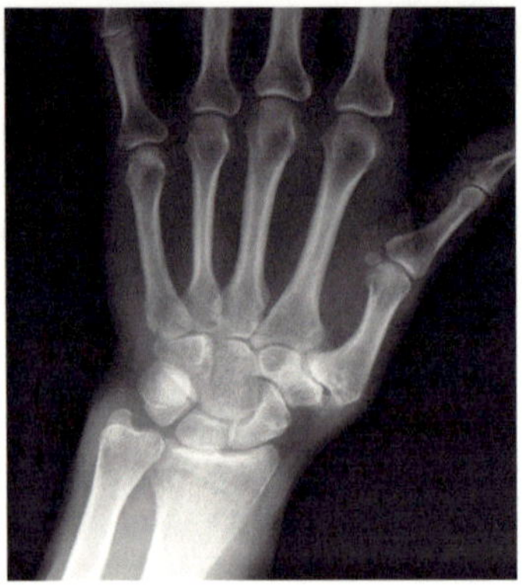

a. Plain radiograph of the hand demonstrating first carpometacarpal joint degenerative change

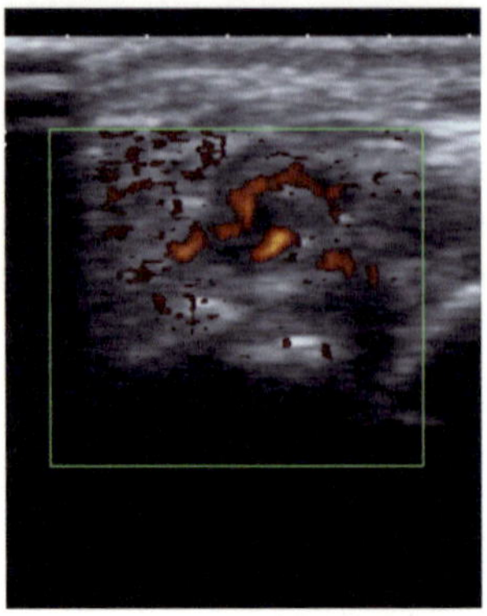

b. First carpometacarpal joint showing synovial thickening and increased vascularity on power Doppler imaging

Fig. 5. Plain x ray and ultrasound power Doppler signal

Validity of measurements of cartilage thickness in the knee using US has shown good reproducibility in normal to moderately damaged cartilage but is less accurate for severely damaged cartilage where the cartilage-soft tissue interfaces become less clear (Keen, Wakefield et al. 2008; Yoon, Kim et al. 2008). Ultrasound properties that can be exploited for assessing cartilage structure include the use of signal intensity which correlates to superficial cartilage integrity, echo duration which correlates to surface irregularity and the interval between signals that correlates to thickness (Kuroki, Nakagawa et al. 2008). High frequency pulsed echo US can be used to assess degeneration of the superficial collagen-rich cartilage zone. It is capable of detecting microstructural changes up to a depth of 500μm (Qvistgaard, Torp-Pedersen et al. 2006).

Hip ultrasound depends on patient size since there is a loss of resolution and poorer penetration of higher frequency probes at depth. Depending on patient size, sometimes only lower frequency curvilinear probes can be used (usually 5-8MHz) with significant loss of detail). In the hip the use of PDS has been found to correlate reliably with vascularity of synovial tissue (Backhaus, Burmester et al. 2001). Ultrasound assessment of femoral head shape, synovial profile, joint effusion and synovial thickening in OA has been shown to be reliable in trained US investigators (Yoon, Kim et al. 2005; Atchia, Birrell et al. 2007). The presence of an effusion or synovial thickening has been assessed by measuring the collum-capsule distance (distance between the neck of the femur and the hip capsule) and comparing it to the asymptomatic side (Atchia, Birrell et al. 2007). When compared with CR Kellgren scores there was a weak correlation to US scoring of osteophytes and femoral head shape (Atchia, Birrell et al. 2007). When associated with pain on activity, there is a highly significant association of global US hip joint evaluation when combined with US synovial thickening as a predictor of pain on activity (Atchia, Birrell et al. 2007).

In summary, there is a reasonable correlation between US measurements of cartilage thickness and histological findings for mild and moderate OA. In the hand US is more sensitive for the detection of osteophytosis but less so for cartilage erosions. In the knee US correlates well with MRI for the detection of effusion, synovial thickening and popliteal cysts but shows poor correlation with a clinical diagnosis of anserine tendinobursitis (Yoon, Kim et al. 2005). In the hip PDS correlates well to increased vascularity of synovial tissue. In the foot and shoulder, there is good correlation between US and CR as well as clinical diagnosis of enthesitis and demonstration of bursitis over the medial aspect of the first metatarsophalangeal joint (Naredo, Acebes et al. 2008; Iagnocco 2010). Further work is still required to standardize definitions, scoring systems and validity (Iagnocco 2010).

5. Vibrational spectroscopy

There is no current validated tool for the diagnosis of symptomatic early OA prior to CR changes (Esmonde-White, Mandair et al. 2009). Chemical changes in synovial fluid and subchondral bone may provide biomarkers of early disease allowing for earlier intervention (Dehring, Crane et al. 2006; Williams and Spector 2008; Sofat 2009). Vibrational spectroscopy can provide detailed chemical information on the interactions between mineral and collagen matrix in cartilage, changes in subchondral bone, changes in the viscosity of synovial fluid and deposition of crystals such as basic calcium phosphate crystals (BCP) (Dehring, Crane et al. 2006).

Atoms in a molecule undergoing periodic motion while the molecule has a constant motion create a vibrational frequency which will depend on the quantity of energy absorbed during vibrational transitions and can produce a characteristic infrared spectra. All biological molecules have a unique spectra which can be measured using a variety of vibrational spectroscopic techniques, each with their own inherent advantages and disadvantages (Lambert, Whitman et al. 2006).

Both near infrared spectroscopy (NIR) and Fourier-transform infra-red (FTIR) spectroscopy have been utilized for the investigation of synovial fluid chemical composition in disease states but cannot identify individual components of synovial fluid (Esmonde-White, Mandair et al. 2009). FTIR uses automated pattern recognition but has the disadvantage that water interferes with certain parts of the spectra which can result in misinterpretation (Yavorskyy, Hernandez-Santana et al. 2008). Raman spectroscopy provides a specific non-invasive, non-destructive and reagentless tool for the investigation of biological tissues (Esmonde-White, Mandair et al. 2009). Water does not interfere with Raman spectroscopy and unique spectra are available for biological molecules (Yavorskyy, Hernandez-Santana et al. 2008). However it is expensive with fewer library spectra available (Yavorskyy, Hernandez-Santana et al. 2008).

Synovial fluid aspirates provide an easy source of biomaterial for the investigation of changes in composition and viscosity in early OA (Esmonde-White, Mandair et al. 2009). Both NIR and FTIR can be used to identify early OA with a classification rate of greater than 95% using the overall chemical composition generated spectral pattern (Esmonde-White, Mandair et al. 2009). Background fluorescence especially from proteins can interfere with the spectra (Yavorskyy, Hernandez-Santana et al. 2008). Further refinement with drop deposition to allow rough component separation and segregation of impurities in conjunction with Raman spectroscopy can improve the diagnostic potential of vibrational spectroscopy (Esmonde-White, Mandair et al. 2009). Correlation of spectral bands with Kellgren and Lawrence grades creates the potential of a future diagnostic tool (Esmonde-White, Mandair et al. 2009).

Crystals such as BCP and calcium pyrophosphate dihydrate (CPPD) are frequently reported in the early stages of OA before changes to subchondral bone are evident (Fuerst, Lammers et al. 2009). BCP crystals are small (1nm) and unlike CPPD (crystals 91-2μm) are not visible using light microscopy unless they clump together (Fuerst, Lammers et al. 2009). Raman spectra can be used to distinguish between crystals and detect their presence in synovial fluid (Yavorskyy, Hernandez-Santana et al. 2008).

Changes in cartilage and subchondral bone can also be detected with vibrational spectroscopy. FTIR has been used to correlate tissue damage with changes in the amide II and III envelopes (part of the spectra) as well as detecting spectral features of proteoglycans and collagen to a spatial resolution of 10μm and collagen degradation in OA knees (Dehring, Crane et al. 2006). Raman spectroscopy can also be used in a non-invasive fashion to investigate the subchondral bone under the non-mineralised layer of articular cartilage providing the potential for a future diagnostic tool in OA (Dehring, Crane et al. 2006).

6. Bone scans

Scintigraphy allows the assessment of the osseous physiology in human joints since it requires a living, metabolically functioning organism (Dye and Chew 1994). Whilst conventional radiography, CT scanning, MRI and ultrasound provide a structural assessment of a joint, bone scanning has the advantage of providing a physiological assessment (Dye and Chew 1994). The main disadvantages of bone scans are that the images are planar with superimposition of a 3D array into 2D and resolution is low for complex joints (Kim 2008).

The indications for performing a bone scan specifically in OA are limited, with scintigraphy used in a clinical setting to differentiate between pathologies. Historically, bone scans were requested to confirm or exclude a diagnosis of inflammatory arthritis, malignancy and fractures in one study (Duncan, Dorai-Raj et al. 1999). OA was the final diagnosis in 11% of scans. However, changes in periarticular uptake have been noted in patients with normal radiographic findings and an unstable bucket handle meniscal tear (Dye and Chew 1994). Potential future application is in the diagnosis of early OA prior to conventional radiographic changes.

Technetium-99m (Tc-99m) is the common gamma emitting radio-isotope used in bone scans. It is linked to methylene diphosphanate (MDP) which is taken up by metabolically active bone. Studies typically consist of a blood flow phase that reflects tissue perfusion, a blood pool phase that reflects vascularity and a final delayed static image phase that reflects a combination of blood supply and tracer extraction by metabolically active bone (Siegel, Donovan et al. 1976).

Newer applications such as single photon emission computed tomography (SPECT) have expanded the role of scintigraphy in bone imaging (Sarikaya, Sarikaya et al. 2001; Kim 2008; Papathanassiou, Bruna-Muraille et al. 2009). SPECT separates into sequential tomographic planes the metabolic activity thus improving image contrast and localization (Sarikaya, Sarikaya et al. 2001). Current clinical applications for SPECT in OA are limited due to the practicalities of low count rates and inefficient use of the camera field-of-view (Collier, Johnson et al. 1985). Bone SPECT has been used in the diagnosis of facet joint OA in the spine with studies showing that it may improve patient selection for therapeutic facet blocks (Holder, Machin et al. 1995; Dolan, Ryan et al. 1996). Conventional radiography and MRI are still the main modes of investigating the painful knee, SPECT has also been used to investigate chronic knee pain. SPECT was more sensitive than bone scintigraphy in detecting articular cartilage damage in the patellofemoral joint (Collier, Johnson et al. 1985). SPECT imaging correlates well with clinical scores and physical examination in patients with OA, even without abnormal radiographic findings which may indicate a future role in the diagnosis of early OA (Kim 2008).

Advances in image alignment software have allowed SPECT imaging to be fused to high resolution CT slices in the region of interest (Papathanassiou, Bruna-Muraille et al. 2009). Whilst technically challenging since patient position must be maintained, it has the advantage of combining high special structural information with highly sensitive functional information (Papathanassiou, Bruna-Muraille et al. 2009). The main disadvantage is the increased radiation dose to the patient of combining both CT and SPECT.

Various radiopharmaceuticals have been described in the literature under development in animals to allow imaging of cartilage as well as bone (Yu, Bartlett et al. 1988; Yu, Shaw et al. 1999). Other radiopharmaceuticals that target inflammation, osteophytes, cysts and sclerosis have also been described in a limited setting in the literature (Merrick 1992; Etchebehere, Etchebehere et al. 1998).

In positron emission spectroscopy (PET), 18-fluorodeoxyglucose (18-FDG) acts as a glucose analogue, taken up in cells within the body which have high glucose requirements. This includes brain and cardiac tissue as well as cells with high metabolic activity. Using CT imaging techniques, the resultant energy from the emitted positrons can be used to produce 3D functional imaging. When combined with CT scanning, the PET and CT images can be co-registered (merged), producing improved resolution and localization of focal of tracer uptake. PET-CT scanning demonstrates increased uptake in OA, (Elzinga, Laken et al. 2007; Omoumi, Mercier et al. 2009) however, the presence of increased of metabolic activity is not specific to this condition. Other isotopes such as 18-Fluoride (18-F) has a high affinity for bone. This isotope PET scan produces high quality bone images within 30 minutes of injection of the tracer (Omoumi, Mercier et al. 2009).

In summary, the current clinical applications of conventional bone scintigraphy in OA are limited to excluding differential diagnoses. Future applications of gamma emitting and positron emitting radiopharmaceuticals may allow imaging of anatomical and physiological changes in joints prior to conventional radiographic changes associated with early OA.

7. Implications of advances in imaging for therapies in OA

It is likely that if treatment interventions become targeted more towards BMLs e.g. with bisphosphonates, that MRI will play a central role in defining the nature and site of BMLs. There is also increasing evidence that synovial thickening is correlated strongly with pain in OA. Ultrasound is becoming increasingly accepted as a useful tool for detecting subclinical synovial thickening and may be used to target therapies to treat local inflammation e.g. corticosteroid injections. Although there are currently no DMOADs (disease-modifying OA drugs) that are effective in the long-term, it is possible that sensitive techniques such as dGEMRIC may be useful in quantifying structural change using novel therapies. In summary, developments in imaging have improved our understanding of OA immensely in recent years and may well play a pivotal role in guiding treatments for the future.

8. References

Altman, R. D. and G. E. Gold (2007). "Atlas of individual radiographic features in osteoarthritis, revised." *Osteoarthritis and Cartilage* 15(Supplement A): A1-56.

Amin, S., M. P. LaValley, et al. (2005). "The relationship between cartilage loss on magnetic resonance imaging and radiographic progression in men and women with knee osteoarthritis." *Arthritis and Rheumatism* 52(10): 3152-3159.

Arrestier, S., C. Rosenberg, et al. (2011). "Ultrasound features of nonstructural lesions of the proximal and distal interphalangeal joints of the hands in patients with finger osteoarthritis." *Joint Bone Spine* 78(1): 65-69.

Atchia, I., F. Birrell, et al. (2007). "A modular, flexible training strategy to achieve competence in diagnostic and interventional musculoskeletal ultrasound in patients with hip osteoarthritis." *Rheumatology* 46(10): 1583-1586.

Backhaus, M., G.-R. Burmester, et al. (2001). "Guidelines for musculoskeletal ultrasound in rheumatology." *Ann Rheum Dis* 60: 641–649.

Bageac, A. C., M. L. Gray, et al. (1999). "Development of an MRI surrogate for immunohistochemical staining of collagen damage in cartilage. " *In 5th international conference on magnetic resonance microscopy. Heidelberg, Germany: Groupement ampere.* 17.

Bagge, E., A. Bjelle, et al. (1991). "Osteoarthritis in the elderly: clinical and radiological findings in 79 and 85 year olds." *Annals of Rheumatology Disease* 50(8): 533-539.

Buckland-Wright, C. (2006). "Which radiographic techniques should we use for research and clinical practice?" *Best Practice & Research Clinical Rheumatology* 20(1): 39-55.

Buckland-Wright, C., D. G. Marfarlane, et al. (1995). "Accuracy and precision of joint space width measurements in standard and macroradiographs of osteoarthritic knees." *Annals of Rheumatology Disease* 54(11): 872-880.

Buckland-Wright, J. C., D. G. MacFarlane, et al. (1995). "Quantitative microfocal radiography detects changes in OA knee joint space width in patients in a placebo controlled trial of NSAID therapy." *Journal of Rheumatology* 22(5): 937-943.

Buckland-Wright, J. C., R. J. Ward, et al. (2004). "Reproducibility of the semi-flexed (metatarsophalangeal) radiographic knee position and automated measurements of medial tibiofemoral joint space width in a multicentre clinical trial of knee osteoarthritis." *Journal of Rheumatology* 31(8): 1588-1597.

Burstein, D., A. Bashir, et al. (2000). "MRI techniques in early stages of cartilage disease." *Investigative Radiology* 35(10): 622-638.

Burstein, D., M. L. Gray, et al. (2009). "Measures in molecular composition and structure in osteoathritis." *Radiologic Clinics of North America* 2009(47): 675-686.

Carballido-Gamio, J., G. B. Joseph, et al. (2011). "Longitudinal analysis of MRI T2 knee cartilage laminar organization in a subset of patients from the osteoarthritis initiative: A texture approach." *Magnetic Resonance in Medicine* 65(4): 1184-1194.

Chan, W. P., M. P. Stevens, et al. (1991). "Osteoarthritis of the knee: comparison of radiography, CT, and MR imaging to assess extent and severity." *American Journal of roentgenology* 157(4): 799-806.

Chao, J., C. Wu, et al. (2010). "Inflammatory characteristics on ultrasound predict poorer longterm response to intra-articular corticosteroid injections in knee osteoarthritis." *The Journal of rheumatology* 37: 650-655.

Collier, B. D., R. P. Johnson, et al. (1985). "Chronic knee pain assessed by SPECT: comparison with other modularities." *Radiology* 157: 795-802.

Crema, M. D., F. W. Roemer, et al. (2011). "Articular Cartilage in the Knee: Current MR Imaging Techniques and Applications in Clinical Practice and Research." *Radiographics* 31: 37-62.

Dehring, K. A., N. J. Crane, et al. (2006). "Identifying chemical changes in subchondral bone taken from murine knee joints using Raman spectroscopy." *Applied Spectroscopy* 60(10): 1134.

Dolan, A. L., P. J. Ryan, et al. (1996). "The value of SPECT scans in identifying back pain likely to benefit from facet joint injection." *British Journal of Rheumatology* 35: 1269-1273.

Duncan, I., A. Dorai-Raj, et al. (1999). "The utility of bone scans in rheumatology." *Clinical Nuclear Medicine* 24(1): 9-14.

Dye, S. F. and M. H. Chew (1994). "The use of scintigraphy to detect increased osseous metabolic activity about the knee." *Instructional Course Lectures* 43: 453-469.

Elzinga, E. H., C. J. Laken, et al. (2007). "2-Deoxy-2-[F-18]fluoro-D-glucose joint uptake on positron emission tomography images: rheumatoid arthritis versus osteoarthritis." *Molecular Imaging and Biology* 9(6): 357-360.

Esmonde-White, K. A., G. S. Mandair, et al. (2009). "Raman spectroscopy of synovial fluid as a tool for diagnosing osteoarthritis." *Journal of Biomedical Optics* 14(3): 034013.

Etchebehere, E. C., M. Etchebehere, et al. (1998). "Orthopaedic pathology of the lower extremities: scintigraphic evaluation in the thigh, knee and leg." *Seminars in Nuclear Medicine* 28(1): 41-61.

Felson, D. T., C. E. Chaisson, et al. (2001). "The association of bone marrow lesions with pain in knee osteoarthritis." *Annals of Internal Medicine* 134: 541-549.

Felson, D. T., S. McLaughlin, et al. (2003). "Bone marrow edema and its relation to progression of knee osteoarthritis." *Annals of Internal Medicine* 139.

Felson, D. T., J. B. Niu, et al. (2007). "Correlation of the development of knee pain with enlarging bone marrow lesions on magnetic resonance imaging." *Arthritis and Rheumatism* 56: 2986-2992.

Fuerst, M., L. Lammers, et al. (2009). "Investigation of calcium crystals in OA knees." *Rheumatology International* 30(5): 623-631.

Hattori, K., Y. Takakura, et al. (2005). "Quantitative ultrasound can assess the regeneration process of tissue-engineered cartilage using a complex between adherent bone marrow cells and a three dimensional scaffold." *Arthritis Research & Therapy* 7: R552-559.

Hayashi, D., A. Guermazi, et al. (2011). "Osteoarthritis year 2010 in review: imaging." *Osteoarthritis and Cartilage*.

Holder, L. E., J. L. Machin, et al. (1995). "Planar and high resolution SPECT bone imaging in the diagnosis of facet syndrome." *Journal of Nuclear Medicine* 36: 37-44.

Hunter, D. J., G. H. Lo, et al. (2008). "The reliability of a new scoring system for knee osteoarthritis MRI and the validity of bone marrow lesion assessment: BLOKS (Boston Leeds osteoarthritis knee score)." *Annals of Rheumatology Disease* 67(2): 206-211.

Iagnocco, A. (2010). "Imaging the joint in osteoarthritis: a place for ultrasound?" *Best Practice & Research Clinical Rheumatology* 24(1): 27-38.

Keen, H. I., R. J. Wakefield, et al. (2009). "A systematic review of ultrasonography in osteoarthritis." *Annals of the Rheumatic Diseases* 68(5): 611-619.

Keen, H. I., R. J. Wakefield, et al. (2008). "Can ultrasonography improve on radiographic assessment in osteoarthritis of the hands? A comparison between radiographic and ultrasonographic detected pathology." *Annals of the Rheumatic Diseases* 67(8): 1116-1120.

Kellgren, J. and J. Lawrence (1957). "Radiological assessment of osteo-arthrosis." *Annals of Rheumatology Disease* 16(4): 494-502.

Kijowski, R., P. Stanton, et al. (2006). "Subchondral bone marrow edema in patients with degeneration of the articular cartilage of the knee joint." *Radiology* 238(3): 943-949.

Kim, H. (2008). "Clinical value of 99mTc-methylene diphosphonate (MDP) bone single photon emission computed tomography (SPECT) in patients with knee osteoarthritis." *Osteoarthritis and Cartilage* 16(2): 212-218.

Kornaat, P. R., R. Y. Ceulmans, et al. (2005). "MRI assessment of knee osteoarthritis: knee Osteoarthritis Scoring System (KOSS) inter-observer and intra-observer reproducibility of compartment-based scoring system." *Skeletal Radiology* 34(2): 95-102.

Kortekaas, M. C., W. Y. Kwok, et al. (2010). "Pain in hand osteoarthritis is associated with inflammation: the value of ultrasound." *Annals of the Rheumatic Diseases* 69(7): 1367-1369.

Koski, J. M., S. Saarakkala, et al. (2006). "Power Doppler ultrasonography and synovitis: correlating ultrasound imaging with histopathological findings and evaluating the performance of ultrasound equipments." *Annals of the Rheumatic Diseases* 65(12): 1590-1595.

Koutroumpas, A. C., I. S. Alexiou, et al. (2010). "Comparison between clinical and ultrasonographic assessment in patients with erosive osteoarthritis of the hands." *Clinical Rheumatology* 29(5): 511-516.

Krishnan, N., S. K. Shetty, et al. (2007). "Delayed gadolinium enhanced magnetic resonance imaging of the meniscus." *Arthritis and Rheumatism* 56(5): 1507-1511.

Kuroki, H., Y. Nakagawa, et al. (2008). "Ultrasound properties of articular cartilage in the tibio-femoral joint in knee osteoarthritis: relation to clinical assessment (International Cartilage Repair Society grade)." *Arthritis Research & Therapy* 10(4): R78.

Lambert, P. J., A. G. Whitman, et al. (2006). "Raman spectroscopy: the gateway into tomorrow's virology." *Virology Journal* 3: 51.

Link, T. M., L. S. Steinbach, et al. (2003). "Osteoarthritis: MR imaging findings in different stages of disease and correlation with clinical findings." *Radiology* 226(2): 373-381.

Mancarella, L., M. Magnani, et al. (2010). "Ultrasound-detected synovitis with power Doppler signal is associated with severe radiographic damage and reduced cartilage thickness in hand osteoarthritis." *Osteoarthritis and Cartilage* 18(10): 1263-1268.

McNally, E. G. (2007). "Ultrasound of the small joints of the hands and feet: current status." *Skeletal Radiology* 37(2): 99-113.

Merrick, M. V. (1992). "Investigating joint disease." *European journal of nuclear medicine and molecular imaging* 19(10): 894-901.

Messent, E. A., R. J. Ward, et al. (2007). "Osteophytes, juxta-articular radiolucencies and cancellous bone changes in the proximal tibia of patients with knee osteoarthritis." *Osteoarthritis and Cartilage* 15(2): 179-186.

Moller, B., H. Bonel, et al. (2009). "Measuring finger joint cartilage by ultrasound as a promising alternative to conventional radiographic imaging." *Arthritis and Rheumatism* 61: 435-441.

Moller, I., D. Bong, et al. (2008). "Ultrasound in the study and monitoring of osteoarthritis." *Osteoarthritis and Cartilage* 16: S4-S7.

Morris, G. A. and A. J. Freemont (1992). "Direct observation of the magnetization exchange dynamics responsible for magnetization transfer contrast in human cartilage in vitro." *Magnetic Resonance Medicine* 28: 97-104.

Naredo, E., C. Acebes, et al. (2008). "Ultrasound validity in the measurement of knee cartilage thickness." *Annals of the Rheumatic Diseases* 68(8): 1322-1327.

Omoumi, P., G. A. Mercier, et al. (2009). "CT arthrography, MR arthrography, PET, and scintigraphy in osteoarthritis." *Radiologic Clinics of North America* 47: 595-615.

Owman, H., T. C.J, et al. (2008). "Association between findings on delayed gadolinium-enhanced magnetic resonance imaging of cartilage and future knee osteoarthritis." *Arthritis and Rheumatism* 58(6): 1727-1730.

Papathanassiou, D., C. Bruna-Muraille, et al. (2009). "Single-photon emission computed tomography combined with computed tomography (SPECT/CT) in bone diseases." *Joint Bone Spine* 76(5): 474-480.

Peterfy, C. G. and H. K. Genant (1996). "Emerging aplications of magnetic resonance imaging in the evaluation of articular cartilage." *Radiologic Clinics of North America* 34(2): 195-213.

Peterfy, C. G., A. Guermazi, et al. (2004). "Whole-organ magnetic resonance imaging score (WORMS) of the knee in osteoarthritis." *Osteoarthritis and Cartilage* 12(3): 177-190.

Potter, H. G., B. R. Black, et al. (2009). "New techniques in articular cartilage imaging." *Clinics in Sports Medicine* 2009(28): 77-94.

Qvistgaard, E., S. Torp-Pedersen, et al. (2006). "Reproducibility and inter-reader agreement of a scoring system for ultrasound evaluation of hip osteoarthritis." *Annals of the Rheumatic Diseases* 65(12): 1613-1619.

Sampson, E. R., C. A. Beck, et al. (2011). "Establishment of an index with increased sensitivity for assessing murine arthritis." *Journal of Orthopedic Research* 29(8): 1145-1151.

Sarikaya, I., A. Sarikaya, et al. (2001). "The role of single photon emission computed tomography in bone imaging." *Seminars in Nuclear Medicie* 31(1): 3-16.

Siegel, B. A., R. L. Donovan, et al. (1976). "Skeletal uptake of 99mTc-diphosphanate in relation to local bone blood flow." *Radiology* 120: 121-123.

Sofat, N. (2009). "Analysing the role of endogenous matrix molecules in the development of osteoarthritis." *International Journal of Experimental Pathology* 90: 463-479.

Wakefield, R. J., P. V. Balint, et al. (2005). "Musculoskeletal ultrasound including definitions for ultrasonographic pathology." *Journal of Rheumatology* 32(12): 2485-2487.

Walther, M., H. Harms, et al. (2002). "Synovial tissue of the hip at Power Doppler US: correlation between vascularity and Power Doppler US signal." *Radiology* 225: 225-231.

Williams, A., L. Sharma, et al. (2005). "Delayed gadolinium-enhanced magnetic resonance imaging of cartilage in knee osteoarthritis: Findings at different radiographic stages of disease and relationship to malalignment." *Arthritis and Rheumatism* 52(11): 3528-3535.

Williams, F. and T. Spector (2008). "Biomarkers in osteoarthritis." *Arthritis Research & Therapy* 10(1): 101.

Wittoek, R., P. Carron, et al. (2010). "Structural and inflammatory sonographic findings in erosive and non-erosive osteoarthritis of the interphalangeal finger joints." *Annals of Rheumatology Disease* 69: 2173-2176.

Wittoek, R., L. Jans, et al. (2010). "Reliability and construct validity of ultrasonography of soft tissue and destructive changes in erosive osteoarthritis of the interphalangeal finger joints: a comparison with MRI." *Annals of the Rheumatic Diseases* 70(2): 278-283.

Xia, Y., T. Farquhar, et al. (1995). Self-diffusion monitors degraded cartilage." *Archives Of Biochemistry and Biophysics* 323(2): 323-328.

Xia, Y., S. Zheng, et al. (2008). "Depth-dependent profiles of glycosaminoglycans in articular cartilage by μMRI and histochemistry." *Journal of Magnetic Resonance Imaging* 28(1): 151-157.

Yavorskyy, A., A. Hernandez-Santana, et al. (2008). "Detection of calcium phosphate crystals in the joint fluid of patients with osteoarthritis - analytical approaches and challenges." *Analyst* 133: 302-318.

Yoon, C.-H., H.-S. Kim, et al. (2008). "Validity of the sonographic longitudinal sagittal image for assessment of the cartilage thickness in the knee osteoarthritis." *Clinical Rheumatology* 27(12): 1507-1516.

Yoon, H. S., S. E. Kim, et al. (2005). "Correlation between ultrasonographic findings and the response to corticosteroid injection in pes anserinus tendinobursitis syndrome in knee osteoarthritis patients." *Journal of Korean Medical Science* 20: 109-112.

Yu, S. W., S. M. Shaw, et al. (1999). "Radionuclide studies of articular cartilage in the early diagnosis of arthritis in the rabbit." *Annals of the Academy of Medicine, Singapore* 28(1): 44-48.

Yu, W. K., J. M. Bartlett, et al. (1988). "Biodistribution of bis-[beta-(N, N-trimethylamino)ethyl]-selenide-75Se diiodide, a potential articular cartilage imaging agent." *International Journal of Radiation Applications and Instrumentation. Part B, Nuclear Medicine and Biology* 15(2): 229-230.

Zanetti, M., E. Bruder, et al. (2000). "Bone marrow edema pattern in osteoarthritic knees: correlation between MR imaging and histologic findings." *Radiology* 2000(215): 835-840.

5

Biomarkers and Ultrasound in the Knee Osteoarthrosis Diagnosis

Sandra Živanović[1], Ljiljana Petrović Rackov[2] and Zoran Mijušković[3]
[1]*Medical Faculty University of Kragujevac, Helth centre of Kragujevac, Rheumatology,*
[2]*Clinique for Rheumatology and Clinical Immunology,*
Military Medical Academy Belgrade,
[3]*Institute for Biochemistry, Military Medical Academy Belgrade,*
Serbia

1. Introduction

This study will present contemporary methods of the knee osteoarthrosis (OA) diagnosis - arthrosonography and biomarkers, which are applied and recommended in the modern practice.

Advantages of ultrasound diagnostics (arthrosonography) and serum biomarkers in rheumatologic diagnostics will be documented through this research which applied these methods. Ultrasound has become an integral part of clinical practice and is applied in many fields of medicine, however, in rheumatology it has not been fully recognized yet. Appliance of biomarkers in knee osteoarthrosis diagnosis is considerably a more expensive method, and has not been usually used for this purpose. It is very precise though in detection of changes in knee joint with osteoarthrosis.

The goal of this study is to affirm the ultrasound diagnostic method for many advantages it has comparing to other methods which have been used as routine, and to recommend it as a important part of clinical rheumatologic checkup.

The following methods are usually used for visualisation of knee joint: radiography, nuclear magnet resonance, computerised tomography, arthroscopy and arthrography. The most commonly applied and routine diagnostic method is radiography. However, the conventional radiography and computerised tomography are the methods without possibility of direct visualisation of the joint cartilage. Narrowing of the joint area is only an indirect indication of a joint damage, and early changes on the cartilage cannot be evaluated (Batalov et al.,2000). Nuclear magnetic resonance provides direct information on changes in different joint tissues, which is why it is nowadays appropriate for the knee osteoarthrosis diagnosis. However, its appliance is limited due to the very expensive medical examination. Methods of direct visualisation of the joint cartilage are arthrography and arthroscopy, which are less used in clinical practice, due to their invasiveness and limited indications.

2. Contemporary diagnostics of the knee osteoarthrosis

Ultrasound examination is non-invasive and much more accessible for evaluation of a large number of patients than other imaging modalities. The European League Against

Rheumatism in the first and second part of the Report from 2005 (D'Agostino et al., 2005, Conaghan et al 2005) recommends ultrasound medical technique as a golden standard in diagnosis of pathological changes in the knee joint, and also recommends arthrosonographic measuring and techniques.

This study will present results of the prospective research, which comprises 88 patients with diagnosis of primary knee osteoarthrosis, according to criteria of the American College of Rheumatology - ACR. Information about pain intensity in the knee was obtained from the patients through anamnesis during the last two weeks, measuring the frequency and intensity of pain during the night, as well as stiffness after a period of rest. Pain intensity was numerically evaluated marking the pain spots on VAS from 0 - 100 mm. Clinical examination of the both knees determined presence or absence of abnormal knee fluid buildup (arthritis) which was evaluated as serious, moderate, minimal or absent, as well as presence or absence of the Baker's cyst. The knee function was evaluated according to the scope of flexion in degrees. Based on HAQ index, the overall health condition of patients was assessed, and the functional ability marked as moderate or serious inability and the need for nursing and assistance. An ultrasound examination of the both knees in the B mode was done by a two rheumatologist on SDU - 1200 device, using a linear probe of 10MHz. Frontal longitudinal view was used to determined presence or absence of synovial inflammation indicators: effusion – defined as the scope of fluid buildup larger than 4mm in the knee suprapatellar, medial or lateral recess (SR, MR, LR); synovitis - defined as thickening of synovial membrane over 4mm.

The maximal depth of effusion and thickness of synovial tissue were measured and presented in mm. Morphologically, effusion was marked as absent or present in suprapatellar, medial or lateral knee recess, while synovitis was marked as absent or present (in nodular, difusal or nodular-difusal mode). Arthrosonography determined existence and size of the Baker's cyst behind the knee joint, as well as existence and thickness of synovitis inside it. Measurement of cartilage thickness was conducted in transversal view at medial and lateral femur condyle, at 90 degree knee bend, and posterior longitudinal view at medial femur condyle when the knee was extended (in mm). The existence and size of osteophytes (denoted as shorter or ≤2mm, and longer or ≥ 2mm) and bone erosions were established by lateral view on femur and tibia medial and lateral condyles. Analysis of serum samples determined concentration of COMP (ng/ml), YKL - 40 (ng/ml) and CTX-I (ng/ml) by ELISA (Enzyme-Linked ImmunoSorbent Assay) methods, using Cartilage Oligo Metric Protein kit (Euro-diagnostica Wieslab tm hCOMP quantitative kit), YKL-40 for Rheumatology and Oncology kit (Quidel, Metra- YKL-40 EIA kit) and Serum Crosslaps (Nordic Bioscience Diagnostica). The research excluded the patients who had the knee damage six months before the research, the patients with the total or partial endoprosthesis or the knee joint osteotomy, with arthroscopy of the knee joint in the past year, and the patients who had been treated with intraarticularly injected corticosteroids or hondroprotective four weeks before enrollment into the research.

Due to appliance of YKL-40 biomarkers, it was also necessary to exclude the patients with rheumatoid arthritis, inflammatory intestinal diseases, bacterial infections, liver fibrosis and malignant diseases. Presentation of these results will be compared with the results of other researches in this field. The advantages of ultrasound diagnostic methods and biomarkers will be documented as contemporary knee osteoarthrosis diagnostic methods in clinical practice.

The mean age of patients was 69,97±9,37 (44 - 88) years. Women prevailed and had even 3,4 times more frequent osteoarthrosis than men, which complies with the data available in literature, according to which osteoarthrosis is more frequent in female subjects (Hart et al., 1999). Duration of the knee osteoarthrosis in the patients enrolled this study was 6,46±6,73 (0,5-37), which indicates initiation of osteoarthrosis in certain patients between 40 and 50 years of age. Epidemiological researches have shown that in the developed countries 50% of population older than 40 can prove arthritic joint changes, but are mainly without symptoms at this age.

2.1 Clinical evaluation of the knee osteoarthrosis deterioration parameters

Knee osteoarthrosis deterioration evaluation is usually done by clinical estimation of the pain intensity according to Dougados (Dougados et al,.1997), which implies estimation of the pain intensity in the knee, estimation of the pain occurring during the night, and presence of fluid buildup (effusion) in knee joint. According to Dougados, estimation of the pain intensity in the knee is done by indication on the part of the patients experiencing the pain, using the pain VAS (0-100 mm) and by clinical estimation of knee osteoarthrosis degree on the part of medical doctors according to VAS for overall estimation of the disease degree (0-100 mm). Mean value of the pain intensity on VAS was 58,86±22,56. The medical doctor's evaluation of the clinical degree of osteoarthrosis on VAS (mm) was 40,45±18,31 average.

Among the subjects, only the patients with deterioration and evaluation on VAS over 30 mm expirienced stiffness longer than 30 min. as well as the night pain. Clinical examination determined knee fluid buildup in 54 (61,3%) of the patients. Fifteen patients (17%) had the Baker's cyst. Based on the clinical evaluation of knee osteoarthrosis deterioration according to Dougados, all the patients were divided in two groups: 74 patients with knee osteoarthrosis deterioration and pain mark over 30 mm on VAS, and 14 patients without deterioration and pain mark below 30 mm on VAS.

Comparing the groups of patients with and without knee osteoarthrosis deterioration, with reference to the years of age (p=0,118) and duration of disease (p=0,211) no significant difference was indicated. The mean age of patients and duration of disease were similar in the both groups of surveyed patients.

Increased body weight, verified by the higher BMI is associated with incidence and progression of knee osteoarthrosis, according to the results of the Rotterdam study (Reijman et al.,2007). Even 81,8% of knee osteoarthrosis patients had the body weight over the optimum. The patients with pain intensity mark over 30mm on the pain VAS had higher body weight - BMI 29,37±1,08 kg/m^2 than the patients with smaller knee pain intensity - BMI 25,04±2,46 kg/m^2 (p=0,000). In this way, it was confirmed that the excessive body weight is the risk factor which contributes to deterioration of knee osteoarthrosis.

The knee fluid buildup is a clinical characteristic of osteoarthrosis, which most commonly occurs in progressive osteoarthrosis, but can also often occur at the initial phases of OA during the periods of disease deteriorating. In the group of patients with the deteriorated knee osteoarthrosis and the pain mark over 30mm on VAS, 29,7% of the patients were without abnormal fluid buildup, while in the group of patients without osteoarthrosis deterioration, there were significantly more patients without fluid buildup (85,71%). Minimal fluid buildup was present at 37,8% of the patients with the pain mark over 30 mm on VAS. The result of moderate fluid buildup was confirmed by a clinical examination of

27% of the patients, and of the serious fluid buildup in 5,4% of the patients, in the group of patients with osteoarthrosis deterioration. In the group of patients without osteoarthrosis deterioration neither moderate nor serious knee fluid buildups were detected. Baker's cyst was diagnosed by clinical examination in 18,1% of the patients with the pain mark over 30 mm on VAS and 7,1% of the patients with lesser pain intensity (Figure 1.). It was concluded that the pain intensity marked on VAS by the patients considerably differed when minimal, moderate or serious knee fluid buildup was found by the clinical examination, or it was absent (p=0,014), which confirms that inflammation contributes to stronger pain in the knee joint (Živanović et al.,2009).

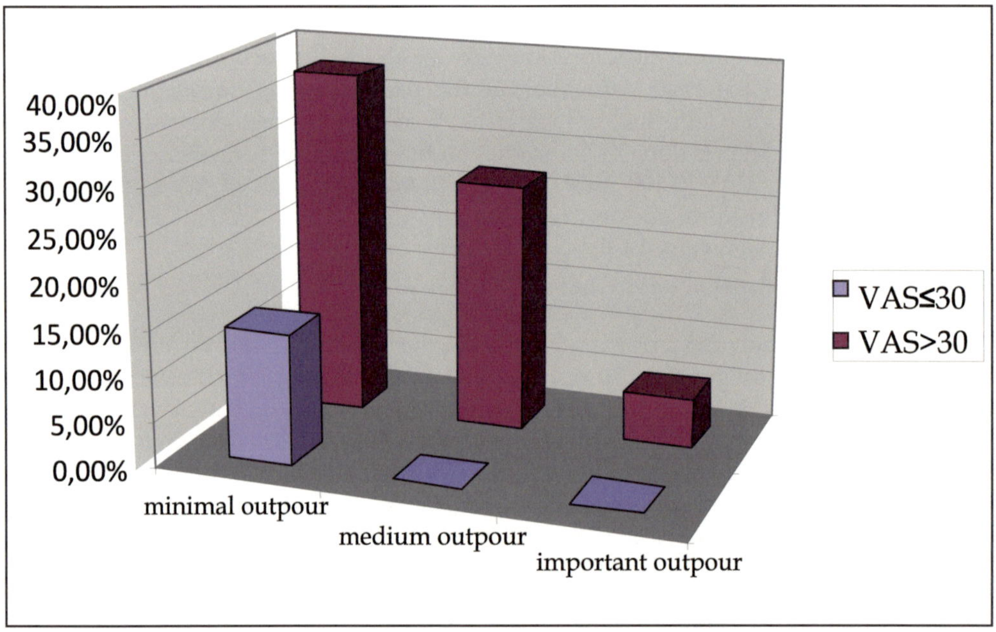

Fig. 1. Comparison of the size of outpour (minimal, medium and important) between the patients with pain scores greater and lower than 30mm on VAS pain scale

The fact was confirmed that small and large crepitations occur in deteriorated osteoarthrosis, with the presence of both stronger pain and synovial inflammation. The patients with deteriorated osteoarthrosis and stronger pain had significantly limited movements in the knee joint, comparing to patients without deterioration, as expected. A survey of the health condition confirmed higher degree of inability in the patients with deteriorated knee osteoarthrosis comparing to the patients without symptoms and indicators of deterioration, which complies with the data obtained from literature.The patients with more intensive pain and problems are more weighty, have limited knee movements and higher degree of inability, and vice versa.

Longer duration of the disease causes more difficult clinical form of the disease, and the bigger body weight is associated with the doctors' estimation of a more difficult form of the disease. In the presence of a serious knee fluid buildup, doctor evaluates osteoarthrosis difficulty with the highest mark, as well as if reduced mobility is detected at a clinical examination and synovitis in suprapatellar recess detected on ultrasound.

2.1.1 Ultrasound diagnostics of inflammatory changes in the knee osteoarthrosis

The average values of the size of effusion and synovitis in osteoarthrosis patients are highest in lateral recess, comparing to the values of same parameters in medial recess and suprapatellar recess. Based on the data that most of patients had effusion in lateral recess, and that clinically established moderate or minimal effusion is arthrosonographically shown as effusion only in lateral recess, it was concluded that inflammation most frequently occurs in this recess (Figure 2.).

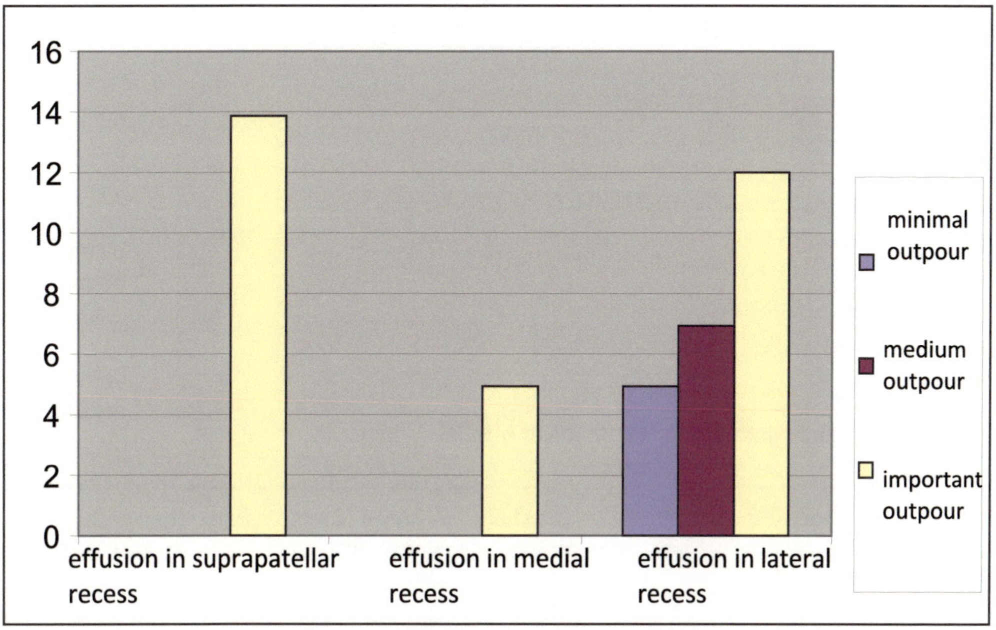

Fig. 2. Comparison of the middle value (median) size of effusion in suprapatellar, medial and/or lateral recess between patients with absent, minimal, medium and important outpour

It was found that synovitis in suprapatellar recess causes serious effusion in all three knee recess and reflects intensive inflammation in the knee joint. Besides, synovitis in medial and lateral recess can cause effusion in the local recess, with suprapatellar extending (Figure 3.) (Živanović et al.,2009).

Duration of disease does not influence appearance, size and locality of synovial inflammation, nor its deterioration in the patients with knee joint osteoarthrosis.

Effusion at the clinical examination was present in 61,3% of the patients, while arthrosonographic examination found effusion in 75,0% of the patients. There is a significant difference between the frequencies of clinically found effusion (the knee fluid buildup) and presence of effusion found by arthrosonography, in the patients with knee osteoarthrosis (p=0,000). Six patients (11,1%) had clinical effusion, but not an ultrasound confirmed effusion. It is also important that in 52,9% of the patients effusion was not clinically found, but ultrasound determined its presence. Based on the facts presented above, it was established that sensitivity of clinical diagnosis of effusion is 73% (percentage of diagnosis of effusion by clinical examination in the group of patients who had effusion proved by ultrasound), while specificity of clinical diagnosis of effusion is 73% (percentage of diagnosis of effusion by clinical checkup in the group of patients who had no effusion proved by ultrasound) (Table 1.) (Živanović et al.,2009).

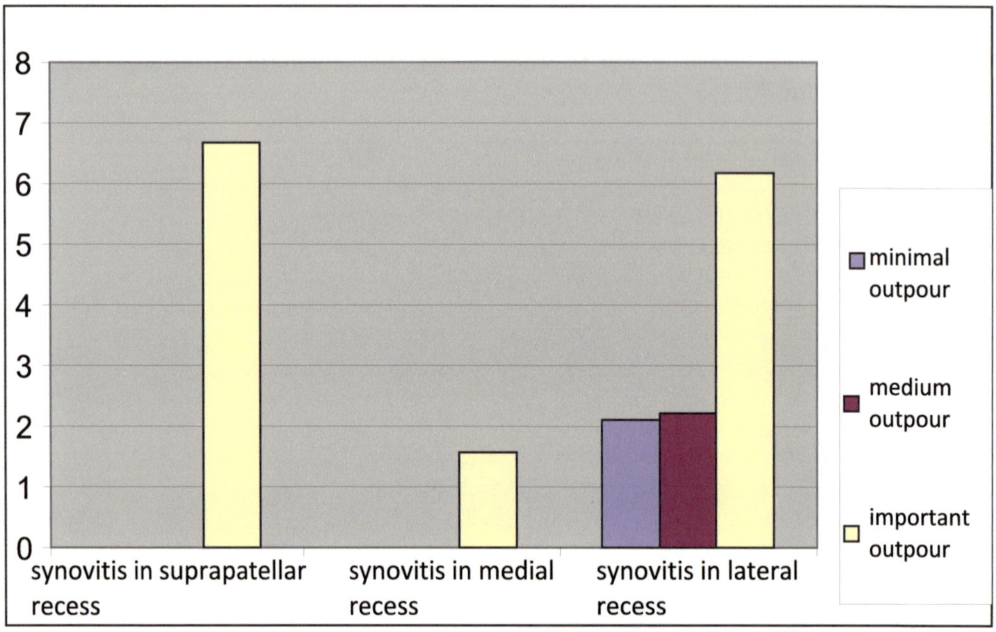

Fig. 3. Comparison of the middle value (median) thicknees of synovitis in suprapatellar, medial and/or lateral recess between patients with absent, minimal, medium and important outpour

clinical findings of effusion	Ultrasound findings of effusion					
	absent		present		total	
	Number of patient	%	Number of patient	%	Number of patient	%
absent	**16**	47,05	**18**	52,94	34	100
present	**6**	11,11	**48**	88,88	54	100
total	22	25,0	66	75,0	88	100
						p=0,000

Table 1. The frequency of clinical findings of effusion, and ultrasound-term findings of effusion in patients with knee OA

Kane et al. recommend arthrosonography as the golden standard, because it is more sensitive than clinical checkup of the joint diseases, and suspect the precision on acurateness of detecting standardised Disease Activity Scores (DAS) based only on a clinical checkup (Kane et al.,2003).

2.1.2 The ultrasound parameter of the knee osteoarthrosis deterioration – Joint effusion and synovial proliferation

Hill's research showed that moderate and serious effusions and synovial proliferation in the joint cause pain in the patients with knee osteoarthrosis (Hill et al.,2001).

The knee pain intensity differs comparing to presence or absence of effusion found by ultrasound, regardless its location. It was established that effusion and synovial inflammation contribute to increase of pain in patients with knee osteoarthrosis.

The average values of effusion size and synovial membrane thickness in the knee recess were higher in group of patients with the signs of knee arthrosis deterioration and the pain mark above 30 mm on VAS (Figure 4.5.).

The largest effusion and synovitis occurred in the lateral recess. It is important that ultrasound also detected effusion in over 63% of patients with osteoarthrosis deterioration, but without clear clinical signs of effusion. The facts presented above indicate that ultrasound is more sensitive method than clinical examination at detection of synovial inflammation, especially in the patients with intensive pain, and without clinical signs of effusion.

In the analyzed group of patients with osteoarthrosis, most of the patients had synovial inflammation in lateral recess and intensity of pain in the knee was related to the size of effusion and synovitis present in lateral recess (Table 2.,3.).

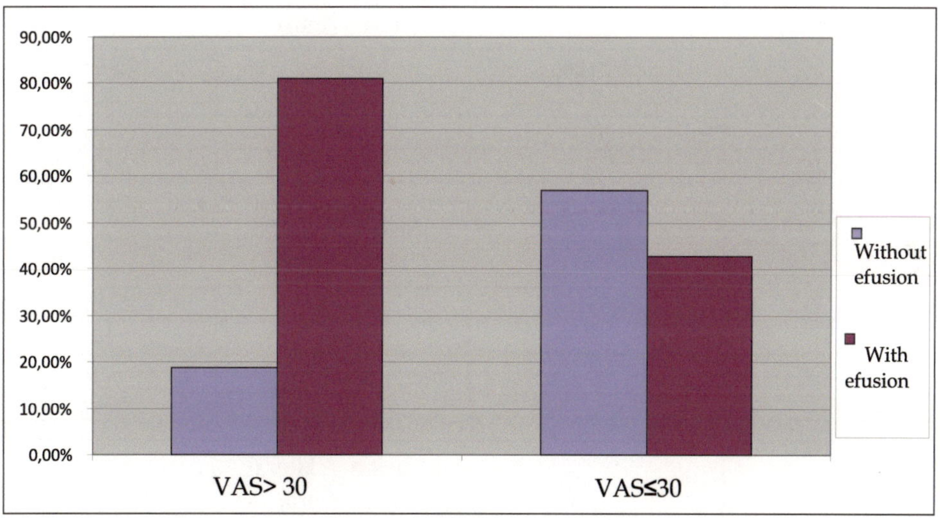

Fig. 4. The presence or absence of effusion in patients with pain score greater than 30 mm on the VAS pain scale and with less than 30 mm on VAS pain scale

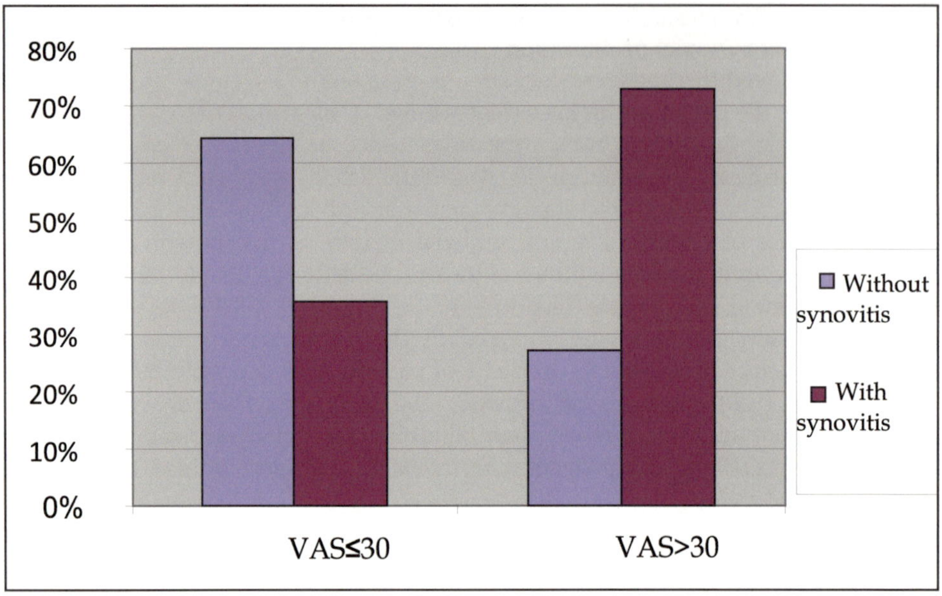

Fig. 5. The presence or absence of synovitis in patients with pain score greater than 30 mm on the VAS pain scale and with less than 30 mm on VAS pain scale

VAS	effusion in suprapatellar recess (mm)		
	25-th per	medijan	75-th per
> 30	0	**0**	**6,12**
≤ 30	0	**0**	**0**
			p=0,123

VAS	effusion in medial recess (mm)		
	25-th per	medijan	75-th per
> 30	0	**0**	**5,09**
≤ 30	0	**0**	**0**
			p=0,015

VAS	effusion in lateral recess (mm)		
	25-th per	medijan.	75-th per
> 30	0	**4,83**	**7,71**
≤ 30	0	**0**	**4,41**
			p=0,010

Table 2. Comparation average value of a quantity of effusion in suprapatellar, medial and lateral recess between the patients with pain scores greater and lower than 30 mm on VAS pain scale

VAS	synovitis in suprapatellar recess (mm)						
	5-ti per	10-ti per	25-ti per	medijan.	75-ti per	90-ti per	95-ti per
> 30	0	0	0	**0**	2,30	4,54	5,45
≤ 30	0	0	0	**0**	0	1,48	0
							p=0,146

VAS	synovitis in medial recess (mm)						
	5-ti per	10-ti per	25-ti per	medijan.	75-ti per	90-ti per	95-ti per
> 30	0	0	0	**0**	0	2,83	3,76
≤ 30	0	0	0	**0**	0	0	0
							p=0,049

VAS	synovitis in lateral recess (mm)						
	5-ti per	10-ti per	25-ti per	medijan.	75-ti per	90-ti per	95-ti per
> 30	0	0	0	**1,88**	3,55	5,82	7,06
≤ 30	0	0	0	**0**	2,52	3,06	
							p=0,054

Table 3. Comparation average value of a quantity of synovitis in suprapatellar, medial and lateral recess between the patients with pain scores greater and lower than 30mm on VAS pain scale

2.1.3 Ultrasound diagnostics of destructive changes in osteoarthrosis

The ultrasound parameters of cartilage and bone destructions are the reduced thickness of cartilage and detected osteophytes and bone erosions.

The cartilage and bone damages progress with the age and the duration of disease.

In the knee osteoarthrosis, cartilage damages primarily and most excessively occur medially, i.e. degenerative changes are the most intensive in the medial condyle, which complies with the data from literature (Pilipović, 2000).

2.1.4 Ultrasound diagnosis of the Baker's cyst

The Baker's cyst is a frequent pathological finding in the knee popliteal area. This research proved that the presence of a Baker's cyst found by a clinical examination depends on the presence and size of effusion. The most frequently, Baker's cyst is found clinically in patients who have serious effusion in the knee. Rarely can the Baker's cyst be palpated and found in the popliteal area and in the patients without effusion. Only 8,82% of patients without effusion had Baker's cyst at the clinical examination, while in over a fourth (26,5%) of the patients without clinical signs of effusion, Baker's cyst was found by ultrasound. Only 20% of patients with clinical diagnosis of the Baker's cyst did not have the cyst at ultrasound examination, while in the majority of patients (80%), it was confirmed by ultrasound. In a considerable number of patients (37%) without clinical signs of Baker's cyst, the cyst was

proved by ultrasound. This large discrepancy in the frequency of diagnosed Baker's cysts in the knees with osteoarthrosis favorises the arthrosonography as the more precise method in detection of soft tissue deviations in popliteal area.
It was calculated that sensitivity of clinical diagnosis of Baker's cyst was 30,77% (percentage of the correct diagnosis of Baker's cyst by clinical examination in the group of patients who indeed had the Baker's cyst proved by ultrasound). Specificity of the clinical diagnosis of Baker's cyst was 93,88% (percentage of diagnosis of Baker's cyst by clinical examination of the group of patients without an ultrasound proven Baker's cyst) (table 4).

Baker cyst clinical diagnosis	Baker cyst - ultrasound diagnosis					
	absent		present		total	
	Number of patient	%	Number of patient	%	Number of patient	%
absent	**46**	63,01	**27**	36,98	73	100
present	**3**	20,0	**12**	80,0	15	100
total	49	55,68	39	44,31	88	100
						p=0,003

Table 4. The relationship of clinical diagnosis of Baker cyst and arthrosonography diagnosis in patients with knee osteoarhrosis

It was shown that the diagnosis of Baker's cyst at clinical examination mostly depends on its area (size) which can be measured by ultrasound (p=0,000), and does not depend on any other clinical nor ultrasound parameters.
It was established that occurrence and size of the Baker's cyst depend on the size of effusion and synovitis in SR and LR.
It was not determined that there is a significant difference in the presence or absence of the Baker's cyst at clinical examination between groups of patients with the pain mark over 30 mm and below 30 mm on VAS (p=0,259). In contrast, it was proved that there is a significant correlation between the evaluation by the patients with knee OA on VAS and the Baker's cyst area measured by ultrasound (r=0,238, p=0,025), which means that the presence of a larger Baker's cyst in popliteal knee area contributes to stronger pain. These results are in complience with the Hill's research in 2001, which determined that the presence of Baker's cyst is associated with occurrence of pain (Hill et al.,2001).

2.2 Predisposing factors of the knee osteoarthrosis deterioration

The main risk factor for knee osteoarthrosis deterioration, apart from overweight and obesity, is occurrence of synovial inflammation, the intensity of which can be measured by arthrosonography, measuring the scope of effusion and synovitis thickness in recessses, especially the lateral recess, as well as by presence and size of Baker's cyst of the bad knee joint.
It was not established that the joint destructions (occurrence of osteophyte and bone erosion on tibia and femur condyle) significantly influence the pain intensity increase, unlike synovial inflammation, effusion and synovitis.

2.3 Biomarkers

Biomarkers (biochemical markers) are molecules or fragments of connective tissue matrix which disperse into biological fluids during tissue metabolism. Their concentration can be measured by immunoassay methods (Garnero et al.,2006). Measuring the concentration of these biomarkers may be complementary with imaging techniques following up the development of diseases such as rheumatoid arthritis and osteoarthrosis (Garnero et al.,2000). It is recommended to measure and simultaneously follow up concentrations of several markers on cartilage, bones and synovial metabolisms, because joining these markers can reflect metabolic changes in all three tissues, showing a better picture of pathophysiological changes in osteoarthrosis (Charni et al.,2005, Garnero et al.,2001). In this research three biomarkers were used: Cartilage Oligomeric Matrix Protein - COMP, human cartilage glycoprotein (YKL-40) known as the Human Cartilage Glycoprotein 39 (HC gp-39 or GP-39) and Collagen type I C - terminal telopeptide (CTX-I).

Cartilage Oligomeric Matrix Protein - COMP is a non-collagen protein of articular cartilage matrix (Clark et al.,1999). It is synthetised by chondrocites and synovial cells after activation of proinflammatory cytokines. This protein is an ingredient of collagen, type II, and it stimulates and regulates fibryllogenesis and stabilises collagen net in cartilage tissue. It is useful as a marker of early cartilage destruction, because it is first emmited in the process of collagen net splitting, which results in cartilage deterioration (Larson et al.,2004).

Human cartilage glycoprotein (YKL-40) is a glycoprotein with molecular mass 38-40 kDa. It has a significant role in tissue remodelling, including the joint cartilage. YKL-40 is synthetised and secreted by hondrocites and synovial cells, also by activated macrophages, liver fibrocytes and colon, breast, lung, ovary and prostate cancer cells (Hakala et al.,1993,Register et al.,2001), as well as osteosarcoma cells (MG-63) (Johansen et al.,1993). It is not known what is the biological function of YKL-40 in malignant tumors, but it has been proven that this glycoprotein stimulates growth of connective tissue cells and chemotaxis. In persons with healthy cartilage, the level of YKL-40 in serum is low, while in the conditions of inflammation or extracellular matrix remodeling, there is a considerable increase in the level of this glycoprotein (Johansen et al.,2001,Volck et al.,1999). For these reasons YKL-40 can be used as a marker of cartilage and synovial tissue metabolism (Harvey et al.,1998). Collagen, type I, and non-collagen proteins are biomarkers of bone tissue metabolism. Researches of Rovetta et al (Rovwtta et al.,2003) showed much higher values of the collagen type I - CTX-I decomposition product in the serum of the patients with the errosive hand osteoarthrosis comparing to the patients with non-errosive hand osteoarthrosis. The study by Berger et al showed that the patients with the rapidly destructive osteoarthrosis have higher values of CTX-I in serum than the patients with slightly progressive osteoarthrosis (Berger et al.,2005).

2.3.1 The knee osteoarthrosis inflammatory change diagnosis by biomarkers

The joint inflammation in osteoarthrosis is usually mild and does not disturb the parameters of inflammation acute phase, but can be proved by the serum markers which indicate synovial activities (Garnero et al.,2001,2003,Kraus,2005). Metabolic changes of cartilage tissues in arthroses imply changes in matrix synthesis and degradation, and matrix molecules are excreted as fragments into the joint liquid, blood and urine, where they can be detected and measured (Lohmander,2004).

In this research, the concentration of the biomarkers COMP, YKL-40 and CTX-I was measured in serum of the patients with knee osteoarthrosis. Comparing to effusion scope (minimal, moderate or serious), considerable difference in average values of COMP, YKL-40 and CTX I biomarker concentration ($p=0,361$, $p=0,690$ and $p= 0,108$, respectively) was not found, probably because of insufficient sensitivity of clinical examination in detection of synovial inflammation.

Significant difference of COMP biomarkers average values in serum was indicated, depending on presence of effusion during ultrasound examination, regardless its location and size. The patients with effusion in the knee have higher COMP concentrations in serum, comparing to the patients without effusion detected by ultrasound (Table5.). That implies that increased COMP concentration in serum can be a good indicator of synovial inflammation in the knee joint arhrosis (Živanović et al.,2009).

EFFUSION	Number of subjects N	Percentage of subjects %	COMP (ng/mL) Median		
			25-th perc.	50-th perc.	75-th perc.
present	22	25.0	44.50	54.00	58.00
absent	66	75.0	48.75	57.00	64.25

***p* = 0.030**

SYNOVITIS	Number of subjects N	Percentage of subjects %	COMP (ng/mL) Median		
			25-th perc.	50-th perc.	75-th perc.
present	29	33.0	45.5	52.0	58.0
absent	59	67.0	50.0	58.0	66.0

***p* = 0.006**

Table 5. Comparison of the median of the concentration of COMP biomarker between patients with present or absent effusion and prolipheration of synovial membrane

It was also found that there was a significant difference in serum COMP biomarker concentration average values between the patients with and without synovial membrane proliferation found by ultrasound, regardless the location and size. This evidence implies the fact that COMP biomarker values increase in serum when the knee joint inflammation is present as synovial membrane hypertrophy. However, COMP biomarker values can only confirm existence of synovial inflammation, i.e. detect it. Its increased concentrations cannot precisely determine inflammation degree (size) nor its location (in recess).

A research related to synovitis type showed that there is a significant difference in COMP average concentrations in serum in patients with nodular, diffusive or nodular-deffusive synovitis. Highest COMP concentrations in serum were determined in patients with diffusive synovitis, which confirms the fact that diffusive proliferative synovitis causes the most intensive inflammation, if it occurs in the knee joint arthrosis (Figure 6.).

The patients with knee artrosis accompanied with knee effusion and synovitis, have higher concentrations of COMP biomarkers in serum, than the patients without ultrasound indicators of synovial inflammation, which confirms that COMP can be a good indicator of synovial inflammation.

During researches of sensitivity and specificity by ROC graph (Receiver Operating Characteristic) it was found that among analysed serum parameters only COMP parameter can be an indicator of effusion in the knee joint. COMP biomarker sensitivity on effusion was 59%, and its specificity 50% (cut off=53,5; area 0,665; p=0,030; confidence interval 0,534-0,776). Cut off value was found to be 53,5 ng/ml, which means that no patients with osteoarthrosis and COMP biomarker concentrations in serum below 53,5 ng/ml have knee joint inflammation, while COMP biomarker values above 53,5 ng/ml indicate presence of inflammation. It means that the Cartilage matrix oligomeric protein have a moderate signifficance at effusion presence estimation (Figure 7.) (Živanović et al.,2011).

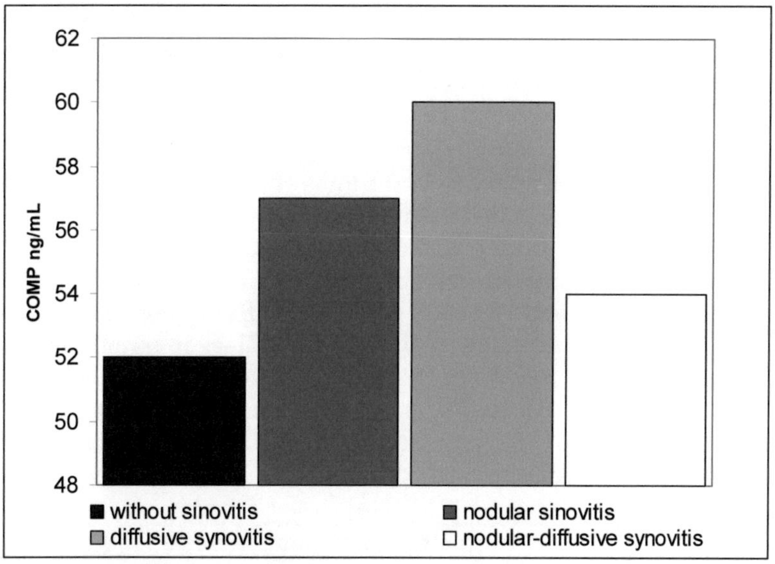

Fig. 6. Comparation of median of COMP biomarker concentration between patients with nodular, diffusive or nodular-difussive synovitis (p=0,014)

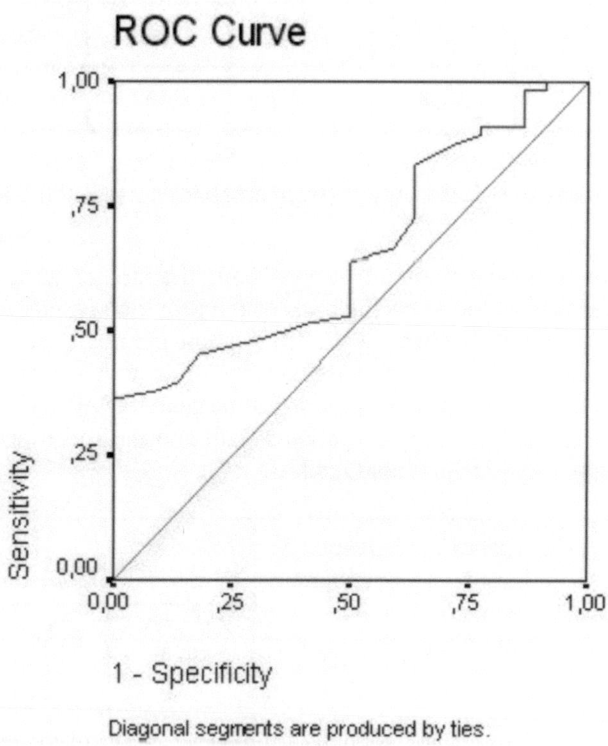

Fig. 7. Cartilage Matrix Oligomeric Protein as a marker of the effusion cut off = 53.5 ng/mL; Area 0.655; p=0.030; confidence interval 0.534-0.776

It was not proved for any of the investigated markers that they could be indicators of the synovial membrane i.e. synovitis proliferation. Presented results of the research did not confirm significant correlation between mean values of YKL-40 and CTX-I biomarkers with inflammation (effusion and/or synovitis) in the knees with arthrosis.

2.3.2 Diagnosis of destructive changes of the knee with osteoarthrosis by biomarkers

The results of this research indicated the negative correlation between YKL-40 values in serum and cartilage thickness on the medial femur condyle (front view). It showed that YKL-40 increased concentrations are associated with reduced thickness of the knee joint cartilage, especially medially, and vice versa (Table 6.). At the finding of a thinning cartilage, especially on the medial femur condyle, high values of YKL-40 in serum can be expected in patients with knee osteoarthrosis. As in the early phase of knee arthrosis the destructive changes on the joint cartilage dominantly occur on the medial tibia and femur condyle, it can be concluded on the bases of the provided results that increased concentrations of YKL-40 in serum can be a good indicator of early damage of joint cartilage (Živanović et al.,2009).

cartilage thickness (mm)	**concentration of biomarkers** (ng/ml)					
	COMP		**YKL 40**		**CTX I**	
	r	p	r	p	r	p
medial.condil (front access)	-0,177	0,099	**-0,249**	**0,019**	-0,043	0,691
medial.condil (back access)	-0,184	0,087	-0,056	0,608	-0,018	0,866
lateral.condil (front access)	-0,067	0,538	-0,080	0,460	-0,087	0,423

Table 6. Correlation between serum concentration of biomarkers COMP, YKL 40 and CTX I with cartilage thickness (mm) in the medial (front and back access) and lateral (front access) femur condyles

Correlation of other biomarkers' concentrations with the size of joint cartilage was not proved, so that it can be concluded on the basis of the provided results that their increased concentrations in the patients' serum cannot be a good parameter for the joint cartilage damage degree in patients with knee joint osteoarthrosis (Živanović et al.,2009).
This research shows that there is a considerable difference in COMP and YKL-40 biomarkers concentration mean values between the patients with shorter and longer osteophytes on tibia and femur condyles (p=0,000) (Table 7.,8.).

OSTEOPHYTES	Number of subjects N	Percentage of subjects %	*mid.value COMP (ng/ml)*		
			25th perc.	Median	*75th perc.*
Shorter	21	23,9	46,5	**55,0**	*59,0*
Longer	67	76,1	48,0	**56,0**	*64,0*
					p = 0,000

Table 7. Comparison of the median of the concentration of biomarker COMP between patients with shorter and longer osteophytes.

OSTEOPHYTES	Number of subjects N	Percentage of subjects %	*mid.value YKL 40 (ng/ml)*		
			25th perc.	Median	*75th perc.*
Shorter	21	23,9	44,5	**62,0**	*90,0*
Longer	67	76,1	80,0	**119,0**	*171,0*
					p = 0,000

Table 8. Comparison of the median of the concentration of biomarker YKL40 between patients with shorter and longer osteophytes.

Osteophytes and bone erosions occur as consequence of damage and loss of cartilage tissue accompanied with cartilage destruction, and indirectly reflect the damage degree. Increased concentration of YKL-40 biomarker can be an indicator of destructive changes degree in the knee osteoarthrosis. That indicates a possibility of using this marker to estimate the joint destruction (Živanović et al.,2009).
Conclusions of this research comply with the results by Johansen et al (Johansen et al.,1996) which showed that in the patients at later stage of knee osteoarthrosis there is an increased level of YKL-40 in serum. Contrary to that, Garnero's study (Garnero,2001) did not prove high concentrations of YKL-40 in patients with the late-stage osteoarthrosis (Figure 8.).

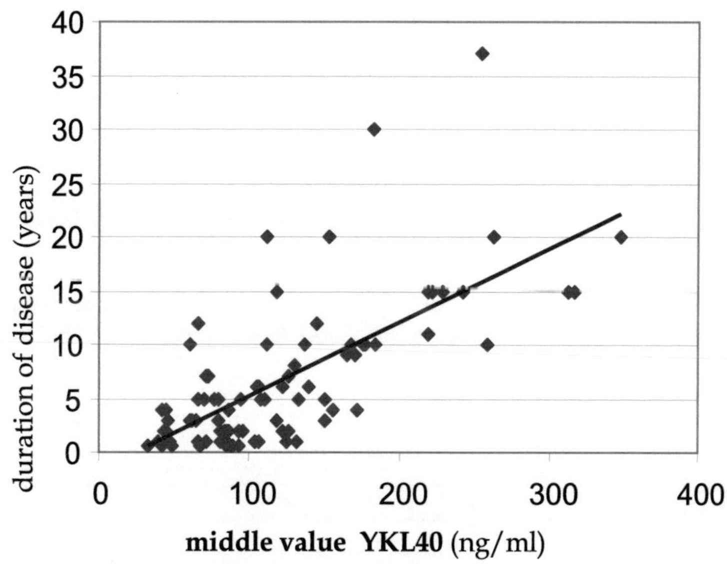

Fig. 8. Link between the middle value (median) of biomarker YKL40 and duration of the knee OA (r = 0,651, p = 0,000)

This research results showed that YKL-40 biomarker can be a highly sensitive marker of occurrence of longer osteophytes. Sensitivity of YKL-40 concentration in serum on occurrence of longer osteophytes on tibia and femur condyles is 79,1%, and its specificity 61,9% (cut off 75,0; area 0,806; p=0,000; confidence interval 0,706-0,906). The cut off value 75,0 ng/ml indicates that all the patients with osteoarthrosis and serum YKL-40 values below 75,0 ng/ml have milder degree of joint destruction comparing to the patients with YKL-40 value above 75,0 ng/ml who have higher-degree joint destruction and the presence of longer osteophytes in the knee joint (Figure 9.) (Živanović et al.,2009).

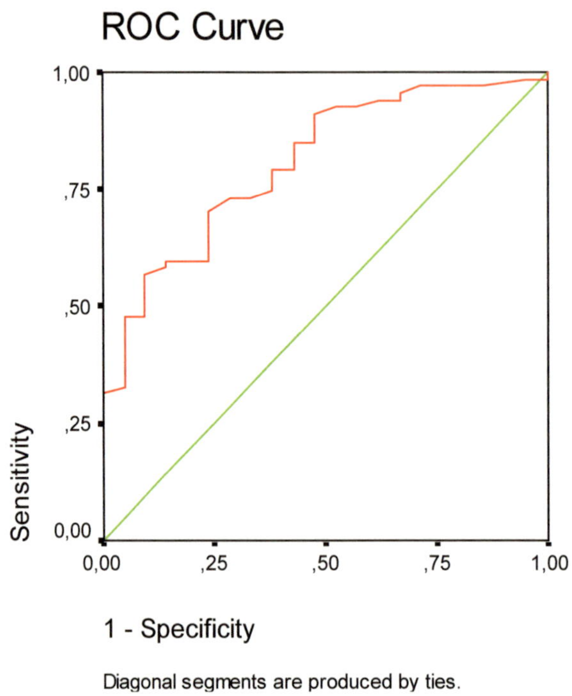

cut off = 75,0; Area 0,806; p=0,000; confidence interval 0,706-0,906

Fig. 9. YKL 40 as a marker for appearance of longer osteophytes at the tibia and femur condyles

It was found that there is a considerable diference of YKL-40 mean values depending on the presence or absence of bone erosions on tibia and femur condyles (Table 9) (Živanović et al.,2010)

	Bone erosion	25-th per	median	75-th per
COMP (ng/ml)	absent	46	55	59,50
	present	48	57	63
				p=0,483
YKL-40 (ng/ml)	absent	46,50	**81**	120,50
	present	79	**111**	171
				p = 0,004
CTX-I (ng/ml)	absent	0,71	0,93	1,10
	present	0,64	0,83	1,11
				p =0,528

Table 9. Comparation of median) concentrations of biomarkers between patients with present or absent bone erosions

Higher concentration of YKL-40 in serum can be found when there is a severe destruction of bones at the joint edges. The highest YKL-40 values were found in patients with erosions on the medial condyles (Figure 10.) (Živanović et al.,2010).
COMP and CTX-I biomarkers are not good indicators (markers) of erosions on tibia and femur condyles, unlike YKL-40 which can be a good indicator of erosions (Figure 11.).
YKL-40 sensitivity on occurrence of erosions on tibia and femur condyles is 69,5%, and its specificity is 51,7% (cut off=84,5; area 0,691; p=0,004; confidence interval 0,574-0,808). It was found that the cut off is 84,5ng/ml, which means that all the patients with osteoarthrosis YKL-40 value below 84,5ng/ml have milder degree of destruction without occurrence of bone erosions, and that YKL-40 values above 84,5ng/ml indicate higher degree of the joint destruction which implies bone erosion (Figure12.) (Živanović et al.,2010).

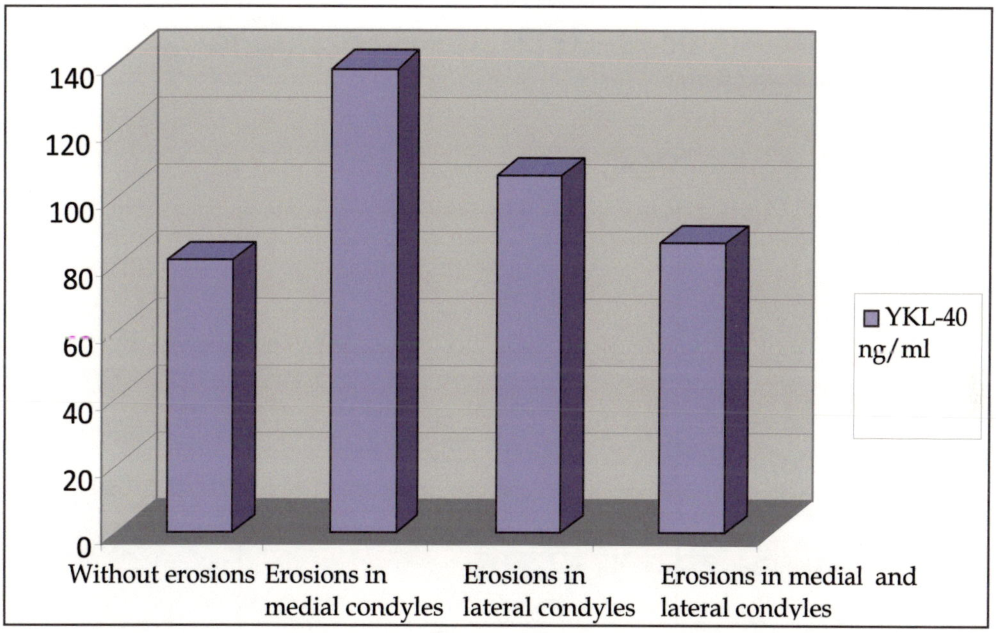

Fig. 10. Differences in mean values (median) of biomarkers YKL-40 concentration in patients with present or absent erossions on the medial and/or lateral the tibia and femoral condyles

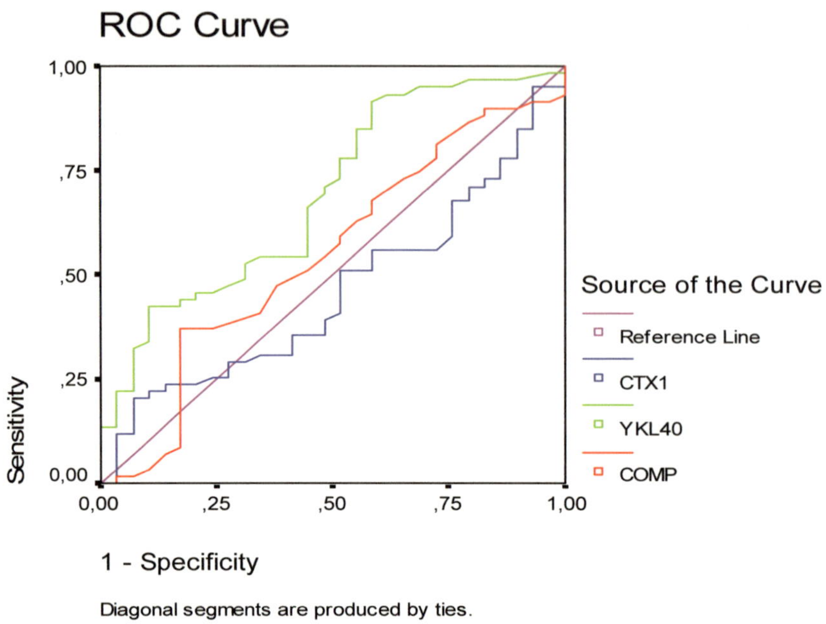

Fig. 11. Biomarkers COMP, YKL-40 and CTX-I as a markers to appear bone erossion in the condyles of the tibia and femur

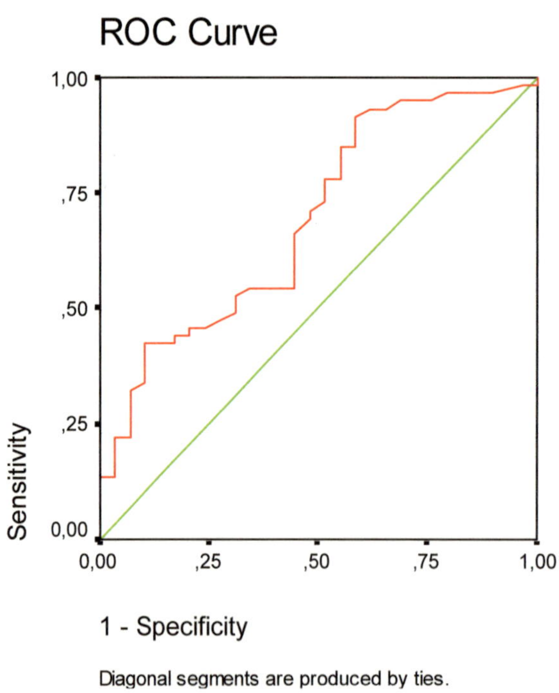

Fig. 12. Biomarker YKL 40 as a marker to appear bone erossion in the condiles of tibia and femur

The results of this research comply with the research results of Morgante et al (Morgante et al.,2001) who determined that YKL-40 is a good prognostic marker of joint destruction. On the other hand, Kawasaki's study showed different evidence related to hip osteoarthrosis. YKL-40 value in serum is a better indicator of synovial inflammantion degree than of the cartilage tissue metabolism (Kawasaki et al.,2001).

In this research the results of multivariant binary logistic regression show that the duration of disease is related to YKL-40 biomarker values in serum. Comparing the YKL-40 concentration mean values with reference to 5, 10, 15 and 20 years duration of the disease, considerable differences were determined (p=0,000). YKL-40 biomarker mean value increases with disease duration (Figure 13.) (Živanović et al.,2009).

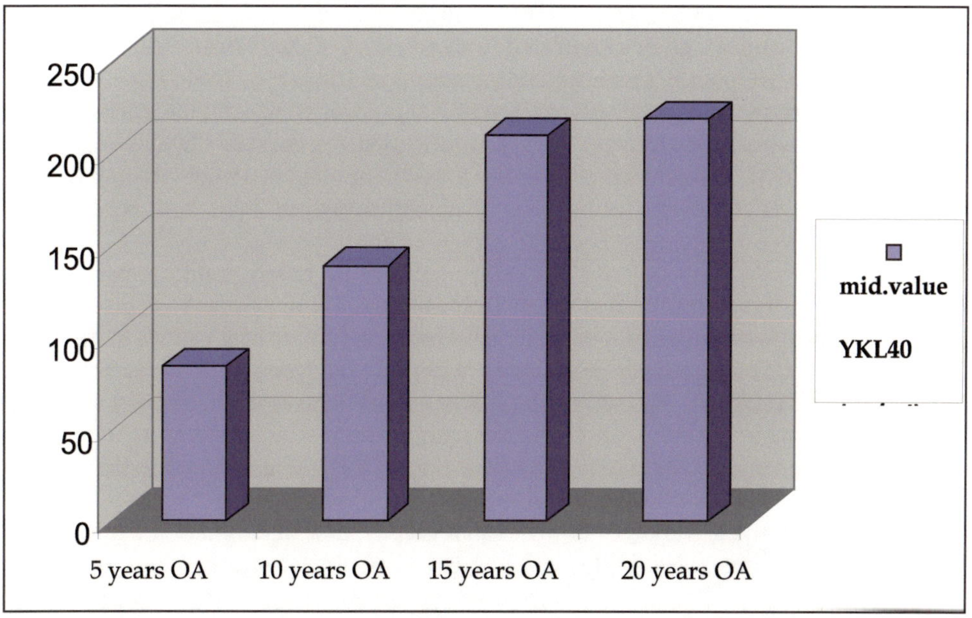

Fig. 13. Increase in concentration of YKL40 for the duration of knee osteoarthrosis (after 5, 10,15 i 20 years)

In the patients with a long-lasting knee arthrosis and with progressed degenerative changes, osteophytes and bone erosions, higher concentrations of YKL-40 can be found in serum. That proves that YKL-40 biomarker can be a valid indicator of knee osteoarthrosis destructive changes (Živanović et al.,2009).

2.3.3 Biomarkers as indicators of the pain degree and knee osteoarthrosis deterioration

Analysis and comparation of the biomarkers concentration in serum between a group of patients with deterioration of knee osteoarthrosis and a group of patients without deterioration have been conducted.

The patients with deterioration of knee osteoarthrosis have similar biomarker concentration values as the patients without symptoms and signs of the disease deterioration. Correlation between VAS mean values and concentration of investigated biomarkers was not proven either. That indicates that values of investigated biomarkers cannot be valid indicators of pain intensity nor manifestation of disease deterioration in patients with knee osteoarthrosis.

3. Conclusion

This study has shown advantages of arthrosonography which distinguish it from the other methods of visualisation, especially at estimation of the knee osteoarthrosis deterioration. The disease deterioration, i.e. sudden intensification of pain the patients undergo is associated with the finding of synovial inflammation at the knee arthrosonography, as well as with presence of the Baker's cyst in the knee popliteal fossa.

It is emphasised that arthrosonography is a more sensitive method than clinical examination at identification of location and size of effusion and synovial proliferation in the knee joint osteoarthrosis, as well as at detection and estimation of Baker's cyst size, especially in patients with intensive pain but without clinical singns of effusion or Baker's cyst existence.

This study presents serum biomarkers as detectors of inflammatory and destructive changes in the knee joint with osteoarthrosis. It is recommended to measure Cartilage Oligomeric Matrix Protein - COMP concentration in serum for estimation of synovial inflammation, and Human Cartilage Glycoprotein 39 - YKL-40 at estimation of joint and bone cartilage damage.

Application of biomarkers as a diagnostic method is much more expensive than arthrosonography, which means that it is not accessible to all the patients. It takes a couple of days to get results on concentration of biomarkers in serum, thus it cannot be said that it is a quick method. Some patients feel uneasy when giving blood sample for tests, which makes the method relatively aggressive and it is not possible to repeat it often. It should also be emphasised that measuring of biomarker concentration in serum does not provide precise data on size and location of inflammatory and destructive changes in the knee joint with osteoarthrosis, but only detects them.

On the other hand, the advantages of arthrosonography that distinguish it from the other diagnostic methods are accessibility and low price, noninvasiveness, quick and precise presentation of both normal and patological soft-tissue structures, as well as possibility of frequent repetitions. The quality of ultrasound examination depends on technical equipment and of the doctor's experience. Anyway, standardisation of the equipment and expert knowledge usually produce a good-quality examination.

This study recommends that arthrosonography should become routine and fundamental method in contemporary rheumatological practice, and a complement to clinical examinations.

4. References

Batalov AZ, Kuzmanova SI, Penev DP. Ultrasonographic evaluation of knee joint cartilage in rheumatoid arthritis patients.Folia Med (Plovdiv). 2000;42(4):23-6.

Berger C,Kröner A,Stiegler H, ThomasLeitha T,Engel A. Elevated levels of serum type I collagen C-telopeptide in patients with rapidly destructive osteoarthritis of the hip. International Ortopaedics. 2005; 29(1):1-5.

Charni N, Juillet F, Garnero P. Urinary type II collagen helical peptide (Helix II) as a new biochemical marker of cartilage degradation in patients with osteoarthritis and rheumatoid arthritis. Arthritis Rheum 2005;52:1081–90.

Clark AG, Jordan JM, Vilim V, Renner JB, Dragomir AD, Luta G, et al. Serum cartilage oligomeric matrix protein reflects osteoarthritis presence and severity. Arthritis Rheum 1999;42:2356-2364.

Conaghan P, D'Agostino MA, Ravaud P, Baron G, Le Bars M, Grassi W, Martin-Mola E, Wakefield R, Brasseur JL, So A, Backhaus M, Malaise M, Burmester G, Schmidely N, Emery P, Dougados M. EULAR report on the use of ultrasonography in painful knee osteoarthritis. Part 2: exploring decision rules for clinical utility. Ann Rheum Dis. 2005 Dec;64(12):1710-4. Epub 2005 May 5.

D'Agostino MA, Conaghan P, Le Bars M, Baron G, Grassi W, Martin-Mola E, Wakefield R, Brasseur JL, So A, Backhaus M, Malaise M, Burmester G, Schmidely N, Ravaud P, Dougados M, Emery P. EULAR report on the use of ultrasonography in painful knee osteoarthritis. Part 1: prevalence of inflammation in osteoarthritis. Ann Rheum Dis. 2005 Dec;64(12):1703-9. Epub 2005 May 5.

Dougados M. La mesure: méthodes d'évaluation des affections rhumatismales. Paris: Expansion Scientifique, 1997.

Garnero P, Delmas PD. Biomarkers in osteoarthritis. Curr Opin Rheumatol 2003;15:641–6.

Garnero P, Piperno M, Gineyts E, Christgau S, Delmas PD, Vignon E. Cross sectional evaluation of biochemical markers of bone, cartilage, and synovial tissue metabolism in patients with knee osteoarthritis: relations with disease activity and joint damage. Ann Rheum Dis 2001;60:619–26.

Garnero P, Rousseau J-C, Delmas P. Molecular basis and clinical use of biochemical markers of bone, cartilage and synovium in joint diseases. Arthritis Rheum 2000;43:953-961.

Garnero P, N Charni, F Juillet, T Conrozier and E Vignon . Increased urinary type II collagen helical and C telopeptide levels are independently associated with a rapidly destructive hip osteoarthritis Annals of the Rheumatic Diseases 2006;65:1639-1644.

Hakala BE, White C, Recklies AD. Human cartilage gp-39, a major secretory product of articular chondrocytes and synovial cells, is a mammalian member of a chitinase protein family. J Biol Chem 1993;293:781-788.

Hart DJ, Doyle DV, Spector TD. Incidence and risk factors for radiographic knee osteoarthritis in middle-aged women, the Chingford Study. Arthritis Rheum 1999;42:17–24.

Harvey, S. et al. Clin. Chem. 44: 509-516, 1998.

Hill CL, Gale DG, Chaisson CE, Skinner K, Kazis L, Gale E, et al. : Knee effusion, popliteal cysts, and synovial thickening: association with knee pain in osteoarthritis. J Rheumatol 2001;28:1330–7.

Johansen JS, Hvolris J, Hansen M, Backer V, Lorenszen I, Price PA. Serum YKL-40 levels in healthy children and adults. Comparison with serum and synovial fluid levels of YKL-40 in patients with osteoarthritis or trauma of the knee joint. Br J Rheumatol 1996;35:553-559.

Johansen JS, Jensen HS, Price PA.A new biochemical marker for joint injury. Analysis of YKL-40 in serum and synovial fluid. Br J Rheumatol. 1993 Nov;32(11):949-55.

Johansen JS, Olee T, Price PA, Hashimoto S, Ochs RL, Lotz M. Regulation of YKL-40 production by human articular chondrocytes. Arthritis Rheum. 2001 Apr;44(4):826-37.

Kane D, Balint PV, Sturrock RD. Ultrasonography is superior to clinical examination in the detection and localization of knee joint effusion in rheumatoid arthritis. J Rheumatol. 2003 May;30(5):966-71 Comment in: J Rheumatol. 2003 May;30(5):908-9.

Kawasaki M, Hasegawa Y, Kondo S, Iwata H. Concentration and localization of YKL-40 in hip joint diseases. J Rheumatol. 2001 Feb;28(2):341-5.

Kraus VB. Biomarkers in osteoarthritis. Curr Opin Rheumatol 2005;17:641–6.

Larsson E, Erlandsson Harris H, Larsson A, Månsson B, Saxne T, Klareskog L. Corticosteroid treatment of experimental arthritis retards cartilage destruction as determined by histology and serum COMP. Rheumatology (Oxford) 2004;43:428–34.

Lohmander LS. Markers of altered metabolism in osteoarthritis. J Rheumatol 2004;31 (Suppl 70) :28–353.

Morgante M, Metelli MR, Morgante D.Observations on the increased serum levels of YKL-40 in patients with rheumatoid arthritis and osteoarthritis Minerva Med. 2001 Jun;92(3):151-3.

Pilipović N. Reumatologija; Beograd 2000.

Register, T.C. et al. Clin. Chem. 47: 2159-2161, 2001.

Reijman M, Pols H A P, Bergink A P, Hazes J M W, Belo JN, Lievense AM, Bierma-Zeinstra S M A Body mass index associated with onset and progression of osteoarthritis of the knee but not of the hip: The Rotterdam Study Annals of the Rheumatic Diseases 2007;66:158-162.

Rovetta G, Monteforte P, Grignolo MC, Brignone A, Buffrini L.Hematic levels of type I collagen C-telopeptide in erosive versus nonerosive osteoarthritis of the hands.Int J Tissue React. 2003;25(1):25-8.

Volck B, Ostergaard K, Johansen JS, Garbarsch C, Price PA.The distribution of YKL-40 in osteoarthritic and normal human articular cartilage. Scand J Rheumatol. 1999;28(3):171-9.

Živanović S, Nikolić S, Jevtić M. Kocić S. Inflamation in knee osteoarthritis - couse worsening traubles, Medical examination, 2010;LXIII(9-10):668-673

Živanović S, Petrović Rackov Lj, Vojvodić D, Vučetić D. Human cartilage glycoprotein 39—biomarker of joint damage in knee osteoarthritis, International Orthopaedics 2009 Aug; Epub 2009 Mar 24. 33(4):1165-70.

Živanović S, Petrović Rackov Lj, Vučetić D, Mijušković Z. Arthrosonography and biomarker Cartilage Oligomeric Matrix Protein in detection of the knee osteoarthrosis effusion, Journal of Medical Biochemistry, 2009; 28(2): 108-15.

Živanović S, Petrović Rackov Lj, Živanović A. Arthrosonography and Biomarkers in the evaluation of destructive knee cartilage osteoarthrosis, Srp. Arch. Celok. Lek. 2009; 137(11-12): 653-8.

Živanović S, Petrović Rackov Lj, Jevtić M, Detection of bone erosiones in knee osteoarthrosis by serum biomarkers, Srp. Arch. Celok. Lek. 2010; 138(1-2): 62-6.

Živanović S, Petrović Rackov Lj, Živanović A, Jevtić M, Nikolić S, Kocić S, Cartilage Oligomeric Matrix Protein - inflamation biomarker in the knee osteoarthritis, Bosnian Journal of Basic Medical Sciences. 2011 Feb;11(1):27-32

Part 3

Biomechanics

6

Biomechanics of Physiological and Pathological Bone Structures

Anna Nikodem and Krzystof Ścigała
Wrocław University of Technology,
Division of Biomedical Engineering and Experimental Mechanics,
Poland

1. Introduction

In 1995 Kuttner and Goldberg defined osteoarthritis as a group of distinct simultaneous diseases, which may have different etiologies but have similar biologic, morphologic, and clinical outcomes. The disease processes does not only affect the articular cartilage, but involve the entire joint, including the subchondral bone, ligaments, capsule, synovial membrane, and periarticular muscles. Ultimately, the articular cartilage degenerates with fibrillation, fissures, ulceration, and full thickness loss of the joint surface (Kuttner & Golderg, 1995).

Osteoarthritis (OA) is also characterised by chronic degradation of articular cartilage and hypertrophy of bone tissue in joint region. OA results from both biological and mechanical causes which lead to instability of bone degradation and remodeling processes of entire joint organ, including the chrondocytes, subchondral bone and synovium articular (Grynpas et al., 1991).

Precise classification of joint degeneration is difficult. For example, American College of Rheumatology (ACR) classifies osteoarthritis as non inflammatory condition despite the fact, that clinical observation show frequent inflammatory reaction (Pelletier et al., 1999; Wang et al., 2002; Malcolm, 2002) although the latter may actually be a manifestation of a superimposed crystalline arthritis. To evaluate degradation of joint cartilage two methods are the most frequently used: Altman scale (Altman et al., 1986) and Kellegren-Lawrence scale. First method differentiates between primary and secondary effects of degradation without taking into account etiological factors which precise identification allows to prevent development of OA. Kellegen-Lawrence defined a five level scale that is used to evaluate changes in tissue structure based on its images. Unfortunately, if computer tomography images are used then only advanced stages of OA disease can be detected.

Origins of OA are not well known but several hypothesis on its etiology were proposed. Hypothesis focus on changes in biochemical composition and physical properties of synovial fluid that debilitates cartilage nutrition, increased friction of joint surface, impaired blood supply as well as increased number of micro-cracks, especially in subchondral bone. When OA affects hip joint then those changes apply to the femoral head and acetabulum. Two, seemingly equivalent hypotheses about the origins and progress of osteoarthritis are presented in the literature (Radin, 1995). According to the first one changes in the articular cartilage cause changes in biomechanical properties of the joint and thus in bone tissue. The second one gives the opposite statement and states that degeneration of cartilage is caused by changes in bone tissue. The common aspect of both hypotheses is a finding that degeneration of joint is related to impaired biomechanics of bone-cartilage system. Changes in mechanical properties of each element of the joint involve changes in their structure (Carter & Hayes, 1977; Rice et al., 1988) while loss of cartilage is mainly caused by reduced capability to self-repair.

2. Changes in biological structures in osteoarthritis

Literature lists loss of cartilage, loss of bone tissue and inflammatory reaction of joint capsule and surrounding soft tissue as a pathomorphologic symptoms of OA disease that soften joint surface and finally lead to collapse. Results of research conducted to investigate origins of osteoarthritis focus separately on identification of changes taking place in cartilage that lead to degradation of subchondral bone, and on modeling of processes related to mechanical friction in joint (Wierzcholski & Miszczak , 2006). Second aspect was addressed in a number of papers that focus on changes in metabolism of cartilage tissue as a function of mechanical load (Glaser & Putz, 2002; Radin et al., 1984). It was observed that loss of articular cartilage is caused by reduced capabilities of self-repairing.

Cartilage is composed of dense crossed structure of type II collagen fibers organised in arcade-like structures. Moreover, it is filled with proteoglycans, water, and chrondocytes. There is less than 10% of total volume of cartilage cells that are responsible for tissue formation and remodeling. Migration of chrondocytes is limited by a dense matrix of collagen fibers, moreover, their proliferation decreases with cell age. Therefore, even in the case of a small, superficial injury, chrondocytes located in the injury area die ensuring there is no bleeding, no infection and no proliferation of new cells. Therefore, matrix defects are not filled (Mow et al., 1994; Frost, 1994; Boyd et al., 2000; Buckwalter et al., 2006). In early osteoarthritis, swelling of the cartilage usually occurs, due to the increased synthesis of proteoglycans. This process reflects effort of chondrocytes to repair cartilage damage. As osteoarthritis progresses, the level of proteoglycans drops and becomes very low, causing the cartilage to soften and lose elasticity, thereby further compromising joint surface integrity. Erosion of the damaged cartilage in an OA joint progresses until the underlying bone is exposed. The increasing stresses exceed the biomechanical yield strength of the bone. The subchondral bone responds with vascular invasion and increased cellularity, becoming thickened and dense (eburnation process) in areas under pressure. Initiated inflammatory reaction stimulates development of subchondral cysts (pseudocysts) that accumulate synovial fluid and focus of osseous metaplasia of synovial connective tissue in subchondral bone (Lozada, 2011; Pelletier et al., 1999; Brishmar, 2003).

Modeling of synovial fluid (Wang et al., 2002; Szwajczak, 2001) as well as description of grease and wear-out of joint (Katta et al., 2008) are another issues often addressed in literature. Synovial fluid is formed through a serum ultrafiltration process by cells that form the synovial membrane (synoviocytes). Synovial cells also manufacture the major protein component of synovial fluid, hyaluronic acid (also known as hyaluronate). Synovial fluid supplies nutrients to the avascular articular cartilage. Synovial fluid is a lubricant that minimises friction and consequently wear-out of articular cartilage surfaces and provides the viscosity needed to absorb shock from slow movements, as well as the elasticity required to absorb shock from rapid movements. Loss of cartilage exposes bone tissue that release mineral content to joint capsule and change its tribological properties (e.g. friction and lubrication) (Glimcher, 1992). Properties of synovial fluid change when lubrication mechanism is altered and simultaneously thickness of the lubrication film is reduced and even reduced in extreme cases (Radin et al., 1995). Since *in vivo* investigation of synovial fluid is difficult to conduct because its properties change quickly after punction. Therefore, there is no satisfactory rheological description.

Third group of investigations concerning OA focus on **determination of mechanical properties of bone tissue and simulation of remodeling processes of bone**, especially subchrondal bone. As a result of changes that take place during osteoarthritis organism tries to do everything possible to countermeasure changes and defects of cartilage. The way to do that is to apply bone remodeling processes that lead to increased bone mass and ossify cartilaginous protrusions lead to irregular outgrowth of new bone (osteophytes) on the cartilage-bone junction (Buckwalter et al., 2006; Chen et al., 2001). Remodeling processes are local and result directly from biomechanics of the joint. Increased mass of bone tissue can be observed in areas where load-bearing conditions are changed, i.e. in subchrondal bone (Grynpas et al., 2001; Glaser & Putz, 2002).

3. Load model of the hip

Osteoarthritis predominantly involves the weight-bearing joints, including the hips, knees cervical and lumbosacral spine. Hip joint is one of the biggest and the most movable part of the human body. Its main purpose it to transfer the weight from lumbar spine to lower limbs. From the view of mechanics, hip joint is composed of two rigid elements: acetabulum and proximal femur that are interconnected with a number of ligaments and muscles. External surface of the bone is covered with compact bone and hyaline cartilage that also covers the surface of acetabulum. Cartilage is up to 3mm thick, has high resistance to load and acts as an absorber of mechanical energy while moving. Proper nutrition of cartilage depends on synovial fluid pressure that results from changing load of the hip.

Value of Neck/Shaft angle is another important parameter of the femur. Its value for healthy people equals 150 degrees for newborn babies, approximately 126-128 degrees for adults and 110 degrees for elder people. Pathology may lead to even bigger changes - even reduction up to 90 degrees was observed (Pauwels, 1976). Value of Neck/Shaft angle is crucial for load distribution, stability of the joint and also depends on load and forces that are applied by muscles (Fig.1). Consequently reduction in angle value increases probability of bone fraction.

From the mechanical point of view, hip joint is at the same time under influence of external and internal loads resulting from gravity, muscles and many others. Consequences of loading depend on load value, type of movement, joint geometry, age of the person and mechanical parameters of cartilage and bone tissue. Proximal femur is filled with trabecular bone tissues, arranged according to load directions. In 1892 Julius Wolf stated that every change in the shape and/or function of bone causes changes to bone architecture and its conformation. Investigation confirms that bones adjust its construction according to min-max rule, which states that bone minimise its mass while maximising load-bearing capabilities at the same time. According to Currey (Currey 1984), remodeling and structure of bone tissue is influenced by pressure resulting from muscle contraction. Capability to maintain upright position is a result of mutual influence of skeleton and muscles and that dynamic pressure resulting from muscle work exceeds static pressure from body mass. According to Currey, correct growth and bone structure development is a result of both dynamic activity of muscles and strength of bone tissue. Consequently, load models of a hip joint presented by several authors (Maquet 1985, Beaupré 1990, Będziński, 1997) take into account loads that result from body mass, muscles and ligaments.

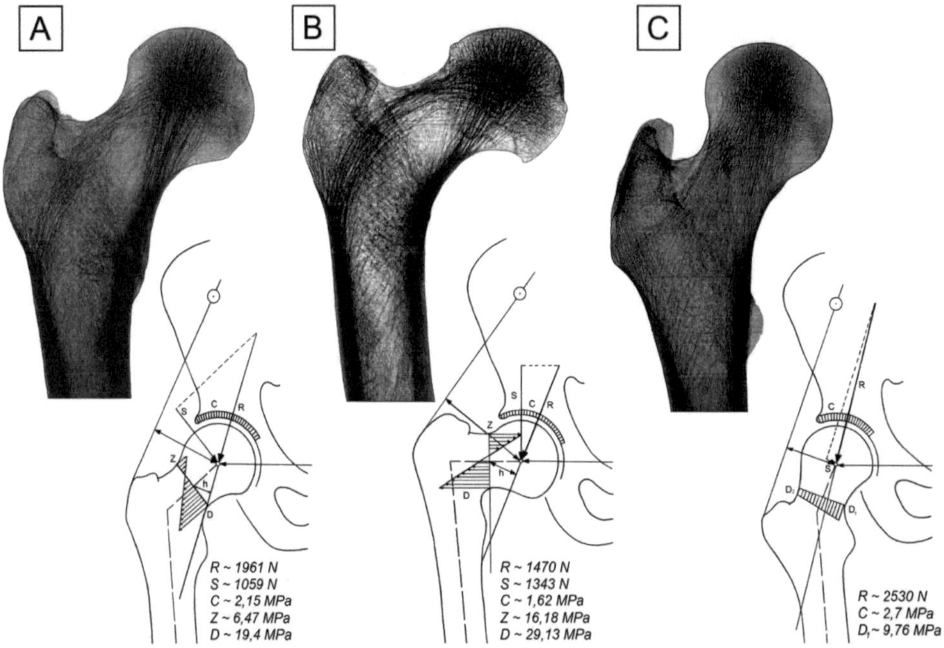

Fig. 1. Cross-section and stress distribution of proximal femur with different Neck/Shaft (CCD) Angle: A. 128°, B. 85°, 150° (Pauwels, 1976)

Capability to adapt bone's structure to load condition may have adverse consequences and lead to pathological changes when balance between processes of bone remodeling is disturbed. Osteoarthritis is characterised with cartilage degradation, necrosis of subchrondal bone that consequently lead to micro-cracks, damage of the joint and inflammation of synovial membrane. Pathological changes lead to structure alteration and result in modification of mechanical parameters.

4. Mechanical properties of cancellous bone

Numerous works (Yamada & Evans, 1970; Cowin, 2001; Huiskes, 2000; An & Draughn, 2000) that analyse mechanical properties of bone tissue showed that no simple and single relationship exist that can comprehensively describe its properties. This is due to strong anisotropy and the fact that values of mechanical parameters depend on numerous factors, among which bone structure (especially cancellous bone) is one of the most important. Cancellous bone tissue is composed of a three-dimensional network of bone trabeculae having different shapes, dimensions, and orientation. The term "cancellous bone tissue structure" means here the method of organisation of the basic tissue-forming elements. The properties of the whole examined bone tissue depend on the properties of the individual bone trabeculae as well as the way and the number of interconnections between them.

Measurements of the structural properties are based on stereological and topographical methods used to quantify bone tissue histology (Hildebrand and al., 1999). Such information concerns both parameters describing the size and the shape of tested objects, as well as parameters describing their orientation (structural anisotropy).
Mechanical properties of bone tissue depend not only on tissue density, but also on structural parameters which determine the organisation of bone tissue in the tested specimen (Tanaka et al., 2001, Nikodem et al., 2009). Description of the structural properties is based on a whole range of parameters (histomorphological properties) defining mass distribution in a bone tissue specimen Tb.Th, BV/TV, Tb.N, Tb.Sp (Parfitt et al, 1987), orientation of the structure, and its character (SMI parameter). Despite the fact that the number of new parameters that are used to describe bone properties are still growing, precise description of the bone structure and dependency between its parameters is still troublesome.
Table 1 contains values of structural parameters measured for samples of normal and OA from 56 femur heads. OA femur heads were taken from patients aged 66 years on average (range 46-91 years) that were treated with alloplastic hip replacement. All cubic samples by dimension (10x10x10) mm were prepared using a rotary electric saw (Accutom-5, Struers). Samples were stored in 4% formalin solution. All samples were scanned using a microcomputed tomography system (μCT-80 Scanco Medical) providing a spatial resolution of 20 μm. Standard 3D algorithms were used to calculate volume density BV/TV, bone surface density BS/TV and Tb.Sp, Tb.Th, Tb.N (Tab. 1).

Variable / sample (n=89)		**physiology (N)**		**osteoarthritis (OA)**	
Structural properties (3D μCT)	Unit	value	SD	value	SD
Bone volume / total volume (BV/TV)	[%]	25,32[a]	5,67	28,71[b]	6,83
Bone surface/bone volume (BS/BV)	[1/mm]	13,38	1,97	12,99	2,64
Trabecular number (Tb.N)	[1/mm]	1,42	0,15	1,47	0,21
Trabecular thickness (Tb.Th)	[mm]	0,18[a]	0,02	0,20[b]	0,04
Trabecular spacing (Tb.Sp)	[mm]	0,67[a]	0,08	0,64[b]	0,09
Connectivity density (ConnD)	[1/mm3]	6,49	2,25	6,08	3,28
Structure model index (SMI)	[1]	1,12[a]	0,08	1,21[b]	0,09
Mineral density	[mgHA/cm2]	211,99	73,43	207,60	75,31

a-b-p<0,05

Table 1. Average value of structural parameters (that can be used to quantify structural anisotropy) and mineral density for healthy and OA bone samples

Using a dedicated software (HISTOMER) and bone samples images, we have determined a fabric ellipse parameter (Fig. 2) and a mean intercept length (MIL) parameter (Whitehouse, 1974, Odgaard, 1997). Resulting MIL values can be used as a measure of structural anisotropy. Results show that as disease progress bone tissue thickens (BV/TV increases), becomes more anisotropic and changes its structure to more plate-like (SMI increases) comparing to healthy tissue.

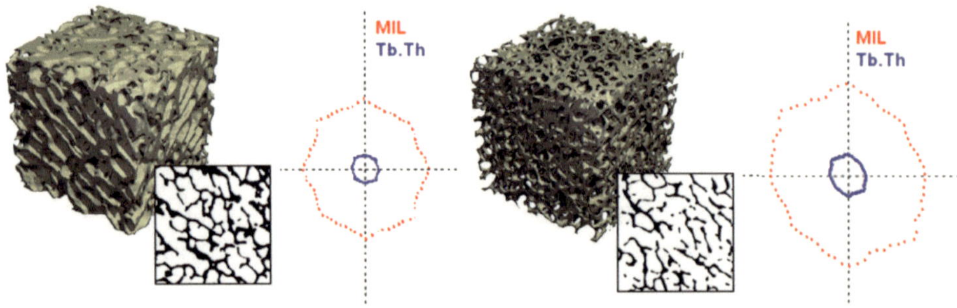

Fig. 2. Structure and fabric ellipse for anatomical and osteoartrotical hip samples

Literature contains a number of papers that compare bone to engineering materials, searching for similarities with properties of bone tissue. Consequently, the literature contains claims that bone can be seen as a two-phase composite material (Carter & Hayes, 1977). That material consists of a mineralised matrix made of collagen fibres characterised by a low elastic modulus and hydroxyapatite (HA) crystals with a high elastic modulus. The modulus of elasticity of two-phase materials is usually located between the values of the elastic modulus of the phases, whereas composite strength is higher than the strength of the components tested individually. Another approach is to compare bones to glass laminate, where fibreglass is the high-modulus material (similarly to the HA crystals), whereas epoxy resin is the low-modulus material (similarly to collagen) (Currey, 1984). According to Jackson, bone belongs to the group of biological ceramics which, like all ceramic materials, are brittle and rigid. Such materials cause measurement problems (samples are difficult to grasp and loading causes small displacements, which require sensitive measuring instruments). However, these approach has several unquestionable advantages, including the ability to use standard theories that assume linear flexibility and the ability to use classic methods of measurement of the mechanical properties, whose results show high repeatability.

Definition of stiffness for trabecular bone is difficult due to the fact that it is composed of 3-dimensional grid of trabeculae and empty space between them. Although, trabeculae itself can be assumed homogenous and has some stiffness (called material stiffness), it is infeasible to measure it as a single trabecula is too small. Therefore, a larger structure, that consists both of several trabeculae and space between them, is usually measured and so called structural stiffness is determined (Turner & Burr, 1993).

Mechanical properties of the bone tissue are usually determined in strength tests conducted in *in vitro* condition. Strength of the tissue is a complex function of multiple parameters such as structure of the tissue, level of organic contents as well as properties of the sample (e.g. sample size and preparation procedure) and tests procedure (e.g. test condition) (Turner & Burr, 1993; Nikodem & Ścigała, 2010). As a result of strength experiments in linear region Young and Kirchoff modulus, Poisson ratio, strain and yield stress can be calculated (Fig.3).

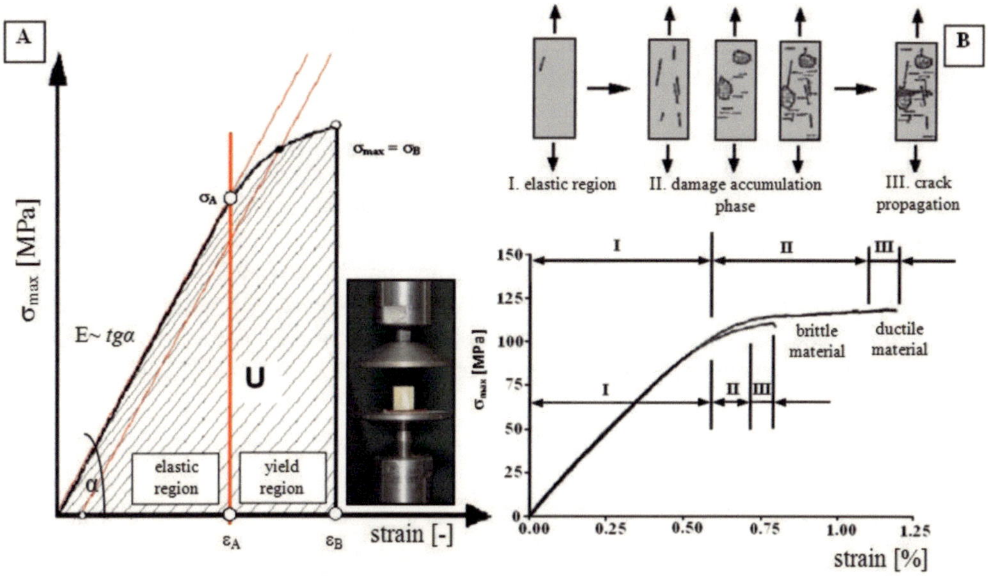

Fig. 3. A. Stress-strain dependency and mechanical parameters such as: Young modulus, ultimate and yield stress and strain energy U, B. changes in integrity of cancellous bone sample during different phase of uniaxial compression test

Table 2 presents selected mechanical parameters (directional stiffness (E1, E2, E3), yield stress and stain energy) evaluated during uniaxial compression testing of femur heads taken from patients that were treated with allopathic hip replacement. It follows that both values of mechanical and structural parameters increase for OA samples.

Variable / sample (n=89)		**physiology (N)**		**osteoarthritis (OA)**	
Mechanical properties	Unit	value	SD	value	SD
Modulus of elasticity (E_1)	[MPa]	147,41	67,60	143,15	81,38
Modulus of elasticity (E_2)	[MPa]	157,36	118,81	89,32	47,15
Modulus of elasticity (E_3)	[MPa]	174,26	131,96	95,48	62,63
Yield strength (σ_{ul})	[MPa]	11,36	3,96	12,68	6,97
Stain energy (U)	[mJ/mm2]	$30{,}98^{a}$	2,15	$27{,}92^{b}$	1,79

a-b-p<0,05

Table 2. Average values of mechanical parameters for samples from both normal and OA bones

Precisely, OA samples are characterised by higher BV/TV, which is caused by more complex and thickened structure (Tb.N, Tb.Th, ConnD). This bone concentration (especially in subchondral region) is relevant to gradual loss of cartilage and change in load bearing conditions. Osteoarthritis has several phases: formation of osteophytes or joint space narrowing, appearance of subchondral cysts, bone deterioration, repair and remodeling. Despite of higher bone volume, lower value of mechanical properties (30%) were observed. In this case, we didn't notice any increase in mineral density proportional to increase in BV/TV value (the average value was even smaller than in control group). Based on measurements we can state that changes in BV/TV (especially in the second phase) are mainly correlated with deterioration of trabeculae and do not depend directly on metabolism of mineral components. Reduction in cartilage mass leads to increased friction between elements of the joint and consequently to irreversible deformation of bones and changes in parameters of bone tissue (Fig. 4).

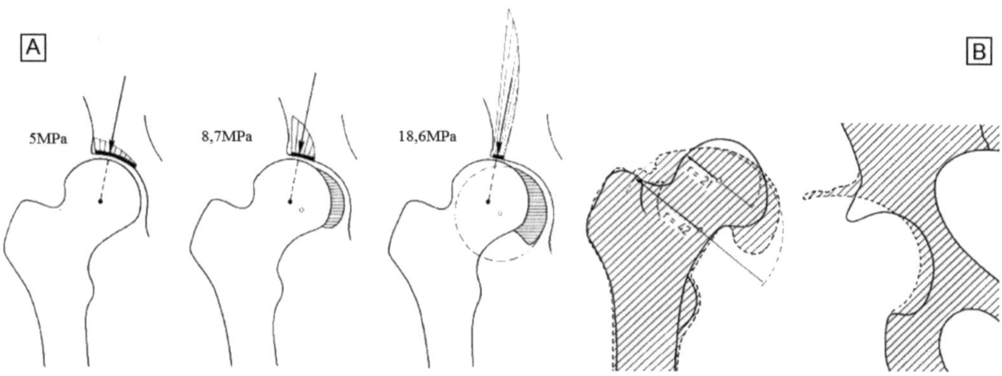

Fig. 4. Changes in stress values for human hip joint (A). and the shape of femur head and acetabulum (B), as a result of osteoarthritis (Pauwels, 1976)

5. Modeling of bone tissue

Modeling of bone structures within the joint, including joints affected by osteoarthritis, is achieved by simulating formation and remodeling of bone tissue. Most often simulations of bone tissue remodeling are based on calculations using finite elements method (Będziński & Ścigała, 2011). Two approaches that differ in presentation of bone tissue are mostly used. Results are used for the same purpose - estimation of how disease influences mechanical behaviour of bone tissue. First approach assumes that bone tissue, can be treated as a continuous material. In that case it is possible to calculate remodeling stimulus as a function of stress or strain distribution in daily time period. Stress and strains can be calculated using fundamental relationships of solid mechanics. In most situations it is assumed that the value of remodeling stimulus is proportional to the density of strain energy (Carter, 1987, Carter et al., 1996; Cheal et al., 1985). Sometimes it is also assumed that this value is a function of principal stress or strain values (Cowin et al, 1985; Hernandez et al., 2001). There are also proposals to make a remodeling stimulus dependent on the signal received by a network of osteocytes deployed in mineralised bone matrix (Huiskes et al., 1987; Weinans, 1999). Simulation of bone remodeling itself is realised by changing density and mechanical properties of each finite element of the model. Value of this change is in some way proportional to the calculated previously stimulus (Carter, 1987; Lanyon, 1987). Models that

fall into this group can be described as macro-scale models and rise several objections (Będziński & Ścigała, 2010). The most important is assumption that the tissue is a continuous material and lack of possibility to extend the model with additional parameters that are structure-related and can stimulate remodeling process. In case of compact bone, that kind of assumption is possible to made without significant restrictions. However in case for cancellous tissue, which is a high porosity material (precisely, it is a complex spatial arrangement of trabeculae), this kind of modeling represents a significant simplification. In real bone tissue control of the remodeling process is realised by a network of bone cells. In that case, osteocytes play a role of sensors, which can detect change of load distribution in whole volume of bone tissue. This signal is next transferred to the network of bone lining cells, and they differentiate in osteoclasts and osteoblasts. Those cells are responsible for change of bone mass and structure, so real remodeling process occurs only at the surface of trabeculae. The mechanical signal that stimulates cells deployed in osteocyte network of compact and cancellous bone trabecula is related to the movement of the inter-osseous fluid that fills cavities and canaliculi of the network (Bagge, 2000; Będziński, 1997; Bartodziej & Ścigała, 2009; Będziński & Ścigała, 2003; Jacobs et al., 1997). By default macro-scale models of bone formation and remodeling do not take these phenomena into account and for some of them, due to restrictions imposed by design, it is even impossible to extended the model.
Second group of models consider actual structure of bone and include a complex system of bone trabeculae and are referred to as micro-scale models (Będziński & Ścigała, 2010). Models from this group usually assume that the stimulus of remodeling process is a function of unequal distribution of stress in bone structure. Gradient of stress is in this case proportional to the stimulus. Stress distribution is calculated only on the surface of trabeculae and changes in bone mass is proportional to the stimulus. Formation and resorption of mass is also modelled on the surface of trabecular bone. In this respect they are more applicable to the rebuilding processes that take place in real bone. On the other hand, this group of models also does not consider influence of inter-osseous fluid flow on bone tissue remodeling processes, however it is possible to take this parameter into account in simulation because of strict definition of trabeculae in model.
Formation and remodeling of bone tissue is closely related to self-repairing processes of tissue structures. Micro-cracks that appear in bone structure are repaired through resorption of bone material in the damage area and formation of new bone structure in this place. Situation changes when bone is overstrained (e.g. due to pathological strains) number of micro-cracks in bone structure may be so large that self-repairing capabilities are insufficient. In such situation micro-cracks accumulate and influence remodeling processes. Process of mechanical degradation of bone tissue should be also considered by micro-scale remodeling models through simulation of micro-cracks of bone trabeculae. For macro-scale models it can be taken into account through extended and more complex representation of remodeling stimulus (Burr, 1985; Doblare & Garcia, 2001; Martin, 2002). Formation and remodeling of bone tissue are slow processes that are influenced by cyclic loads. Therefore, in most simulations of both processes, the models of stress and strain are evaluated for relatively long time periods. Assuming simulation is an iterative process the most frequently used time period equals 24 hours. This is due to the fact, that one day is a period of time when processes related to long-time stresses, such as creep and relaxation, occur. These processes should be taken into account when calculating stress and strain values for successive iterations of the simulation, irrespectively from the bone model used.

6. Simulation of formation and remodeling of bone structure

Micro-scale simulation procedures usually use an algorithm based on Tsubota model of remodeling processes (Ścigała et al., 2004; Będziński & Ścigała, 2011; Tsubota et al., 2002). The main factor that influences the value of remodeling stimulus in this model is uneven distribution of stress. This model assumes that value of this stimulus can be calculated as:

$$\Gamma = \ln\left(\frac{\sigma_c}{\sigma_d}\right) \tag{1}$$

where σ_c is a stress value in point C (that is currently analysed), and σ_d is a value that depends on stress in a precisely defined neighbourhood of point C.

This model also assumes that only stress on the surface of bone trabeculae is vital for remodeling processes. In other words, the osteocytes network, is evenly distributed in volume of trabeculae. However signal collected by those cells is proportional only to the distribution of stresses on surface of trabeculae. Assumption is justified, as cell processes (bone formation and deposition) that are elementary of remodeling of bone mineral matrix take place only on the surface of trabeculae. Additional assumptions determine the area of bone tissue that contain cells that will respond to remodeling stimulus. According to Tsubota (Tsubota et al., 2002) this area is assumed to have a circular or spherical (for 3D analysis) shape of radius L_L (Fig.5). Response of bone cells to the signal is limited in distance and radius of presented circular area. This is basically maximal distance from which bone cells can detect signal for remodeling.

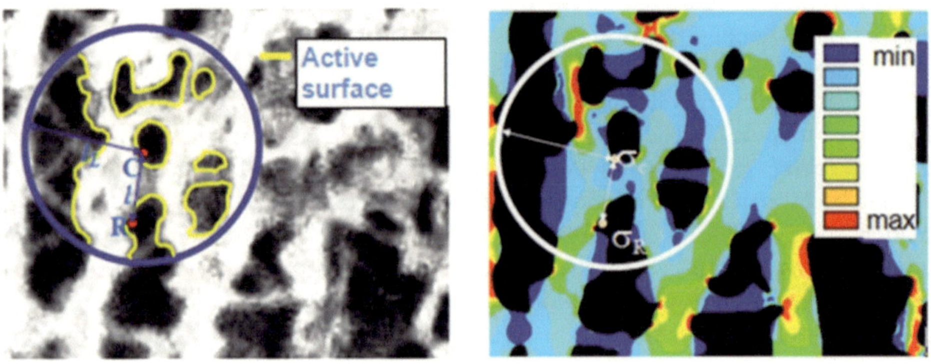

Fig. 5. Determination of local distribution of stress stimulus Γ

As described above analysis focus only on the surface of bone trabeculae and inner area of circular/spherical shape. Value of remodeling stimulus in point *C* depends on stress in each point *R* of the analysed area. Each point *R* influences the value of stimulus with different coefficient that depends on the distance between points *C* and *R*. Presented model determines this coefficient using a linear weight function that takes maximal value in point *C* and minimal value for points located on the edge of circular region:

$$\sigma_d = \frac{\int_S w(L)\sigma_R dS}{\int_S w(L) dS}, \quad w(L) = \begin{cases} 1 - \frac{L}{L_L} & \text{where} \quad 0 < L < L_L \\ 0 & \text{where} \quad L > L_L \end{cases} \tag{2}$$

where S is the analysed area, L is a distance between C and R points, σ_R is a stress value in point R and L_L is a radius of the analysed area.
Initial finite element model (FEM) that is used to simulate remodeling processes is composed of a regular grid of finite elements where two groups of elements can be differentiated: bone trabeculae and space between bone trabeculae. For each type of element a different material model was defined. For elements forming trabeculae we use a linear elasticity material with properties typical for bone mineral matrix. Elements that form inter trabecular spaces are assumed to be composed of linear elasticity material, with mechanical properties of very low values (actually as low as possible without model instability). Model is constructed by ring shaped patterns randomly placed over this grid. Each ring element represents bone trabeculae, while its inner, empty area models space between trabeculae. Random and dense placement according to this pattern creates an initial model that has isotropic and homogenous pseudo-trabeculae structure (Fig.6).

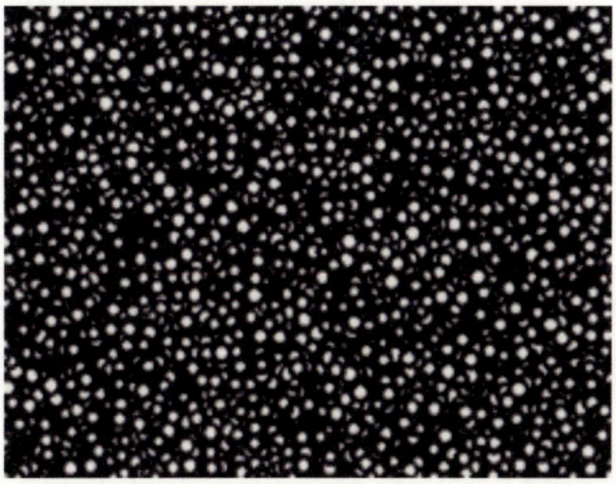

Fig. 6. Example of a initial model used in FEM modeling to simulate cancellous bone remodeling

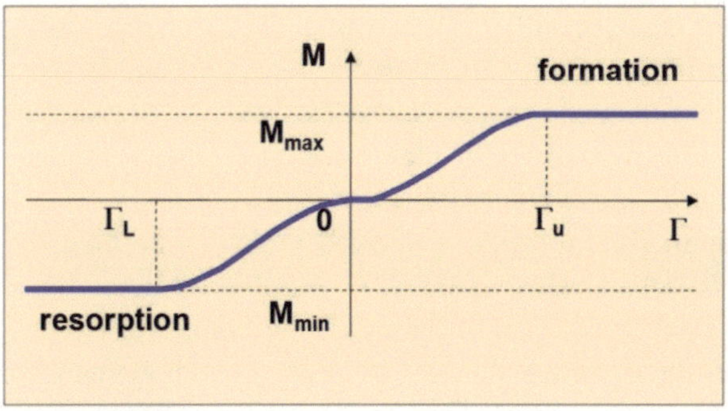

Fig. 7. Formation and resorption procedures (M) as a function of remodeling stimulus (Γ)

A typical simulation procedure that models remodeling processes takes an initial FEM model and calculates value of remodeling stimulus Γ for each finite element that coincident with surface of bone trabecula. Verification is the next step of a modeling procedure. In Tsubota model, it is assumed that formation and resorption processes are initiated when the value of remodeling stimulus exceeds the threshold (Fig. 7).

When value of the remodeling stimulus for a finite element is greater than Γ_U, then bone formation processes are initiated and new bone material is created on the trabeculae surface. On the other hand, when remodeling stimulus is smaller than Γ_L threshold, bone degradation processes are started and trabeculae material degrades. In FEM model both processes are implemented through changes in material of the finite element. For the first case (i.e. bone formation), material of the neighbouring elements is changed from space between trabeculae to bone trabeculae. For the second case, material of currently analysed element is changed to space between trabeculae. If remodeling stimulus is between thresholds Γ_L and Γ_U then no changes to the structure are made (Fig. 8).

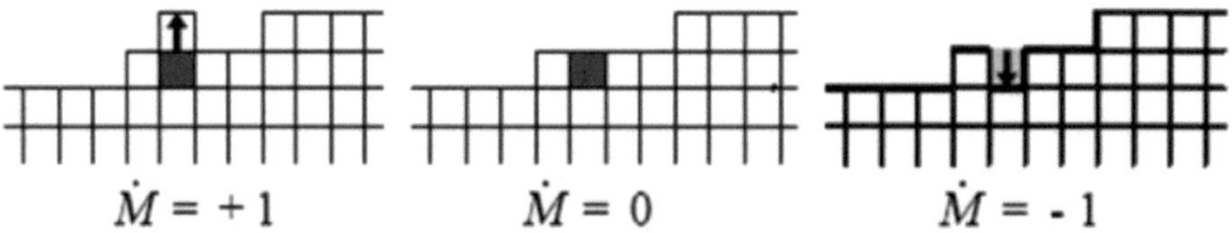

Fig. 8. Implementation of bone formation and resorption processes in FEM model (Tsubota et al., 2002)

Figure 9 presents scheme of a basic simulation procedure used to model processes that happen in cancellous bone. During each analysis of formation and remodeling of cancellous bone all the loads that characterise daily physical activity are determined but only these are taken into account that have cyclic character. Simulator takes initial bone model with isotropic and homogenous trabeculae structure and applies selected loads. It is worth to note that every cyclic load is substituted with a few static loads that are selected in order to follow changes that are specific to cyclic load simulated and model it with desired precision. In each case calculations are conducted using the FEM method and applied to finite elements selected from the model (as described above calculations only involve trabeculae from the bone surface). For each element selected, value of von Mises stress is calculated. Calculated data is stored in a table, that relates finite element with its stress value. The next step selects radius of circular (or spherical) area that is used to determine finite elements that will be taken into account when mechanical stimulus of remodeling is calculated. The selection of radius depends on the size of the FEM model. For each element in the aforementioned table parameters σ_c, σ_d and value of mechanical stimulus Γ are calculated and stored.
Next step of the simulation procedure decides which finite element bone material (i.e. trabeculae or space between trabeculae) will be modified due to stimulus. Elements stored in the table are analysed once again and for each of them, it is verified whether calculated stimulus exceeds threshold values Γ_L or Γ_U. If for a given element threshold is exceeded, element is put to the a set of elements for which bone formation or resorption processes will occur. After this procedure mechanical properties of all the selected elements and consequently, structure of the trabeculae, are modified. Modified bone model is then used as an initial model in the next iteration of the simulation procedure. Iterations are run as long as number of elements selected for bone formation or resporption process (number of elements in aforementioned set) is smaller than the threshold assumed. Threshold value depends on the complexity of the model and total number of finite elements.

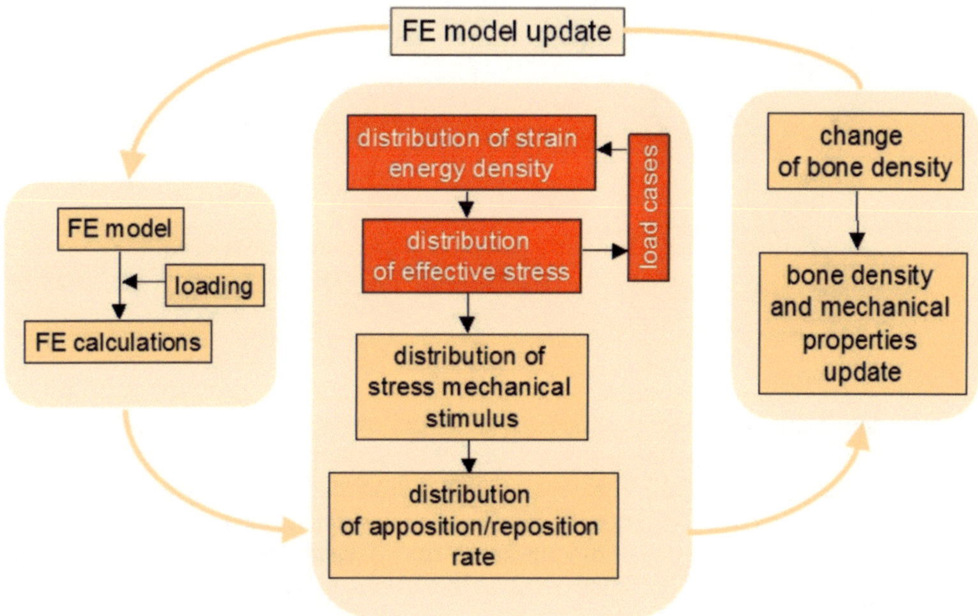

Fig. 9. Scheme of the basic simulation procedure for FEM model

Simulation procedure described above contains adaptive functions that modify distribution of mechanical stimulus on the surface of trabeculae, based on inter-osseous fluid flow. Basic parameters calculated from analysis of fluid flow include significant differences in flow pressure near the ends and middle of trabecula. According to the assumption that intensity of remodeling processes depends on stress values resulting from fluid pressure that influences bone cells in each trabecula, value of remodeling stimulus should depend on that pressure and be different for cells located in different regions of the same trabecula.

In the simulation procedure first module is responsible for evaluation of changes in stimulus values related to inter-osseous fluid flow. At the beginning this module carry out identification of elements at the ends of each trabecula. First each element on the surface of trabeculae is identified using previously prepared table and all surrounding elements are selected (see Fig. 10). For each element from selected group it is verified what kind of material it represents. If most of surrounding elements are defined as material of trabecula, central element is assumed to be at the end of trabecula. In other case, when surrounding elements are mostly inter-trabecular space, it is decided that the central element is located in the middle of trabecula. Number of surrounding elements investigated was estimated experimentally, by carrying numerous simulations with various trabecular structures.

The simulation procedure presented above enables to analyse formation and remodeling processes of bone trabeculae comprehensively. However, this simulation method has large computational overhead which makes this approach impractical for large bones and extended trabeculae structures.

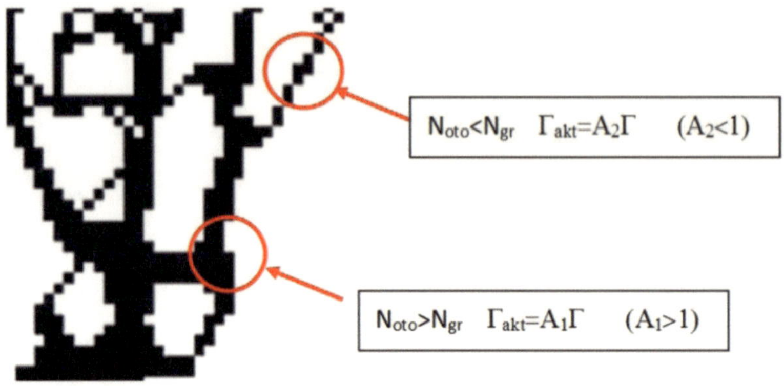

Fig. 10. Correction of value of stimulus of remodeling

Aforementioned approach can be simplified in several ways. The example presented here simplifies simulation procedure by modifying the way deformations and stresses in trabeculae are analysed. Initial model was created as described previously and has isotropic and homogenous structure. Next this model was used to simulate loading from the top edge while bottom edge was fixed (i.e. mounted). Measured values of force varied from high values on one side of the sample to the small on the other side (Fig. 11).

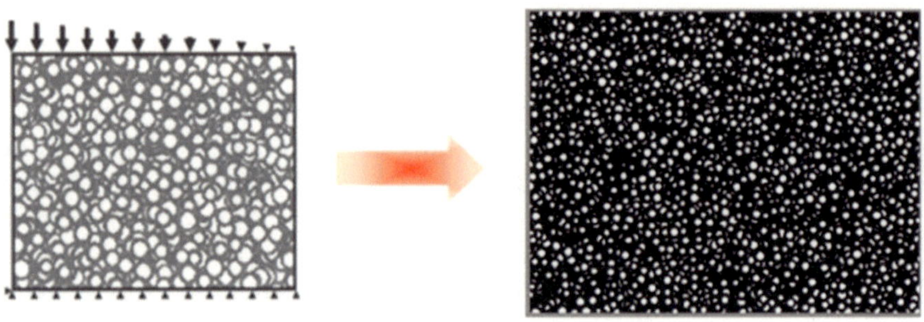

Fig. 11. Loading model and FE model of bone tissue rectangular sample

As a result of analytical analysis of the model and using Huber-von Mises hypothesis, distribution of reduced stress was calculated. Values of stress was then modified in a similar way as was used for values of remodeling mechanical stimulus - i.e. to take into account distribution of inter-osseous fluid pressure.
Figure 12 presents results of these computations. Analysis of the resulting distribution lead to the observation that stress values are proportional to the remodeling stimulus calculated in the simulations. This means that it is possible to point out areas of the bone model that will be affected with bone formation and bone resorption.The area on the right side of the model is characterised with low values of von Mises stress because of low values of forces applied to the right upper corner of the sample. Values of stress increase gradually from right to left according to applied load. Looking at Fig. 12 it is obvious that element with high values of von Mises stress form structures very similar to the real trabecular structures. It is possible to observe structures similar to the thick, strong trabecular structures near to the left part of model, mostly directed vertically. In the middle part of the model, thickness of trabeculae decrease and more inter trabecular spaces can be observed. Trabeculae are not

only vertically arranged but we can also observe inclined structures and small disconnected structures near the right side of the sample.

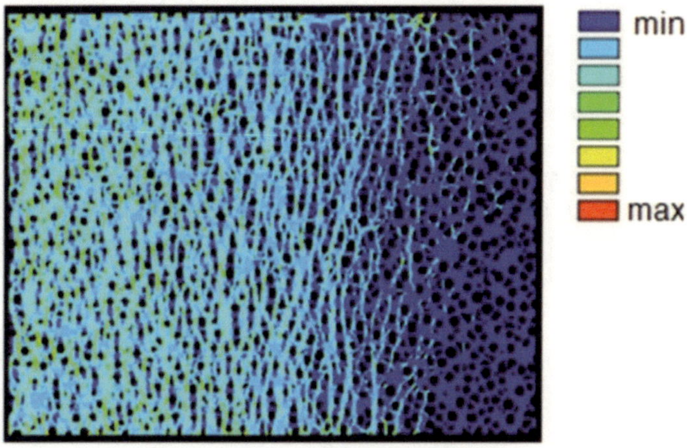

Fig. 12. Von Mises stress distribution of analysed structure

Above analysis shows that von Mises stress value is a good parameter for description of trabecules loading. Group of elements characterised with von Mises stress value higher than minimal value estimated previously contains almost all the elements that exist in real trabecular structure. This gives an opportunity to simplify computational complexity of the simulation by using different method of calculating remodeling stimulus. This approach requires defining quantitative relation between load-bearing structure of trabecular bone determined with basic (also taking into account flow of inter-osseous fluid) and simplified procedure.

We have carried on several analyses to evaluate this relation. This was done with different bone models that were composed of a small number of elements in order to speed up computations. Basic result of this approach, for the case of a rectangular model loaded in exactly the same way as described previously, is presented in Fig. 13. Using both standard and simplified methods very similar structures of trabeculae were obtained. Both structures have two main and one additional load-bearing structure. Vertical bearing structure, composed of thick trabeculae, can be found in the area that was relatively heavily loaded (A). Second of the main bearing structures is composed of two trabeculae - diagonal (B) and vertical (C). This is a result of maximizing capacity to carry stress and reducing the mass simultaneously. Diagonal trabecula carry stress from the right side of the bone model through one single and tight structure. Additional load-bearing structure is an auxiliary structure that is composed of trabeculae of small size and mostly horizontal arrangement (D); only some trabeculae are arranged vertically and only few have diagonal orientation.

Analysis show that all the trabeculae that exist in bone structure generated with standard simulation method also appear in structure calculated using simplified simulation. Location of end points of all trabeculae from both simulation procedures differs slightly, by no more ten two finite elements. Since in FEM models grid of finite elements is dense and trabeculae are relatively large comparing to a single element (A, B and C structures), it is justified to state that error of using simplified simulation method is small and negligible. For trabeculae of relatively small size (structure D) error in location of trabeculae ends is even smaller and only in some situation exceeds size of a single finite element. Thickness of trabeculae resulting from both simulation approaches differ mainly in the basic structures with the biggest difference in B and C and small in A structure. The biggest differences concern basic structures with complex shape that carry relatively low load. For a small spread load standard definition of a mechanical stimulus allows for more precise definition of real element structures that are responsible for load-bearing. Using simplified definition it is always needed to be aware of slight overestimations of load-bearing size. In a final description of the structure those overestimates will not have significant influence on load-bearing properties - some areas of the resulting structure will be characterised with slightly smaller values of stress but will still serve mechanical function in exactly the same way as in structures resulting from standard simulation method.

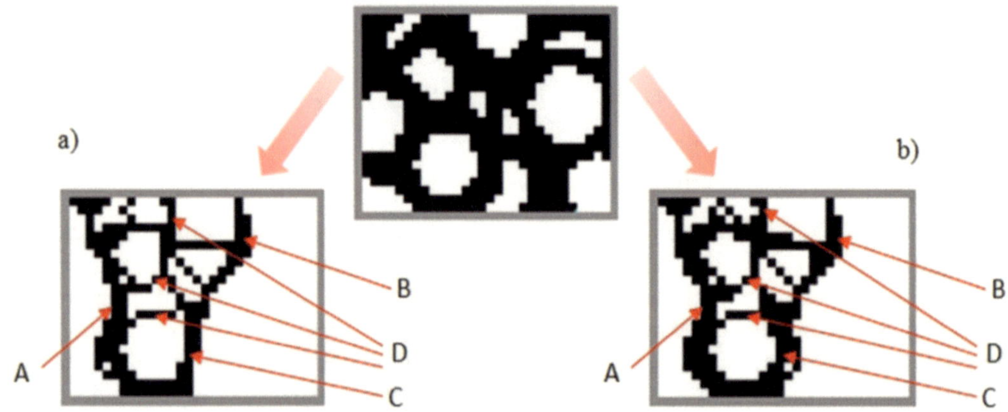

Fig. 13. Comparison of structures developer form the same initial model with classic and simplified algorithm

The result depends significantly on the density of ring-shaped structures deployed in initial model and the density of finite elements grid. Density of the grid for all the models presented in this chapter was high - each pixel from the figures presenting trabecular bone structure represents a single finite element. In case of three-dimensional models density of spheres is significantly smaller, so this small density is only result of great number of element in three-dimensional models and long time of calculations. Ratio of the size of ring-shaped structure versus size of the whole model is a significant parameter that influence simulations.

Figure 14 compares results of remodeling simulations run for the same bone model but different total number of finite elements in the FEM model. In each case model was loaded with the same load but different load-bearing structure were formed. For all cases load-bearing structure was created in the part of the model that was heavy loaded. For models that used sparse grid of finite elements (A and B) this structure consist of thick, long and vertically or diagonal oriented trabeculae. For models with dense grid (C and D) structure is also composed of similar trabeculae but number of trabeculae is much larger. Diagonal trabeculae dominate in parts of the model that were less loaded with separate (unconnected) elements for the case when dense grid of finite elements was used.

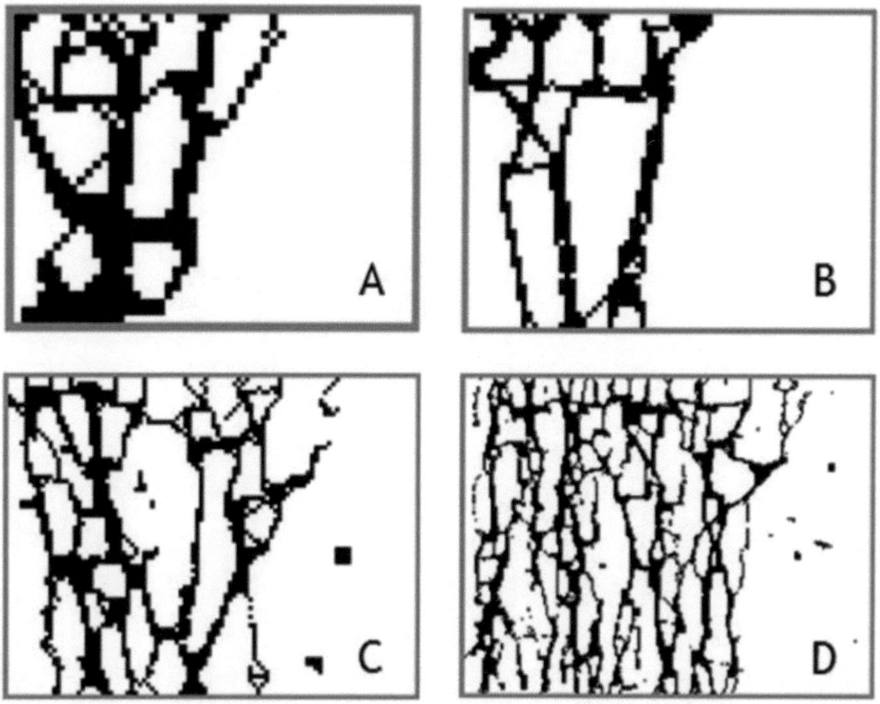

Fig. 14. Comparison of structures from the same initial model with various density of finite elements mesh and initial rings (A - 50 elements along longer side of model, B - 75 element, C - 100 elements, D - 200 elements)

Use of simplified procedure for modeling formation and remodeling processes of trabecular bone is justified, possible and gives correct results. However, in order to get correct results simulation procedure has to meet several initial conditions and be constantly monitored. Precisely:

1. initial FEM model should be composed of a large number of finite elements and the ring-shaped structure with size similar to size of real tabeculae,
2. density of the initial model has to be large, which means that number of elements that represent bone trabeculae has to be much larger than the number of elements that represent space between trabeculae. Complying this requirement will allow to get load-bearing structures without the need for additional bone mass being add to the model during simulation. This is also important from the practical point of view as modification of the model extend simulation time,
3. threshold value of the stress that is used to decide which elements are kept or removed from the model should be selected on the individual basis for each model. It is recommended to run a standard simulation procedure for a few iterations and save it for comparison. Then simplified procedure should be run with different value of this parameter until the resulting structure has no significant differences from the one saved. When proper value of the parameter is found successive iterations are run,
4. simplified procedure requires use, of an additional correction module that will allow to eliminate unconnected structures from the model, as these have no influence on the load-bearing.

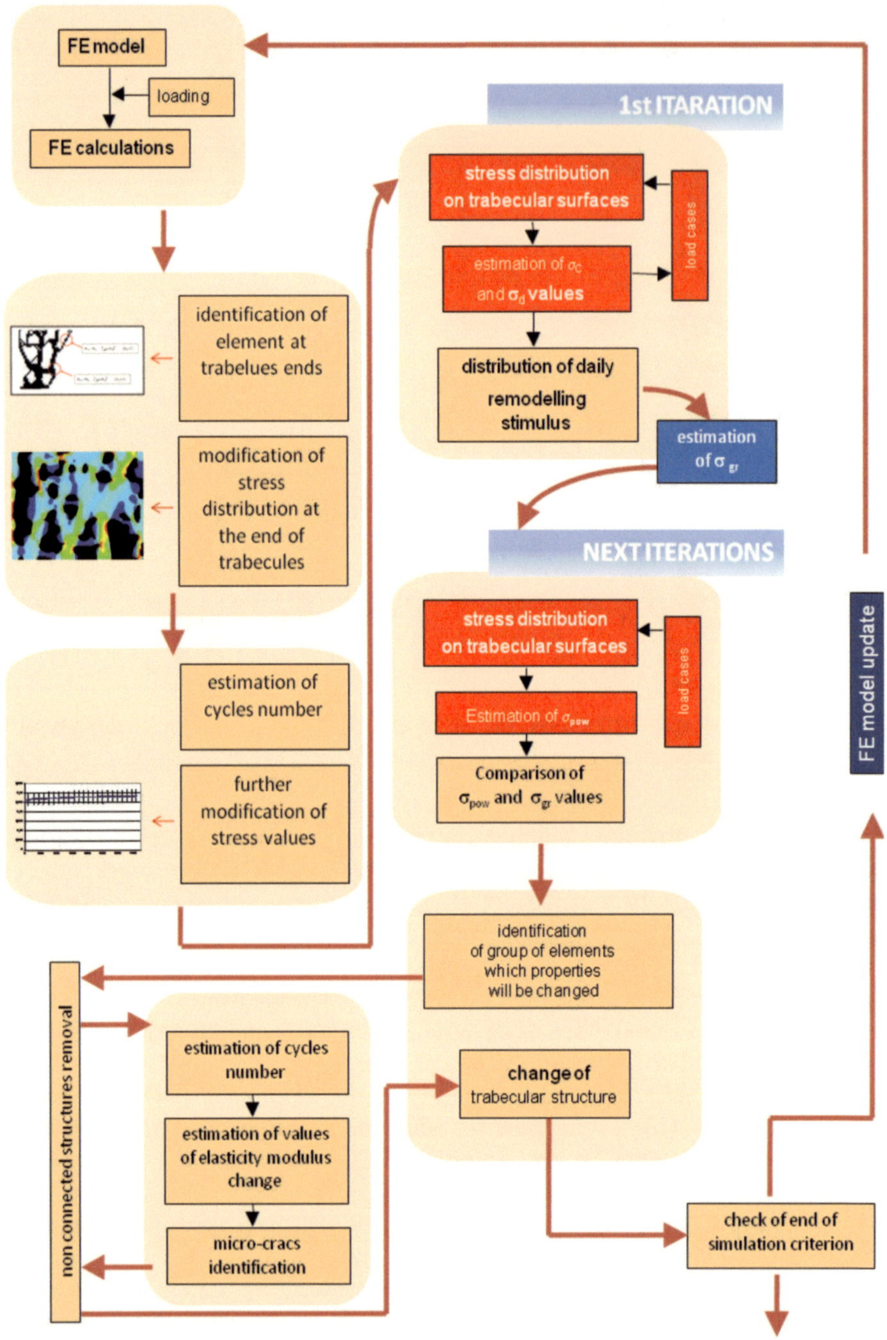

Fig. 15. Algorithm of bone remodeling simulation

Figure 15 presents a general structure of the simplified procedure for simulation of formation and remodeling of trabecular bone structures. Figure presents all the computational units required with correction and micro-cracks analysis modules that are additional with respect to standard Tsubota model. Correction module is designed to take into account creep and relaxation of stress in bone structure. This is based on the analysis of number of load iterations that were already applied to the modelled structure and resulting range of deformation and stress changes. Number of load iteration is calculated assuming that each cycle of loading procedure consist of constant number of load iterations, represents full period of time and it is possible to determine number of iterations of particular type. Change in the deformation values is calculated based on the number of iterations and using Currey model for creep while change in stress results from stress relaxation model by Sasaki (Currey, 1965; Sasaki & Enyo, 1995). Second module is responsible for analysing origins and accumulation of cracks in trabecular structure and also draws from information about total number of load iterations already applied to the model.

At the beginning of each iteration the total number of cycles from the beginning of simulation is calculated and stored in a table that also contains finite element identifiers and stress value calculated for last iteration performed. This table only stores information about elements that characterize bone material. At the end of each iteration, elasticity modulus value (that is related to damage accumulation) is calculated based on stress value and number of cycles. New value of elasticity modulus is calculated for each stored in the table.

Next, examination of new elasticity modulus value allows determination of group of elements to which analysed element belongs to. This is based on threshold value of elasticity modulus that is typical for bone tissue. If actual value of elasticity modulus is lower than threshold, status of the element is changed and material properties are changed so that element will now represent inter trabecular space. In that way, micro-cracks can be introduced into the model and in further iterations damage accumulation may progress.

Process of mechanical degradation can develop further in three different ways:

1. micro-crack in a bone trabeculae may lead to increased load in that trabeculae and possibly in neighbouring trabeculae. In such a case stress values increase leading to increased mechanical stimulus of bone remodeling. When value of stimulus exceeds upper threshold defined in Tsubota model, bone formation process is initiated on the trabeculae surface and usually also in the vicinity of the micro-crack. Consequently, bone repairs itself and trabeculae are reconstructed in a shape that is very similar to the original one (prior to crack). In real remodeling processes reconstructed element is a new bone material. Therefore, in simulations we erase information about number of load iterations that were applied to the finite element that contains reconstructed bone. This is a self-remodeling scenario,
2. creation of a micro-crack may not lead to significant change in stress in affected trabeculae nor in neighbouring ones. If this happens then self-remodeling processes are not initiated and no new bone material is created in the vicinity of the crack. However, stress values near the crack have increased and speed up wear-out of neighbouring bone material with consecutive load iterations. Consequently, value of elasticity modulus for elements located near the crack decrease and crack evolves. This usually leads to excessive load of neighbouring trabeculae and new micro-cracks that spread across them. As number of micro-cracks increases remodeling processes are initiated from time to time. Usually, degradation of bone structure progresses faster than remodeling leading to accumulation of micro-cracks,

3. several micro-cracks may appear simultaneously leading to significant change in elasticity modulus in several neighbouring elements. In such a case crack evolves immediately across the single of a few, neighbouring trabeculae. When trabeculae brakes, both parts are relieved and values of stress in finite elements that model them drops to minimal values. This initiates resorption processes and in successive iterations elements will represent space between bone material. Such situation also increases stress in neighbouring trabeculae that in turn initiates bone formation processes and leads to creation of new bone trabeculae. New trabeculae have different shape compared to trabeculae that broke. In some cases, when several micro-cracks appear in neighbouring trabeculae, some part of the bone mass may become disconnected from the load-bearing structure. Such structure is detected by dedicated module of the simulation procedure and removed from the model (elements that represent this mass are modified to represent space between bone mass). Relatively large cavity in the bone structure of this type, initiates formation of new bone mass in surrounding trabeculae and construction of new load-bearing structures. This scenario presents a remodeling of bone structure stimulated by mechanical degradation.

Analysis of formation and remodeling of trabecular structures was carried out using model of normal femur bone. Model of femur proximal epiphysis was created using the same algorithm as in previous case. Loading that is typical for stance phase of gait (according to Beaupré) was applied to the model.

Analysis of remodeling process for model of intact femur bone shows significant deposition of trabecular structures in the proximal part of grater trochanter - region marked as A (Fig. 16). Bone reposition in this area results from simplified loading model in which muscle force (from hip abductors) was applied to the middle part of lateral surface of greater trochanter. In real hip joint there are several muscle forces. One of the muscles is attached in the upper part of this surface. Because of that in real bone that kind of low density trabecular structure are not observed.

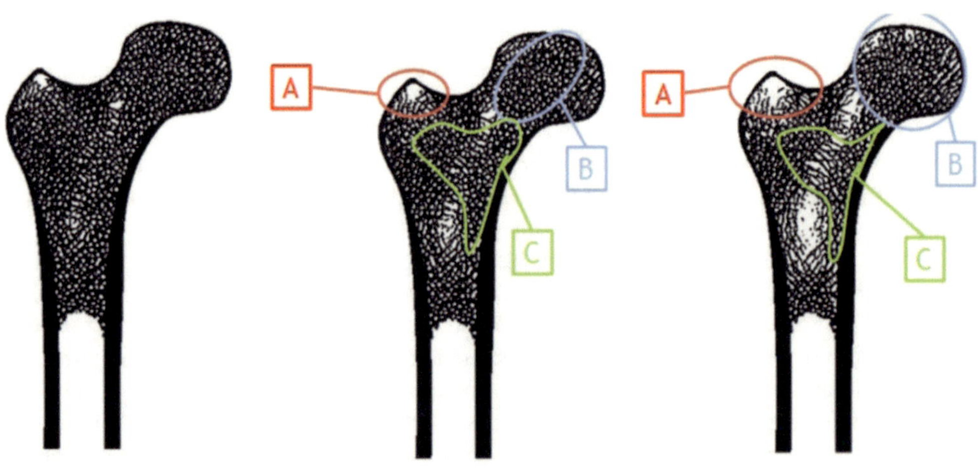

Fig. 16. Successive iterations (from left to right) of bone formation and remodeling processes for trabecular structures in model of femur bone

Trabecular structures in femur head (marked as B on Fig. 16) changed significantly. This is clearly seen for trabeculae located close to articular surface as they become longer and diagonal arranged. In the central part of the femur head directed structures are not so well visualized. Trabecular structures in the region of lesser trochanter (marked as C in the Fig. 16) also changed significantly and two main load-bearing structures can be seen. First of them is a structure placed in the close range form layer of compact bone. It's a dense structure with almost even distribution of trabeculae. Second structure, is characterised by highly directed trabeculae - this structure connects greater and lesser trochanter. Trabeculae can be characterised as inclined structures and, in case of supportive structure, trabeculae are directed horizontally.

In the case of pathologically deformed femur, we can observe significant differences in trabecular structures distribution in comparison to the model of intact femur bone.

In first part of simulation we can observe significant deposition of trabecular structures in the distant part of the model, especially in central region (Fig. 17 A). Deposition of that kind can be observed also in the proximal part of grater trochanter, as well as in the lower part of femur head (Fig. 17 B). Trabecular structures in the femur head and most part of proximal epiphysis of femur are not modified significantly, still ring shaped structures from initial trabeculae distribution are visible (Fig. 17 C). During remodeling the trabecular structures in the femur head become more directed (Fig. 17 D). However, trabecular structures are still dense. Most of trabeculae are significantly thicker than in other areas and length of those trabeculae is small. In upper and central part of femur neck, small deposition of trabecular structures can be observed (Fig. 17 E). In the main part of inter - trochanter region it is possible to observe gradual deposition of directed structures, in form of two arches crossing each other and connecting lateral and middle part of bone (Fig. 17 F). After next step of simulation it is possible to observe clearly formed marrow cave (Fig. 17 G). Directed structures in the inter - trochanter region are also clearly formed (Fig. 17 H). Similarly, in the head of femur we can observe more and more directed trabecular structures.

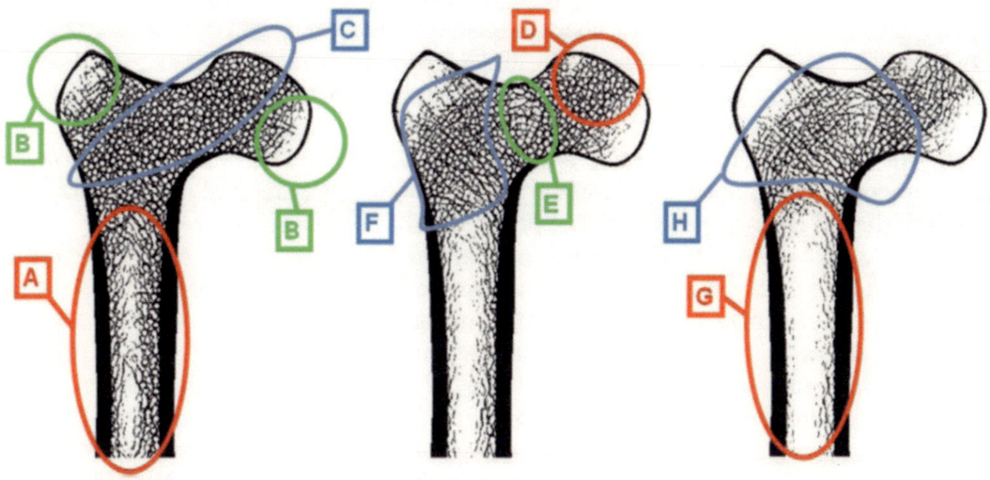

Fig. 17. Successive iterations (from left to right) of bone formation and remodeling processes for trabecular structures in model of pathologically deformed femur bone

It follows that in the case of deformed femur, pathological distribution of trabecular structures can be characterised by much more directed structures than in case of intact femur. In most parts of the bone deposition of trabeculae can be observed. However cancellous tissue is still dense in the head of femur. In some parts of this area porosity, of trabecular structures is even lesser than in model of intact bone.

7. Conclusion

Presented work consists both experimental and numerical analysis. Value of each part can't be underestimated. Experimental investigations are essential for understanding of connection between trabecular structure and mechanics. First look at any bone tissue leads to conclusion that it is really complicated result of biological processes of tissue differentiation and formation. Details of this complicated structure, which have significant influence on bone properties, can be analysed at different levels - whole bone, bone tissue, bone structure, bone trabecule, trabecula internal structure, bone cells. One way to understand and describe processes that take place in bone tissue on different levels is to introduce new parameters and relationships between them. Unfortunately, in many cases, number of measured parameters - structural and mechanical - is so large that the bone description becomes so complex that people start to wonder if it is still useful and necessary. However, the amount of data is priceless for preparation of bone models and simulation of biological processes that take place inside of bone tissue. Moreover, detailed description of structure is necessary to understand bone tissue mechanics, which is needed in case of surgical treatment, and to understand mechanics of pathology. From that point of view, we are unable to understand in details, complex behaviour of bone without experimental investigations, and we are unable to simulate trabecular structures comprehensively without data collected during experiment.

Numerical simulations give us a wider view at bone tissue as a living organ. Number of processes that we can model nowadays allow us to observe changes in structure as a result of changes in loading conditions. Simulations allow introduction of patient related disturbances to modelled process easily (e.g. deformation of bone, changes in daily physical activity, changes in mass of patient, changes related to treatment, etc.). We can predict with some precision what kind of structures will exist in bone and whether they will lead to pathology or recovery. Observation how trabecular structures form give us perspective an how our skeleton develops and an how it is influenced by mechanical parameters.

Finally such analysis, should develop analytical models of bone tissue. Both, experimental and numerical work, take significantly long time to prepare and to conduct. Full understanding of ongoing process will be possible at the level of generalized model.

Presented results show how different is mechanical behaviour and internal structure of pathological bone tissue in femur bone comparing to healthy. Changes are not only related to the values of parameters evaluated for both intact and pathological bone, but also bone structure is affected significantly. Clearly there is a relationship between bone structure and mechanics that can be described using the same functions for both healthy and OA bones, however parameters and constants in those functions will be different for both cases. Numerical simulations allow analysis of how distribution of mechanical parameters lead to different structure in case of intact and pathological bone. We can observe details of process of forming 'correct' and pathological structures. We can easily detect regions in bone where changes are significant, and the regions where changes are irrelevant. It is even possible to

analyze relationship between change in particular mechanical parameters and bone response to that changes which enables estimation of loading conditions which will result in bone structure changes that will be the most dangerous to patient.
Changes in bone structure and behaviour during development of osteoarthritis are not fully understand. Presented research is strongly focused on biomechanics of bone tissue, and in simulations mostly biomechanical parameters were taken into consideration. Relationships, between bone structure and mechanics, loading and structure formation or remodeling were described as equations or models.

8. Acknowledgment

This work has been supported by the National Science Centre grant no. N 518 505139. The authors wish to thank to *Bert van Rietbergen* from Technische Universiteit Eindhoven for help and an opportunity to use the micro-CT system.

9. References

Altman R., Asch E., Bloch D. (1986). Developement of criteria for the classification and reporting of osteoarthritis: classification of osteoarthritisof the knee. *Arthritis & Rheumatism*, Vol. 29, No. 8 (Aug), pp. 1039-1049, ISSN: 0004-3591

An, Y.H., Draughn R.A. (2000). *Mechanical testing of bone and bone-implant interface,* CRC Press LLC , ISBN: 0-8493-0266-8, Boca Raton, FL

Bagge M. (2000). A model of bone adaptation as an optimisation process. *Journal of Biomechanics,* Vol. 33, No. 11 (Nov), pp. 1349 - 1357, ISSN: 0021-9290

Bartodziej J., Ścigała K. (2009). Analysis of trabecular structure remodeling for pathological load case. *Proceedings of IV Internatinal Conference on Computational Bioengineering,* Bertinoro, Italy, 16-18 September

Beaupré G.S., Orr T.E., Carter D.R. (1990). An approach for time-dependent bone modeling and remodeling theoretical development. *Journal of Orthopedic Research,* Vol. 8, No. 8 (Sep), pp. 651-661, ISSN: 0736-0266

Będziński R. (1997). *Biomechanika inżynierska: zagadnienia Wybrane,* Wydawnictwo Politechniki Wrocławskiej, ISBN: 83-7085-240-8, Wrocław, Poland

Będziński R., Ścigała K. (2003). FEM analysis of strain distribution in tibia bone and its relationship between strains and adaptation of bone tissue. *CAMES (Computer Assisted Mechanics and Engineering Sciences),* Vol. 10, No. 3, pp. 353 - 368, ISSN: 1232-308X

Będziński R., Ścigała K. (2010). Biomechanical basis of tissue - implant interactions, In: *Computer Methods in Mechanics: Lectures of the CMM 2009, Series Advanced Structured Materials,* Kuczma M., Wilmanski K. (Eds), pp. 379-390, Springer-Verlag, ISBN: 3-6420-5240-1, New York, LLC

Będziński R., Ścigała K. (2011). Metody numeryczne I doświadczalne w biomechanice, In: *Biomechanika,* Będziński R. (Eds), pp. 77-178, Wydawnictwo PAN, ISBN: 978-83-89687-61-6, Warszawa

Boyd S.K., Müller R., Matyas J.R., Wohl G.R., Zernicke R.F. (2000). Early morphometric and anisotropic change in periarticular cancellous bone in a model of experimental knee osteoarthritis quantified using microcomputed tomography. *Clinical biomechanics (Bristol, Avon),* Vol. 15, No. 8, pp. 624–631, ISSN: 1879-1271

Brishmar H. (2003). *Morphological and molecular changes in developing guinea pig osteoarthritis.* Karolinska University Press, ISBN: 91-7349-456-9, Stockholm

Buckwalter J.A., Martin J.A., Brown T.D. (2006). Perspectives on chondrocyte mechanobiology and osteoarthritis. *Biorheology,* Vol. 43, No. 3-4, pp. 603– 609, ISSN: 0006-355X

Burr D.B., Martin R.B., Schaffler, M.B., Randin E. L. (1985). Bone remodeling in response to in vivo fatigue microdamage. *Journal of Biomechanics,* Vol. 18, No. 3, pp. 189 - 200, ISSN: 0021-9290

Carter D.R. (1987). Mechanical Loading History and Skeletal Biology. *Journal of Biomechanics,* Vol. 20, No. (11-12), pp. 1095-1109, ISSN: 0021-9290

Carter D.R., Hayes W.C. (1977). Bone compressive behavior of bone as a two–phase porous structure. *American Journal of Bone and Joint Surgery,* Vol. 59, No. 7 (Oct.), pp. 954-962, ISSN: 00219355

Carter D.R., van der Meulen M.C.H., Beaupré G.S. (1996). Mechanical Factors in bone growth and development. *Bone,* Vol. 18, No. 1, pp. 5-10, ISSN: 8756-3282

Cheal E.J., Hayes W.C., White A.A. (1985). Stress Analysis of Compression Plate Fixation and its Effects on Long Bone Remodeling. *Journal of Biomechanics,* Vol. 18, No. 2, pp. 141-150, ISSN: 0021-9290

Chen S.S., Falcovitz Y.H., Schneiderman R., Maroudas A., Sah R.R. (2001). Depth-dependent compressive properties of normal aged human femoral head articular cartilage: relationship to fixed charge density. *Osteoarthritis and Cartilage,* Vol. 9, No.6 (Aug), pp. 561–569, ISSN: 1063-4584

Cowin S.C, Hart R.T., Balser J.R., Kohn D.H. (1985). Functional Adaptation in Long Bones: Establishing in vivo Values for Surface Remodeling Rate Coefficients. *Journal of Biomechanics,* Vol. 18, No. 9, pp. 665-684, ISSN: 0021-9290

Cowin S.C. (2001). *Bone Mechanics Handbook,* CRC Press, ISBN: 0-8493-9117-2, Boca Raton, FL

Currey J.D. (1965). Anelasticity in Bone and Echinoderm Skeletons. *Journal of Experimental Biology.* Vol. 43, pp. 279-292, ISSN: 0022-0949

Currey J.D. (1984). Comparative Mechanical Properties and Histology of Bone. *American Zoologist,* Vol. 24, No.1, pp. 5–12, ISSN: 0003-1569

Doblare M., Garcia J.M. (2001). Application of an anisotropic bone remodelling model based on a damage-repair theory to the analysis of the proximal femur before and after total hip replacement. *Journal of Biomechanics,* Vol. 34, No. 9, pp. 1157-1170, ISSN: 0021-9290

Frost H.M. (1994). Wolff's Law and bone's structural adaptations to mechanical usage: an overview for clinicians. *Angle Orthodontist,* Vol. 64, No. 3, pp. 175-188, ISSN: 0003-3219

Glaser C., Putz R. (2002). Functional anatomy of articular cartilage under compressive loading: Quantitative aspects of global, local and zonal reactions of the collagenous network with respect to the surface integrity. *Osteoarthritis and Cartilage,* Vol. 10, No.2 (Feb), pp. 83-99, ISSN: 1063-4584

Glimcher M.J. (1992). The structure of mineral component of bone and the mechanism of calcification, In: *Disorders of bone and mineral metabolism,* Coe F.L., Favus M.J, pp. 265-286, Raven Press, ISBN: 0-88167-749-3, New York

Grynpas M.D., Alpert B., Katz I., Lieberman I., Pritzker K.P.H. (1991). Subchondral bone in osteoarthritis. *Calcified Tissue International,* Vol. 49, No.1, pp. 20-26, ISSN: 0171-967X

Hernandez C. J., Beaupre G.S., Marcus R., Carter D.R. (2001). A theoretical analysis of the contributions of remodeling space, mineralization and bone balance to changes in bone mineral density during alendronate treatment. *Bone,* Vol. 29, No. 6 (Dec), pp. 511 - 516, ISSN: 8756-3282

Hildebrand T., Laib A., Müller R., Dequeker J., Rüegsegger P. (1999). Direct three-dimensional morphometric analysis of human cancellous bone: microstructural data from spine, femur, iliac crest and calcaneus. *Journal of Bone and Mineral Research,* Vol.14, No. 7, pp. 1167–1174, ISSN: 1523-4681

Huiskes R., Weinans H., Grootenboer H.J., Dalstra M., Fundala B., Slooff T.J. (1987). Adaptive bone-remodeling theory applied to prosthetic design analysis. *Journal of Biomechanics,* Vol. 20, No. (11-12), pp. 1135-1150, ISSN: 0021-9290

Huiskes R. (2000). If bone is the answer, then what is the question? *Journal of Anatomy,* Vol. 197, No.2, pp.: 145–156, ISSN: 1469-7580\

Jacobs C.R., Simo J.C., Beaupre G.S., Carter D.R. (1997). Adaptive bone remodeling incorporating simultaneous density and anisotropy considerations. *Journal of Biomechanics,* Vol. 30, No. 6 (Jun), pp. 603-613, ISSN: 0021-9290

Katta J., Jin Z., Ingham E., Fisher J. (2008). Biotribology of articular cartilage—A review of the recent advances. *Medical Engineering & Physics,* Vol. 30, No. 10 (Dec), pp. 1349–1363, ISSN: 1350-4533

Kuttner K.E., Golderg V.M. (1995). Osteoarthritis disorders. *American Academy of Orthopedic Surgeons,* pp. 21–255, Rosemont, IL

Lanyon L.E. (1987). Functional strain in bone tissue as an objective, and controlling stimulus for adaptive bone remodeling. *Journal of Biomechanics,* Vol. 20, No. (11-12), pp. 1083-1093, ISSN: 0021-9290

Lozada C.J. (22.07.2011). Osteoarthritis, In: *Medscape,* 15.06.2011, Available from: <http://emedicine.medscape.com/article/330487-overview>

Malcolm A.J. (2002). Mini-Symposium: non-neoplasticosteoarticular pathology: Metabolic bone disease. *Current Diagnostic Pathology,* Vol. 8, pp. 19-25, ISSN: 0968-6053

Maquet P.G. (1985). *Biomechanics of the hip: As applied to osteoarthritis and related conditions,* Springer-Verlag, ISBN: 0387132570, Berlin and New York

Martin R. (2002). Is all cortical bone remodeling initiated by microdamage? *Bone,* Vol. 30, No. 1 (Jan), pp. 8-13, ISSN: 8756-3282

Mow V.C., Bachrach N.M., Setton L.A., Guilak F. (1994). Stress, strain, pressure and flow fields in articular cartilage and chondrocytes, In: *Cell mechanics and cellular egineering.,* Mow V.C., pp. 345-379, Springer, ISBN: 0-387-94307-2, New York

Nikodem A., Będziński R., Ścigała K., Dragan S. (2009). Mechanical and structural anisotropy of human cancellous femur bone. *Journal of Vibroengineering,* Vol. 11, No. 3, pp. 571-576, ISSN 1392-8716

Nikodem A., Ścigała K. (2010). Impact of some external factors on the values of the mechanical parameters determined in tests of bone tissue. *Acta of Bioengineering and Biomechanics,* Vol. 12, No. 3, pp. 85-93, ISSN 1509-409X

Odgaard A. (1997). Three dimensional methods for quantification of cancellous bone architecture. *Bone,* Vol. 20, No.4, pp. 315–328, ISSN: 8756-3282

Parfitt A.M., Drezner M.K., Glorieux F.H., Kanis J.A., Malluche H., Meunieur P.J., Ott S.M., Recker R.R. (1987). Bone Histomorphometry : Standardization of nomenclature, symbols, and units. *Journal of Bone and Mineral Research,* Vol. 2, No.6 (Dec), pp. 595–610, ISSN: 1523-4681

Pauwels F. (1976). *Biomechanics of the normal and diseased hip. Theoretical foundation, technique and results of treatment,* Springer-Verlag, ISBN: 0-3870-7428-7, New York

Pelletier J.M., Battista J.D., Lajeunesse D. (1999). Biochemical factors in joint articular tissue degradation in osteoarthritis. In: *Osteoarthritis. Clinical and experimental aspects,* Reginster J.Y., et al., pp. 156-187, Springer, ISBN: 3-5406-5127-6, Berlin

Radin E.L. (1995). Osteoarthrosis--the orthopedic surgeon's perspective. *Acta orthopaedica Scandinavica. Supplementum,* Vol. 266, pp. 6-9, ISSN: 0300-8827

Radin E.L., Martin R.B., Burr D.B., Caterson B., Boyd R.D., Goodwin C. (1984). Effects on Mechanical Loading on the Tissues on the Rabbit Knee. *Journal of Orthopedic Research,* Vol. 2, No.3, pp. 221–234, ISSN: 1554-527X

Rice J.C., Cowin S.C., Bowman J.A. (1988). On the dependence of elasticity and strength of cancellous bone on apparent density. *Journal of Biomechanics,* Vol. 21, No.2, pp. 155-168, ISSN: 0021-9290

Sasaki N, Enyo A. (1995). Viscoelastic properties of bone as a function of water content. *Journal of Biomechanics* Vol. 28, No.7 (Jul), pp. 809-815, ISSN: 0021-9290

Ścigała K., Kiełbowicz A., Słowiński J. (2004). Symulacja numeryczna procesu tworzenia się struktury beleczkowej kości gąbczastej. *Systems : journal of transdisciplinary systems science,* Vol. 9, No. 2, pp. 827-832, ISSN: 1427-275X

Szwajczak E., Kucaba-Piętal A., Telega J.J. (2001). Liquid crystaline properties of synovial fluid. *Engineering Transactions,* Vol. 49, No. (2-3), pp. 315-358, ISSN: 67-888X

Tanaka T., Sakurai T., Kashima I. (2001). Structuring of parameters for assessing vertebral bone strength by star volume analysis using a morphological filter. *Journal of Bone and Mineral Metabolism,* Vol. 19, No.3, pp. 150–158, ISSN: 0914-8779

Tsubota K., Adachi T., Tomita Y. (2002). Functional adaptation of cancellous bone in human proximal femur predicted by trabecular surface remodeling simulation toward uniform stress state. *Journal of Biomechanics,* Vol. 35, No. 12 (Dec), pp. 1541-1551, ISSN: 0021-9290

Turner C.H., Burr D.B., (1993). Basic Biomechanical Measurements of Bone: A Tutorial. *Bone,* Vol. 14, No.4 (Jul-Aug), pp. 595–608, ISSN: 8756-3282

Wang J., Liu X., Li F., Yao L. (2002). Rheumatoid arthritis is auto-immunoreaction to collagen II in cartilage happened in synovial tissue. *Medical Hypotheses,* Vol. 59, No. 4, pp. 411–415, ISSN: 306-9877

Weinans H. (1999). Growth, Adaptation and Aging of the Skeletal System. *Journal of Theoretical and Applied Mechanics,* Vol. 37, No. 3, pp. 729 - 741, ISSN: 0079-3701

Whitehouse W.J. (1974). The quantitative morphology of anisotropic trabecular bone. *Journal of Microscopy,* Vol. 101, No.3 (Jul), pp. 153–168, ISSN: 1365-2818

Wierzcholski K., Miszczak A. (2006). *Tom II: Analityczne i numeryczne wyznaczanie ciśnienia, sił nośnych i tarcia w odkształcalnej szczelinie stawu człowieka.* Fundacja Rozwoju Akademii Morskiej, ISBN: 83-87438-89-8, Gdynia

Yamada H., Evans F.G. (1970). *Strength of biological materials,* Williams & Wilkins, ISBN: 0-6830-9323-1, Baltimore MD

7

Subchondral Bone in Osteoarthritis

David M. Findlay
Discipline of Orthopaedics and Trauma, University of Adelaide, Adelaide, Australia

1. Introduction

Osteoarthritis (OA) is characterised by progressive degenerative damage to articular cartilage, but ultimately the disease affects the whole joint, with important implications for the affected limb and the entire body (Martel-Pelletier and Pelletier, 2010; Edmonds, 2009). There has been an ongoing debate regarding the origins of OA, and specifically whether it initiates in the bone or the cartilage. The debate is somewhat artificial because it assumes that the answer must be one or the other of these possibilities. More likely, OA has multiple etiologies, which converge to produce the recognized manifestations of joint pain and stiffness and degeneration of articular cartilage. Genetic and environmental risk factors for OA, such as increased weight, female sex, joint dysplasias and malalignment, and injury, clearly contribute to the establishment and progression of this condition (Felson, 1988). However, it is most important to consider all possibilities for the underlying cause(s) for OA because our current level of understanding has failed to produce treatments for this condition that offer much more than palliation, with many sufferers proceeding to joint replacement in end stage disease.

There are well described changes that are observed in both articular cartilage and subchondral bone in OA (Martel-Pelletier and Pelletier, 2010; Edmonds, 2009; Goldring and Goldring, 2010; Kwan et al., 2010). Changes in the bone include sclerotic changes, typified by increased subchondral plate thickness and osteophyte formation, and the development of bone marrow lesions that can be visualized by MR imaging, and which seem to precede, temporally and spatially, bone cysts in the subchondral compartment (Tanamas et al., 2010). The subchondral bone does much more than provide a substrate on which the articular cartilage sits. While it does give support to the cartilage, it also offers complementarity of shape to the opposite side of the articulation, with important consequences for the joint when this congruency is lost. In addition, the predominantly trabecular structure of the subchondral bone gives compliance and shock absorption to the joint (Madry et al., 2010). It was thought that the sclerotic changes in the subchondral bone in OA made it stiffer and less compliant, resulting in increased loading of the cartilage (Radin et al., 1982) but later work showed that the bone in OA may actually be less mineralised and therefore less stiff (Day et al., 2001). The price paid for the shock absorption role of subchondral bone is the production of damage within the bone matrix by repeated loading. This bone matrix damage is repaired by bone turnover and remodeling, which are highly developed functionalities of bone cells: osteocytes to detect the damage, osteoclasts to remove the damage and osteoblasts to replace sites of damage with healthy new bone (Eriksen, 2010). A characteristic of OA is that the process of subchondral remodeling is increased (Tat et al., 2010), as visualized, for example, with bone scintigraphy (Dieppe et al., 1993). The subchondral compartment also carries essential infrastructure for the joint: it has a rich nervous supply, consistent with it being a major source of pain in joint pathology such as OA, and abundant vasculature, suggesting a significant negative impact on joint health if blood supply to this site is reduced.

2. Bone structure as a cause of OA

2.1 Bone micro-architecture in OA

Changes in the microstructure of bone in OA, particularly the subchondral plate and the trabecular bone, have been well described (Madry et al., 2010; Fazzalari and Parkinson, 1998, Shen et al, 2009, Blain et al., 2008). In human OA subjects, changes consistently include thicker trabeculae and a higher trabecular BV/TV than for normal or osteoporotic subchondral bone. In severe OA, a reduced hardness of trabecular bone from the femoral head, compared with normal subjects, was found (Dall'Ara et al., 2011). All these changes have been measured in bone taken at late stage disease, at which time they may relate to the skeleton broadly because they have been found in bone from the inter-trochanteric region of the proximal femur, which is separated by several centimeters from the affected joint (Kumarasinge et al., 2010), and in bone from the iliac crest. Nevertheless, it is not known when in human disease these changes appear and whether they are in some way causative of the disease process or simply describe it. Animal models for the most part show that changes in the subchondral bone parallel cartilage degradation (for example, Moodie et al., 2011). A recent comprehensive study by Stok et al. used longitudinal high resolution imaging to compare over time the joints of two mouse strains, one which spontaneously develops OA of the knee, and one which does not (Stok et al., 2009). The susceptible mice developed more trabecular bone, in a region specific manner, and particularly in the tibial compartment, in parallel with arthritic changes in the articular cartilage. Even in this very comprehensive study, the authors were unable to assign initiation of disease to either bone or cartilage.

2.2 Bone shape changes leading to OA

It is clear that shape deformities in bone can lead to OA in some joints, most obviously and commonly the hip and knee. There are a large number of ways in which bone shape can become sub-optimal for joint articulation and load bearing. These can be either congenital, developmental, or due to disease or fracture. Examples include malalignment of the knee (Hunter et al., 2009a) and the dysplastic hip, whether this occurs as a result of perinatal dislocation or congenitally incorrect morphology of the acetabulum or femoral head. Untreated hip dysplasia can manifest as joint laxity or impingement and decreased joint range of motion, and can result in degenerative changes, often accompanied with pain, and in OA at an early age (Mechlenburg, 2008). Genetics are likely to play a major role in OA that has bone deformity as its underlying cause. Waarsing et al. (2011a) have reported in abstract on the changes in femoral shape that occur across the lifetime of rats. The implications of their data are that deformity can develop over time, driven by genes or environment of interaction between these. Indeed, in recently published work from the same group, a range of shape 'modes' are described for the proximal femur, several of which predispose to OA, but only in carriers of susceptibility alleles of genes that associate with OA (Waarsing et al., 2011b). In human subjects, it was shown that the shape of the proximal femur, in particular the relative size of the femoral head and neck, was associated with the risk of OA (Lynch et al., 2009). Diseases such as Paget's disease of bone, or deficiency of factors essential for skeletal development and health, such as in vitamin D-dependent Rickets, can also cause bone deformities and malalignment of bones that alter the biomechanics of joints and lead to OA (Ralston, 2008). Finally, fractures that involve articular cartilage can destroy the congruency of the joint, leading to the development of OA. This is typically seen in pelvic fractures that involve the acetabulum and in tibial plateau fractures when good reduction of the fracture has not been achieved (Honkonen, 1995). All of these shape changes alter the biomechanics of joints, which is then transduced in ways that are still poorly understood into cellular and biochemical changes that lead to inflammation and eventually cartilage loss.

3. Differential gene expression in OA bone

In addition to structural changes in bone in OA, gene expression in bone from OA individuals is quite different from that in age and sex-matched controls or osteoporotic individuals. Taking RNA from trabecular bone at the intertrochanteric region of the femur, a site distal from the articular surface of the femur, Kuliwaba et al. (2000) showed that IL-6 and IL-11 mRNA were significantly less abundant in an OA group than in an age-matched control group. Osteocalcin mRNA expression was significantly greater in OA and increased significantly with age in the OA group but not in controls. Hopwood et al. (2005, 2007) performed gene microarray analysis on bone from the same region of the femur and identified a large number of differentially expressed genes in OA compared with control or osteoporotic bone. In some cases, variance of gene expression was greater in the OA bone than control or osteoporotic bone and for other genes the variance was less. For some genes, there was a clear gender-related difference. A substantial number of the top-ranking differentially expressed genes are known to play roles in osteoblasts, osteocytes and osteoclasts. Many of these genes are targets of either the WNT or the TGF-beta/BMP signalling pathways and a subset is involved in osteoclast function. The authors suggested that altered expression of these sets of genes may in part explain the altered bone remodelling observed in OA. Increased insulin-like growth factor types I and II and TGF-beta protein was reported in OA cortical bone from the iliac crest, consistent with an increased anabolic stimulus in OA bone (Dequeker et al., 1993). Also consistent with this are the observations of Truong et al. (2006), of differential expression in OA of genes encoding bone anabolic factors in trabecular bone from the proximal femur. Those data revealed elevated mRNA for alkaline phosphatase, osteocalcin, osteopontin, COL1A1, and COL1A2 in OA bone compared to control, which the authors suggested reflect possible increases in osteoblastic biosynthetic activity and/or bone turnover at the intertrochanteric region of the femur in OA. Interestingly, in the controls but not in the OA samples, positive associations were observed between a number of the molecular and histomorphometric parameters, suggesting, firstly, that the measured expression of genes in bone relates to remodeling mechanisms and, secondly, that these bone regulatory processes may be altered in OA. These data were supported by more recent work, again showing strong associations between the expression of genes, such as CTNNB1 and TWIST1 and structural and remodeling indices in control bone but not in OA and the converse with genes such as

MMP25 (Kumarasinghe et al., 2010). Gene expression has also been explored in osteoblasts taken from OA subchondral bone. Interestingly, these cells appear to retain in culture differences, compared with control cells, in the expression of important regulatory genes, with a very recent example showing increased TGF-beta in OA cells inducing increased DKK-2 (Chan et al., 2011). Silencing of either TGF-beta or DKK2 in these cells was reported to normalize the OA phenotype, including the decreased mineralization, in untreated OA osteoblasts. Strong associations were found between the ratio of RANKL/OPG mRNA and the indices of bone turnover, ES/BS and OS/BS, but only in trabecular bone from control individuals and not in OA bone (Fazzalari et al., 2001), again suggesting that bone turnover may be regulated differently in this disease. Truong et al. (2006) further speculated that the finding of differential gene expression, as well as architectural changes and differences between OA and controls at a skeletal site distal to the active site of joint degeneration, supports the concept of generalised involvement of bone in the pathogenesis of OA. The above data invite the speculation that altered expression of the genes that direct bone turnover leads to differences in bone, subchondrally or generally, which increases the risk of OA or initiates or progresses the disease. However, the limitation of the work to date is that it has all been performed in bone from end-stage disease. What is urgently required in order to better understand OA, and the role of bone in it, is longitudinal data describing gene expression and its relationship to bone turnover, across the OA disease process. It should be acknowledged that a great deal of effort has been made to identify genetic risk factors for OA through gene association studies (Spector and McGregor, 2004). Genes implicated in these association studies include VDR, AGC1, IGF-1, ER alpha, TGF-beta, cartilage matrix protein, cartilage link protein, and collagen II, IX, and XI. While some of these genes might appear to relate more to cartilage than bone, genes such as VDR, IGF-1 and TGF-beta could well be involved in the regulation of bone growth and remodeling. In discussion, these authors describe OA as a complex disease, in which genes may operate differently at different body sites and on different disease features within body sites. In addition, it is not known at what stage of development OA-related genes might influence the skeleton.

4. Vascular pathology

There is now a great deal of evidence to support the concept that vascular pathology might be directly involved in skeletal pathology (reviewed in Findlay, 2007). In particular, venous stasis, hypertension, and altered coagulability have all been reported in both animal models of OA, and in the human disease (Arnoldi et al., 1994). Since bone is highly vascular, particularly at the ends of long bones, and cartilage is avascular, vascular pathology can directly affect bone (and other tissues in the joint) but cannot directly affect articular cartilage. Some of the evidence for changes in vascularity and/or blood flow in the subchondral bone having a causal role in OA is presented below.

4.1 Impaired venous blood flow and increased intraosseous pressure in OA

Impaired venous blood flow (venous stasis) and consequent decreased outflow of blood from the articular ends of long bones, resulting in increased intraosseous pressure, has long been proposed as one causal factor in osteoarthritis. Long bones have multiple feeding and draining vessels, but the ability of the system to drain the blood is compromised once the larger draining vessels, for example the femoral vein, are blocked. Patients with severe degenerative osteoarthritis of the hip are reported to have impaired venous drainage from the juxtachondral cancellous bone across the cortex (Lucht et al., 1981). Brookes and Helal (1968) further investigated the concept that defective venous drainage is generally present in OA. Their work was based on the assumptions that there is a disturbance of osteogenesis in OA and that vascular factors are involved in normal bone turnover. They used phlebography to examine the subchondral vasculature in a large group of knee osteoarthritic patients compared with individuals with no OA symptoms. They found that the subchondral medullary sinusoids were distended only in the patients with primary OA and the contrast agent was cleared more slowly from affected knees, suggesting a more sluggish cancellous circulation. The patients with sinusoidal engorgement all had a history of diffuse aching pain in the affected bone and, for those patients treated by osteotomy, relief of pain was concomittent with resolution of the vascular engorgement. Anecdotally, the affected bone was softer than normal, as judged by ease of insertion of a needle, suggesting decreased mineral in the bone. The patient data are interesting but, since they relate to established OA, they give little clue to cause and effect. However, in the same publication, the authors described an experiment in rats, in which they ligated the draining veins from the knee and produced venous engorgement in the hind limb bones. An increased amount of trabecular bone was noted in the tibial and femoral epiphyses of these animals and both the subchondral bone plate and the calcified zone of the articular cartilage were also thickened. These very interesting observations led Brookes and Helal (1968) to propose that osteoarthritis can be promoted by venous congestion resulting in impeded microcirculation. Arnoldi wrote extensively on the role of vascular pathology in osteoarthritis and suggested a continuum of vascular changes and joint disease from OA to osteonecrosis (Arnoldi, 1994). He concluded that intact arterial inflow combined with increased resistance to venous outflow is responsible for the intraosseous venous hypertension frequently observed in established osteoarthritis, as well as in nontraumatic ischemic necrosis of bone. He further showed that increasing the intraarticular pressure in rabbits increased intraosseous pressure. This is because the drainage veins from the ends of the long bones in general lie within the joint capsule. For example, the drainage veins from the femoral neck emerge at the edge of the cartilage and are initially within the joint capsule. Thus, even small increases in articular pressure are sufficient to collapse these thin walled vessels and decrease the flow of blood. These findings suggest that increased intra-articular pressure, produced by obesity or intra-articular inflammation, could be one of the mechanisms for producing intraosseous hypertension in OA, either as a primary event in the disease or as an exacerbating factor. Kiaer et al. (1990) showed increased intraosseous pressure and hypoxia in the femoral head of hips with early osteoarthritis and in ischemic necrosis of bone. They concluded that necrosis of bone trabeculae and marrow are early manifestations of both osteoarthritis and ischemic necrosis of bone. Lee et al. (2009) used modern imaging techniques to explore the relationship between fluid dynamics in subchondral bone and OA progression. Using dynamic contrast-enhanced (DCE) MRI, they described the temporal and spatial perfusion patterns in subchondral bone in relation to the development of bone and cartilage lesions, in the Dunkin-Hartley guinea pig model of OA. They obtained evidence for decreased perfusion of the subchondral bone and fluid stasis in that model, likely due to outflow obstruction, and that these changes temporally precede, and spatially localise at, the same site as eventual bone and cartilage lesions. These data support, in a spontaneous animal model that mirrors many of the changes seen in human disease, a role for vascular changes in the subchondral bone as drivers for OA disease.

4.2 Consequences of decreased bone blood perfusion in the subchondral bone

Arnoldi (1994) discussed the concept that decreased bone blood perfusion, and the consequent decreased interstitial fluid flow in the subchondral bone, lead to ischaemia and bone death. This idea related primarily to vascular necrosis of bone, but there is some evidence that episodes of ischaemia in the subchondral bone compartment might occur also in OA. Thus, there are two potential outcomes of venous stasis in subchondral bone. The first is that poor perfusion in the subchondral bone may also result in a decrease in nourishment to the overlying cartilage, as proposed by Imhof et al. (1997). More recently, Pan et al. (2009) were one of several groups to show that small molecules can penetrate into the calcified cartilage from the subchondral bone. In elegant experiments, they used fluorescence and photobleaching methods to demonstrate that fluorescein can diffuse between subchondral bone and articular cartilage, and that these compartments form a functional unit with biochemical as well as mechanical interactions. Secondly, the mechanical strength of the subchondral bone may be adversely affected by episodes of ischaemia. What is commonly observed in both established OA and in early OA, in individuals with painful joints (Mandalia et al., 2005), are areas of subchondral bone that appear bright with magnetic resonance (MR) imaging, which are often termed bone marrow lesions (BML) (reviewed in Bassiouni, 2010 and Daheshia and Yao, 2011). Longitudinal studies have shown that the presence of BML is a potent risk factor for structural deterioration in knee OA (Felson et al., 2003; Hunter et al., 2006; Garnero et al, 2005; Zhai et al., 2006; Carrino et al., 2006; Dore et al., 2010) and future joint replacement (Tanamas et al., 2010). Enlargement of these bone marrow lesions has been strongly associated with increased cartilage loss (Mandalia et al., 2005). Conversely, a reduction in the extent of bone marrow abnormalities on MRI is associated with a decrease in cartilage degradation (Hunter et al., 2006). It has recently been shown that subchondral cysts, which are characteristic of established and severe OA, arise at the same sites as BML (Crema et al, 2010). A number of studies point to possible causal factors for BML, including mechanical loading (Bennell et al., 2010), dietary fatty acid intake (Wang et al., 2009) and total serum cholesterol and triglycerides (Davies-Tuck et al., 2009), disturbances in the latter having well established vascular implications. BML have been described as containing bone that is sclerotic, but which has reduced mineral density, perhaps rendering the area mechanically compromised (Hunter et al., 2009). Consistent with this, is the finding that BMLs are strongly associated with subchondral bone attrition (Roemer et al., 2010). Thus, episodes of venous stasis in OA may lead to loss of osteocyte viability in the corresponding regions of subchondral bone. It has been shown that loss of osteocyte viability causes increased bone turnover in order to repair damaged and necrotic bone tissue, due to activation of osteoclastic resorption (Noble et al., 2003; Cardoso et al., 2009). There may be a stage in this process, during which bone attrition leads to compromised structural support for the overlying articular cartilage.

There is good histological and biochemical evidence of increased bone remodelling in subchondral bone containing BML (Plenk et al., 1997). In addition, increased subchondral bone remodeling, detected by bone scans, has been well described in established OA, where it has been reported to predict joint space narrowing (Berger et al., 2003; MacFarlane et al., 1993). Whether the increased bone turnover is cause or effect cannot be determined in human OA, however several animal models of OA are interesting in this regard. Muraoka et al. (2007) reported that in Hartley guinea pigs, the subchondral cancellous bone was fragile before the onset of cartilage degeneration. In the rat anterior cruciate ligament transection model of OA, increased subchondral bone resorption is associated with early development of cartilage lesions, which precedes significant cartilage thinning and subchondral bone sclerosis (Hayami et al., 2006). Significantly, treatment with the anti-resorptive bisphosphonate, alendronate, in that model suppressed both subchondral bone resorption and the later development of OA symptoms in the knee joint (Hayami et al., 2004), suggesting that subchondral bone remodeling plays an important role in the pathogenesis of OA. Similarly, calcitonin reduced the levels of circulating bone turnover markers and the severity of OA lesions in the dog model of ACLT (Manicourt et al., 1999). Thus, it is likely that events in the subchondral bone have a direct effect on the overlying cartilage. Amin et al. (2009) reported on very interesting experiments in which chondrocyte survival was assessed in bovine cartilage explants in the presence or absence of subchondral bone in the explant culture. Although the authors noted several limitations of their experiments and cautioned against over-interpretation, they made several observations. They found that excision of subchondral bone from articular cartilage resulted in an increase in chondrocyte death at seven days, mainly in the superficial zone. However, the presence of the excised subchondral bone in the culture medium abrogated this increase in chondrocyte death, most likely due to soluble mediator(s) released from the subchondral bone. Amin et al. (2009a) also reported in abstract on an experiment, using the same model, but comparing normal and OA human osteochondral explants. In that experiment, chondrocyte death increased in cartilage after excision of the subchondral bone but inclusion of healthy excised bone in culture protected the cartilage. In contrast, chondrocytes were not protected by the inclusion of sclerotic OA subchondral bone. Neither the cells nor the molecules responsible for chondrocyte survival or death were identified in these experiments, and this information is required. Nevertheless, it is known that active osteoclasts produce cytokine products that are catabolic for chondrocytes, such as IL-1 beta (O'Keefe et al., 1997), and osteocytes have been shown capable of assuming a catabolic phenotype (Atkins et al., 2009). Therefore, active remodeling in the juxta-articular bone could promote a catabolic phenotype in chondrocytes in the overlying articular cartilage.

4.3 Prevalence of hypertension in OA

Patients with end-stage hip OA exhibit a high prevalence of vascular-related comorbidities (Kiefer et al., 2003) and a causal link between the progression of OA and atheromatous vascular disease and hypertension has recently been proposed (Huang et al., 1995). Uncontrolled hypertension is a strong risk factor, not only for cardiovascular disease, but also numerous end-organ morbidities. There is evidence that the consequences of hypertension are due to endothelial cell damage or dysfunction (Tektonidou et al., 2004; Korompilias et al., 2007; Zhang et al., 2007). Because both coagulation and fibrinolysis are regulated by vascular endothelial cells, hypertension is associated with increased risk of thrombotic disorders. The potential importance of altered coagulability is discussed below. There appears to be a higher incidence of hypertension in individuals with OA, although it is difficult to dissect a direct contribution of one to the other. It has been reported that generalized osteoarthrosis is significantly more common in older males with high than with low diastolic blood pressure (Lawrence et al., 1975). In the cohort described in that publication, the relationship between hypertension and osteoarthrosis was independent of obesity. Osteoarthrosis of the knee in females was reported as more frequent in hypertensive individuals, again independent of obesity. However, many of those patients were overweight or obese, as commonly observed in OA cohorts. Weinberger et al. (1989) reported that 75% of a cohort of patients with OA had symptoms associated with hypertension and heart disease, which is probably higher than an age-matched population. These data do not provide a strong link between hypertension and the initiation or progression of OA and it would be of interest to explore this relationship more in similar populations treated or untreated for their hypertension. In attempting to elucidate whether hypertension is a causal factor in OA, it is important to determine whether it is truly involved in the disease or is simply a component of the disease cluster of the 'metabolic syndrome', which includes increased BMI and obesity, hypertension, and a compilation of factors characterized by insulin resistance and the identification of 3 of the 5 criteria of abdominal obesity, elevated triglycerides, decreased high-density lipoprotein level, elevated blood pressure, and elevated fasting plasma glucose (Steinbaum, 2004).

4.4 Coagulation abnormalities in OA

Coagulation abnormalities have been described in patients with hip osteonecrosis (ON), resulting in investigation in OA as well. Intravascular coagulation, activated by a variety of underlying diseases, has been postulated as the common link leading to ischaemic insult, intraosseous thrombosis and bone necrosis. Patients with hip ON were investigated for the presence of a spectrum of thrombophilic disorders to assess whether their presence is associated with an increased risk of ON (Korompilias et al., 2004). More than 80% of these patients had a thrombotic abnormality and the authors speculated that ON may result from repetitive thrombotic or embolic phenomena that occur in the vulnerable vasculature of the femoral head. In a rabbit model of steroid-associated femoral ON, micro-angiography of the subchondral bone showed clear evidence of thrombus-blocked and leaking blood vessels (Zhang et al., 2007). Understanding of the relationship between hypercoagulable states and ON may allow pharmacologic intervention to prevent this process. The work of Cheras and Ghosh showed that changes in coagulability of the blood might also predispose to OA (Cheras et al., 1997; Ghosh and Cheras, 2001). Cheras *et al.* (1993) observed intraosseous intravascular lipid and thrombosis, particularly in the venous microvasculature, in femoral heads from patients with degenerative osteoarthritis, but not in non-osteoarthritic femoral heads. A study of femoral heads from OA patients showed frequent widespread loss of osteocyte viability, and led to the suggestion that episodic osteocyte death and elevated bone remodeling, as discussed above, could be a cause rather than a result of at least some forms of OA (Cheras et al., 1993). Intriguingly, Ghosh and Cheras (1997) found significant differences in serum fibrinogenic and fibrinolytic parameters, and lipid profiles, between an osteoarthritis group and a control group. Their data are consistent with hypercoagulability and hypofibrinolysis in OA. They described increased pro-coagulant factors in individuals with a comparatively recent diagnosis of OA and proposed that the findings of coagulation and lipid abnormalities support a possible relationship between the etiology of osteoarthritis and ischemic necrosis of bone. Interestingly, the coagulability changes were associated with evidence of increased bone turnover, possibly due to increased bone repair in OA. A potential consequence of ischemia in the subchondral bone is the loss of interstitial fluid flow that leads to cell death of osteocytes (Bakker et al., 2004). If an increased propensity for intravascular coagulation has a role in OA, treatments that normalize clotting would be expected to reduce the symptoms of OA. Although this possibility has not been well researched, Ghosh and Cheras (1997) described a study, which utilized large breed dogs with or without radiologically confirmed hip OA. The dogs were given subcutaneous Calcium Pentosan Polysulphate (CaPPS) for 4 weeks. Prior to treatment, platelet aggregability was increased in the OA group, which, like the human OA group described above, also displayed hypofibrinolysis. Interestingly, CaPPS treatment normalized these parameters and the dogs showed clinical improvement with respect to their OA symptoms. Qualitatively similar results were seen in a 24-week study in human OA subjects treated with CaPPS, although interpretation of this study was complicated by a strong placebo response. In a more recent study, sodium pentosan polysulphate was given to patients with OA of grade Kellgren-Lawrence 1 to 3 (Kumagia et al., 2010). At a dose of drug that increased INR significantly, OA symptoms improved rapidly and for the period of the study. Despite such studies, the role of this class of compound in human OA is controversial, with the possible reasons for different findings being that they are perhaps not, in fact, efficacious, or that they have been given to inappropriate cohorts, with advanced OA, or that there is variability of drug quality and potency, or the already mentioned placebo response that is common in OA. However, the basic science continues to be supportive of a therapeutic role for these compounds in OA. A recent study in a mouse model of collagenase-induced OA showed that glucosamine hydrochloride treatment inhibited destructive changes in cartilage and bone erosion and prevented osteophyte formation (Ivanovska and Dimitrova, 2011). These observations occurred in parallel with decreased expression of the bone anabolic molecule, BMP-2, in the subchondral bone and increased expression of the anti-anabolic Wnt inhibitor, DKK-1. In attempting to account for these effects, there is a large literature describing the anti-inflammatory effects of the glucosamine class of compounds, in particular with anti-inflammatory and anti-atherosclerotic effects on vascular endothelial cells (Ju et al., 2008; Largo et al., 2009). The concept that protection of vascular endothelial cells can have a beneficial effect in subchondral bone and joints is supported by the study mentioned above using a rabbit model of steroid-associated femoral ON (Zhang et al., 2007). Micro-angiography of the subchondral bone showed clear evidence of thrombus-blocked and leaking blood vessels in this disorder, which was prevented in this model by coadministration of flavinoid vascular protective agents. It has not been determined whether hypercoagulability and hypofibrinolysis precede or cause OA, or whether they are a consequence of the disease. However, familial studies by Glueck et al. (1994), in patients with ischemic necrosis of bone, indicated that genetically linked hypofibrinolysis associated with raised PAI-1 may be a major cause of osteonecrosis. Similar familial studies in osteoarthritis are indicated, in addition to prospective studies of individuals with hypercoagulability or hypofibrinolysis.

5. Summary

OA is clearly a disease that intimately involves bone, in ways that include altered gene expression in bone, altered bone structure, altered blood flow and altered biomechanics. The extent of involvement of various joint components is likely to be different in different joints and in different disease causations. In some joints, notably hips and knees, there are bone shapes, either congenital or acquired, that predispose to OA. To that extent, OA can be said to initiate in the bone. Longitudinal studies are required to investigate the causes of bone shape abnormalities and whether there might be an opportunity to intervene to maintain, particularly in hip joints, their optimal shape. What role the bone plays in the initiation and progression of 'idiopathic' or 'general' OA is still not clear, although changes can be observed in subchondral bone from its earliest manifestations. There is also evidence that agents that are known to act on bone and not directly on cartilage, such as bisphosphonate anti-resorptives, can inhibit the course of OA, at least experimentally. The data reviewed here suggest the value of investigating other agents that address bone turnover, and promote the health of the subchondral vasculature, in OA. These approaches could accompany other current management, such as weight loss, exercise programs and intra-articular lubricants, starting as early in the disease as possible. In evaluation of approaches that target the bone in OA, endpoints will benefit from new imaging modalities that are much more informative of all the compartments of the joint, cartilage, synovium, tendon and muscle, and bone.

6. Acknowledgements

Funding from the National Health and Medical Research Council of Australia is gratefully acknowledged, as is the support of the Department of Orthopaedics and Trauma at the Royal Adelaide Hospital, Adelaide, SA, Australia and the University of Adelaide.

7. Abbreviations

OA: osteoarthritis, MRI: magnetic resonance imaging, BML: bone marrow lesions, ON: osteonecrosis, BMI: body mass index, ES/BS: eroded surface/bone surface, OS/BS: osteoid surface/bone surface, RANKL: receptor activator of nuclear factor kappa B ligand, OPG: osteoprotegerin

8. References

Amin AK, Huntley JS, Simpson AH, Hall AC. Chondrocyte survival in articular cartilage: the influence of subchondral bone in a bovine model. J Bone Joint Surg Br. 2009 91:691-9.

Amin AK, Huntley JS, Simpson AH, Hamish, A, Hall AC. Bone-Cartilage Interactions: The Survival of Human Articular Chondrocytes is Influenced by Subchondral bone. Transactions 2009a ORS meeting, http://www.ors.org/web/Transactions/55/0973.PDF

Arnoldi CC. Vascular aspects of degenerative joint disorders. A synthesis. Acta Orthop Scand Suppl. 1994 261:1-82.

Atkins GJ, Welldon KJ, Holding CA, Haynes DR, Howie DW, Findlay DM. The induction of a catabolic phenotype in human primary osteoblasts and osteocytes by polyethylene particles. Biomaterials. 2009 30:3672-81.

Bakker A, Klein-Nulend J, Burger E. Shear stress inhibits while disuse promotes osteocyte apoptosis. Biochem Biophys Res Commun 2004 320:1163-8.

Bassiouni HM.Bone marrow lesions in the knee: the clinical conundrum. Int J Rheum Dis. 2010 13:196-202.

Bennell KL, Creaby MW, Wrigley TV, Bowles KA, Hinman RS, Cicuttini F, Hunter DJ. Bone marrow lesions are related to dynamic knee loading in medial knee osteoarthritis. Ann Rheum Dis. 2010 69:1151-4.

Berger CE, Kroner AH, Minai-Pour MB, Ogris E, Engel A. Biochemical markers of bone metabolism in bone marrow edema syndrome of the hip. Bone 2003 33:346-51.

Blain H, Chavassieux P, Portero-Muzy N, Bonnel F, Canovas F, Chammas M, Maury P, Delmas PD. Cortical and trabecular bone distribution in the femoral neck in osteoporosis and osteoarthritis. Bone. 2008 43:862-8.

Brookes M, Helal B. Primary osteoarthritis, venous engorgement and osteogenesis. J Bone Joint Surg Br. 1968 50:493-504.

Cardoso L, Herman BC, Verborgt O, Laudier D, Majeska RJ, Schaffler MB. Osteocyte apoptosis controls activation of intracortical resorption in response to bone fatigue. J Bone Miner Res. 2009 24:597-605.

Carrino JA, Blum J, Parellada JA, Schweitzer ME, Morrison WB. MRI of bone marrow edema-like signal in the pathogenesis of subchondral cysts. Osteoarthritis Cartilage 2006 14:1081-5.

Chan TF, Couchourel D, Abed E, Delalandre A, Duval N, Lajeunesse D. Elevated Dickkopf-2 levels contribute to the abnormal phenotype of human osteoarthritic osteoblasts. J Bone Miner Res. 2011 26:1399-410.

Cheras PA, Freemont AJ, Sikorski JM. Intraosseous thrombosis in ischemic necrosis of bone and osteoarthritis. Osteoarthritis Cartilage 1993 1:219-32.

Cheras PA, Whitaker AN, Blackwell EA, Sinton TJ, Chapman MD, Peacock KA. Hypercoagulability and hypofibrinolysis in primary osteoarthritis. Clin Orthop 1997 334:57-67.

Crema MD, Roemer FW, Zhu Y, Marra MD, Niu J, Zhang Y, Lynch JA, Javaid MK, Lewis CE, El-Khoury GY, Felson DT, Guermazi A. Subchondral cystlike lesions develop longitudinally in areas of bone marrow edema-like lesions in patients with or at risk for knee osteoarthritis: detection with MR imaging- the MOST study. Radiology. 2010 256:855-62.

Daheshia M, Yao JQ. The bone marrow lesion in osteoarthritis. Rheumatol Int. 2011 31:143-8.

Dall'Ara E, Ohman C, Baleani M, Viceconti M. Reduced tissue hardness of trabecular bone is associated with severe osteoarthritis. J Biomech. 2011 44:1593-8.

Davies-Tuck ML, Hanna F, Davis SR, Bell RJ, Davison SL, Wluka AE, Adams J, Cicuttini FM. Total cholesterol and triglycerides are associated with the development of new bone marrow lesions in asymptomatic middle-aged women - a prospective cohort study. Arthritis Res Ther. 2009 11:R181.

Day JS, Ding M, van der Linden JC, Hvid I, Sumner DR, Weinans H. A decreased subchondral trabecular bone tissue elastic modulus is associated with pre-arthritic cartilage damage. J Orthop Res. 2001 19:914-8.

Dequeker J, Mohan S, Finkelman RD, Aerssens J, Baylink DJ. Generalized osteoarthritis associated with increased insulin-like growth factor types I and II and transforming growth factor beta in cortical bone from the iliac crest. Possible mechanism of increased bone density and protection against osteoporosis. Arthritis Rheum. 1993 36:1702-8.

Dieppe P, Cushnaghan J, Young P, Kirwan J. Prediction of the progression of joint space narrowing in osteoarthritis of the knee by bone scintigraphy. Ann Rheum Dis. 1993 52:557-63.

Dore D, Martens A, Quinn S, Ding C, Winzenberg T, Zhai G, Pelletier JP, Martel-Pelletier J,

Abram F, Cicuttini F, Jones G. Bone marrow lesions predict site-specific cartilage defect development and volume loss: a prospective study in older adults. Arthritis Res Ther. 2010 12:R222.

Edmonds S. Therapeutic targets for osteoarthritis. Maturitas. 2009 63:191-4.

Eriksen EF. Cellular mechanisms of bone remodeling. Rev Endocr Metab Disord. 2010 11:219-27.

Fazzalari NL, Parkinson IH. Femoral trabecular bone of osteoarthritic and normal subjects in an age and sex matched group. Osteoarthritis Cartilage. 1998 6:377-82.

Fazzalari NL, Kuliwaba JS, Atkins GJ, Forwood MR, Findlay DM. The ratio of messenger RNA levels of receptor activator of nuclear factor kappaB ligand to osteoprotegerin correlates with bone remodeling indices in normal human cancellous bone but not in osteoarthritis. J Bone Miner Res. 2001 16:1015-27.

Felson DT. Epidemiology of hip and knee osteoarthritis. Epidemiol Rev. 1988 10:1-28

Felson DT, McLaughlin S, Goggins J, LaValley MP, Gale ME, Totterman S, Li W, Hill C, Gale D. Bone marrow edema and its relation to progression of knee osteoarthritis. Ann Intern Med. 2003; 139:330-6.

Findlay DM. Vascular pathology and osteoarthritis. Rheumatology (Oxford). 2007 46:1763-8.

Garnero P, Peterfy C, Zaim S, Schoenharting M. Bone marrow abnormalities on magnetic resonance imaging are associated with type II collagen degradation in knee osteoarthritis: a three-month longitudinal study. Arthritis Rheum 2005 52:2822-9.

Ghosh P, Cheras PA. Vascular mechanisms in osteoarthritis. Best Pract Res Clin Rheumatol 2001 15:693-709.

Glueck CJ, Glueck HI, Welch M, Freiberg R, Tracy T, Hamer T, Stroop D. Familial idiopathic osteonecrosis mediated by familial hypofibrinolysis with high levels of plasminogen activator inhibitor. Thromb Haemost 1994 71:195-8.

Goldring MB, Goldring SR. Articular cartilage and subchondral bone in the pathogenesis of osteoarthritis. Ann N Y Acad Sci. 2010 1192:230-7

Hayami T, Pickarski M, Wesolowski GA, McLane J, Bone A, Destefano J, Rodan GA, Duong L. The role of subchondral bone remodeling in osteoarthritis: reduction of cartilage degeneration and prevention of osteophyte formation by alendronate in the rat anterior cruciate ligament transection model. Arthritis Rheum 2004 50:1193-206.

Hayami T, Pickarski M, Zhuo Y, Wesolowski GA, Rodan GA, Duong le T. Characterization of articular cartilage and subchondral bone changes in the rat anterior cruciate ligament transection and meniscectomized models of osteoarthritis. Bone 2006 38:234-43.

Hopwood B, Gronthos S, Kuliwaba JS, Robey PG, Findlay DM, Fazzalari NL. Identification of differentially expressed genes between osteoarthritic and normal trabecular bone from the intertrochanteric region of the proximal femur using cDNA microarray analysis. Bone. 2005 36:635-44.

Hopwood B, Tsykin A, Findlay DM, Fazzalari NL. Microarray gene expression profiling of osteoarthritic bone suggests altered bone remodelling, WNT and transforming growth factor-beta/bone morphogenic protein signalling. Arthritis Res Ther. 2007 9:R100.

Huang PL, Huang Z, Mashimo H, Bloch KD, Moskowitz MA, Bevan JA, Fishman MC. Hypertension in mice lacking the gene for endothelial nitric oxide synthase. Nature 1995 377:239-42.

Hunter DJ, Zhang Y, Niu J, Goggins J, Amin S, LaValley MP, Guermazi A, Genant H, Gale D, Felson DT. Increase in bone marrow lesions associated with cartilage loss: a longitudinal magnetic resonance imaging study of knee osteoarthritis. Arthritis Rheum 2006 54:1529-35.

Hunter DJ, Gerstenfeld L, Bishop G, Davis AD, Mason ZD, Einhorn TA, Maciewicz RA, Newham P, Foster M, Jackson S, Morgan EF. Bone marrow lesions from osteoarthritis knees are characterized by sclerotic bone that is less well mineralized. Arthritis Res Ther. 2009 11:R11.

Hunter DJ, Sharma L, Skaife T. Alignment and osteoarthritis of the knee. J Bone Joint Surg Am. 2009a 91 Suppl 1:85-9.

Imhof H, Breitenseher M, Kainberger F, Trattnig S. Degenerative joint disease: cartilage or vascular disease? Skeletal Radiol 1997 26:398-403.

Ivanovska N, Dimitrova P. Bone resorption and remodeling in murine collagenase-induced osteoarthritis after administration of glucosamine. Arthritis Res Ther. 2011 13:R44.

Ju Y, Hua J, Sakamoto K, Ogawa H, Nagaoka I. Modulation of TNF-alpha-induced endothelial cell activation by glucosamine, a naturally occurring amino monosaccharide. Int J Mol Med. 2008 22:809-15.

Kiaer T, Pedersen NW, Kristensen KD, Starklint H. Intra-osseous pressure and oxygen tension in avascular necrosis and osteoarthritis of the hip. J Bone Joint Surg Br. 1990 72:1023-30.

Kiefer FN, Neysari S, Humar R, Li W, Munk VC, Battegay EJ. Hypertension and angiogenesis. Curr Pharm Des 2003 9:1733-44.

Korompilias AV, Ortel TL, Urbaniak JR. Coagulation abnormalities in patients with hip osteonecrosis. Orthop Clin North Am 2004 35:265-71.

Kuliwaba JS, Findlay DM, Atkins GJ, Forwood MR, Fazzalari NL. Enhanced expression of osteocalcin mRNA in human osteoarthritic trabecular bone of the proximal femur is associated with decreased expression of interleukin-6 and interleukin-11 mRNA. J Bone Miner Res. 2000 15:332-41.

Kumagai K, Shirabe S, Miyata N, Murata M, Yamauchi A, Kataoka Y, Niwa M. Sodium pentosan polysulfate resulted in cartilage improvement in knee osteoarthritis--an open clinical trial. BMC Clin Pharmacol. 2010 10:7.

Kumarasinghe DD, Perilli E, Tsangari H, Truong L, Kuliwaba JS, Hopwood B, Atkins GJ, Fazzalari NL. Critical molecular regulators, histomorphometric indices and their correlations in the trabecular bone in primary hip osteoarthritis. Osteoarthritis Cartilage. 2010 18:1337-44.

Kwan Tat S, Lajeunesse D, Pelletier JP, Martel-Pelletier J. Targeting subchondral bone for treating osteoarthritis: what is the evidence? Best Pract Res Clin Rheumatol. 2010 24:51-70.

Largo R, Martínez-Calatrava MJ, Sánchez-Pernaute O, Marcos ME, Moreno-Rubio J, Aparicio C, Egido J, Herrero-Beaumont G. Effect of a high dose of glucosamine on systemic and tissue inflammation in an experimental model of atherosclerosis aggravated by chronic arthritis. Am J Physiol Heart Circ Physiol. 2009 297:H268-76.

Lawrence JS Hypertension in relation to musculoskeletal disorders. Ann Rheum Dis 1975 34:451-56.

Lee JH, Dyke JP, Ballon D, Ciombor DM, Rosenwasser MP, Aaron RK. Subchondral fluid dynamics in a model of osteoarthritis: use of dynamic contrast-enhanced magnetic resonance imaging. Osteoarthritis Cartilage. 2009 17:1350-5.

Lucht U, Djurhuus JC, Sørensen S, Bünger C, Sneppen O The relationship between increasing intraarticular pressures and intraosseous pressures in the juxtaarticular bones. An experimental investigation in dogs. Acta Orthop Scand. 1981 52:491-5.

Lynch JA, Parimi N, Chaganti RK, Nevitt MC, Lane NE; Study of Osteoporotic Fractures Research Group. The association of proximal femoral shape and incident radiographic hip OA in elderly women. Osteoarthritis Cartilage. 2009 17:1313-8.

Macfarlane DG, Buckland-Wright JC, Lynch J, Fogelman I. A study of the early and late 99technetium scintigraphic images and their relationship to symptoms in osteoarthritis of the hands. Br J Rheumatol 1993 32:977-81.

Madry H, van Dijk CN, Mueller-Gerbl M. The basic science of the subchondral bone. Knee Surg Sports Traumatol Arthrosc. 2010 18:419-33.

Mandalia V, Fogg AJ, Chari R, Murray J, Beale A, Henson JH. Bone bruising of the knee.Clin Radiol 2005; 60:627-36.

Manicourt DH, Altman RD, Williams JM, Devogelaer JP, Druetz-Van Egeren A, Lenz ME, Pietryla D, Thonar EJ. Treatment with calcitonin suppresses the responses of bone, cartilage, and synovium in the early stages of canine experimental osteoarthritis and significantly reduces the severity of the cartilage lesions. Arthritis Rheum 1999 42:1159-67.

Martel-Pelletier J, Pelletier JP. Is osteoarthritis a disease involving only cartilage or other articular tissues? Eklem Hastalik Cerrahisi. 2010 21:2-14.

Mechlenburg I. Evaluation of Bernese periacetabular osteotomy: prospective studies examining projected load-bearing area, bone density, cartilage thickness and migration. Acta Orthop Suppl. 2008 79:4-43.

Moodie JP, Stok KS, Müller R, Vincent TL, Shefelbine SJ. Multimodal imaging demonstrates concomitant changes in bone and cartilage after destabilisation of the medial meniscus and increased joint laxity. Osteoarthritis Cartilage. 2011 19:163-70.

Muraoka T, Hagino H, Okano T, Enokida M, Teshima R. Role of subchondral bone in osteoarthritis development: a comparative study of two strains of guinea pigs with and without spontaneously occurring osteoarthritis. Arthritis Rheum. 2007 56:3366-74.

Noble BS, Peet N, Stevens HY, Brabbs A, Mosley JR, Reilly GC, Reeve J, Skerry TM, Lanyon LE. Mechanical loading: biphasic osteocyte survival and targeting of osteoclasts for bone destruction in rat cortical bone. Am J Physiol Cell Physiol. 2003 284:C934-43.

O'Keefe RJ, Teot LA, Singh D, Puzas JE, Rosier RN, Hicks DG. Osteoclasts constitutively express regulators of bone resorption: an immunohistochemical and in situ hybridization study. Lab Invest. 1997 76:457-65.

Pan J, Zhou X, Li W, Novotny JE, Doty SB, Wang L. In situ measurement of transport between subchondral bone and articular cartilage. J Orthop Res. 2009 27:1347-52.

Plenk H Jr, Hofmann S, Eschberger J, Gstettner M, Kramer J, Schneider W, Engel A. Histomorphology and bone morphometry of the bone marrow edema syndrome of the hip.Clin Orthop Relat Res 1997 334:73-84.

Radin EL, Swann DA, Paul IL, McGrath PJ. Factors influencing articular cartilage wear in vitro. Arthritis Rheum. 1982 25:974-80.

Ralston SH. Pathogenesis of Paget's disease of bone. Bone. 2008 43:819-25.

Roemer FW, Neogi T, Nevitt MC, Felson DT, Zhu Y, Zhang Y, Lynch JA, Javaid MK, Crema MD, Torner J, Lewis CE, Guermazi A. Subchondral bone marrow lesions are highly associated with, and predict subchondral bone attrition longitudinally: the MOST study. Osteoarthritis Cartilage. 2010 18:47-53.

Shen Y, Zhang ZM, Jiang SD, Jiang LS, Dai LY. Postmenopausal women with osteoarthritis and osteoporosis show different ultrastructural characteristics of trabecular bone of the femoral head. BMC Musculoskelet Disord. 2009 10:35.

Spector TD, MacGregor AJ. Risk factors for osteoarthritis: genetics. Osteoarthritis Cartilage. 2004 12 Suppl A:S39-44.

Steinbaum SR. The metabolic syndrome: an emerging health epidemic in women. Prog Cardiovasc Dis 2004 46:321-36.

Stok KS, Pelled G, Zilberman Y, Kallai I, Goldhahn J, Gazit D, Müller R. Revealing the interplay of bone and cartilage in osteoarthritis through multimodal imaging of murine joints. Bone. 2009 45:414-22.

Tanamas SK, Wluka AE, Pelletier JP, Martel-Pelletier J, Abram F, Wang Y, Cicuttini FM. The association between subchondral bone cysts and tibial cartilage volume and risk of joint replacement in people with knee osteoarthritis: a longitudinal study. Arthritis Res Ther. 2010 12:R58.

Tektonidou MG, Anapliotou M, Vlachoyiannopoulos P, Moutsopoulos HM. Presence of systemic autoimmune disorders in patients with autoimmune thyroid diseases. Ann Rheum Dis 2004 63:1159-61.

Truong LH, Kuliwaba JS, Tsangari H, Fazzalari NL. Differential gene expression of bone anabolic factors and trabecular bone architectural changes in the proximal femoral shaft of primary hip osteoarthritis patients. Arthritis Res Ther. 2006 8:R188.

Waarsing JH, Botter SM, Gabriëls S, Van der Pluijm I, Weinans H. The Life-Course of Femoral Shape in Mice. Transactions 2011a ORS meeting, http://www.ors.org/web/Transactions/57/0369.PDF

Waarsing JH, Kloppenburg M, Slagboom PE, Kroon HM, Houwing-Duistermaat JJ, Weinans H, Meulenbelt I. Osteoarthritis susceptibility genes influence the association between hip morphology and osteoarthritis. Arthritis Rheum. 2011b 63:1349-54.

Wang Y, Davies-Tuck ML, Wluka AE, Forbes A, English DR, Giles GG, O'Sullivan R, Cicuttini FM. Dietary fatty acid intake affects the risk of developing bone marrow lesions in healthy middle-aged adults without clinical knee osteoarthritis: a prospective cohort study. Arthritis Res Ther. 2009 11:R63.

Weinberger M, Tierney WM, Booher P. Common problems experienced by adults with osteoarthritis. Arthritis Care Res 1989; 2:94-100.

Zhai G, Blizzard L, Srikanth V, Ding C, Cooley H, Cicuttini F, Jones G. Correlates of knee pain in older adults: Tasmanian Older Adult Cohort Study. Arthritis Rheum 2006 55:264-71.

Zhang G, Qin L, Sheng H, Yeung KW, Yeung HY, Cheung WH, Griffith J, Chan CW, Lee KM, Leung KS. Epimedium-derived phytoestrogen exert beneficial effect on preventing steroid-associated osteonecrosis in rabbits with inhibition of both thrombosis and lipid-deposition. Bone. 2007 40:685-92.

8

The Relationship Between Gait Mechanics and Radiographic Disease Severity in Knee Osteoarthritis

Ershela L. Sims et al.[1,2*]
[1]*Department of Biological Anthropology and Anatomy, Duke University*
[2]*Applied Science Department, NC School of Science and Mathematics*
USA

1. Introduction

Osteoarthritis (OA) is a multifactorial degenerative joint disease affecting more than 10% of adults over the age of 55 (Baliunas et al., 2002; Miyazaki et al., 2002). Radiographic indications of OA can be found in at least one joint in most people over 65; with prevalence rates as high as 80% in people over the age of 75, depending on the joint (Helmick et al., 2008; Lawrence et al., 2008; Lawrence et al., 1998; Sangha, 2000). Systematic autopsy studies reveal near universal pathological signs of OA in people over age 65 (Sangha, 2000). It is the most prevalent type of arthritis (Lawrence et al., 2008) and the knee is one of the most commonly affected joints. Symptomatic knee OA affects 4.3M adults over age 60 (Dillon et al., 2006). Moreover, OA of the knee is particularly debilitating in terms of normal locomotor activity and as such has devastating physical and psychological effects (Maly et al., 2006; Nebel et al., 2009).

Characterized by pain and lack of mobility, osteoarthritis of the knee may have a profound influence on gait patterns. Among the most commonly reported differences are slower walking speeds, shortened step lengths, larger double support times (the period of time in the gait cycle when both feet are in contact with the ground), as well as decreased hip range of motion and knee range of motion angles as compared to a non-arthritic population (Al-Zahrani & Bakheit, 2002; Andriacchi et al., 1977; Baliunas et al., 2002; Brinkmann & Perry, 1985; Kaufman et al., 2001; Messier et al., 2005a; Messier et al., 1992). Patients also exhibit decreased knee angular velocity (Messier, 1994; Messier et al., 1992), a change compensated for by increased hip angular velocity (Messier, 1994). In addition, patients with knee OA have been shown to demonstrate both altered ground reaction forces and increased dynamic

*Francis J. Keefe[3], Daniel Schmitt[1], Virginia B. Kraus[4], Mathew W. Williams[5], Tamara Somers[3], Paul Riordan[3] and Farshid Guilak[6]
[1]*Department of Biological Anthropology and Anatomy, Duke University, USA*
[3]*Department of Psychiatry and Behavioral Science, Duke University, USA*
[4]*Department of Rheumatology and Immunology, Duke University, USA*
[5]*Department of Emergency Medicine, Wake Forest Baptist Medical Center, USA*
[6]*Department of Surgery, Duke University, USA*

loads on the medial compartments of the knee as characterized by the external knee adduction moment compared to healthy, age-matched controls (Al-Zahrani & Bakheit, 2002; Baliunas et al., 2002; Messier et al., 1992; Mundermann et al., 2005). Research has determined that disability is a major consequence of lower limb OA (Creamer et al., 2000). The pain, stiffness, and decreased range of motion associated with OA often interfere with activities of daily living; of the 10% of Americans over 55 years old who are affected by knee OA, a quarter have clinically significant disability (Baliunas et al., 2002). In fact, knee OA has been referred to as the leading cause of impaired mobility in the elderly (Guccione et al., 1994).

The etiology of knee OA is not entirely clear. In the past, the scientific community dismissed OA as the inevitable age-related wear-and-tear of articular cartilage. However, given the debilitating effects of the disease on the general population, this area of research has grown and studies indicate that OA is a dynamic process with a multifactorial etiology that is more complex than suggested by the age-related wear-and-tear model (Anderson-MacKenzie et al., 2005; Andriacchi et al., 2004; Senior, 2000). OA research has identified a number of risk factors for knee OA. These include obesity, gender, age, repeated trauma to joint tissues, and lower extremity injuries. Obesity has been found to be a risk factor for both the development (Davis et al., 1989; Felson et al., 1997; Hart & Spector, 1993) and progression of OA (Reijman et al., 2007; Sharif et al., 1995). Women have a significantly greater risk of developing knee OA than men (Srikanth et al., 2005), with the ratio of women to men affected by knee OA as high as 4:1 (Sangha, 2000). A study by Lohmander et al., determined that previous ACL injury in female soccer players was associated with a high prevalence of knee OA (Lohmander et al., 2004). As previously mentioned, people with osteoarthritis of the knee exhibit aberrant gait patterns compared to their non-arthritic counterparts. Some gait changes observed in knee OA may be indicative of compensatory mechanisms, while others are associated with the onset and development of disease. Multiple studies have that suggested many of the associated gait abnormalities attempt to compensate for joint instability (Al-Zahrani & Bakheit, 2002) or seek to minimize loading of the affected joint and thus mitigate pain (Baliunas et al., 2002; Kaufman et al., 2001; Manetta et al., 2002; Mundermann et al., 2005; Mundermann et al., 2004). In order to better understand the variety of factors influencing OA as well as its progression, researchers have systematically examined a number of variables that might explain variations in gait and mobility in persons with knee OA (Cooper et al., 2000; Hurwitz et al., 2002; Lohmander et al., 2004; Nebel et al., 2009; Syed & Davis, 2000). Among the variables that have been examined are: static knee alignment (Hurwitz et al., 2002), body composition (Messier, 1994; Messier et al., 2005b; Syed & Davis, 2000), pain and psychosocial variables (Maly et al., 2005; Nebel et al., 2009; Somers et al., 2009), previous lower extremity injury (Lohmander et al., 2004) and even gait biomechanics (Miyazaki et al., 2002; Teichtahl et al., 2003). Some studies further investigated these relationships to determine which factors influence gait variation by sex (McKean et al., 2007; Sims et al., 2009a) and by race (Sims et al., 2009b). One such study found that radiographic disease severity accounted for 21% of the variance in knee adduction moment in men, while it did not contribute at all in women (Sims et al., 2009a).

It has long been hypothesized that changes in gait and joint biomechanics impact the onset and progression of OA. Mechanical factors such as joint loading and knee adduction moment during walking have been linked to the progression of knee OA (Hurwitz et al., 2002; Miyazaki et al., 2002; Mundermann et al., 2005). A study by Miyazaki et al., found that baseline knee adduction moment could predict radiographic OA progression (Miyazaki et al., 2002). Alteration of mechanical loads, often through ligament abnormality, has been linked to the development of OA and pathological changes associated with the disease. Studies have shown that cartilage dynamically responds and adapts to mechanical stimuli (Smith et al., 2000). With this in mind, Andriacchi and colleagues proposed a model of the disease with two stages: initiation and progression (Andriacchi et al., 2004). In the initiation phase, a physical injury that may be chronic or traumatic such as ACL injury causes a significant shift in the load bearing contact site of the joint surface. Unaccustomed to frequent loading and unable to adapt due to time constraints or aging, the newly stressed cartilage becomes damaged. In the progression phase, the degeneration of the cartilage passes an irreversibility threshold that leaves the tissue vulnerable to further loads and progressive damage (Andriacchi et al., 2004). Kinetically, the pathogenesis of OA is strongly associated with the knee adduction moment (Amin et al., 2004; Baliunas et al., 2002; Hurwitz et al., 2002). Individuals with increased knee adduction moment are more likely to develop chronic knee pain, which is most frequently associated with OA (Amin et al., 2004) and OA subjects with greater knee adduction moments tend to have more severe OA (Mundermann et al., 2005; Mundermann et al., 2004; Sharma et al., 1998).

The relationship between joint mechanics and radiographic disease severity is not yet fully understood. Some previous research has shown that radiographic OA correlates poorly with functional limitation (Summers et al., 1988), while other research has found that change in radiographic OA is related to the incidence of severe functional limitation (White et al., 2010). Nebel and colleagues found that radiographic disease severity accounted for as much as 18% of the variance in knee range of motion and 23% of the variance in peak vertical ground reaction force (Nebel et al., 2009). One factor that might explain these varied results is study design. Studies differ with regard to the level(s) of radiographic disease being examined as well as the particular lower extremity biomechanics that are investigated. Many investigations of the biomechanics of gait in persons with knee OA have been based on a population of patients with moderate and/or severe OA (Baliunas et al., 2002; Kaufman et al., 2001; Landry et al., 2007). Studies that focus solely on OA patients with severe disease have provided beneficial information on gait changes associated with end stage disease. Unfortunately, however, these studies tell us little about the progression of OA or how mild and moderate stages differ from end stage disease. Investigations of gait mechanics across multiple levels of disease severity (mild, moderate, and severe) can provide needed information on the mechanical processes of OA disease progression. Some studies have investigated the effect of increasing levels of radiographic osteoarthritis disease severity on gait parameters (Astephen et al., 2008; Sharma et al., 1998; Wilson et al., 2011; Zeni & Higginson, 2010). However, these studies have largely focused on biomechanical variables associated with joint loading. Sharma and colleagues found that there is a significant relationship between the adduction moment and radiographic OA disease severity, even after controlling for age, sex, and pain level (Sharma et al., 1998). Another study found that the magnitude of the knee adduction moment during stance and the magnitude of the knee flexion angle during gait are associated with structural knee OA severity measured from radiographs in patients clinically diagnosed with mild to moderate levels of disease (Wilson et al., 2011). Finally, a study of patients with moderate and severe radiographic OA found that OA patients had significantly lower knee and ankle joint moments, joint excursion, and ground reaction forces when walking at self selected speeds (Zeni & Higginson, 2010). However, when they accounted for speed in the statistical analysis, the only significant difference was knee joint excursion. The current study seeks to add new data to this discussion by not only investigating variables associated with loading of the knee, but also spatiotemporal variables that are often reduced in patients with knee OA (Györy et al., 1976).

While our group has published other studies on gait mechanics of an OA population (Nebel et al., 2009; Sims et al., 2009a; Sims et al., 2009b; Somers et al., 2009) that involve radiographic findings, this study examines that link in much more detail. The purpose of this study was to further our understanding of the relationship between radiographic disease severity and gait patterns in persons with knee OA. This study not only focused on gait variables in patients with severe OA, it also examined gait variables in patients across all severity levels (mild, moderate, and severe). We predicted that more severe knee OA would correlate positively with increased gait disability measured through slower walking speed, shorter strides, lower peak vertical forces, greater knee adduction moments, smaller loading rates and a more limited knee range of motion. We further hypothesized that significant differences in gait mechanics would exist between the three radiographic disease severity levels, even after controlling for speed.

2. Methods

2.1 Participants

A total of 189 (46 men, 143 women) patients with radiographic OA in at least one knee and persistent knee pain participated in this study. Study entry required that patients meet the American College of Rheumatology criteria for osteoarthritis of the knee (Altman et al., 1986), along with the following inclusion criteria: body mass index (BMI) greater than 25 kg/m^2 and less than 42 kg/m^2, chronic knee pain, and no other weight bearing joint affected by OA as assessed by clinical examination. Exclusion criteria included: a significant medical conditions that would increase risk of an adverse experience (e.g. myocardial infarction), already involved in regular exercise, an abnormal cardiac response to exercise, a non-OA inflammatory anthropathy, and regular use of corticosteroids. All data presented were collected as part of a baseline evaluation of a subset of the participants enrolled in an ongoing randomized trial (OA Life #NCT00305890) evaluating the separate and combined effects of 1) lifestyle behavioral weight management and 2) pain coping skills training interventions for knee OA. Data were collected at the baseline evaluation prior to randomization to treatment conditions. The study was approved by the Duke University Medical Center Institutional Review Board, and all participants provided informed consent.

Weight-bearing, fixed-flexion (30 degrees) posteroanterior radiographs of both knees were taken with the SynaFlexer™ X-ray positioning frame (Synarc, San Francisco, CA) (Peterfy et al., 2003). The x-rays were scored by a grader with high intra- and inter-rater reliability (Addison et al., 2009), and radiographic disease severity was established using the Kellgren and Lawrence (K/L) radiographic grading system (Kellgren & Lawrence, 1957). This system rates the level of disease on a scale of 0-4, with a score of 0 representing no disease, 1 representing mild disease, 2 representing moderate disease, 3 representing moderate to severe disease, and 4 representing severe disease. In addition to the standard system, OA severity levels were created for the current study, and designated as follows: mild (K/L =1), moderate (K/L= 2 or 3), and severe (K/L = 4); limbs with K/L<1 were excluded from analyses. For subjects with bilateral knee OA, the limb with the highest K/L grade was recorded as the most affected limb and was the only limb used in all data analyses. The breakdown of participants with unilateral versus bilateral knee OA was 149 bilateral and 40 unilateral.

2.2 Protocol

Three-dimensional kinematic data were collected using a motion analysis system (Motion Analysis Inc, Santa Rosa, CA). In preparation for data collection, patients completed three practice trials along a 30 meter walkway at two speeds: the speed at which they normally perform their daily walking activities (normal) and the maximum speed they felt comfortable achieving (fast). These two speeds were chosen in order to assess the speed at which the participants are most comfortable and to determine how their gait mechanics changed when presented with a challenge. Gait velocity was measured using two wireless infrared photocell timing devices (Brower Timing Systems, Draper Utah) positioned 5 meters apart and the patient's target walking velocity for each speed was determined. Following the practice trials, kinematic data were collected at 60Hz. Reflective markers were placed bilaterally at the following landmarks: anterior superior iliac spine, thigh, lateral knee (at the joint line), shank, lateral malleolus, calcaneus, and foot (2nd webspace). A marker was also placed at the superior aspect of the L5-sacral interface to aid in defining the pelvis. In addition, markers were placed bilaterally on the medial femoral condyle and medial malleolus for collection of a static trial. After completion of the static trial, the 4 medial markers were removed. Patients performed five walking trials along the walkway at each of the self-selected speeds.

Time synchronized ground reaction force data were collected at 1200Hz using AMTI force platforms (Advanced Medical Technologies Inc., Watertown, MA). Variability in walking velocity for each speed was restricted to ±5%; trials outside of this range or trials during which the subject did not contact at least one of the force plates cleanly were repeated. EvaRT (Motion Analysis Inc, Santa Rosa CA) software was used to track the reflective markers and condition the data. The raw data were smoothed using a 4th order, recursive Butterworth filter with a 6Hz cutoff frequency. Three trials at each speed in which all markers were identified and the subject had clean contact with the force plate were averaged to yield kinetic and kinematic data. The following variables were measured: velocity, stride frequency, stride length, support time, peak vertical ground reaction force, knee range of motion across the entire gait cycle, and peak knee adduction moment. Loading rate and time to peak vertical ground reaction force were also determined from measured ground reaction forces. These outcome measures were computed using OrthoTrak 6.3 (Motion Analysis Inc, Santa Rosa CA). Stride length data were normalized to subject height, ground reaction force data was normalized to body weight, and the adduction moment data was normalized to height and weight. Since the current study does not include a control population for the basis of comparison, mean values the gait measures will be compared to control data acquired from the literature. Both sets of control kinematic data were collected at 60Hz using a Motion Analysis system and kinetic data were collected using two force platforms.

2.3 Statistical analysis

Statistical analysis was performed using SPSS (version 12.0.1 for windows, SPSS, Inc Chicago IL). Correlation between level of OA and the gait variables was evaluated using

Pearson's correlation coefficient (r), and significance level was adjusted accordingly to $p<0.005$ (Bonferroni's adjustment). This analysis was performed at each speed (normal and fast). A 1x3 analysis of variance was used to compare means for velocity and knee range of motion for the different levels of radiographic disease severity at each speed ($\alpha=0.05$). Since it has been reported that support time is influenced by walking speed (Andriacchi et al., 1977), a 1x3 analysis of covariance was used to compare means for support time for the different levels of radiographic disease severity at each speed ($\alpha=0.05$). Since previous research has also determined that the magnitude of the vertical ground reaction force is affected by walking speed (Andriacchi et al., 1977), means for peak vertical ground reaction force, loading rate, and time to peak were compared to level of radiographic disease severity at each speed level using an analysis of covariance as well. Post-hoc testing (LSD) was performed when necessary.

3. Results

Descriptive statistics for subject demographics are presented in Table 1 and gait characteristics for the OA subjects at both speeds are given in Table 2. Demographics and gait mechanics were characteristic of a population of overweight OA patients with varying degrees of radiographic severity (Table 3).

Variable	Mean (SD)	% (n)
Age (years)	58.54 (9.72)	
Height (m)	1.67 (0.081)	
Weight (kg)	94.74 (16.22)	
BMI (kg/m²)	34.17 (4.36)	
Sex:		
Female		76 (143)
Male		24 (46)
Race:		
Black		35 (66)
White		63 (119)
Other		2 (4)
Disease severity:		
Mild		12 (23)
Moderate		61 (116)
Severe		27 (50)

Table 1. Descriptive Statistics for Subject Demographics. BMI: Body Mass Index.

Variable	Normal Speed	Fast Speed
Velocity (m/s)	1.123 (0.190)	1.504 (0.301)
Stride Frequency	0.903 (0.086)	1.111 (0.122)
Stride Length (m)	1.193 (0.172)	1.374 (0.221)
Support Time (%)	63.17 (3.37)	60.77 (3.77)
KROM (degrees)	57.85 (9.36)	59.64(8.58)
PVF (BW)	1.047 (0.077)	1.154 (0.126)
KAM(%BW*HT)	0.367(0.200)	0.380 (0.197)
Loading Rate (%BW/s)	9.26 (3.46)	15.11 (7.47)
Time to Peak (s)	0.204 (0.056)	0.137 (0.035)

Table 2. Gait mechanics at self selected normal and fast speeds. All values are mean (SD). KROM: knee range of motion; PVF: peak vertical ground reaction force; KAM: knee adduction moment.

Variable	Current Study	Messier 1992	Zeni 2009	Kaufman 2001
Velocity (m/s)	1.123 (0.190)	1.097 (0.359)		1.090 (0.11)
Stride Length (m)	1.193 (0.172)	1.196 (0.251)		
Support Time (%)	63.17 (3.37)	64.01 (0.43)		
KROM (degrees)	57.85 (9.36)			54.00 (7.00)
PVF (BW)	1.047 (0.077)		1.048 (0.05)	
KAM(%BW*HT)	0.367(0.20)	0.150 (0.03)		0.39 (0.28)
Loading Rate (%BW/s)	9.26 (3.46)	20.61 (2.34)	8.33 (1.44)	

Table 3. Comparison of the gait mechanics from the current study, at a normal self-selected walking speed, to data from the literature (Kaufman et al., 2001; Messier et al., 1992; Zeni & Higginson, 2010). All values are mean (SD). KROM: knee range of motion; PVF: peak vertical ground reaction force; KAM: knee adduction moment.

Variable	Current Study		Messier, 2005	Kaufman, 2001
Velocity (m/s)	1.123 (0.190)	↓	1.296 (0.084)*	1.17 (0.14)
Stride Length† (m)	1.193 (0.172)	↓	1.307 (0.050)†	
Support Time (%)	63.17 (3.37)	↑	61.14 (0.65)**	
KROM (degrees)	57.85 (9.36)			60.0 (4.0)
KAM (%BW*HT)	0.367(0.200)			0.360 (0.36)
Loading Rate (%BW/s)	9.26 (3.46)	↓	20.13 (2.48) ‡	

Table 4. Comparison of gait mechanics of OA patients at a normal self-selected walking speed to control subject data from the literature (Kaufman et al., 2001; Messier et al., 2005a). All values are mean (SD). KROM: knee range of motion; PVF: peak vertical ground reaction force; KAM: knee adduction moment. Statistically significant differencs: † denotes $p<0.05$, * denotes $p<0.005$ and denotes ‡ $p<0.0001$. **For support time: $p<0.06$

OA patients in this study walked slower, had a shorter stride length, smaller knee range of motion, spent more time in the support phase and had a smaller loading rate than their counterparts without OA (Table 4).

3.1 Correlations

None of the spatiotemporal variables showed a strong correlation with radiographic disease severity. However, a few variables had a weak statistically significant correlation with K/L grade (Table 4). Knee range of motion (KROM) was inversely correlated with radiographic disease severity ($p<0.001$) at both self selected speeds and peak vertical ground reaction force was inversely correlated with radiographic disease severity ($p<0.005$) at both speeds. Stated another way, subjects in this study with more severe radiographic disease severity walked with a smaller knee range of motion and had smaller ground reaction forces than their counterparts with less severe radiographic disease severity.

Variable	Normal Speed	Fast Speed
KROM (degrees)	r = -0.306†	r = -0.307†
PVF (% BW)	r = -0.240*	r = -0.230*

Table 5. Correlations of radiographic disease severity with gait data. All correlations were significant ($p<0.005$)* and ($p<0.001$) †. KROM: knee range of motion; PVF: peak vertical ground reaction force.

3.2 Analysis of variance

The results of the analysis of variance for velocity by level of radiographic disease severity (Figure 1) demonstrated that there was a significant difference in walking velocity between mild and severe OA and moderate and severe OA at the fast speed. There were no significant differences in mean walking velocity by severity level at the normal walking speed. Differences in mean knee range of motion and mean peak vertical ground reaction force by level of OA severity existed at both speeds (Figures 2 and 3). Patients with severe OA had the smallest knee range of motion and the smallest peak vertical ground reaction force in all instances. The statistical analysis revealed significant differences in knee range of motion between patients with mild and severe OA at the normal and fast speeds as well as moderate and severe OA at the normal and fast speeds (Figure 2). The analysis of variance for stride length did not show any differences by OA severity level at either speed.

The results of the analyses of covariance for support time, knee adduction moment and loading rate did not reveal any significant differences between the different levels of radiographic disease severity at either speed. While not significantly different from the other groups, patients with moderate OA spent the least amount of time in the support phase of the gait cycle at the normal walking speed. At the fast speed, the more severe the level of OA, the more time spent in support. While these differences were not statistically significant, loading rate at the normal self selected speed was greater in patients with mild OA and decreased with increasing level of OA. At the fast speed, variation in loading rate by OA severity was inconsistent. Again, while not significantly different, mean knee adduction moment decreased with increasing radiographic severity at the normal walking speed and it increased with increasing radiographic severity at the fast speed. The analysis of covariance for peak vertical ground reaction force (Figure 3) determined that there was a statistically significant difference between moderate and mild OA and moderate and severe OA at the fast speed. Statistically significant differences in mean peak vertical ground reaction force also existed between the levels of radiographic OA at the normal speed.

The analysis of covariance for the time to peak vertical reaction force (Figure 4) did not reveal any differences in time to peak for the different levels of radiographic disease severity.

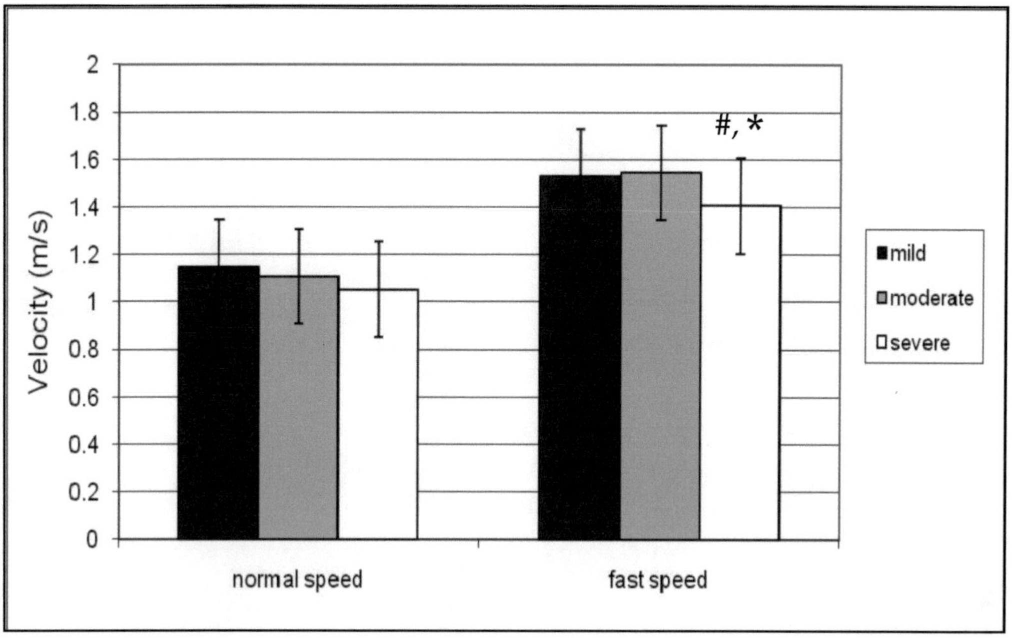

Fig. 1. Analysis of variance results for velocity (# denotes a significant difference from mild OA and * denotes significant difference from moderate OA)

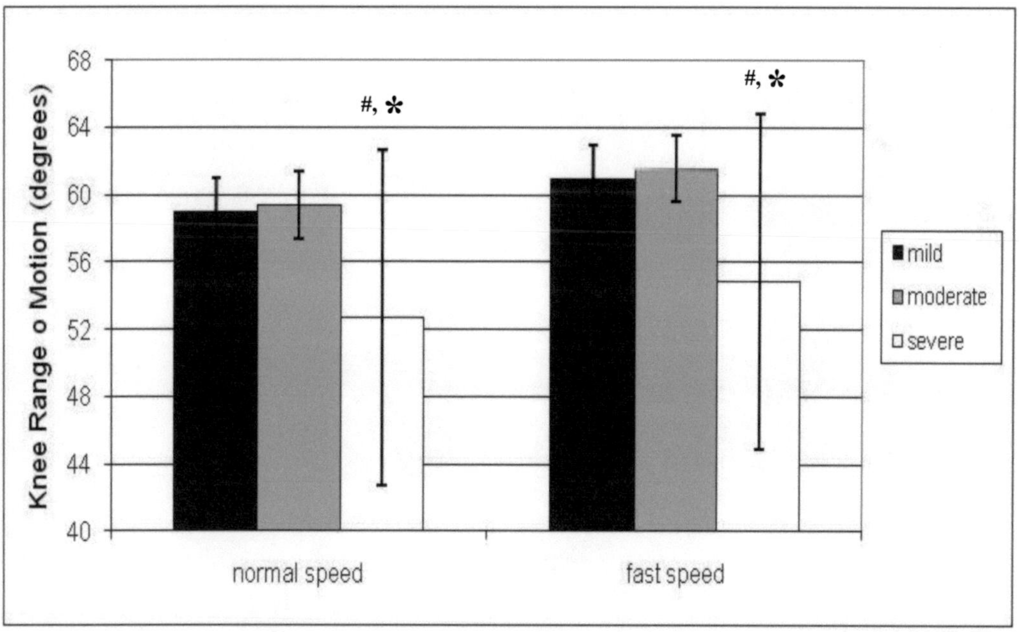

Fig. 2. Analysis of variance results for knee range of motion. # denotes significant difference from mild OA, * denotes significant difference from moderate OA

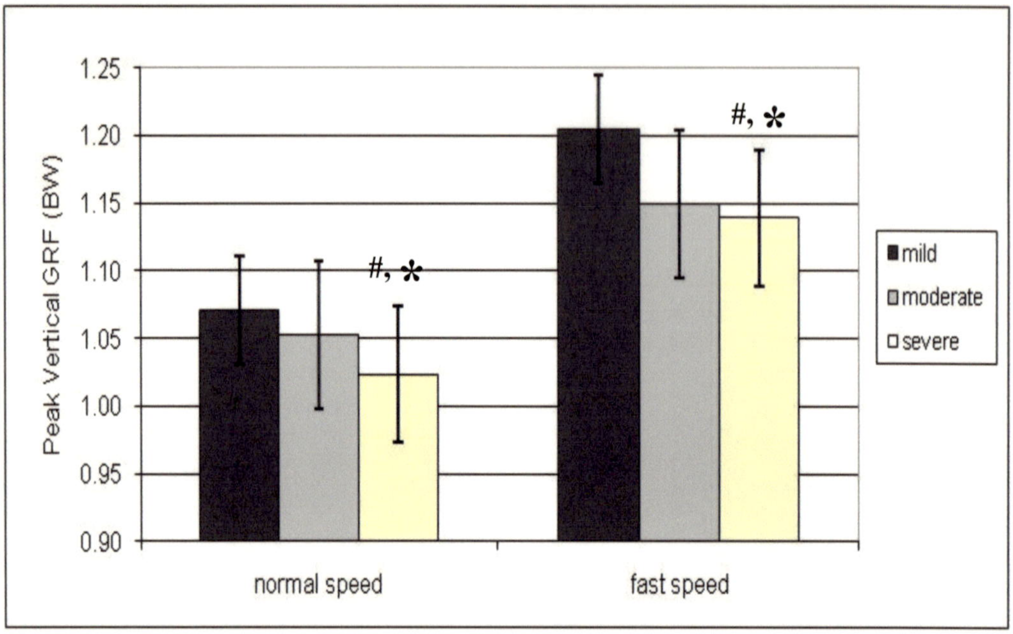

Fig. 3. Analysis of covariance results for peak vertical ground reaction force; # denotes significant difference from mild OA and * denotes significant difference from moderate OA

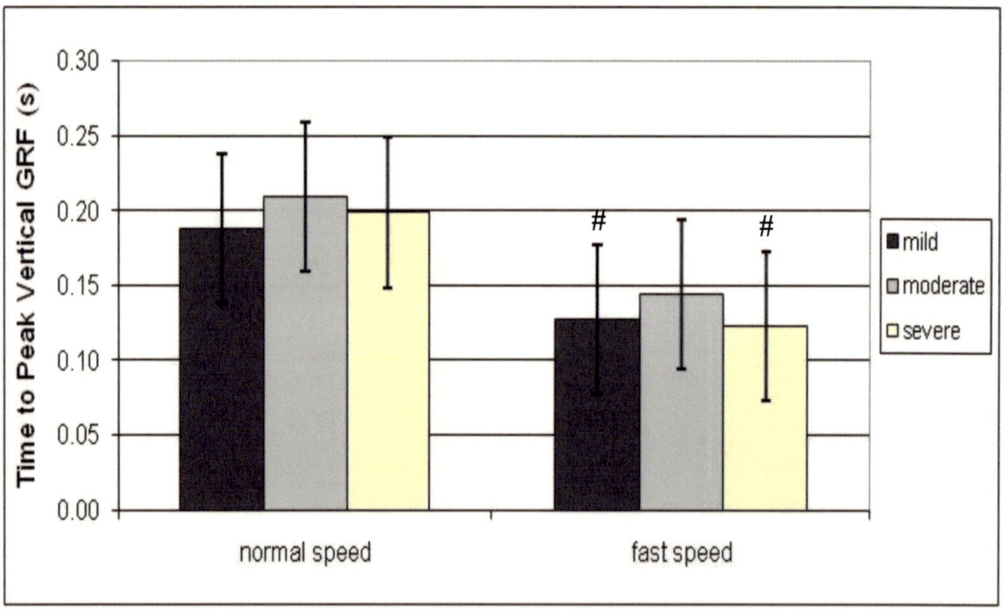

Fig. 4. Analysis of covariance results for time to peak vertical ground reaction force; # denotes a significant difference from moderate OA at the normal speed, however at the fast speed there was a significant difference between mild and moderate and moderate and severe levels of radiographic disease severity.

4. Discussion

Given the conflicting results of previous studies, the purpose of this study was to further examine the relationship between radiographic disease severity and gait patterns in persons with knee OA by not only looking at radiographic grade, but by looking at gait patterns in subjects grouped by severity level. This study expanded on previous work by investigating differences in gait mechanics across all levels of radiographic severity (mild, moderate, and severe). The current study investigated joint mechanics, as well as spatiotemporal gait characteristics.

It was predicted that more severe levels of knee OA would correlate positively with increased gait disability measured through slower walking velocity, shorter strides, lower peak vertical forces, greater knee adduction moments, smaller loading rates and a more limited knee range of motion. The results showed that four of these measures of gait disability differed significantly in patient groups having different levels of radiographic disease severity. It was further hypothesized that significant differences in gait mechanics would exist between the three radiographic disease severity levels, even after controlling for speed. This hypothesis was supported in that both peak vertical ground reaction force and time to peak vertical ground reaction force varied with radiographic disease severity independent of walking speed.

The gait biomechanics of the subjects in this study are consistent with previous reports. OA patients had a shorter stride length, slower walking velocity, lower stride frequency, a longer support time, and smaller loading rate than their counterparts without OA (Al-Zahrani & Bakheit, 2002; Brinkmann & Perry, 1985; Messier et al., 2005a; Messier et al., 1992). Furthermore, mean peak knee adduction moment and mean KROM were consistent with previous reported values in persons with OA (Baliunas et al., 2002; Kaufman et al., 2001; Messier et al., 2005a; Messier et al., 1992). When broken down by radiographic severity, subjects with more severe OA walked more slowly, with stiffer knees and loaded their limbs less.

Knee OA is the most common cause of disability in community dwelling elderly adults (Guccione et al., 1994) and these altered gait mechanics can potentially influence progression of OA and quality of life. For example, the typical mean walking speed for adults is 1.3 m/s and in general a reduction in walking velocity by 12% has clinical significance. The mean walking velocity in this study at the normal speed is at about a 14% reduction and for the patients with severe OA it is a 21% reduction. Given the increase in gait disability with increased OA severity found in this study, patients with severe radiographic disease may be unable to easily execute activities of daily living such as ambulation, and they may also be unable to complete the physical activities prescribed as part of the treatment plan for their OA disease.

As others studies have reported (Nebel et al., 2009; White et al., 2010; Wilson et al., 2011), the present study found that there was only a modest relationship between K/L grade and gait mechanics. Knee range of motion and peak vertical ground reaction force was inversely correlated with radiographic disease severity at both speeds. Each of these variables, as well as velocity, stride frequency, loading rate, knee adduction moment and time to peak vertical ground reaction force, were also examined by level of severity. Statistically significant differences were seen in four of these gait variables. As predicted, patients with severe OA had the smallest knee range of motion and the smallest peak vertical ground reaction force at both speeds. The influence of radiographic disease severity on knee range of motion is understandable given that severe erosion of cartilage and presence of osteophytes as well as joint space narrowing could limit knee range of motion (Holla et al., 2011). It was expected that patients with severe OA would not load their limbs as much and load them more slowly to alleviate pain. Peak vertical ground reaction force decreased with increasing OA severity at both speeds. This alteration in gait mechanics is consistent with the notion that patients are seeking to reduce loading at the knee. Finally, time to peak vertical GRF was greatest in patients with moderate OA; the differences were statistically significant at the fast speed. It is important to note that, in this study, differences related to peak vertical ground reaction force were not a function of slower walking speed. This is in contrast to previous work that has suggested alterations in gait variables may arise partially as a result of altered walking speed (Mundermann et al., 2004; Zeni & Higginson, 2010). In this study, walking velocity did not differ as a function OA disease severity at the normal walking speed. However when challenged to walk at a fast speed, patients with severe OA walked significantly slower than patients with mild and moderate OA. Given that the external KAM during walking has been associated with radiographic disease severity (Sharma et al., 1998; Zeni & Higginson, 2010), it was expected that such a correlation would be observed in the current study, however, it was not. Some trends for knee adduction moment were revealed though. At the normal speed knee adduction moment decreased with increasing level of severity and the exact opposite was true at the fast walking speed; knee adduction moment increased with increasing radiographic severity. The trend at the fast speed was consistent with previous studies (Miyazaki et al., 2002; Wilson et al., 2011). A similar trend was observed for loading rate. While differences in loading rate were not statistically significant, loading rate decreased with increasing radiographic severity at the normal speed and it increased with increasing level of severity at the fast speed.

Based on the variables that differed by radiographic severity: velocity, knee range of motion, peak vertical ground reaction force, and time to peak vertical ground reaction force, it appears that subjects may have altered their gait mechanics as part of a compensatory strategy. These alterations may also be the result of altered control strategies (e.g. increased time to peak vertical ground reaction force) that may result in damaging gait patterns. Factors such as obesity, pain severity, and helplessness have been suggested to be important determinants of physical limitation in patients with knee OA (Creamer et al., 2000). Perhaps the compensatory strategies exhibited by the patients in this study are related to pain they experience with increasing disease severity. While the current study did not investigate the influence of pain on gait mechanics, a previous study by this group did find that pain accounted for as much as 24% of the variance in walking speed in patients with knee OA after controlling for demographics and disease severity (Somers et al., 2009). Another possible explanation for the compensatory gait mechanisms is kinesiophobia, or pain-related fear of movement, which refers to the fear of movement and injury due to consequent pain (Somers et al., 2009). If the patients with more severe OA are experiencing more pain, then it may be affecting their movement. Findings by Heuts et al., 2004 in which they found self-reported level of pain to be significantly correlated with functional limitations support this theory. Furthermore, there is increasing interest in the role of pain cognitions, specifically pain catastrophizing and pain-related fear in predicting adjustment to OA disease (Heuts et al., 2004; Somers et al., 2008; Somers et al., 2009). Somers and colleagues found that pain-related fear and pain catastrophizing explained a significant amount of variance in walking velocity and that pain catastrophizing was a significant individual predictor of walking velocity (Somers et al., 2009). Thus further investigation of the influence of pain and pain cognitions on the relationship between OA severity and additional gait variables (knee range of motion, peak vertical ground reaction force, and time to peak vertical ground reaction force), might be beneficial.

5. Conclusion

The purpose of this study was to examine the relationship between radiographic disease severity and gait patterns in persons with knee OA by looking at gait mechanics and joint loading in subjects across all severity levels. The results indicate that variation in gait could not be fully explained by K/L grade; although, when K/L grade was used to form different levels of radiographic disease severity, significant differences did exist. The results showed that significant differences existed in peak vertical ground reaction force and time to peak vertical ground reaction force by level of radiographic severity, even after controlling for walking speed. This study continues to point to osteoarthritis of the knee as a multifactorial disease. While radiographic disease severity is related to changes in gait biomechanics, the aberrant gait patterns could be a combination of radiographic disease severity and the pain experienced at a given severity. It may even be related to a combination of pain cognitions and radiographic disease severity. The authors suggest that future work should be done to look at the influence of pain and pain related fear of movement or other pain cognitions on gait mechanics within each severity group.

6. Acknowledgements

The authors would like to thank Sarah Jaffe, Dr. Mary Beth Nebel, Alicia Abbey, and Bryan Gibson for their contributions to this work. This research was supported by NIH grants AR50245 and AG15768.

7. References

Addison, S., Coleman, R., S Feng, McDaniel, G., & Kraus, V. (2009). Whole-body bone scintigraphy provides a measure of the total-body burden of osteoarthritis for the purpose of systemic biomarker validation. *Arthritis and Rheumatism, 60*(11), 3366-3373.

Al-Zahrani, K.S., & Bakheit, A.M.O. (2002). A study of the gait characteristics of patients with chronic osteoarthritis of the knee. *Disability and rehabilitation, 24*(5), 275-280.

Altman, R., Asch, E., Bloch, D., Bole, G., Borenstein, D., Brandt, K., Christy, W., Cooke, T.D., Greenwald, R., Hochberg, M., Howell, D., Kaplan, D., Koopman, W., Longley III, S., Mankin, H., McShane, D.J., Medsger Jr, T., Meenan, R., Mikkelsen, W., Moskowitz, R., Murphy, W., Rothschild, B., Segal, M., Sokoloff, L., & Wolfe, F. (1986). Development of criteria for the classification and reporting of osteoarthritis. Classification of osteoarthritis of the knee. Diagnostic and Therapeutic Criteria

Committee of the American Rheumatism Association. *Arthritis Rheum, 29*(8), 1039-1049.

Amin, S., Luepongsak, N., McGibbon, C.A., LaValley, M.P., Krebs, D., & Felson, D.T. (2004). Knee adduction moment and development of chronic knee pain in elders. *Arthritis and Rheumatism, 51*(3), 371-376.

Anderson-MacKenzie, J., Quasnichka, H., Starr, R., Lewis, E., Billinghan, M., & Bailey, A. (2005). Fundamental subchondral bone changes in spontaneous knee osteoarthritis. *International Journal of Biochemistry & Cell Biology, 37*(1), 224-236.

Andriacchi, T., Mundermann, A., Smith, R.L., Alexander, E.J., Dyrby, C.O., & Koo, S. (2004). A framework for the in vivo pathomechanics of osteoarthritis at the knee. *Annals of Biomedical Engineering 32*(3), 447-457.

Andriacchi, T., Ogle, J., & Galante, J. (1977). Walking speed as a basis for normal and abnormal gait measurements. *J. Biomechanics, 10*, 261-268.

Astephen, J.L., Deluzio, K.J., Caldwell, G.E., Dunbar, M.J., & Hubley-Kozey, C.L. (2008). Gait and neuromuscular pattern changes are associated with differences in knee osteoarthritis severity levels. *J Biomechanics, 41*, 868-876.

Baliunas, A.J., Hurwitz, D.E., Ryals, A.B., Karrar, A., Case, J.P., Block, J.A., & Andriacchi, T.P. (2002). Increased knee joint loads during walking are present in subjects with knee osteoarthritis. *Osteoarthritis and cartilage, 10*(7), 573-579.

Brinkmann, J.J.R., & Perry, J.J. (1985). Rate and range of knee motion during ambulation in healthy and arthritic subjects. *Physical therapy, 65*(7), 1055-1060.

Cooper, C., Snow, S., McAlindon, T.E., Kellingray, S., Stuart, B., Coggon, D., & Dieppe, P.A. (2000). Risk factors for the incidence and progression of radiographic knee osteoarthritis. *Arthritis Rheum, 43*(5), 995-1000.

Creamer, P., Lethbridge-Cejku, M., & Hochberg, M.C. (2000). Factors associated with functional impairment in symptomatic knee osteoarthritis. *Rheumatology (Oxford), 39*(5), 490-496.

Davis, M.A., Ettinger, W.H., Neuhaus, J.M., Cho, S.A., & Hauck, W.W. (1989). The association of knee injury and obesity with unilateral and bilateral osteoarthritis of the knee. *American Journal of Epidemiolgy, 130*(2), 278-288.

Dillon, C.F., Rasch, E.K., Gu, Q., & Hirsch, R. (2006). Prevalence of knee osteoarthritis in the United States: arthritis data from the Third National Health and Nutrition Examination Survey 1991-94. *Journal of Rheumatology, 33*(11), 2271-2279.

Felson, D.T., Zhang, Y., Hannan, M., Naimark, A., Weissman, B., Aliabadi, P., & Levy, D. (1997). Risk Factors for Incident Radiographic Knee Osteoarthritis in the Elderly. The Framingham Study. *Arthritis & Rheumatism, 40*(4), 728-733.

Guccione, A.A., Felson, D.T., Anderson, J.J., Anthony, J.M., Zhang, Y., Wilson, P.W., Kelly-Hayes, M., Wolf, P.A., Kreger, B.E., & Kannel, W.B. (1994). The Effects of Specific Medical Conditions on the Functional Limitations of Elders in the Framingham Study. *American Journal of Public Health, 84*(3), 351-358.

Györy, A.N., Chao, E.Y., & Stauffer, R.N. (1976). Functional evaluation of normal and pathologic knees during gait. *Archives of physical medicine and rehabilitation, 57*(12), 571-577.

Hart, D.J., & Spector, T.D. (1993). The relationship of obesity, fat distribution and osteoarthritis in women in the general population: the Chingford Study. *The Journal of rheumatology, 20*(2), 331-335.

Helmick, C.G., D.T. Felson, Lawrence, R.C., Gabriel, S., R., H., & H., M.K. (2008). Estimates of the prevalence of arthritis and other rheumatic conditions in the United States. Part I. *Arthritis and Rheumatism, 58*, 15-25.

Heuts, P.H., Vlaeyen, J.W., Roelofs, J., de Bie, R.A., Aretz, K., van Weel, C., & van Schayck, O.C. (2004). Pain-related fear and daily functioning in patients with osteoarthritis. *Pain, 110*(1-2), 228-235.

Holla, J.F., Steultjens, M.P., van der Leeden, M., Roorda, L.D., Bierma-Zeinstra, S.M., den Broeder, A.A., & Dekker, J. (2011). Determinants of range of joint motion in patients with early symptomatic osteoarthritis of the hip and/or knee: an exploratory study in the CHECK cohort. *Osteoarthritis Cartilage, 19*(4), 411-419. doi: S1063-4584(11)00026-4 [pii] 10.1016/j.joca.2011.01.013

Hurwitz, D.E., Ryals, A.B., Case, J.P., Block, J.A., & Andriacchi, T.P. (2002). The knee adduction moment during gait in subjects with knee osteoarthritis is more closely correlated with static alignment than radiographic disease severity, toe out angle and pain. *J Orthop Res, 20*(1), 101-107.

Kaufman, K.R., Hughes, C., Morrey, B.F., Morrey, M., & An, K.N. (2001). Gait characteristics of patients with knee osteoarthritis. *Journal of biomechanics, 34*(7), 907-915.

Kellgren, J.H., & Lawrence, J.C. (1957). Radiological assessment of osteoarthritis. *Ann Rheum. Disease, 16*, 494-501.

Landry, S.C., McKean, K.A., Hubley-Kozey, C.L., Stanish, W.D., & Deluzio, K.J. (2007). Knee biomechanics of moderate OA patients measured during gait at a self-selected and fast walking speed. *J Biomech, 40*(8), 1754-1761.

Lawrence, R.C., Felson, D.T., Helmick, C.G., Arnold, L.M., Choi, H., Deyo, R.A., Gabriel, S., Hirsch, R., Hochberg, M., Hunder, G., Jordan, J., Katz, J., Kremers, H.M., & Wolfe, F. (2008). Estimates of the prevalence of arthritis and other rheumatic conditions in the United States: Part II. *Arthritis and Rheumatism, 58*(1), 26-35.

Lawrence, R.C., Helmick, C.G., Arnett, F.C., Deyo RA, Felson DT, & Giannini EH. (1998). Estimates of the prevalence of arthritis and selected musculoskeletal disorders in the United States. *Arthritis and Rheumatism, 41*, 778-799.

Lohmander, L.S., Östenberg, A., Englund, M., & Roos, H. (2004). High prevalence of knee osteoarthritis, pain, and functional limitations in female soccer players twelve years after anterior cruciate ligament injury. *Arthritis and Rheumatism, 50*(10), 3145-3152.

Maly, M.R., Costigan, P.A., & Olney, S.J. (2005). Contribution of psychosocial and mechanical variables to physical performance measures in knee osteoarthritis. *Physical Therapy, 85*, 1318-1328.

Maly, M.R., Costigan, P.A., & Olney, S.J. (2006). Determinants of Self Efficacy for Physical Tasks in People with Knee Osteoarthritis. *Arthritis Care & Research, 55*(1), 94-101.

Manetta, J., Franz, L.H., Moon, C., Perrell, K., & Fang, M. (2002). Comparison of hip and knee muscle moments in subjects with and without knee pain. *Gait and Posture, 16*(3), 249-254.

McKean, K.A., Landry, S.C., Hubley-Kozey, C.L., Dunbar, M.J., Stanish, W.D., & Deluzio, K.J. (2007). Gender differences exist in osteoarthritic gait. *J. Clin. Biomech, 22*, 400-409.

Messier, S.P. (1994). Osteoarthritis of the knee and associated factors of age and obesity: effects on gait. . *Medicine and Science in Sports and Exercise 26*(12), 1446-1452.

Messier, S.P., DeVita, P., Cowan, R.E., Seay, J., Young, H.C., & Marsh, A.P. (2005a). Do older adults with knee osteoarthritis place greater loads on the knee during gait? A preliminary study. *Archives of physical medicine and rehabilitation, 86*(4), 703-709.

Messier, S.P., Gutekunst, D.J., Davis, C., & DeVita, P. (2005b). Weight loss reduces knee-joint loads in overweight and obese older adults with knee osteoarthritis. *Arthritis Rheum, 52*(7), 2026-2032.

Messier, S.P., Loeser, R.F., Hoover, J.L., Semble, E.L., & Wise, C.M. (1992). Osteoarthritis of the knee: effects on gait, strength, and flexibility. *Archives of physical medicine and rehabilitation, 73*(1), 29-36.

Miyazaki, T., Wada, M., Kawahara, H., Sato, M., Baba, H., & Shimada, S. (2002). Dynamic load at baseline can predict radiographic disease progression in medial compartment knee osteoarthritis. *Annals Rheumatic Disease, 61*(7), 617-622.

Mundermann, A., Dyrby, C.O., & Andriacchi, T.P. (2005). Secondary gait changes in patients with medial compartment knee osteoarthritis: increased load at the ankle, knee, and hip during walking. *Arthritis Rheum, 52*(9), 2835-2844.

Mundermann, A., Dyrby, C.O., Hurwitz, D.E., Sharma, L., & Andriacchi, T.P. (2004). Potential strategies to reduce medial compartment loading in patients with knee osteoarthritis of varying severity: reduced walking speed. *Arthritis Rheum, 50*(4), 1172-1178. doi: 10.1002/art.20132

Nebel, M.B., Sims, E.L., Keefe, F.J., Kraus, V.B., Guilak, F., Caldwell, D.S., Pells, J.J., Queen, R., & Schmitt, D. (2009). The relationship of self-reported pain and functional impairment to gait mechanics in overweight and obese persons with knee osteoarthritis. *Archives of Physical Medicine and Rehabilitation, 90*, 1874-1879.

Peterfy, C., Li, J., Siam, S., Duryea, J., Lynch, J., & Miaux, Y. (2003). Comparison of fixed-flexion positioning with fluoroscopic semi-flexed positioning for quantifying radiographic joint-space width in the knee: test-retest reproducibility. *Skeletal Radiol, 32*, 128-132.

Reijman, M., Pols, H., Bergink, A., Hazes, J., Belo, J., Lievense, A., & Bierma-Zeinstra, S. (2007). Body Mass Index associated with onset and progression of osteoarthritis of the knee but not of the hip: The Rotterdam Study. . *Annals of Rheumatic Disease, 66*(158-162).

Sangha, O. (2000). Epidemiology of rheumatic diseases. *Rheumatology, 39*(Suppl 2), 3-12.

Senior, K. (2000). Osteoarthritis research: on the verge of a revolution? *Lancet, 355*(9199), 208.

Sharif, M., George, E., Shepstone, L., Knudson, W., Thonar, E.J., Cushnaghan, J., & Dieppe, P. (1995). Serum hyaluronic acid level as a predictor of disease progression in osteoarthritis of the knee. *Arthritis and rheumatism, 38*(6), 760-767.

Sharma, L., Hurwitz, D.E., Thonar, E.J., Sum, J.A., Lenz, M.E., Dunlop, D.D., Schnitzer, T.J., Kirwan-Mellis, G., & Andriacchi, T.P. (1998). Knee adduction moment, serum hyaluronan level, and disease severity in medial tibiofemoral osteoarthritis. *Arthritis and Rheumatism, 41*, 1233-1240.

Sims, E.L., Carland, J.M., Keefe, F.J., Kraus, V.B., Guilak, F., & Schmitt, D. (2009a). Sex Differences in Biomechanics Associated with Knee Osteoarthritis. *Journal of Women & Aging, 21*, 159-170.

Sims, E.L., Keefe, F.J., Kraus, V.B., Guilak, F., Queen, R.M., & Schmitt, D. (2009b). Racial differences in gait mechanics associated with knee osteoarthritis. *Aging Clin Exp Res, 21*(6), 463-469. doi: 6832 [pii]

Smith, R.L., Lin, J., Trindale, M., Shida, J., Kajiyama, G., Vu, T., Hoffman, A., Meulen, M.v.d., Goodman, S., Schurman, D., & Carter, D. (2000). Time-dependent effects of intermittent hydrostatic pressure on articular chondrocyte type II collagen and aggrecan mRNA expression. . *Journal of Rehabilitation Research and Development, 37*(2), 153-162.

Somers, T.J., Keefe, F.J., Carson, J.W., Pells, J.J., & Lacaille, L. (2008). Pain catastrophizing in borderline morbidly obese and morbidly obese individuals with osteoarthritic knee pain. *Pain Res Manag, 13*(5), 401-406.

Somers, T.J., Keefe, F.J., Pells, J.J., Dixon, K.E., Waters, S.J., Riordan, P.A., Blumenthal, J.A., McKee, D.C., LaCaille, L., Tucker, J.M., Schmitt, D., Caldwell, D.S., Kraus, V.B., Sims, E.L., Shelby, R.A., & Rice, J.R. (2009). Pain catastrophizing and pain-related fear in osteoarthritis patients: relationships to pain and disability. *J Pain Symptom Manage, 37*(5), 863-872.

Srikanth, V.K., Fryer, J.L., Zhai, G., Winzenberg, T.M., Hosmer, D., & Jones, G. (2005). A meta-analysis of sex differences prevalence, incidence and severity of osteoarthritis. *Osteoarthritis and Cartilage 13*(9), 769-781.

Summers, M.N., Haley, W.E., Reveille, J.D., & Alarcon, G.S. (1988). Radiographic assessment and psychologic variables as predictors of pain and functional impairment in osteoarthritis of the knee or hip. *Arthritis Rheum, 31*(2), 204-209.

Syed, I.Y., & Davis, B.L. (2000). Obesity and osteoarthritis of the knee: hypotheses concerning the relationship between ground reaction forces and quadriceps fatigue in long-duration walking. *Medical Hypotheses, 54*(2), 182-185.

Teichtahl, A., Wluka, A., & Cicuttini, F. (2003). Abnormal biomechanics: a precursor or result of knee osteoarthritis? . *British Journal of Sports Medicine, 37*(4), 289-290.

White, D., Zhang, Y., Niu, J., Keysor, J., Nevitt, M., Lewis, C.E., Torner, J., & Neogi, T. (2010). Do worsening knee radiographs mean greater chances of severe functional limitation? *Arthritis Care & Research, 62*, 1433-1439.

Wilson, J.L.A., Deluzio, K.J., Dunbar, M.J., Caldwell, G.E., & Hubley-Kozey, C.L. (2011). The association between knee joint biomechanics and neuromuscular control and moderate knee osteoarthritis radiographic and pain severity. *Osteoarthritis and Cartilage, 19*, 186-193.

Zeni, J.A., & Higginson, J.S. (2010). Differences in gait parameters between healthy subjects and persons with moderate and severe knee osteoarthritis: A result of altered walking speed? *Clinical Biomechanics, 24*(4), 372-378.

9

Osteoarthritis in Sports and Exercise: Risk Factors and Preventive Strategies

Eduard Alentorn-Geli and Lluís Puig Verdié
Department of Orthopedic Surgery, Hospital del Mar i l'Esperança, Parc de Salut MAR, Barcelona, Spain

1. Introduction

Osteoarthritis in people participating in sports have considerably increased over the last decades (Hunter DJ & Eckstein F, 2009; Wolf BR & Amendola A, 2005). Sports have many psychological, social and health benefits (Hunt A, 2003; Maffulli N et al., 2011), but individuals with past exposure to maintained vigorous exercise may have an increased risk of developing articular cartilage degeneration (Buckwalter JA, 2003; Kujala UM et al., 2003). Mechanical loading is crucial for an adequate growth and development of articular cartilage (Darling EM & Athanasiou KA, 2003). While too high of a mechanical load can damage normal articular cartilage, some stimulation is necessary to promote chondrogenesis (Darling EM & Athanasiou KA, 2003). Articular cartilage that is not mechanically stimulated will become thinner and will atrophy with time (Vanwanseele B et al., 2002). Given that the cartilage responses to mechanical loading, any type of physical activity may play a role in either the etiology or the protection against osteoarthritis. Where is the threshold at which exercise is no longer hazardous for articular cartilage but instead provides the exact stimulus for its homeostasis? There is no easy answer to this question as each individual has a unique response to each stimulus based on his own genetics but also on many associated factors that have been linked to cartilage damage.

Osteoarthritis is a clinical syndrome caused by joint degeneration that results in permanent and often progressive joint pain and dysfunction (Buckwalter JA, 2003). Osteoarthritis has a multifactorial etiology with the influence of both systemic and local factors (Zhang Y & Jordan JM, 2010). Older age, female gender, obesity, osteoporosis, genetic factors, history of traumatic joint injuries, repetitive use of joints at high loads (either in sports, occupational work, or recreational exercise), muscle weakness, poor neuromuscular control, joint laxity, joint instability, lower extremity malalignment, or leg-length discrepancy may contribute to osteoarthritis (Astephen Wilson JL et al., 2011; Blagojevic M et al., 2010; Bosomworth NJ, 2009; Harvey WF et al., 2010; Neogi T & Zhang Y, 2011; Pietrosimone BG et al., 2011; Roos EM et al., 2011; Sharma L et al., 2010; Zhang Y & Jordan JM, 2010). The knowledge of these risk factors is of great relevance to implement adequate preventive strategies for a highly debilitating disease with a clear impact on the patient's quality of life (Guccione AA et al., 1994). Prevention is also crucial because patients with osteoarthritis have an overall higher risk of death compared with the general population (Nüesch E et al., 2011).

The purpose of this chapter is to review the existing literature regarding the risk factors for osteoarthritis, paying special attention to past exposure to sports and exercise and also to prior joint injury and neuromuscular disorders. This chapter also reports proposed or potential preventive strategies for the development or progression of osteoarthritis.

2. Overview of risk factors for osteoarthritis

This chapter is focused on the risk of exercise and sports participation in the development and progression of osteoarthritis. In addition, there are many other identified risk factors that should be covered in order to better understand the problem of osteoarthritis and offer effective preventive measures. There are several recognized risk factors for developing osteoarthritis (Bosomworth NJ, 2009): older age, female sex, obesity, osteoporosis, occupation, sports activities, previous trauma, muscle weakness or dysfunction, proprioceptive deficit, lower limb malalignment, leg-length inequality, and genetic factors. Age, sex, and genetic factors are non-modifiable, whereas the others may be modified by an appropriate intervention. This chapter will be focused on the analysis of history of joint injury, neuromuscular dysfunction, and exercise and sports participation as risk factors for osteoarthritis.

Each body's tissue looses its optimum properties with ageing, which may contribute to any disorder. Older age is a well accepted risk factor for osteoarthritis (Bosomworth NJ, 2009; Hunter DJ & Sambrook PN, 2002; Stevens-Lapsley JE & Kohrt WM, 2010; Thelin N et al., 2006; Vrezas I et al., 2010; Ward MM et al., 1995). In fact, osteoarthritis is rare among young individuals. Articular cartilage changes with aging have been well documented both clinically and experimentally (Bosomworth NJ, 2009; Hardingham T & Bayliss M, 1990; Horton WE et al., 2006; Hunter DJ & Sambrook PN, 2002). This is a non-modifiable risk factor the prevention of its influence should begin in early ages and continue throughout the rest of the life. Obviously, this factor is always related to subject exercising or participating in sports. Thus, any investigation dealing with a certain risk factor must be adjusted for age.

Females have been reported to have an increased risk of osteoarthritis (Bosomworth NJ, 2009; Hunter DJ & Sambrook PN, 2002; Jordan JM et al., 1996; Stevens-Lapsley JE & Kohrt WM, 2010). It was suggested that this difference from males would be explained by the influence of sex hormones, primarily estrogen (Hunter DJ & Sambrook PN, 2002; Riancho JA et al., 2010; Rosner IA et al., 1986; Stevens-Lapsley JE & Kohrt WM, 2010). The risk of osteoarthritis between males and females is similar under 50 years old, but significantly increases above this age in females (Felson DT et al., 1995; Oliveria SA et al., 1995). Thus, in postmenopausal women the risk of osteoarthritis is increased with respect to an age-matched cohort of males (Hunter DJ & Sambrook PN, 2002). A potential preventive pharmacological strategy with estrogen replacement therapy has been proposed for these patients (Spector TD et al., 1997). However, a recent systematic review concluded that there is some evidence for a protective effect of this therapy for hip, but not for knee osteoarthritis (de Klerk BM et al., 2009). De Klerk and colleagues stated that heterogeneity between the hormones used and outcome measurements made statistical data pooling impossible (de Klerk BM et al., 2009). Relationship between the exogenous hormone use and osteoarthritis was not clearly observed. They concluded that other aspects, yet to be determined, may play a role in the increased incidence in women aged over 50 years (de Klerk BM et al., 2009). Hunter and Sambrook suggested randomized, prospective clinical trials to clarify the effects of hormone replacement therapy on the development of osteoarthritis (Hunter DJ & Sambrook PN, 2002).

One of the most accepted risk factors for developing osteoarthritis is obesity (Hunter DJ & Sambrook PN, 2002). Increased weight may overload joints and alter the normal physiology of cartilage (Pallu S et al., 2010). Obesity is a clear modifiable risk factor, so there is an evident preventive measure that can be offer to patients. Weight loss would not only reduce the risk of osteoarthritis by unloading joints, but also by the fact that exercise would be of benefit for joints if performed through an adequate progression, beginning with non-weight-bearing exercises until the weight has been reduced (Felson DT et al., 1992). There are a lot of studies concluding on the increased risk of osteoarthritis in patients with obesity (Anderson JJ & Felson DT, 1988; Chaganti RK & Lane NE, 2011; Hart DJ & Spector TD, 1993; Kohatsu ND & Schurman DJ, 1990). The combination of risk factors may elicit a further increased risk of osteoarthritis, as exemplified by obesity and physical activity among elderly patients (odds ratio of 13 for developing knee osteoarthritis) (McAlindon TE et al., 1999), or obesity and female sex (Davis MA et al., 1988). The risk of osteoarthritis in obese patients is higher for knee and hand joints than for the hip joints (Grotle M et al., 2008). Interestingly, men with overweight during their 20's had higher rate than those who became overweight during their 40's on the incidence of self-reported osteoarthritis (Gelber AC et al., 1999). Hunter and Sambrook have concluded that there is consistent and conclusive evidence demonstrating the association between obesity and osteoarthritis (Hunter DJ & Sambrook PN, 2002).

Osteoporosis has been considered a risk factor for osteoarthritis (Bosomworth NJ, 2009; Hannan MT et al., 1993; Hunter DJ & Sambrook PN, 2002; Nevitt MC et al., 1995; Zhang Y et al., 2000). Although some initial studies suggested that osteoporosis would decrease the incidence of this disorder (Hunter DJ & Sambrook PN, 2002), more recent studies demonstrated that an increase in bone mineral density of 5%-10% is consistently related to both hip and knee osteoarthritis (Hannan MT et al., 1993; Nevitt MC et al., 1995). Low bone mineral density is associated with the incidence, but decreased progression of radiographic knee osteoarthritis (Zhang Y et al., 2000). The relationship between bone mineral density and osteoarthritis has been linked to vitamin D (McAlindon TE et al., 1996). Both low intake and low serum levels of vitamin D have been related to the progression of knee osteoarthritis (McAlindon TE et al., 1996).

Special attention is required for occupational osteoarthritis. Physical workload has been shown to be an important risk factor for the development of articular cartilage degeneration (Aluoch MA & Wao HO, 2009; Maetzel A et al., 1997). It is not the purpose of this chapter to review in detail the association between osteoarthritis and exposure to occupational physical activity. For a deeper knowledge of this risk factor, the reader is referred to the comprehensive review performed by Aluoch and Wao (Aluoch MA & Wao HO, 2009). Essentially, there is a strong relationship between high physical workload (frequent knee bending, heavy lifting, frequent stair climbing, and prolonged squatting) and risk of hand, hip, knee, and foot osteoarthritis (Aluoch MA & Wao HO, 2009). Jobs involved in occupational osteoarthritis include construction, agriculture, forestry, fishing, transportations, mining, and manufacturing (Aluoch MA & Wao HO, 2009). Occupational osteoarthritis is a modifiable risk factor. Measures aimed to prevent new cases of osteoarthritis or to decrease its progression should be taken (Hunter DJ & Sambrook PN, 2002).

Lower limb malalignment and leg-length inequality would also be risk factors for progression, but not onset, of osteoarthritis (Brouwer GM et al., 2007; Golightly YM et al., 2007; 2010; Hunter DJ et al., 2007). Both factors may not initiate or cause osteoarthritis, but just worsen the already damaged articular cartilage. Knee varus malalignment but not knee valgus was associated with both onset and progression of osteoarthritis (Brouwer GM et al., 2007). This observation was particularly applicable to obese individuals, again showing the bad consequences of having various risk factors associated in the same subject. Unfortunately, this finding has not been reproducible (Hunter DJ et al., 2007). Leg-length inequality was associated with progression of radiographic knee osteoarthritis, but not with incident radiographic knee or hip osteoarthritis, progression of chronic knee symptoms, and incident and progression of chronic hip symptoms (Golightly YM et al., 2010). Both factors may be modifiable by surgery or raised insoles (Neogi T & Zhang Y, 2011).

Genetics, epigenetics, and genomics are probably the most promising areas to be developed in relation to the study of osteoarthritis. The study of these areas is yielding valuable insights into the etiology of osteoarthritis but there is still much to know (Meulenbelt I et al., 2011). It is likely that individuals with a genetic predisposition would have osteoarthritis in many joints (Felson DT et al., 2000). Genetic factors may account for at least 50% of cases of osteoarthritis in the hands and hips, and a smaller percentage in the knees (Spector TD et al., 1996a). Overall, Loughlin considers that the search for osteoarthritis susceptibility loci has been limited (Loughlin J, 2011). Genes affected for most common forms of osteoarthritis would include vitamin D receptor gene, insulin-like growth factor I gene, cartilage oligomeric protein genes, and HLA region (Felson DT et al., 2000). Genetics may contribute to osteoarthritis to a different extend depending on each individual. The heterogeneous nature of the disease in terms of potential causes and presentation may explain why genetics are not the only aspect to consider. In other words, genetic and environmental factors must be considered altogether for an adequate prevention of osteoarthritis.

3. History of joint injury

Any kind of physical activity implies a chance of injury. Former athletes have a high rate of joint injury (Krajnc Z et al., 2010). Individuals with a history of joint injury have a higher risk of developing osteoarthritis (Hunter DJ & Eckstein F, 2009). The role of joint injury in the development of osteoarthritis has been mainly studied in the knee joint. Previous knee injury may be one of the most important modifiable risk factors for subsequent knee osteoarthritis in men, and second only after obesity in women (Felson DT et al., 2000; Hunter DJ & Sambrook PN, 2002). Knee injuries typically occur in the younger population thus causing prolonged disability and high economic costs (Hunter DJ & Sambrook PN, 2002; Yelin E & Callahan LF, 1995). Knee joint injuries increase the risk of osteoarthritis by increasing tibiofemoral contact area and pressures in meniscal injuries, by causing joint instability in ligament injuries, by chondral lesions itself, or by impairing the neuromuscular system.

The menisci are responsible for load-bearing, shock-absorption, joint stability, joint lubrication, and joint congruity (King D, 1936). All these functions contribute to the preservation of articular cartilage, which may be injured whenever meniscal disorders develop. Meniscal tears may be classified in acute-traumatic or chronic-degenerative. Acute-traumatic tears mainly occur in young patients, usually participating in sports, and increase the risk of developing knee osteoarthritis (Englund M et al., 2003). Acute tears mainly occur in patients with no previous cartilage injuries. Long-term consequences of acute-traumatic meniscal tears in terms of osteoarthritis may be influenced by length of follow-up, age at the time of injury, sex, and associated injuries (Lohmander LS et al., 2007). In contrast, chronic-degenerative tears may affect one third of the general population over 50 years after no trauma at all (Englund M et al., 2008; Lohmander LS et al., 2007), and are associated with pre-existing and progression of knee osteoarthritis (Englund M et al., 2003). These meniscal injuries are more commonly associated with pre-existing joint cartilage damage than acute-traumatic tears (Christoforakis J et al., 2005; Englund M & Lohmander LS, 2004). The pre-existing osteoarthritis is worsened by meniscal tears (Hunter DJ et al., 2006; Raynauld JP et al., 2006). Therefore, their risk of osteoarthritis in chronic-degenerative meniscal injuries is explained by two factors; that is, the presence of prior cartilage injury, and the meniscus tear itself. The "double" mechanism of osteoarthritis in these injuries may explain the worst long-term radiographic and clinical outcomes compared to acute-traumatic tears (Englund M et al., 2001; 2003; 2004).

Repetitive increased loading in a patient with unrepaired meniscal tear also increases the risk of developing knee osteoarthritis (Lohmander LS et al., 2007). Also, articular cartilage degeneration is produced when meniscectomy is performed. Partial or total meniscectomies increase the tibiofemoral contact area and increase the joint contact pressures (Baratz M et al., 1986; Burke DL et al., 1978; Fairbank TJ, 1948; Seedhom BB & Hargreaves DJ, 1979), thus explaining the early onset knee osteoarthritic changes (Hoser C et al., 2001; Jorgensen U et al., 1987; Roos H et al., 1998). The contralateral healthy knee is also affected although to a lesser degree (Englund M & Lohmander LS, 2004). The greater the area of meniscectomy, the greater the mechanical distress on the knee, and a greater chondral deterioration can be expected. Meniscal resection of only 15% to 34% increases the contact pressure more than a 350%, whereas a total meniscectomy increases the contact load on the cartilage up to a 700% (Ahmed AM & Burke DL, 1983; Fukubayashi TK & Kurosawa H, 1980). Roos and colleagues compared the risk of knee osteoarthritis in a cohort of 123 patients 21 years after total meniscectomy (Roos H et al., 1998). The relative risk of developing knee osteoarthritis after total meniscectomy was 14 (95% confidence interval 3.5-121.2), using age- and sex-matched pairs for comparison. Forty eight percent of patients in the meniscectomy group had grade II or more radiographic osteoarthritis with the Kellegren-Lawrence classification compared to only a 7% in the control group. In addition, knee symptoms were reported twice as often in meniscectomized patients compared to controls (Roos H et al., 1998). The authors found no relationship with knee osteoarthritis depending on the localization of the compartment or type of meniscus tear. In contrast, Lohmander and colleagues stated in their review that the symptoms and functional outcomes of lateral meniscectomy in relation to knee osteoarthritis were worst compared to medial meniscectomy (Lohmander LS et al., 2007). In accordance with Roos and colleagues, Neuman and colleagues observed that the primary risk factor for tibiofemoral osteoarthritis was a prior meniscectomy after prospectively evaluating the occurrence of knee osteoarthritis 15 years after non-operative treatment of anterior cruciate ligament injury (Neuman P et al., 2008). Cooper and colleagues found that patients with previous knee injury had 3 times more risk of knee osteoarthritis compared to uninjured subjects. This risk was increased 4-fold if meniscectomy had to be performed (Cooper C et al., 1994). Specifically, meniscectomy was a strong risk factor for medial tibiofemoral osteoarthritis. In their excellent review article about the long-term consequences of anterior cruciate ligament and meniscal tears, Lohmander and colleagues found that some 50% of patients undergoing meniscectomy 15 to

20 years earlier had radiographic knee osteoarthritis, with an odds ratio of about 10 compared to age- and sex-matched controls (Lohmander LS et al., 2007). The authors stated that symptoms and functional outcomes of meniscectomy were worst if other risk factors were present (i.e., women and obesity). Also, Hunter and Sambrook stated that older age at the time of injury predicts a more rapid progression to knee osteoarthritis (Hunter DJ & Sambrook PN, 2002). Patients with finger joint osteoarthritis at the time of meniscectomy had a higher risk of developing knee osteoarthritis compared to patients without finger osteoarthritis (Englund M et al., 2004). This may indicate the potential relationship between genetic predisposition and osteoarthritis. Lohmander and colleagues considered that studies assessing radiographic osteoarthritic changes after meniscus tears had large variations in sample sizes, patients lost at follow-up, age and sex distribution, and, overall, they had concerns on the quality of study designs. The review performed by Lohmander and colleagues did not provide support of meniscus suture or meniscus allograft transplantation to prevent future development of knee osteoarthritis (Lohmander LS et al., 2007).

Anterior cruciate ligament tears also occur more commonly in young patients, usually under 30 years old (Lohmander LS et al., 2007). Therefore, these injuries explain a large number of early-onset knee osteoarthritis cases with associated pain, functional limitations, and decreased quality of life in the individuals between 30 and 50 years (Lohmander LS et al., 2004; 2007; von Porat A et al., 2004). Radiographic knee osteoarthritis following an anterior cruciate ligament injury ranges from 10% to 90% at 10 to 20 years of follow-up (Gillquist J & Messner K, 1999; Lohmander LS & Roos H, 1994). Such a wide range may be explained by differences in the assessment method of radiographic osteoarthritis, sample size, loss of patients to, and length of, follow-up, sex distribution, age at the time of injury, and associated knee injuries (Lohmander LS et al., 2007). Lohmander and colleagues reported an approximate rate of radiographic knee osteoarthritis of more than 50% after 10 to 20 years of anterior cruciate ligament injury (Lohmander LS et al., 2007). The great majority of their reviewed studies using the Lysholm score had a mean follow-up values around 90 (good or excellent) (Lohmander LS et al., 2007). Scores for quality of life and sport and recreation after anterior cruciate ligament rehabilitation and/or surgery were found to be at its best at 1 to 2 years of follow-up, gradually deteriorating afterwards (Lohmander LS et al., 2007). After 12 years of an anterior cruciate ligament rupture with a mean age at follow-up of 31 years, 75% of female soccer players had a significant impairment of knee-related quality of life and 42% symptomatic radiographic knee osteoarthritis (Lohmander LS et al., 2004). Similar consequences were reported in male soccer players 14 years after this injury, with a mean age at follow-up of 38 years (von Porat A et al., 2004).

Anterior cruciate ligament injuries are often associated with other knee injuries. Keays and colleagues found that concomitant meniscal and chondral damage significantly increased the risk of tibiofemoral osteoarthritis in patients undergoing anterior cruciate ligament reconstruction (Keays SL et al., 2010). Partial meniscectomy at the time of reconstruction significantly increases the risk of developing knee osteoarthritis compared to those with normal menisci (Magnussen RA et al., 2009). If complete meniscectomy is needed, then patients will develop radiographic knee osteoarthritis in near 100% of cases at 5-to-10-year follow-up (Magnussen RA et al., 2009). Meniscal repair was found to have inconsistent influence on the prevention of developing knee osteoarthritis after anterior cruciate ligament reconstruction (Magnussen RA et al., 2009). The presence of cartilage injury at the time of a meniscus tear requiring operation accelerates knee osteoarthritis in patients under 40 years old undergoing anterior cruciate ligament reconstruction (Ichiba A & Kishimoto I,

2009). Although improvements in knee function were observed up to 15 years after ligament reconstruction, combined injuries (ACL, menisci, and chondral injuries) led to a higher risk of knee osteoarthritis compared with isolated anterior cruciate ligament tears (Oiestad BE et al., 2010a).

The technique of anterior cruciate ligament reconstruction has conflicting evidence regarding the influence on the development of knee osteoarthritis (Keays SL et al., 2010; Vairo GL et al., 2010). The use of bone-patellar tendon bone would seem to increase the risk of knee osteoarthritis compared to the use of hamstring tendons autograft (Keays SL et al., 2010; Vairo GL et al., 2010). However, other authors have reported that at a median of 7 years after ligament reconstruction with either autograft, the prevalence of osteoarthritis as seen on standard weight-bearing radiographs and the clinical outcomes was comparable (Lidén M et al., 2008).

Overall, there is a clear consensus that meniscal, ligament, and chondral injuries increase the risk of knee osteoarthritis (Ichiba A & Kishimoto I, 2009; Keays SL et al., 2010; Lidén M et al., 2008; Lohmander LS et al., 2007; Maffulli N et al., 2003; Magnussen RA et al., 2009; Neuman P et al., 2008; Oiestad BE et al., 2010a; 2010b; Roos H et al., 1998). Anterior cruciate ligament and menisci injuries increase the risk of joint degeneration whether or not being surgically treated (Lohmander LS et al., 2004; 2007; von Porat A et al., 2004). In addition, a past history of knee surgery is associated with a rapid progression to knee arthroplasty (Riddle DL et al., 2011). Therefore, prevention of injuries should be considered as one of the most important parts of training programs in athletes or subjects who wish to participate in sports (Roos H et al., 1998).

4. Muscle weakness and afferent sensory dysfunction

The neuromuscular system is crucial to prevent joint damage. Muscles provide dynamic stability, aid in shock absorption, and provide adequate force transmission across joints (Brandt KD, 1997; Mikesky AE et al., 2000; Palmieri-Smith RM & Thomas AC, 2009). Therefore, deconditioned muscles or poor neuromuscular control may increase the risk of osteoarthritis (Roos EM et al., 2011). Impairment of the neuromuscular system may be caused by inadequate training or joint injuries. Preventive programs aimed to improve this system are essential to reduce the risk of osteoarthritis (Keays SL et al., 2010; Neuman P et al., 2008; Roos EM et al., 2011; Segal NA et al., 2010). Muscle weakness is considered a predictor of knee osteoarthritis onset, but there is no clear consensus regarding its role in osteoarthritis progression. In contrast, afferent sensory dysfunction has been related to progression, but not onset, of osteoarthritis (Roos EM et al., 2011).

Anterior cruciate ligament injuries may cause muscle inhibition, muscle atrophy, and changes in activation patterns and knee kinematics (Berchuck M et al., 1990; Palmieri-Smith RM & Thomas AC, 2009; Snyder-Mackler L et al., 1993; Suter E & Herzog W, 2000). Oiestad and colleagues did not detect association between quadriceps weakness after anterior cruciate ligament reconstruction and knee osteoarthritis as measured 10-15 years later (Oiestad BE et al., 2010b). However, it is accepted that muscle weakness and neuromuscular impairment do exist after anterior cruciate ligament injuries (Berchuck M et al., 1990; Palmieri-Smith RM & Thomas AC, 2009; Roos EM et al., 2011). Palmieri-Smith and Thomas used the term arthrogenic inhibition to refer to the neurological "shutdown" of muscles surrounding an injured joint, preventing full activation, reducing strength, and promoting atrophy (Palmieri-Smith RM & Thomas AC, 2009). Neuromuscular impairment following anterior cruciate ligament injuries would also cause knee instability and a loss of smooth control of agonist and antagonist muscle interaction, contributing to the accelerated degeneration of the joint (Brandt KD, 1997; Herzog W & Longino D, 2007; Roos EM et al., 2011).

Neuman and colleagues observed the incidence of radiographic osteoarthritis in a cohort of patients with unilateral, acute anterior cruciate ligament tears undergoing non-operative treatment with neuromuscular training and early activity modification after 10-to-15 years (Neuman P et al., 2008). The authors found that all patients developing knee osteoarthritis were previously meniscectomized. None of the remaining non-meniscectomized patients had radiographic signs of knee osteoarthritis at 10-to-15 years of follow-up. Sixty-eight percent of patients had asymptomatic knees. The authors concluded that non-operative treatment of anterior cruciate ligament tears by means of neuromuscular training and early activity modification might also have been related to the low prevalence of radiographic knee osteoarthritis (Neuman P et al., 2008). Ageberg and colleagues reported a longitudinal prospective cohort study of 100 anterior cruciate ligament-deficient patients undergoing conservative treatment with neuromuscular training and activity modification (Ageberg E et al., 2007). The majority of patients in this study demonstrated good functional performance and knee muscle strength throughout the 15-year study with this treatment without undergoing reconstructive surgery. The main concern of this study was the lack of a matched comparative group. If reconstruction of anterior cruciate ligament is performed, Keays and colleagues found that the restoration of quadriceps-to-hamstring strength balance was associated with less osteoarthritis (Keays SL et al., 2010). Therefore, protection of articular cartilage when anterior cruciate ligament injury occurs may be more related to the neuromuscular training than the reconstruction of the torn ligament itself (Keays SL et al., 2010; Lohmander LS et al., 2007; Neuman P et al., 2008). Thus, early activity modification and neuromuscular knee rehabilitation after anterior cruciate ligament injury may be a very important aspect to decrease the impairment of the neuromuscular system.

Quadriceps and hip muscles weakness are common in patients with knee osteoarthritis (Felson DT et al., 2000; Hinman RS et al., 2010). Roos and colleagues suggested that muscle weakness might be a risk factor related to all of the most important risk factors for osteoarthritis, as muscle strength is lower in women than in men, is reduced following injury, decreases with age and is lower relative to overall body mass in obese individuals (Roos EM et al., 2011). Taking into account this relationship, the study of the isolated role of muscle weakness in osteoarthritis may be difficult. The combination of muscle weakness with other risk factors would increase the risk of osteoarthritis more than muscle weakness alone (Roos EM et al., 2011). It has been argued that muscle weakness would be the consequence of atrophy due to minimized use of painful joints (Felson DT et al., 2000). However, it is also present in patients with knee osteoarthritis who have no history of joint pain (Felson DT et al., 2000), so it would be a risk factor for structural damage to the joint and not only a consequence of a painful joint (Slemenda C et al., 1998). Thus, muscle weakness may be considered an independent risk factor for knee osteoarthritis (Roos EM et al., 2011). Slemenda and colleagues evaluated the baseline knee extensor strength in a cohort of women without radiographic knee osteoarthritis (Slemenda C et al., 1998). After 30 months, radiographs were taken from this sample and results demonstrated that those women with radiographic knee osteoarthritis had lower baseline strength values compared to subjects without it (Slemenda C et al., 1998). For each 10-lb-ft increase in knee extensor strength, Slemenda and colleagues found a 20% reduction in the odds ratio of prevalent radiographic knee osteoarthritis and a 29% reduction in the odds ratio of symptomatic knee osteoarthritis (Slemenda C et al., 1997). In an experimental animal model study, Longino and colleagues induced quadriceps muscle weakness by injecting botulinum toxin A into muscles (Longino D et al., 2005). Only 4 weeks after the induction of muscle weakness, the authors found retropatellar cartilage degeneration in the experimental rabbits compared to control rabbits. Segal and colleagues found that greater knee extensor strength protected against development of incident symptomatic, but not radiographic, knee osteoarthritis in both sexes (Segal NA et al., 2009; 2010). Subjects with greater quadriceps strength also had less knee pain and better physical function over follow-up (Amin S et al., 2009). Some of the benefits of neuromuscular training on knee osteoarthritis may be explained by induced changes in glycosaminoglycan content (Roos EM & Dahlberg LE, 2005). While there seems to be a protective effect of muscle strengthening against the onset of osteoarthritis, that seems to be controversial for osteoarthritis progression (Roos EM et al., 2011). Further well-designed studies are needed to elucidate if muscle strengthening would prevent osteoarthritis progression.

The afferent somatosensory system comprises the receptors, afferent neurons and central processing centers that permit the detection of environmental sensory inputs, including the tactile sense, proprioception, temperature, and nociception (Roos EM et al., 2011). Proprioception, including the sense of position in space, underlies the ability to maintain erect posture, control joint movements and respond to perturbations (Roos EM et al., 2011). The link between proprioception and osteoarthritis is not only based on theoretical reasoning. Patients with knee osteoarthritis had significantly worse proprioceptive capacities than age-matched, normal individuals (Koralewicz LM & Engh GA, 2000; Pai YC et al., 1997; Roos EM et al., 2011; Sharma L, 1999). Impaired proprioception contributes to articular cartilage damage (Roos EM et al., 2011; Sharma L & Pai YC, 1997). Functional consequences of impaired proprioception include lower gait velocity, shorter stride length, and slower stair walking time (Sharma L & Pai YC, 1997). The study of long-term influence of proprioception impairment on osteoarthritis has a major confounding factor, as proprioception declines with age (Hurley MV et al., 1998; Pai YC et al., 1997), and older age is the most important risk factor for developing osteoarthritis (Roos EM et al., 2011). Proprioception would have a role as a risk factor for osteoarthritis progression (Roos EM et al., 2011), but not for osteoarthritis onset (Felson DT et al., 2009). Unfortunately, the relationship between afferent somatosensory system and protective or damaging muscle activity has been minimally evaluated in the setting of osteoarthritis (Sharma L & Pai YC, 1997).

Roos and colleagues summarized their extensive review of this factor in two main issues. First, exercise training interventions should address both muscle weakness and afferent sensory dysfunction (Roos EM et al., 2011). Second, exercise regimens that aim to achieve modification of joint loading or cartilage structure seem to be more promising in at-risk individuals or those with early disease (Roos EM et al., 2011).

5. Exercise and sports participation

Professor Joseph A. Buckwalter established a clear differentiation between the occurrences of osteoarthritis after exercise and sports exposition in normal or previously injured joints (Buckwalter JA, 2003; 2004). The investigation of the link between sports and osteoarthritis should not take into account athletes with significant joint injuries, as osteoarthritis may be a consequence of the injury instead of the exposition to exercise itself. Professor Buckwalter differentiated between activities like running and others with higher impact and torsional loads (Buckwalter JA & Martin JA, 2004), as higher impact loads produce a higher cartilage deformation compared to lower loads (Eckstein F et al., 2005). Although running may be the main action of many sports, this type of exercise will be differentiated from cutting sports because of his different prognosis with respect to osteoarthritis (Buckwalter JA & Martin JA, 2004). Following this distinction, an up-to-date review of the existing literature is presented in chronological order throughout the coming paragraphs.

5.1 Running

All identified studies dealing with the association between running and osteoarthritis are summarized in Table 1. As shown, 39 articles were found but only 15 were specifically conducted to assess the risk of running in the development of osteoarthritis (Fries JF et al., 1994; Konradsen L et al., 1990; Kujala UM et al., 1999; Lane NE et al., 1986; Lane NE et al., 1987; Lane NE et al., 1990; Lane NE et al., 1993; Lane NE et al., 1998; Marti B et al., 1989; McDermott M & Freyne P, 1983; Panush RS et al., 1986; Panush RS et al., 1995; Puranen J et al., 1975; Wang BW et al., 2002; Ward MM et al., 1995). The other 24 studies have combined the exposure of running and other sports to assess the risk of osteoarthritis or general disability. Among these studies, some have included subjects exposed to running and other sports (Cheng Y et al., 2000; Imeokparia RL et al., 1994; Kettunen JA et al., 2001; Kohatsu ND & Schurman DJ, 1990; Krampla WW et al., 2008; Rogers LQ et al., 2002; Spector TD et al., 1996b; Sutton AJ et al., 2001; Vingard E et al., 1998; Wijayaratne SP et al., 2008), and others have included runners compared to subjects performing other sports (Chakravarty EF et al., 2008; Dahaghin S et al., 2009; Felson DT et al., 2007; Hart DJ et al., 1999; Hootman JM et al., 2003; Kettunen JA et al., 2000; Kujala UM et al., 1994; Kujala UM et al., 1995; Lau EC et al., 2000; Manninen P et al., 2001; Raty HP et al., 1997; Sohn RS & Micheli LJ, 1985; Vingard E et al., 1993; Vrezas I et al., 2010). Of all studies dealing with running, 10.2% studied general disability and 10.2% spine, 7.7% hand, 46% hip, 74.3% knee, and 10.2% ankle osteoarthritis. All but 4 studies concluded that running was not associated with an increased risk of osteoarthritis. Four studies found that running increased the risk of hip and knee osteoarthritis (Cheng Y et al., 2000; Marti B et al., 1989; McDermott M & Freyne P, 1983; Spector TD et al., 1996b), but 2 of them involved subjects exposed to more physical activities (Cheng Y et al., 2000; Spector TD et al., 1996b). No studies have demonstrated a clear increase in the risk of spine, hand or ankle osteoarthritis after running exposure. Most common sources of bias in these reviewed studies were recall and selection bias, and lack of control of other potential risk factors for osteoarthritis. In fact, many of them did not adjusted the analysis for previous joint injury, body mass index or occupational workload (Table 1). Fifteen studies may be classified as Level II-evidence (38%), 19 as Level III-evidence (49%), and 5 as Level IV-evidence (13%).

5.2 Sports participation

Sports with higher impact and torsional loads may increase the risk of osteoarthritis more than straight-ahead sports or exercise. Theoretically, sports such as cycling, swimming, or golf may not be considered among those with higher risk of osteoarthritis. For a complete classification of sports depending on the intensity of joint impact and torsional loads, the reader is directed towards the article by Buckwalter and Martin (Buckwalter JA & Martin JA, 2004).

Author	Type of study	Study / Patient characteristics	Exercise	Exposure to running	Joints	Results	Confounding factors considered	Observations	Conclusions
Puranen et al., 1975	Case-control, Cross-sectional study, Level III evidence	74 ex-élite runners (mean age 55y, range 31-81) and 115 controls (mean age 56, range 40-75);	Running	Élite running: starting age 15y (range 12-25), total participation 21y (range 8-50)	Hip	Hip OA changes: runners 4% (controls 8.6% Osteophyte formation only: runners 9.5%, controls 14.8% (none had hip pain). Clear OA changes associated with more hip pain	Control of main confounding factors not reported: sex, BMI, occupational load, other exposure to sports, history of joint injury, etc.	No statistics reported Lack of control of confounding factors Controls might have been exposed to run	Running was not associated with increased risk of hip OA
McDermott and Freyne 1983	Case series, Level IV evidence	20 male middle and long distance runners with at least 3 months of knee pain Clinical and radiological knee OA	Running	Miles/week: mean between 41-62 in all runners. Years of running: mean 12-19 in all runners	Knee	All subjects with OA had genu varum 4/6 subjects with OA (3/14 in the group without OA) had previous injury Knee OA associated with injury and genu varum Miles/week: mean 62 in runners with, and 41 in runners without knee OA. Years of running: 19 in runners with, and 12 in runners without knee OA ($p<0.05$)	Control of main confounding factors not reported: sex, BMI, occupational load, exposure to sports, etc. History of joint injury and malalignment not isolated	No control group Joint injury and genu varum influenced the development of OA Small sample size	Longer exposure in years of running may increase the risk of knee OA
Sohn and Micheli, 1985	Case-control, Level III evidence	504 former runners (mean age 57y, range 23-77) compared to 287 ex-swimmers; mean follow-up 55y (range 2-25). Clinical hip and knee OA	Running Swimming	Running: miles/week by age: >70y 18, 60-69y 18, 50-59y 30, 40-49y 33, 0-40y 58; number of years running by age: >70y 8, 60-69y 9, 50-59y 12, 40-49y 14, 0-40y 10	Hip Knee	Severe hip or knee pain: 2% runners, 2.4% swimmers; any kind of hip or knee pain: 15% runners, 19 swimmers ($p>0.05$); no differences in pain between groups for any age range. Surgery for pain (mainly arthroplasties): runners 0.8%, swimmers 2.1%. Runners with higher miles run per week had not significantly more pain nor runners with higher cumulative years of running.	Age, sex, weight, educational level, socioeconomic status, cardiovascular fitness and attitude towards exercise-matched Control of occupational workload, exposure to other sports, BMI not reported	Runners response 76%, swimmers 58% Comparative group was not sedentary. Swimmers with history of running excluded No radiographs taken, pain may not be explained by OA	There was no association between middle- and long-distance running and risk of hip or knee OA
Lane et al., 1986	Cross-sectional, Level III evidence	41 long-distance runners (aged 50-72y) compared to 41 matched controls Clinical and radiological lumbar, knee and hands OA	Running	Running: min/week 224, years run 8.5, mean total miles run 9552	Lumbar spine Knee Hands	Female, but not male, runners had more sclerosis and spur formation in spine and knee, but not hand, radiographs. No differences in JSN, crepitation, joint stability, or symptomatic OA between groups	Age, sex, education, and occupation-matched controls. Control for history of joint injury in the analysis not reported	Controls heavier than runners Controls also exposed to running, although significantly less	Running was not associated with increased risk of lumbar spine, knee and hand OA

Author	Type of study	Study / Patient characteristics	Exercise	Exposure to running	Joints	Results	Confounding factors considered	Observations	Conclusions
Panush et al., 1986	Cross-sectional, Level III evidence	17 male runners (mean age 56y, range 50-74) compared to 18 male non-runners (mean age 61y, range 50-74) (no differences in age, height, weight). Clinical and radiological hip, knee, and ankle OA	Running	Runners: mean years running 12y (range 5-27); mean miles/week 28 (range 20-40); mean lifetime mileage 17343 (range 6500-49140)	Hip Knee Ankle	Runners vs non-runners: Hip pain 26% vs 11%, knee pain 29% vs 22%, ankle pain 12% vs 5%. Runners vs non-runners: Osteophytes per subject hip 0.6 vs 0.9, knee 3.9 vs 4.8, ankle 2.2 vs 1.8; cartilage thickness mm hip 4.65 vs 4.3, knee medial 5 vs 5 and lateral 5.8 vs 5.6, ankle 3 vs 3.1; degeneration % hip 0 vs 0, knee 0.06 vs 0.17, ankle 0 vs 0 (all differences p>0.05).	Not controlled for occupational load and history of joint injury.	Controls not exposed to exercise/sports. Small sample size Joint injury and occupational load influenced OA	Running was not associated with hip, knee and ankle OA
Lane et al., 1987	Cross-sectional, Level III evidence	498 long-distance runners (mean age 58y, SEM 0.3, male ratio 0.86, mean BMI 22.8) compared to 365 controls (mean age 63y, SEM 0.4, male ratio 0.56, mean BMI 24.3). General musculoskeletal disability	Running	Exercise: min/week mean 322 (SEM 20). Running: min/week mean 228 (SEM 11), miles run per week 25 (1), years run 11 (1.5)	General physical disability	Runners less physical disability than age-matched controls. Runners had greater functional capacity, sought medical care less frequently, and weighted less than controls.	Age, sex, education, and occupation-matched controls. Control for history of joint injury in the analysis not reported	Controls also exposed to running and exercise (less than runners) Runners significantly different than controls in age, sex, and BMI No targeted to OA	Running was related to improved general musculo-skeletal health
Marti et al., 1989	Case-control, Level III evidence	27 former elite long-distance runners (mean age 42y) 9 former bobsleigh riders (mean age 42y), and 23 controls (mean age 35y. Clinical and radiological hip OA	Running	Running: mean 97km/week Bobsleigh riders: mean 12km/week	Hip	Hip OA index (computed by summing JSN, sclerosis and osteophyte): mean 1.37 (0.76-1.98 95% CI) in runners, 0.33 (-0.05-0.72) in bobsleigh, and 0.32 (0-0.64) in controls (p=0.006). Runners more osteophyte and sclerosis compared to controls. Hip pain: 30% in runners, and 0% in bobsleigh and controls. Adjusting for age: runners more hip OA. Adjusting for mileage: runners not more hip OA	Analysis not adjusted for sex, BMI, occupational workload or history of joint injury. Adjusted for age and mileage	Participation 92% Small sample size Radiological blinding Controls and bobsleigh also exposed to running No baseline x-rays Reference values of OA in community not known	Running was associated with an increased risk of OA
Konradsen et al., 1990	Cross-sectional, Level III evidence	27 male orienteering runners (median age 58y, range 50-68; median weight 71kg, range 60-81) and 27 matched controls (median age 57y, range 53-65; median weight 75kg, range 55-82). Clinical and radiological OA	Running	Running: median ages 40y (range 32-50); median km/week <30y: 42 (range 20-65); 31-40y: 34 (15-65); 41-50y: 30 (13-63); 51-60y: 28 (13-63); >61y: 21 (13-43)	Hip Knee Ankle	No significant differences between runners and controls with regard to OA and osteophytosis of hip, knee, ankle. No differences in joint alignment, range of motion, or complaints of pain between groups. 22% of runners had pain during running, with no radiological differences compared to subjects without pain.	Age, height, weight, and occupational load-matched controls No major joint injuries in the sample, except 3 subjects, 1 of them excluded for the analysis	Participation 90% Controls were sedentary Statistics not much detailed Runners no longer active excluded Small sample size	Running at a recreational level was not associated with hip, knee, and ankle OA

Author	Type of study	Study / Patient characteristics	Exercise	Exposure to running	Joints	Results	Confounding factors considered	Observations	Conclusions
Kohatsu and Schurman, 1990	Case-control, Level III evidence	46 subjects (cases) with knee OA (mean age 71y, 60% females, BMI 27, years of school 14) and 46 matched controls (mean age 71y, 60% females, BMI 27, years of school 14) Diagnosed knee OA in patients undergoing TKA	Running Walking Team sports Racquet sports Others	Not reported	Knee	Similar exposure to running, team sports, racquet sports, and other sports in cases compared to controls (4.5% vs 8.7%, 12.2% vs 17.4%, 15.8% vs 22.2%, 59.5% vs 65.2%, respectively). Cases less exposed to walking compared to controls (35.7% vs 56.5%, $p<0.01$)	Age, gender, and educational-matched controls Unmatched for BMI Cases participated in heavier work for ages between 30 to 49y compared to controls Cases had more history of knee injuries ($p<0.01$)	Participation 68% Cases had higher BMI ($p<0.0001$) Subjects exposed to different sports Running not quantified	General leisure-time physical activity was not associated with significant risk of knee OA
Lane et al. 1990	Cohort study, Level II evidence	34 runners (mean age 59.8y, 62% males, BMI 22.7) vs 34 matched controls (mean age 59.1y, 62% males, BMI 24.2) Clinical and radiological OA at baseline and 2 years later	Running	Runners (mean values): exercise (min/week) 336, running (min/week) 173, miles/week 21.6	Lumbar spine Knee Hands	Runners had lower disability score ($p<0.05$) Lumbar OA: similar progression for JSN and sclerosis between groups; runners more progression of spurs in males. Knee OA: more progression of spurs in runners compared to controls Hand OA: more progression of JSN and sclerosis in runners, similar progression of spurs	Age, sex, occupation, and years of school-matched controls. Injuries collected but not reported (only reports on joint pain in those subjects who stopped running).	Follow-up 83% Controls higher BMI than runners, $p<0.01$ Controls also exposed to running JSN and sclerosis for knee OA unknown Spurs alone not enough for OA	Running was not associated with increased risk of lumbar spine, knee, and hands OA
Lane et al., 1993	Cohort study, Level II evidence	33 runners (mean age 63.3y, 60% males, weight 67.8kg) vs 33 matched controls (mean age 63.5y, 60% males, weight 73.1kg) Clinical and radiological OA at baseline and 5 years later	Running	Runners (mean values): exercise (min/week) 304, running (min/week) 185	Lumbar spine Knee Hands	Lumbar OA: both groups progressed in spurs. Knee OA: runners had no progression of spurs and combined JSN, sclerosis and spurs; controls had progression of both parameters. Hand OA: both groups progressed in spurs and combined JSN, sclerosis and spurs. No differences in age, sex, weight, exercise, running and disability between subjects with and without hand and knee OA. Running was not predictive of lumbar spine, knee or hand OA.	Age, sex, occupation, and years of school-matched controls. Injuries collected but its influence not reported	Follow-up 80% Controls were heavier than runners, $p<0.05$ Sample also exposed to other exercises (cycling, swimming, racquet sports) Controls increased min/week of exercise during the follow-up Spurs alone not enough for OA	Running was not associated with increased risk of lumbar spine, knee, and hands OA

Author	Type of study	Study / Patient characteristics	Exercise	Exposure to running	Joints	Results	Confounding factors considered	Observations	Conclusions
Vingard et al., 1993	Case-control, Level III evidence	233 cases with hip replacement because of OA and 302 controls, aged 50-70y.	Running, soccer, track and field, ice hockey, racquet sports, golf, bowling, cycling, swimming, handball,…	Not detailed for each sport. Reported as low, medium or high exposure. Collected: hours/week, week per year, total years, and level achieved.	Hip	Running: risk of hip OA in moderated and high exposure compared to low exposure: RR 1.7 (0.4-6.9) and 2.1 (0.6-6.8), respectively.	Controls were age, education, smoking, and BMI-matched Sports analysis adjusted for age, BMI, occupational work load, and different kind of sports simultaneously.	Participation: 92% cases, 77% controls. Subjects likely participated in different kind of sports. Controls also exposed to sports. No conclusive information on specific sports	Running was not associated with hip OA
Imeokparia et al., 1994	Case-control, Level III evidence	239 cases (85 men, 154 women) with knee OA vs 239 age and sex-matched controls, mean age 66y for both Radiographic knee OA	Running, cycling, swimming, racquet, soccer, golf, bowling	Not reported; Most subjects doing moderate (dance, weight lift, tennis, basketball) or light activities (volleyball, golf)	Knee	Sports exposure (cases): running 22%, cycling 84.5%, swimming 83.7%, racquet 51.5%, soccer 25.9%, Golf 62.7%, bowling 82.9% High physical activity only increased risk of knee OA in women OR 1.74 (1.01-3) adjusting for age, education, marital status and BMI. After adjusting by age, BMI, education, knee injuries, no association remained significant	Controlled for education level, BMI, age, smoking, hormone use, history of knee injury (12% cases and 2.5% controls) Confounders controlled in 2 analysis: age, education, marital status and BMI, and age, BMI, education, and knee injury	Limited to cases with < grade 3 OA Confounders controlled in 2 analyses Subjects exposed to different sports Running not isolated	Running not clearly associated with knee OA in women
Kujala et al., 1994	Cohort study, Level II evidence	2448 male ex-elite athletes representing Finland in sport events from 1920-1965 vs 1712 healthy age-matched controls at age 20y; Follow-up in 1970: 2049 athletes available, mean age 46y (range 21-85), 1403 in controls, mean age 44y (range 24-86); Follow-up in 1990: 1436 athletes available, 959 in controls. Study through questionnaires Athletes 3 groups: endurance, mixed sports, power sports Study compares admissions to hospitals because of hip, knee and ankle OA	Endurance: Running Cross-country ski; Mixed sports: Soccer Ice hockey Basketball Track & field; Power sports: Boxing Wrestling Weight lifting Throwing	Not reported; Former athletes at an elite level: Olympic games, World championships, European championships	Hip Knee Ankle	More admissions for hip, knee, ankle OA in athletes (5.9%) than controls (2.6%) ($p<0.0001$) Endurance (long-distance running): hip OA 5.2% (95% CI 2.6-10.2), knee OA 2.5% (0.7-6.3%), ankle OA 0%, compared to 1.4% (0.9-2.2), 1.3% (0.8-2), and 0% in the control group, respectively. OR for hip, knee, or ankle OA in runners compared to controls: 1.84 (95% CI 0.93-3.61). Adjusted OR for hip, knee, or ankle OA in runners compared to controls: 2.42 (1.26-4.68) Mean age at first admission: higher in endurance than others: 70.6y compared to 58.2y, 61.9y, and 61.2y in mixed sports, power sports, and controls, respectively.	Adjusted for age, weight and occupation History of joint injury not controlled	P value not reported for some comparison Only considering admission may hide other patients with OA at lower stages Exposure not quantified Endurance mixes running and cross-country skiing	Running was not associated with increased risk of hip, knee, or ankle OA Endurance athletes had admissions for hip, knee, or ankle OA at older ages

Author	Type of study	Study / Patient characteristics	Exercise	Exposure to running	Joints	Results	Confounding factors considered	Observations	Conclusions
Fries et al., 1994	Cohort study, Level II evidence	451 long-distance runners (mean age 58y, males 83%, mean BMI 22.7) compared to 330 controls (mean age 61y, male 56%, mean BMI 24.1). General musculoskeletal disability at 8 years of follow-up	Running	Runners: mean 16859 miles run over 12.4y before study Running (min/week): runners 118 vs controls 6.6 Other vigorous exercise (min/week): runners 160 vs controls 117 Past running: runners 98% vs controls 24% Currently running: runners 62% vs controls 5%	General physical disability	After 8 years, runners had a lower progression of disability compared to controls (p<0.001). The difference was consistent for men and women.	Analysis adjusted for age, sex, BMI, baseline disability, smoking, history of arthritis. There were between-group differences in musculoskeletal complaints and injuries, and analysis only adjusted for history of arthritis. Analysis not adjusted for occupational workload.	Follow-up 84% runners, 78% controls All subjects also exposed to other vigorous exercises (runners 262 and controls 118 min/week Runners significantly different than controls in age, sex, smoke, and BMI No targeted to OA	Running was related to slower development of general musculoskeletal disability
Panush et al., 1995	Cohort study, Level II evidence	12 male runners (mean age 63y, SD 6) compared to 10 male non-runners (mean age 68y, SD 8) (no differences in age, height, weight). Clinical and radiological hip, knee, and ankle OA at 8-year follow-up	Running	Runners: mean years running 22y (SD 14); mean miles/week 22 (SD 11); lifetime mileage 25168; 42% marathoners	Hip Knee Ankle	Runners vs non-runners: Hip pain 9% vs 10%, knee pain 0% vs 0%, ankle pain 0% vs 10%. No differences in hip, knee, and ankle OA between runners and non-runners.	Adjustment of analysis for age, sex, BMI, occupation and history of joint injury not known.	Statistics poorly reported Small sample size Joint injury and occupational load influenced OA 20% of runners and 10% of non-runners participated in other type of exercises	Running was not associated with hip, knee and ankle OA

Author	Type of study	Study / Patient characteristics	Exercise	Exposure to running	Joints	Results	Confounding factors considered	Observations	Conclusions
Kujala et al., 1995	Case series, Level IV evidence	Ex-elite athletes from 1920-1965 ages 45-68y; 28 runners (long-distance), 31 soccer, 29 WL, 29 shooters; subjects interviewed for weight and height at age 20y Clinical and radiographic OA	Running, Soccer, WL, Shooters	Runners: endurance training for 31y (range 4-68y), total hours 9408 (1300-18752); Soccer: team sport training for 17y (0-41), total hours 2607 (0-9936); WL: power sport training for 15y (0-69), total hours 2269 (0-8483); Shooters: endurance training for 20y (0-46), total hours 2845 (0-8536)	Knee	Knee injuries: runners 10%, soccer 38%, WL 20%, shooters 3% Knee OA: runners 14%, soccer 29%, WL 31%, shooters 3%. Runners not significantly different. TF OA runners 4%, soccer 26%, WL 17%, shooters 0%. Runners not different. PF OA: runners 11%, soccer 16%, WL 28%, shooters 3%. Runners not different. Monthly knee pain: runners 21%, soccer 45%, WL 28%, shooters 17%. Runners not different. Knee disability: runners 11%, soccer 35%, WL 24%, shooters 7%. Runners not different. Age-adjusted OA compare to shooters: runners OR 4.8 Age-adjusted risk of OA with hours spent in training: endurance OR 1.06 (0.94-1.2)	Age-, BMI-, occupation-, and injured-adjusted Leisure-time activity controlled Exposure to exercise highly detailed Interviews, physical exam and radiography by independent investigator Comparison of knee OA between groups in non-injured subjects not detailed	Participation 80% Data on weight and height under risk of recall bias Runners and WL more exposed to occupational workload Number of runners and shooters with OA was low (risk type II error) No control group	Runners exposed to lower risk of OA compared to other types of sports
Ward et al., 1995	Cohort study, Level II evidence	454 runners (mean age 58y (range 50-85), male 82%, smokers 1.5%) and 292 non-runners (mean age 62y (range 50-83), male 54%, smokers 6.2%) General physical disability	Running	Runners: mean minutes of vigorous exercise per week 293 (vs 90 in non-runners); mean years of running 10.6; mean miles run per week 25.6y; mean minutes of running per week 224	General physical disability	Some physical disability: runners 49% vs non-runners 77% Major risk factors for physical disability were: arthritis symptoms, older age, greater BMI, strenuous work-related physical activity, use of more medication.	Several risk factors considered Similar baseline proportion of family history of arthritis, arthritis symptoms, lower extremity injury, history of bone fracture, and occupation workload between groups.	Former runners included in the non-runners group Non-runners also participating in other vigorous exercises Both groups exposed to other risk factors Study not targeted towards study of effects of running on OA	Running was not associated with increased risk of physical disability compared to non-runners
Spector et al., 1996	Case-control study, Level III evidence	81 ex-elite female athletes (67 long-distance runners and 14 tennis players) aged 52y (SD 6), BMI 22 (SD 2.8) and 977 age-matched female controls Clinical and radiological OA	Running Tennis	Mean competition for 15y in runners and 19y in tennis; mean hours of vigorous weight-bearing sports per week: runners 2.6, tennis 5.7; mean miles per week of running 14.6; mean hours per week of tennis player 5.2	Hip Knee	Adjusted risk of TF osteophytes and JSN in ex-athletes: OR 3.57 (1.89-6.71), OR 1.17 (0.71-1.94), respectively. Adjusted risk of PF osteophytes and JSN in ex-athletes: OR 3.5 (1.8-6.81), OR 2.97 (1.15-7.67), respectively. Adjusted risk of hip osteophytes and JSN in ex-athletes: OR 2.52 (1.01-6.26) and OR 1.6 (0.73-3.48), respectively. Adjusted mean joint space of subjects without OA greater in ex-athletes.	Age, sex, height, and weight-adjusted analysis For knee, analysis adjusted also for knee injuries, knee pain, smoking, menopause, BMI. Knee pain: ex-athletes 33%, controls 25% Knee injury: ex-athletes 3.7%, controls 13.7% ($p<0.05$) Hip pain: 18.5% both groups Occupational workload not controlled	Participation 71% Ex-athletes were younger, taller, lighter and less smokers than controls Athletes participated in running and tennis Controls also exposed to exercise	Running and tennis in women was associated with a 2-3-fold increase in the risk of radiological OA

Author	Type of study	Study / Patient characteristics	Exercise	Exposure to running	Joints	Results	Confounding factors considered	Observations	Conclusions
Raty et al., 1997	Case series, Level IV evidence	Ex-elite athletes from 1920-1965; 29 runners mean age 59y (long-distance), 30 soccer mean age 56y, 27 WL mean age 59y, 28 shooters mean age 61y	Running, Soccer, WL, Shooters	Median lifetime train (h): runners 9650; soccer 9120; WL 8410; shooters 2750. Mean years in elite level: runners 9.7y, soccer 13.4y, WL 11.7y, shooters 14.5y	Lumbar spine	Lumbar pain: current: runners 0%, soccer 7%, WL 3%, shooters 4% (p=0.6); past year: runners 48%, soccer 37%, WL 38%, shooters 64% (p=0.13); > 10 episodes lifetime: runners 7%, soccer 23%, WL 28%, shooters 29% (p=0.2). ROM: runners 55°, soccer 53°, WL 55°, shooters 51° (p=0.41)	Age- and occupation-adjusted History of back pain reported, but not past lumbar injuries Interviews, physical exam and radiography by independent investigator No control group	Not clear information on lumbar OA Lumbar injuries not reported Extreme lumbar ROM not involved in included sports	Lumbar mobility was not impaired in runners
Lane et al., 1998	Cohort study, Level II evidence	28 runners mean age 66y (range 60-77), 60% males, mean BMI 23.6, and 27 non-runners mean age 66y, 74% males, mean BMI 24.7. Clinical and radiological OA at 9 years of follow-up	Running	Runners: mean 279 min/week of exercise; mean 107 min/week running; mean miles run/week 18; mean years running 17	Hip Knee	Hip joint: osteophytes, JSN, total hip score not significantly different between both groups. Knee joint: both groups significantly progressed in osteophytes; only controls significantly progressed in JSN; only runners significantly progressed in total knee score	Age, sex, education and occupation-adjusted History of injury not clearly controlled	Controls participated in mean 169 min/week of exercise Small sample size Potential risk of selection bias.	Running was not associated with increased risk of hip OA and progression of knee OA
Vingard et al., 1998	Case-control, Level III evidence	230 (cases) women aged 50-70y with hip OA compared to 273 age-matched controls	Running, and many other sports: handball, soccer, tennis, badminton, track and field, cross-country skiing, and others	Details not reported Exposure to sports to the age of 50y: hours per week, weeks per year, how many years. Exposure graded as: low (total of <100h), medium (total of 100-800h), high exposure (total of >800h).	Hip	Hip OA: left 26%, right 35%, both 39% Hip OA: high vs low exposure RR 2.3 (1.5-3.7), medium vs low exposure RR 1.5 (0.9-2.5). Match of sports and occupational load: risk only increased in the following combination: Medium exposure to sports and high exposure to work load RR 2.7 (1.1-7), high exposure to sports and medium exposure to work load RR 2.7 (1.2-5.9), and high exposure to both RR 4.3 (1.7-11)	Adjusted for age, BMI, occupational load, number of children, smoking, and hormone therapy. Not controlled for history of hip injury	Participation 95% cases, 89% controls Controls have been exposed to sports Subjects exposed to different sports at various intensities Only women included Overall low participation in sports Running not isolated Low number of running cases	Exposure to sports was not associated with increased risk of hip OA in women alone, but in combination to work load.

Author	Type of study	Study / Patient characteristics	Exercise	Exposure to running	Joints	Results	Confounding factors considered	Observations	Conclusions
Kujala et al., 1999	Cohort study, Level II evidence	264 male orienteering runners (mean age 58y, range 47-71; mean BMI 23) compared to 188 male non-smoking controls (mean age 60y, range 50-71; mean BMI 25). Clinical OA at 11 years of follow-up	Running	Not specified	Hip Knee	Hip OA: running OR 0.78 (0.35-1.73) Knee OA: running OR 1.79 (1.1-3.54) Hip pain: running OR 0.74 (0.37-1.46) Knee pain: running OR 1.75 (0.96-3.18) Hip pain in stairs: running OR 0.47 (0.2-1.08) Knee pain in stairs: running OR 0.78 (0.4-1.4) Runners: 23.5% had ligament or meniscus injury (vs 16.8% in controls); 38% of runners with knee injuries had OA (vs 7% without injury)	Age, sex, and area of residence-adjusted analysis Not adjusted for BMI and occupational workload. History of previous knee injury likely influencing development of OA	Exposure to running not quantified 11% of controls have participated in other physical activities Differences in weight and BMI	Overall, running was not associated with greater lower-limb disability, except for knee OA
Hart et al., 1999	Cohort study, Level II evidence	830 women (mean age 54y, BMI 24, knee injury 12.7%, knee pain 24%) assessed for risk factors for incidence of radiological knee OA at 4 years of follow-up.	Walking Sports	Not reported	Knee	Osteophytes: walking OR 0.6 (0.22-1.71); sports OR 1.23 (0.54-2.81). JSN: walking OR 0.38 (0.15-0.93); sports: OR 0.98 (0.42-2.3)	Adjusted hysterectomy, ERT, smoking, physical activity, knee pain, social class. History of knee injury and occupational load collected but adjustment in the analysis unknown	Participation 83% Poorly detailed exposure to physical activity Specific effects of running unknown Short follow-up	Physical activity was not associated with incident knee OA
Cheng et al., 2000	Cohort study, Level II evidence	16961 subjects aged 20-87y (median age 44y for men (76%) and 43y for women (24%)) followed-up for a mean of 10.9y for incidence of hip and knee OA. Self-reported physician-diagnosed hip and knee OA	Running, walking, other physical activity	Physical activity: high (walking or jogging >20 miles/week), moderate (between 10-20 miles/week), low (<10 miles/week), other (other activities than walkin/jogging)	Hip Knee	439 incident cases in men (3.4%) and 162 in women (3.9%); subjects >50y: incident OA higher in women; subjects <50y: incident OA similar between men and women Physical activity <50y: men high HR 2.4 (1.5-3.9), moderate 1.2 (1-1.4), low 1 (0.6-1.5), other 1.4 (0.9-2); women high HR 1.5 (0.4-5.1), moderate 1.2 (0.9-1.5), low 0.8 (0.4-1.6), other 1.1 (0.6-2). Physical activity >50y: men high HR 1.2 (0.6-2.3), moderate 1 (0.8-1.2), low 1.3 (0.9-1.8), other 1.1 (0.7-1.5); women high HR 1.4 (0.4-4.6), moderate 1.2 (0.9-1.5), low 0.6 (0.3-1.2), other 0.7 (0.4-1.3).	Adjusted for age, gender, BMI, smoking and ethanol and caffeine use. History of joint injury and occupational workload not controlled in the analysis.	Kappa agreement 0.68 between self-reported physician-diagnosed OA and chart review for OA Subjects participated in running and other kind of exercises	High levels of physical activity were associated with increased incidence of self-reported physician-diagnosed hip and knee OA in men < 50y, but not in the rest of the sample

Author	Type of study	Study / Patient characteristics	Exercise	Exposure to running	Joints	Results	Confounding factors considered	Observations	Conclusions
Kettunen et al., 2000	Case series, Level IV evidence	Ex-elite athletes from 1920-1965; 28 runners mean age 59y (range 51-67y) (long-distance), 31 soccer mean age 56y (45-67y), 29 WL mean age 59y (46-66y), 29 shooters mean age 61y (50-687) Hip pain, disability, occupation and athletic loading	Running, Soccer, WL, Shooters	Runners: median lifetime endurance training (h): 8980 (range 1300-18752); team sport training 0 (range 0-3072); power training 0 (0-1280)	Hip	Hip OA: runners 12%, soccer 12%, WL 20%, Shooters 24%; Hip pain: runners 21%, soccer 13%, WL 7%, Shooters 17%; Hip disability: runners 7%, soccer 3%, WL 3%, Shooters 3% In hip OA, more disability but not necessarily more pain	Age- and occupation-adjusted History of hip injury not reported Interviews, physical exam and radiography by independent investigator	No control group Small sample Only includes worst grades of hip OA Study not targeted towards hip OA; Statistics for between-groups differences in hip OA not reported Runners also exposed to other types of exercise	Running was not associated with increased risk of hip OA compared to other kind of sports
Lau et aL, 2000	Case-control, Level III evidence	138 subjects with hip OA and 414 controls. 658 subjects with knee OA, 658 controls. Clinical and radiological hip and knee OA	Running, badminton, soccer, gymnastics, kung fu	Not detailed	Hip Knee	Hip OA: Low number of cases in all sports, except gymnastics in women; Knee OA: Low number of cases except running, soccer in men, and running, gymnastics, kung-fu in women. Hip OA: men: running OR 0.7 (0.2-2.3), soccer 1.3 (0.3-5.4), gymnastics 1.2 (0.2-6.9), kung-fu 0.8 (0.08-6.7); women: running 0.9 (0.2-3.3), badminton 1 (0.2-5), gymnastics 6 (2.1-17.6). Knee OA: men: running OR 0.6 (0.3-1.4), soccer 1.3 (0.6-2.8), gymnastics 2 (0.8-5.3), kung-fu 1.4 (0.4-4.4); women: running 1.4 (0.7-2.8), badminton 0.5 (0.1-2.7), gymnastics 7.2 (3.1-16.8), kung-fu 20 (2.7-149).	Age-, sex-, weight-, occupation-, hip/knee injuries-controlled, but analysis only differentiating for sex	Only includes worst grades of OA Too high risk of type II error in sports with low number of cases No data on number of injuries in each group or sport	Running was not associated with increased risk of hip and knee OA in both men and women

Author	Type of study	Study / Patient characteristics	Exercise	Exposure to running	Joints	Results	Confounding factors considered	Observations	Conclusions
Kettunen et al., 2001	Case-control, Level III evidence	Initial sample: 2448 male ex-elite athletes representing Finland in sport events from 1920-1965 vs 1712 healthy age-matched controls at age 20y; Follow-up in 1995: 1321 athletes available, 814 in controls. Hip and knee OA in <45y / >45y Study through questionnaires Athletes of endurance, track and field, mixed and power sport Mean age: endurance 68y, track and field 64y, team sports 61, Power sport 64y, Shooters 70y, controls 62y	Endurance: Running Cross-country ski; Track & field; Other sports (team and power sports)	Not reported; Former athletes at an elite level: Olympic games, World championships, European championships	Hip Knee	For age, weight, occupation-adjusted analysis (only significant results showed): -Hip disability: endurance OR 0.35 (0.14-0-85), Track and field OR 0.3 (0.12-0.73), All sports OR 0.54 (0.36-0.82) -Knee disability: Team sport OR 1.76 (1.03-3) -Hip OA: no differences. -Knee OA: Team sport OR 2.04 (1.35-3.07) -Hip pain: Endurance OR 0.32 (0.17-0.61), Shooting OR 0.32 (0.12-0.87), all sports OR 0.66 (0.5-0.88) -Knee pain: Team sports OR 1.56 (1.07-2.28)	Adjusted for age, weight and occupation History of joint injury not excluded from the analysis of OA	Exposure not quantified Likely influence of injury on hip and knee pain, disability, and OA	Running was not associated with increased risk of hip or knee OA Running associated with decreased risk of hip disability
Manninen et al., 2001	Case-control, Level III evidence	281 cases undergoing TKA for knee OA (men 55, women 226, mean age 28y) and 524 age-, sex-matched controls	Running, cross-country skiing, biking, track and field, volleyball, tennis, baseball, and others	Only few at competitive level. Exposure: hours per week, month per year, total years, cumulative hours of physical exercise. High exposure: >8654h in men, >6862h in women. Low exposure lower than these values.	Knee	Men with high cumulative exercise were protected against knee OA compared to low exposure OR 0.28 (0.08-0.96) for all ages. Women with high exposure were protected against knee OA in age ranges 30-49y, and >49y compared to low exposure OR 0.51 (0.23-1.15) and 0.59 (0.3-1.16), respectively. Running: men OR 0.26 (0.05-1.3), women OR 0.7 (0.48-1.02)	Analysis adjusted for age, BMI, physical work stress, knee injury, and smoking.	Participation 70% Subjects participated in more than 1 sport. Controls exposed to same sports. Specific sport exposure not provided.	Running was not associated with increased risk of knee OA in men and women

Author	Type of study	Study / Patient characteristics	Exercise	Exposure to running	Joints	Results	Confounding factors considered	Observations	Conclusions
Sutton et al., 2001	Case-control, Level III evidence	216 cases (66 men, 150 women) mean age 57y (range 40-96) and 864 age, and sex-matched controls. Sports: Vigorous (team sports, boxing, weight lift, skiing, running, martial arts, racquet sports, etc.), moderate (swimming, cricket, gymnastics, aerobics, sailing, horse riding, etc.), gentle (shooting, golf, yoga, motor sports, fishing, etc.).	Running but many other sports, grades as vigorous, moderate, and gentle activities	Exposure detailed, but reported as number of activities instead of details on training parameters. Exposure to sports considered for 2 time periods: 5-14y before, and 15-24y before the age of diagnosis.	Knee	Neither activity level in any of the 2 periods elicited a significant increased risk of knee OA. Walking for both time periods had a risk of knee OA: OR 1.7 (1.1-2.4) and OR 2.1 (1.5-3), respectively. Performing lot of exercise increased the risk of knee OA OR 1.8 (1-3) for exposure 15-24y. Being physically active did not increase the risk of knee OA in either period.	Analysis adjusted for knee injuries and BMI. Use of age-, and sex-matched controls. Occupational load not assessed.	Subjects participated in more than 1 sport. Controls exposed to same sports. Specific sport exposure not provided Knee OA was self-reported; knee replacement cases not collected. No details in average time spent in sports per week/month. Running not isolated	Increased levels of regular physical activity throughout life did not increase the risk of knee OA.
Rogers et al., 2002	Case-control, Level III evidence	415 cases (men 306, women 109) with diagnosis of hip/knee OA at follow-up compared to 1995 controls (men 1521, women 474). Self-reported hip and knee OA	Running, walking, treadmill, cycling, swimming, aerobic, weight train, racquet sports, soccer, basketball	Not detailed. Sports categorized in low and moderate/high joint stress	Hip Knee	Activities associated with moderate/high joint stress were associated with the lowest risk of hip/knee OA in both men and women: men OR 0.62 (0.43-0.89); women OR 0.24 (0.11-0.52).	Analysis adjusted for age, BMI, history of knee or hip injury, and years of follow-up.	Minimum 2y follow-up Minimum exposure to sports 3 months. Controls not exposed to sports Combination of moderate and high joint stress activities. Hip/knee OA not disclosed Running not isolated	Physical activity in terms of sports may reduce the risk of hip/knee OA, especially in women.
Wang et al., 2002	Cohort study, Level II evidence	370 runners mean age 58y (82% men, 18 women) and 249 controls mean age 60y (56% men, 44% women) General disability assessed through Health Assessment Questionnaire	Running	Runners: mean 10.8y running with average 25851Km; 235 min/week (19 in controls); other vigorous exercise 76 min/week (83 in controls); mean distance run 2203Km/year (200 in controls)	General disability	Runners significantly lower disability levels. Loss of disability delayed in runners. Running protected against mortality.	Not much details in adjusted variables. Sex-adjusted. Age-matched controls. History of joint injury collected but unknown if considered for analysis.	Controls also exposed to running (1374Km in 2.2y) Running not isolated	Running and other aerobic exercise in elderly persons protected against disability.

Author	Type of study	Study / Patient characteristics	Exercise	Exposure to running	Joints	Results	Confounding factors considered	Observations	Conclusions
Hootman et al., 2003	Cohort study, Level II evidence	5284 prospectively followed for incident hip and knee OA in relation to physical activity levels, mean follow-up 12.8y Self-reported physician-diagnosed hip and knee OA	Running Walking Other sports	Women 13.2 miles/week (range 2-48); men 13.8 miles/week (range 1-70)	Hip Knee	Hip/knee OA: miles/week of running: 10-20 OR 0.83 (0.52-1.31), 20-30 OR 1 (0.49-2.05), 30-40 0.67 (0.14-3.12), >40 OR 1.16 (0.3-4.43); min/mile 1.02 (0.92-1.13); sessions/week 0.99 (0.86-1.15)	Adjusted for training parameters, gender, age, BMI, previous hip and knee injury and surgery, smoking status, and comorbid conditions. Occupational workload not adjusted (although subjects had no heavy works)	Running not isolated Subjects participated in other sports	Physical activity was not associated with increased risk of hip and knee OA
Szoeke et al., 2006	Cohort study, Level II evidence	224 women assessed for hand and knee OA 11y after inclusion in a prospective study. Radiological hand and knee OA.	General physical activity	Not detailed. Baseline: 25% daily physical activity, 20 no physical activity; Follow-up: 40% daily physical activity, 13% no physical activity	Knee hand	Overall OA 56%: 21% knee OA, 44% hand OA. Physical activity not associated with hand OA. Physical activity at ages 20-29y associated with higher risk of knee OA (p=0.03): daily exercise 10 times greater (0.3-13.1), exercise 2-6 times a week 8 times greater (0.3-13.1), once a week 7 times greater (0.1-7.3), and few times per month 1.8 times greater (0.04-4).	Controlled for age, BMI, hormone use and smoking. Occupational load and joint injuries not controlled.	Participation 51% Subjects exposed to many sports. Intensity not reported Sports not reported. Sports involving hand use not known Running not isolated	High physical activity was associated with knee, but not hand, OA.
Felson et al., 2007	Cohort study, Level II evidence	1279 subjects (mean age at baseline 53.2y) followed-up for a mean of 8.75y for incident clinical and radiographic knee OA	Running Walking	Not detailed Walking: divided in walking <6 or >6 miles/week	Knee	Neither recreational walking, jogging, nor high activity levels were associated with an increased risk of knee OA.	Adjusted by age, sex, BMI, and history of joint injury. Not adjusted by occupational workload	Follow-up of 75% of subjects Large sample, prospective study Sample size of runners too small Running not clearly evaluated	Recreational exercise in middle-to-elderly subjects was not associated with increased knee OA
Krampla et al., 2008	Case series, Level IV evidence	8 ex-long-distance runners (mean age 46y) evaluated at 10y of follow-up for MRI-based knee OA	Running Other sports	Runners completed total of 34 races, mean race time 3'5h, mean min/km 5'5; runs of >20Km 435	Knee	Signs of knee OA based on MRI studies in 37.5%, all with associated meniscal tears. All subjects with knee OA demonstrated a progression of the disease in the follow-up (no new cases)	Not adjusted for age, sex, BMI, family history of OA, knee injuries and occupational workload	Follow-up 80% No statistics reported Small sample size Subjects exposed to other kind of sports	Running was not clearly associated with knee OA
Chakravarty et al., 2008	Cohort study, Level II evidence	45 long-distance runners (mean age 71y, 65% men, 44% previous knee injury, BMI 23) and 53 age-, education-, and occupation-matched controls (mean age 72y, 70% men, 36% previous knee injury, BMI 25) followed for nearly 2 decades for radiographic knee OA	Running Other sports	Vigorous exercise: runners 293 min/week, controls 199 min/week Running: runners 95 min/week, controls 1 min week	Knee	Knee OA: runners 20%, controls 32% (p=0.2). Severe knee OA: runners 2.2%, controls 9.4% (p=0.2) Knee OA associated with BMI, initial radiographic damage and longer follow-up. Knee OA not associated with gender, education, previous knee injury, and mean exercise time.	Adjusted for age, gender, BMI, education, previous knee injury, and initial radiographic and disability scores. Not clearly adjusted for occupational workload.	Subjects performed other kind of exercises Running not isolated Controls also exposed to running earlier in life	Running was not associated with accelerated radiographic knee OA

Author	Type of study	Study / Patient characteristics	Exercise	Exposure to running	Joints	Results	Confounding factors considered	Observations	Conclusions
Wijayaratne et al., 2008	Cohort study, Level II evidence	148 women (mean age 53y, BMI 27) followed for 2y for modification of MRI-based patella cartilage volume changes	Running, walking, aerobics, swimming, others	Not reported	Knee	Fortnightly exercise for at least 20 minutes tended to be associated with a reduced rate of patella cartilage volume loss (p=0.09).	Adjusted for age, height, weight, initial patella cartilage volume, and patella bone volume. Not adjusted for occupational workload	Subjects with previous joint injury excluded Life-long exposure to exercise not assessed	Running was not associated with increased risk of patellofemoral OA
Dahaghin et al., 2009	Case-control, Level III evidence	480 cases with knee OA (mean age 57y SD 12y) and 490 controls without knee OA (mean age 46y SD15y) (p<0.00001); 70% women in cases, 65% in controls; BMI 30 cases, 27 controls (p<0.00001)	Running, Body-building, Soccer, Volleyball, Others	Not reported	Knee	Participation in sports: 32% cases, 40% controls Running OR 1.05 (0.7-1.58)	Age, sex, and BMI-adjusted History of knee injuries not reported Occupational workload collected Adjustment of knee OA in runners depending on workload not known	Subjects exposed to different sports Minimum exposure to sports = 6 months Low participation in sports in both groups Controls also exposed to sports	Running was not associated with increased risk of knee OA
Vrezas et al., 2010	Case-control, Level III evidence	295 male cases with knee OA and 327 male controls, aged 25-70y Radiographic knee OA	Running, cycling, swimming, soccer, ball games, gymnastics, weight lifting, body building	Running: exposure from 0h to 3530h	Knee	Running, swimming, body-building, weight lifting: not increase risk of knee OA Exposure to running: 0-700h OR 0.8 (0.4-1.7), 700-1695h OR 1 (0.5-2.3), 1695-3530h 1.9 (0.8-4.1), >3530h 1.9 (0.8-4.3)	Age, sex, BMI and occupation History of joint injury not reported	Participation 55-61% Mild OA not included Isolation of running not known Potential effect of joint injury on OA	Running was not associated with increased risk of knee OA

y, years; OA, osteoarthritis; BMI, body mass index; min, minutes; JSN, joint space narrowing; vs, versus; SEM, Standard error of the mean; kg, kilogram; TKA, total knee arthroplasty; Kcal, kilocalories; OR, odds ratio (95% interval confidence); RR, relative risk (95% interval confidence); SD, standard deviation; WL, weight lifters; TF, tibiofemoral; PF, patellofemoral; h, hours; ERT, estrogen replacement therapy; HR, hazard ratio (95% interval confidence); km, kilometre; MRI, magnetic resonance imaging.

Table 1. Summary of studies evaluating the risk of osteoarthritis after exposure to running.

Table 2 summarizes all identified studies regarding the association between sports and osteoarthritis. As shown, 53 articles were found but 34 of them included different sports in the same study. In 13 of the 53 studies the exercise in which subjects had participated was not reported in detail (Cooper C et al., 2000; Eastmond CJ et al., 1979; Felson DT et al., 1997; Juhakoski R et al., 2009; Lane NE et al., 1999; McAlindon TE et al., 1999; Ratzlaff CR et al., 2011; Sutton AJ et al., 2001; Szoeke CE et al., 2006; Verweij LM et al., 2009; Vingard E, 1991; Wang Y et al., 2011; White JA et al., 1993). Of the 19 studies conducted specifically for a certain sport, 12 involved soccer (64%), 2 ballet (11%), and 1 baseball (5%), 1 track and field (5%), 1 Australian football (5%), 1 javelin throw (5%), and 1 high jump (5%). Of all 53 studies, 1 was not joint-specific (Turner AP et al., 2000), and 4 (7.7%) assessed spine (Raty HP et al., 1997; Sortland O et al., 1982; Vingard E et al., 1995; White JA et al., 1993), 2 (3.8%) shoulder (Schmitt H et al., 2001; Vingard E et al., 1995), 2 (3.8%) elbow (Adams JE, 1965; Schmitt H et al., 2001), 1 (1.9%) hand (Szoeke CE et al., 2006), 25 (48%) hip (Andersson S et al., 1989; Cooper C et al., 1998; Drawer S & Fuller CW, 2001; Eastmond CJ et al., 1979; Juhakoski R et al., 2009; Kettunen JA et al., 2000; Kettunen JA et al., 2001; Klunder KB et al., 1980; Kujala UM et al., 1994; Lane NE et al., 1999; Lau EC et al., 2000; Lindberg H et al., 1993; Ratzlaff CR et al., 2011; Rogers LQ et al., 2002; Schmitt H et al., 2004; Shepard GJ et al., 2003; Solonen KA, 1966; Spector TD et al., 1996b; Van Dijk CN et al., 1995; Vingard E, 1991; Vingard E et al., 1993; Vingard E et al., 1995; Vingard E et al., 1998; Wang Y et al., 2011; White JA et al., 1993), 34 (65.4%) knee (Andersson S et al., 1989; Chantraine A, 1985; Cooper C et al., 2000; Dahaghin S et al., 2009; Deacon A et al., 1997; Drawer S & Fuller CW, 2001; Eastmond CJ et al., 1979; Elleuch MH et al., 2008; Felson DT et al., 1997; Frobell RB et al., 2008; Hart DJ et al., 1999; Imeokparia RL et al., 1994; Kettunen JA et al., 2001; Klunder KB et al., 1980; Krajnc Z et al., 2010; Kujala UM et al., 1994; Kujala UM et al., 1995; Lau EC et al., 2000; Manninen P et al., 2001; McAlindon TE et al., 1999; Rogers LQ et al., 2002; Roos H et al., 1994; Sandmark H, 2000; Sandmark H & Vingärd E, 1999; Solonen KA, 1966; Spector TD et al., 1996b; Sutton AJ et al., 2001; Szoeke CE et al., 2006; Thelin N et al., 2006; Verweij LM et al., 2009; Vingard E et al., 1995; Vrezas I et al., 2010; Wang Y et al., 2011; White JA et al., 1993), 7 (13.5%) ankle (Andersson S et al., 1989; Brodelius A, 1961; Drawer S & Fuller CW, 2001; Kujala UM et al., 1994; Schmitt H et al., 2003; Solonen KA, 1966; Van Dijk CN et al., 1995), and 3 (5.8%) foot (Andersson S et al., 1989; Van Dijk CN et al., 1995; Vingard E et al., 1995) osteoarthritis. Ten studies may be classified as Level II-evidence (18.8%), 33 as Level III-evidence (62.4%), and 10 as Level IV-evidence (18.8%). Most common sources of bias were recall and selection bias, and lack of control of other potential risk factors like body mass index, history of knee injury and occupational workload. In addition, many control subjects were also exposed to some type of sport in their life (Table 2).

6. Preventive strategies for osteoarthritis

Preventive strategies against osteoarthritis require a knowledge of risk factors that influence the initiation of the disorder and its subsequent progression (Cooper C et al., 2000). Principal risk factors for osteoarthritis were older age, female sex, obesity, osteoporosis, occupation, sports activities, previous trauma, muscle weakness or dysfunction, proprioceptive deficit, and genetic factors. Only age, sex, and genetic factors are non-modifiable. Therefore, there is a potential to prevent osteoarthritis from all modifiable risk factors. Surprisingly, prevention of osteoarthritis has not been the focus of most of the existing references. In fact, there is a scarcity of studies aimed to assess prevention measures for osteoarthritis.

Author	Type of study	Study / Patient characteristics	Exercise	Exposure to sport	Joints	Results	Confounding factors considered	Observations	Conclusions
Brodelius, 1961	Cross-sectional, Level III evidence	34 male soccer players (mean age 27y, range 21-46y), 16 female dancers (aged 18-39y), and 195 controls Radiographic OA assessed	Soccer, Dance	Soccer mean 12y (range 5-20y) Dance > 3-30y	Ankle	OA higher in athletes Controls: OA increases with age but not related to sex Soccer: 33/34 had ankle OA; 13/15 players with previous injury had ankle OA Dancers: 14/16 ankle OA	Previous injury and age controlled No information on control of other risk factors Age related to OA in all groups	No statistical analysis reported; Volunteers enrolment in soccer players Only radiographic OA assessed	Overuse and injury may cause ankle OA
Adams, 1964	Cross-sectional, Level III evidence	162 baseball players aged 9-14y (pitchers and non-pitchers) and Radiographic elbow OA	Baseball	Not reported; mean length of play in pitchers 3y	Elbow	Elbow soreness 45%; Accelerated growth and fragmentation of medial epicondylar epiphysis: 95% pitchers, 15% non-pitchers, 8.5% controls; Fragmentation of medial epicondylar epiphysis: 48%, non-pitchers 12%, controls 6%; Osteochondritis 7.5%, 0% in others	Prior fracture, infection or deformity not included No control of potential confounders, although patients were young and probably pretty homogeneous	Cross-sectional study at young ages (patients may develop OA later in life). No statistics reported	Baseball participation elicits elbow radiographic changes in young players
Solonen, 1966	Cross-sectional, Level III evidence	60 male soccer players compared to 40 non-soccer matched controls Soccer aged 18 to 37y (mean 26y), controls aged 18 to 88y (mean 41y) Clinical and radiographic OA assessed	Soccer	Amateur soccer mean 13y (range 5-23y)	Hip Knee Ankle	No hip disorders; Knee: chondromalacia 30%, ligament insufficiency 13%, PF OA 28% (21% in controls); Ankle: OA in 92% (20% in controls)	Age and other risk factors uncontrolled History of knee / ankle injuries in both groups Soccer: 18 players sprained knee, 20 rupture of ligament, 6 meniscus tear; 48 players ankle sprain, 5 ankle LCL rupture, 3 malleolus fracture	No statistical analysis reported; Controls with joint injuries; Reasons not to participate not reported	No hip OA in soccer Ankle OA more common than knee OA
Eastmond et al., 1979	Cross-sectional, Level III evidence	364 female physical education teachers aged 46-60y, and 527 controls from the general population aged 45-64y Radiographic hip and knee OA	General sports	Not reported; 51% of teachers playing at least twice weekly	Hip Knee	68.5% still participating in sports; non-competitive tennis the most common sport; Hip OA (46-54y): Teachers grades 2-46.7% vs 3.9% controls; Hip OA (55-64y): Teachers grades 2-4 9.1% vs 8.3% Knee OA (46-54y): Teachers grades 0-1 93.2% vs 81.6%; grades 2-4 6.8% vs 18.4%, respectively; ($p<0.001$); Knee OA (55-64y): Teachers grades 0-1 89.4% vs 48.7% controls; grades 2-4 10.6% vs 51.3%, respectively.	Only partially controlled by age. Not controlled by other risk factors, including history of joint injury	Participation 76% Controls obtained from reference values Subjects exposed to different sports	Exposure to general sports at a non-competitive level does not increase the risk of hip and knee OA

Author	Type of study	Study / Patient characteristics	Exercise	Exposure to sport	Joints	Results	Confounding factors considered	Observations	Conclusions
Klunder & Hansen, 1980	Cross-sectional, Level III evidence	57 former soccer players vs 57 age- and weight-matched controls Soccer mean age 56y (range 40-79y), weight 78kg (61-104kg) in both groups; Controls mean age 56y (42-80y) Radiographic OA assessed	Soccer	Mean playing hours/week 6.7 (3-10); Mean years played 22.8y (11-41y)	Hip Knee	Soccer more OA compared to controls (53% vs 33%) ($p<0.05$) Hip OA: More in soccer 49% than controls 26% ($p<0.05$) Knee OA: Soccer 14%, Controls 12% (n.s.)	Controlled by main risk factors Age- and weight-matched controls No hip/knee injuries in controls at the time of evaluation; 3 (5%) controls had history of lower extremity injury, 13 (22%) in soccer Exposure to soccer detailed Exposure to heavy job: soccer 26%, controls 47%	Gender of soccer players not specified (assumed all men) Low number of knee OA cases Statistics not used controlling for injury & occupation Only radiographic OA assessed	Hip, but not knee, OA in soccer
Sortland et al., 1982	Cross-sectional, Level III evidence	43 former soccer players mean age 49y; 43 age-matched controls mean age 50y Clinical and radiographic OA assessed	Soccer	Competitive level; Mean 26 international (range 2-104), 326 national matches (120-626)	Cervical spine	Both groups: cervical OA in lower part affecting discs and uncovertebral joints; Soccer higher cervical OA in upper part ($p<0.02$), and lower part in intervertebral joints ($p<0.02$) No difference headers or not	Controls no history of neck trauma 21% of soccer players with cervical injuries, not isolated in the analysis	Gender of soccer players not specified (assumed all men) OA influenced by injuries in 21% of players	Soccer increases the risk of early development cervical OA
Chantraine, 1985	Case series, Level IV evidence	81 (162 knees) former players mean age 48y (range 40-74y) Clinical and radiographic OA assessed	Soccer	Competitive level for mean 19y (range 6-25y)	Knee	Overall 56% knees with OA: only 30% symptomatic Operated (meniscectomized) knees = 100% OA Not operated knees = 41% OA: age 40-49y = 32% OA, 50-59y = 43% OA, 60-69 60% OA, >70y 83% OA	Exposure highly detailed Players with cruciate ligament injury excluded 28% knees prior meniscectomy (10-27y before the study) Natural history of disease not controlled	Poor control of important confounders Knee injuries not isolated No control group Poor causal-effect relationship	Knee OA increased in former soccer players Meniscectomy increases risk of OA
Andersson et al., 1989	Case series, Level IV evidence	42 dancers of high level, mean age 57y (range 44-80); 35% men, 65% women	Classic ballet dance	Mean 18y of exposure (range 10-57y)	Hip Knee Ankle 1MTTP	13% hip OA all symptomatic (higher than general population); 9% of TF OA and 9% PF OA (and 14% with osteophytes) all symptomatic; 2.3% ankle OA; 54% 1MTTP OA all symptomatic	Not compared to control group, lack of control for potential confounders	Only compared to reference values (many not available) No control group Radiographic OA only considered if joint space narrowing	Ballet may increase the risk of 1MTTP joint OA, but not hip, knee and ankle
Vingard E, 1991	Case-control, Level III evidence	239 men with THR and 302 controls without THR, compared for BMI, aged 20-50y Radiographic hip OA	General sports	Not reported	Hip	Relative risk of hip OA as a function of BMI did not change after adjusting for sports activity	Controlled for age, smoking, occupation, but not for injuries	Subjects exposed to different sports Study not aimed to study sports-OA	Adjusting BMI-induced hip OA is not affected by sports

Author	Type of study	Study / Patient characteristics	Exercise	Exposure to sport	Joints	Results	Confounding factors considered	Observations	Conclusions
Lindberg et al., 1993	Case-control, Level III evidence	286 former soccer players mean age 55y (range 40-88y), and 572 age-matched controls Radiographic OA assessed	Soccer	71 players elite level, 215 amateur level Soccer exposure at least to the age of 25y	Hip	Hip OA higher in soccer: 5.6% vs 2.8%; OR 2.1 (1-4.2); bilateral hip OA equal in both groups (25%); no differences in type & severity Hip OA: Elite players 14%, all others 4.2% Elite players > risk of hip OA than amateur: OR 3.7 (1.4-10.1); no differences amateurs & controls; for 40-64y elite players more risk of hip OA than amateurs: OR 5.6 (2.5-20)	Age controlled Poor control of other potential confounding factors Only radiographic OA assessed	Exposure to soccer in controls not known	Soccer higher risk of hip OA Elite soccer much more risk of hip OA compared to amateurs
White et al., 1993	Cross-sectional, Level III evidence	12 year-follow-up of the postal survey from original sample Eastmond et a., 1979. 248 female physical education teachers aged 48-60y and 301 female controls aged 48-73y, divide in middle-aged (45-59y) and elderly (60-74y); 12 Clinical OA	General sports	Not reported; 21% sports at international level	Hip Knee Lumbar spine	70% of those with OA at middle age had played representative sport vs 9% in controls. No differences between subjects with moderate-severe and nil-minimal radiographic OA in the study of 1979 with respect to sports duration and number of activities participated. Control women had more any joint joint stiffness and pain in both ages (48-60y, 61-73y) compared to teachers	Controlled by age, occupation, prior fractures, BMI, family history of arthritis, but no information on past history of other injuries.	Participation 68% Subjects exposed to different sports. Physical activity and sports participation also in controls No radiographs	Active women participating in general sports have less pain and joint stiffness compared to less active controls
Imeokparia et al., 1994	Case-control, Level III evidence	239 cases (85 men, 154 women) with knee OA vs 239 age and sex-matched controls, mean age 66y for both Radiographic knee OA	Running, cycling, swimming, racquet, soccer, golf, bowling	Not reported; Most subjects doing moderate (dance, weight lift, tennis, basketball) or light activities (volleyball, golf)	Knee	Sports exposure (cases): running 22%, cycling 84.5%, swimming 83.7%, racquet 51.5%, soccer 25.9%, Golf 62.7%, bowling 82.9% High physical activity only increased risk of knee OA in women OR 1.74 (1.01-3) adjusting for age, education, marital status and BMI. After adjusting by age, BMI, education, knee injuries, no association remained significant	Controlled for education level, BMI, age, smoking, hormone use, history of knee injury (12% cases and 2.5% controls) Confounders controlled in 2 analysis: age, education, marital status and BMI, and age, BMI, education, and knee injury	Limited to cases with < grade 3 OA Confounders controlled in 2 separate analysis Subjects exposed to different sports at various intensities	Women are at increased risk of knee OA after high intensity sports, but not if adjusting for knee injuries

Author	Type of study	Study / Patient characteristics	Exercise	Exposure to sport	Joints	Results	Confounding factors considered	Observations	Conclusions
Vingard et al., 1993	Case-control, Level III evidence	233 cases with hip replacement because of OA and 302 controls, aged 50-70y.	Running, soccer, track and field, ice hockey, racquet sports, golf, bowling, cycling, swimming, handball, etc.	Not detailed for each sport. Reported as low, medium or high exposure. Collected: hours/week, week per year, total years, and level achieved.	Hip	Sports more common in younger years. Risk of hip OA compared to low exposure: Exposure <29y RR medium exposure 2 (1-2-3.2), high exposure RR 3.5 (2.2-5.6); >49y RR 2.6 (1.5-4.5), RR 4.5 (2.7-7.6), respectively. Significant risk factors for hip OA: Racquet and track and field for high exposure (compared to low exposure): RR 3.3 (1.2-12.7) and RR 3.7 (1.1-13.2), respectively. Combination sports & workload: high exposure to both factors in men RR of hip OA 8.5 (4-18).	Controls were age, education, smoking, and BMI-matched Sports analysis adjusted for age, BMI, occupational work load, and different kind of sports simultaneously.	Participation: 92% cases, 77% controls. Subjects likely participated in different kind of sports. Controls also exposed to sports. No conclusive information on specific sports	Long-term exposure to sports participation increases the risk of hip OA, especially if added to high workloads.
Kujala et al., 1994	Case-control, Level III evidence	2448 male ex-elite athletes representing Finland in sport events from 1920-1965 vs 1712 healthy age-matched controls at age 20y; Follow-up in 1970: 2049 athletes available, mean age 46y (range 21-85), 1403 in controls, mean age 44y (range 24-86); Follow-up in 1990: 1436 athletes available, 959 in controls. Study through questionnaires Athletes 3 groups: endurance, mixed sports, power sports Study compares admissions to hospitals because of hip, knee and ankle OA	Endurance: Running Cross-country ski; Mixed sports: Soccer Ice hockey Basketball Track & field; Power sports: Boxing Wrestling Weight lifting Throwing	Not reported; Former athletes at an elite level: Olympic games, World championships, European championships	Hip Knee Ankle	More admissions for hip, knee, ankle OA in athletes (5.9%) than controls (2.6%) (p<0.0001) OA athletes vs controls: Hip 3.3 vs 1.4%, knee 2.4 vs 1.3%, ankle 0.4 vs 0% (p unknown) Hip OA: Endurance 5.3%, Mixed sports 2.5%, Power sports 3.5%, Controls 1.4% (p unknown) Knee OA: Endurance 2.5%, Mixed sports 1.9%, Power sports 3%, Controls 1.3% (p unknown) Ankle OA: Endurance 0%, Mixed sports 0.6%, Power sports 0.4%, Controls 0% (p unknown) OA adjusted for age, weight and occupation: Endurance OR 2.42 (1.26-4.68) (p=0.011); Mixed sports OR 2.37 (1.32-4.24) (p=0.002); Power sports OR 2.68 (1.5-4.7) (p=0.0005); All sport OR 2.5 (1.5-4.1) (p=0.0001); Control OR 1 Mean age admission: higher in endurance than others; Median days in hospital higher in power sports than others (p=0.02)	Adjusted for age, weight and occupation Ice hockey and basketball players lower age History of joint injury not controlled	Ice hockey, basketball & weight lifters had no matched controls P value not reported for some comparison Only considering admission may hide other patients with OA at lower stages Exposure not quantified	Ex-elite athletes have a higher risk of hospital admission for hip and knee OA Endurance athletes have admissions at older ages

Author	Type of study	Study / Patient characteristics	Exercise	Exposure to sport	Joints	Results	Confounding factors considered	Observations	Conclusions
Roos et al., 1994	Case-control, Level III evidence	286 former soccer players (71 elite, 215 non-elite), and 572 age-matched controls (whole-sample mean age 55y (range 40-88y); mean age elite 62y, non-elite 53y Radiographic OA assessed	Soccer	71 players elite level. 215 amateur level Soccer exposure at least to the age of 25y	Knee	Knee OA in soccer 7% vs 1.6% controls; Knee OA: Elite 15.5% vs age-matched non-elite (4.2%) and controls (2.8%). Knee OA: elite vs non-elite OR 3.7 (1.5-9.3); non-elite vs controls OR 2.7 (1-6.8). Mean age at diagnosis: soccer 45y, controls 49y. Knee OA in non-injured subjects: elite 10.7%, non-elite 2.7%, controls 1.2%; Elite: 11 knee OA (5 in injured subjects); Non-elite 9 OA (4 in injured); Controls: 9 OA (2 in injured). Knee injuries: elite 33%, age-matched non-elite 7%, controls 2.1% Joint injury: increases risk of knee OA x3 in elite, x4 in non-elite, x13 In controls	Age and history of injury controlled History of sports participation poorly detailed for the control group	Exposure to exercise in controls only reported for those with knee OA Statistical analysis not reported for injured vs non-injured subjects	Elite, but not amateur, soccer increases risk of knee OA Joint injury increases the risk of OA in all groups, especially in controls
Kujala et al., 1995	Case series, Level IV evidence	Ex-elite athletes from 1920-1965 ages 45-68y; 28 runners (long-distance), 31 soccer, 29 weight lifters (WL), 29 shooters; subjects interviewed for weight and height at age 20y Clinical and radiographic OA	Running, Soccer, WL, Shooters	Runners: endurance training for 31y (range 4-68y), total hours 9408 (1300-18752); Soccer: team sport training for 17y (0-41), total hours 2607 (0-9936); WL: power sport training for 15y (0-69), total hours 2269 (0-8483); Shooters: endurance training for 20y (0-46), total hours 2845 (0-8536)	Knee	Knee injuries: runners 10%, soccer 38%, WL 20%, shooters 3% Knee OA: runners 14%, soccer 29%, WL 31%, shooters 3%; soccer and WL significantly higher than shooters (p<0.05). TF OA runners 4%, soccer 26%, WL 17%, shooters 0%: soccer significantly higher that shooters (p<0.05). Soccer significantly more knee disability and extension deficit than shooters (p<0.01) Higher knee OA with higher BMI (p=0.0002); Higher knee OA with injuries (p=0.0003) Age-adjusted OA compare to shooters: soccer OR 12.3 (1.35-111), WL OR 12.9 (1.47-113), runners OR 4.8; Age-adjusted risk of OA with hours spent in training: team sport OR 1.14 (1.03-1.27), power training OR 1.12 (1-1.25), endurance OR 1.06 (0.94-1.2); Hours of team sports increase risk of TF (OR 1.2 (1.03-2.29)) but not PF OA	Age-, BMI-, occupation-, and injured-adjusted Leisure-time activity controlled Exposure to exercise highly detailed Interviews, physical exam and radiography by independent investigator Runners and WL exposed to much more years of heavy work WL exposed to much more years of kneeling/squatting at work Comparison of knee OA between groups in non-injured subjects not detailed	Participation 80% Data on weight and height under risk of recall bias Runners and WL more exposed to occupational workload Number of runners and shooters with OA was low (risk type II error) No control group	Soccer and WL more knee OA than runners and shooters Risk of OA in soccer largely due to injuries Running low risk of knee OA

Author	Type of study	Study / Patient characteristics	Exercise	Exposure to sport	Joints	Results	Confounding factors considered	Observations	Conclusions
Van Dijk CN et al., 1995	Cross-sectional study, Level III evidence	19 ex-ballet dancers (mean age 59 aged 50-66y) vs 19 female controls	Ballet dance	Mean duration career 37y (range 13-54); mean dance time per week 45h (range 10-70)	Hip Ankle Subtalar 1MTTP	Hip OA: No differences between 2 groups Subtalar OA: 18% cases, 0% controls ($p=0.04$) Ankle and 1MTTP OA: Higher in cases ($p<0.05$)	Age-, Height-, Weight-matched controls. Not controlled for occupation in cases All ballet dancers had joint injuries Some controls with history of sports	47% controls had been involved in recreational sports (average 2h/week for 8y)	Dancers more ankle and 1MTTP OA compared to controls
Vingard et al., 1995	Case-control, Level III evidence	114 ex-elite men aged 50-80y and 355 age-matched controls Musculoskeletal disorders	Track and field	Not reported; ex-elite athletes	Spine Shoulder Hip Knee Feet	No increase in spine, shoulder, feet and knee OA in ex-elite athletes Hip OA higher in ex-elite athletes compared to controls PR 3.6 (1.4-9.3)	Age-adjusted analysis Information on other risk factors collected but not used for the statistical analysis	Not specific for OA No radiographs Not control of confounders	Track and field may increase the risk of hip OA
Spector et al., 1996	Case-control study, Level III evidence	81 ex-elite female athletes (67 long-distance runners and 14 tennis players) aged 52y (SD 6), BMI 22 (SD 2.8) and 977 age-matched female controls Clinical and radiological OA	Running Tennis	Mean competition for 15y in runners and 19y in tennis; mean hours of vigorous weight-bearing sports per week: runners 2.6, tennis 5.7; mean miles per week of running 14.6; mean hours per week of tennis player 5.2	Hip Knee	Adjusted risk of TF osteophytes and joint space narrowing in ex-athletes: OR 3.57 (1.89-6.71), OR 1.17 (0.71-1.94), respectively. Adjusted risk of PF osteophytes and joint space narrowing in ex-athletes: OR 3.5 (1.8-6.81), OR 2.97 (1.15-7.67), respectively. Adjusted risk of hip osteophytes and joint space narrowing in ex-athletes: OR 2.52 (1.01-6.26) and OR 1.6 (0.73-3.48), respectively. Adjusted mean joint space of subjects without OA greater in ex-athletes. No significant differences in tennis players compared to ex-runners with respect to TF, PF and hip osteophytes, and PF JSN.	Age, sex, height, and weight-adjusted analysis For knee, analysis adjusted also for knee injuries, knee pain, smoking, menopause, BMI. Knee pain: ex-athletes 33%, controls 25% Knee injury: ex-athletes 3.7%, controls 13.7% ($p<0.05$) Hip pain: 18.5% both groups Occupational workload not controlled	Participation 71% Ex-athletes were younger, taller, lighter and less smokers than controls Athletes participated in running and tennis Controls also exposed to exercise	Running and tennis was associated with a 2-3-fold increase in the risk of radiological OA. Tennis was not associated with greater risk of OA compared to ex-runners

Author	Type of study	Study / Patient characteristics	Exercise	Exposure to sport	Joints	Results	Confounding factors considered	Observations	Conclusions
Deacon A et al., 1997	Case-control, Cross-sectional study, Level III evidence	50 retired Australian football players (mean age 53y range 34-85) and 50 controls (mean age 55y range 35-79) Clinical and radiological knee OA	Australian football	Participation in sports (excluding football): players mean 25y controls 39y Number of football games: mean 360 over mean 19y	Knee	Knee injuries: 62% players (46% meniscal and 26% cruciate ligaments), 6% controls. Players had higher functional knee OA OR 10 (3.7-28), and higher radiographic knee OA OR 4 (1.9-8) compared to controls No differences in functional, and radiographic knee OA (after adjusting for weight) between injured and non-injured players. Players with cruciate and menisci injuries had higher risk of OA compared to players with other knee injuries and to controls	3 Controls had prior knee injuries Similar family history of OA Adjusted for age, height, weight, BMI, knee injuries	Participation 78% Players had higher BMI, height, and weight (p<0.0001), and were excluded from the regression analysis Controls had participated in sports	Ex-elite Australian football players had a higher risk of clinical and radiological knee OA compared to controls
Felson et al., 1997	Cohort study, Level II evidence	Framingham study cohort: 598 participants without knee OA in whom risk factors for developing the disease were studied: mean age 70y (SD 5), 63% women, mean BMI 26, prior knee injury 6%	Not reported Sports probably mixed & not reported	Not reported. Level of physical activity through the Framingham Physical Activity Index (considers number of hours of physical activity during a typical day and Kcal spent with those activities)	Knee	Adjusted risk of physical activity level for knee OA: 1st quartile OR 1, 2nd quartile 2.4 (1-5.3), 3rd quartile 3.1 (1.4-6.9), 4th quartile 3.3 (1.4-7.5). Adjusted risk of physical activity level for knee OA by sex (1st quartile vs 4th quartile): men 3.8 (0.9-17.3); women 3.1 (1.1-8.6). Adjusted risk of physical activity level for knee OA by knee symptoms (1st, 2nd, 3rd, 4th quartile): presence of symptoms: OR 1, OR 13.7 (0.5-362), OR 6.4 (0.1-320), OR 57 (1.6-2107), respectively; no symptoms: OR 1, OR 2.4 (1-5.3), OR 3.1 (1.4-6.9), OR 3.3 (1.4-7.5), respect.	Adjusted for age, sex, BMI, weight, smoking, knee injuries, chondrocalcinosis, and hand OA, simultaneously in the same analysis Not adjusted for occupation and family history.	Grade I radiographic OA not considered knee OA at baseline Subjects developing grade I in the follow-up not considered incident cases Not aimed to assess long-term effects of specific sports on knee OA	Most physically active subjects are at increased risk of developing knee OA
Raty et al., 1997	Case series, Level IV evidence	Ex-elite athletes from 1920-1965; 29 runners mean age 59y (long-distance), 30 soccer mean age 56y, 27 weight lifters (WL) mean age 59y, 28 shooters mean age 61y	Running, Soccer, WL, Shooters	Median lifetime train (h): runners 9650; soccer 9120; WL 8410; shooters 2750. Mean years in elite level: runners 9.7y, soccer 13.4y, WL 11.7y, shooters 14.5y	Lumbar spine	Lumbar pain: current: runners 0%, soccer 7%, WL 3%, shooters 4% (p=0.6); past year: runners 48%, soccer 37%, WL 38%, shooters 64% (p=0.13); > 10 episodes lifetime: runners 7%, soccer 23%, WL 28%, shooters 29% (p=0.2). ROM: runners 55°, soccer 53°, WL 55°, shooters 51° (p=0.41)	Age- and occupation-adjusted History of back pain reported, but not past lumbar injuries Interviews, physical exam and radiography by independent investigator No control group	Not clear information on lumbar OA Lumbar injuries not reported Extreme lumbar ROM not involved in included sports	Lumbar mobility not impaired in running, soccer, WL, shooters

Author	Type of study	Study / Patient characteristics	Exercise	Exposure to sport	Joints	Results	Confounding factors considered	Observations	Conclusions
Cooper et al., 1998	Case-control, Level III evidence	611 subjects waiting for hip replacement because primary OA compared to paired 611 controls; Cases: mean age 70y; men (34%) and women (66%) similar age, pain duration, and severity of OA	Tennis, swimming, soccer, cricket, golf	At least weekly for 3 months each year for 10 years since leaving school	Hip	Risk hip OA in with injury: Men OR 24.8 (3-199), women OR 2.8 (1.4-5.8), all OR 4.3 (2.2-8.4). Risk of hip OA significantly higher for tennis & swimming in women (OR 1.6 (1.1-2.2) and 1.5 (1.1-2), respectively), but not in men. Risk hip OA in all: soccer OR 1.1 (0.7-1.6), cricket OR 0.9 (0.5-1.4), golf OR 1.4 (0.9-2.3), any sport participation OR 1.2 (0.9-1.6)	Age-, sex-, and family physician-adjusted Risk of OA in sports not analyzed excluding injured subjects	Exposure to sports heterogeneous and not much detailed Injuries influencing hip OA in subjects with history of sports	Risk of hip OA not increased because in sports Women more risk of hip OA in tennis and swimming
Vingard et al., 1998	Case-control, Level III evidence	230 (cases) women aged 50-70y with hip OA compared to 273 age-matched controls	Handball, soccer, tennis, badminton, track and field, bowling, running, orienteering, cross-country skiing, skating, swimming, gymnastics, horse ride, golf, and others	Details not reported Exposure to sports to the age of 50y: hours per week, weeks per year, how many years. Exposure graded as: low (total of <100h), medium (total of 100-800h), high exposure (total of >800h).	Hip	Hip OA: left 26%, right 35%, both 39% Hip OA: high vs low exposure RR 2.3 (1.5-3.7), medium vs low exposure RR 1.5 (0.9-2.5). Match of sports and occupational load: risk only increased in the following combination: Medium exposure to sports and high exposure to work load RR 2.7 (1.1-7), high exposure to sports and medium exposure to work load RR 2.7 (1.2-5.9), and high exposure to both RR 4.3 (1.7-11)	Adjusted for age, BMI, occupational load, number of children, smoking, and hormone therapy. Not controlled for history of hip injury	Participation 95% cases, 89% controls Controls have been exposed to sports Subjects exposed to different sports at various intensities Only women included Overall low participation in sports	Exposure to sports does not increase risk of hip OA in women alone, but in combination to work load.
Hart et al., 1999	Cohort study, Level II evidence	830 women (mean age 54y, BMI 24, knee injury 12.7%, knee pain 24%) assessed for risk factors for incidence of radiological knee OA at 4 years of follow-up.	Walking Sports	Not reported	Knee	Osteophytes: walking OR 0.6 (0.22-1.71); sports OR 1.23 (0.54-2.81). Joint space narrowing: walking OR 0.38 (0.15-0.93); sports: OR 0.98 (0.42-2.3)	Adjusted hysterectomy, estrogen replacement therapy, smoking, physical activity, knee pain, social class. History of knee injury and occupational load collected but adjustment in the analysis unknown	Participation 83% Poorly detailed exposure to physical activity Specific effects of running unknown Short follow-up	Physical activity was not associated with incident knee OA

Author	Type of study	Study / Patient characteristics	Exercise	Exposure to sport	Joints	Results	Confounding factors considered	Observations	Conclusions
Lane et al., 1999	Cohort study, Level II evidence	5818 subjects evaluated for radiographic hip OA at baseline (aged 65y or above) Clinical and radiological hip OA	Many sports	Details not reported. Times per week and year exposed to many activities during teenagers, age 30 and 50y. Results reported as: 1) general physical activity; 2) Only weight-bearing activities	Hip	Hip OA: grades 0-I 88%, grade II 7%, grades III-IV 5%. Patients with grade III-IV were significantly older, taller and with higher BMI compared to others. General physical activity: Patients with grades III-IV and grades <II of hip OA had greater past exposure to physical activity (times/week) as teenagers and at 50y. Weight-bearing activities: Subjects with grades III-IV hip OA showed greater exposure (times/week) compared to others. Risk of radiographic hip OA was higher in quartile 4 of exposure at age 30y and quartile 3 at 50y (OR 1.4 for both). Clinical hip OA was higher in quartile 4 at teenagers (OR 1.7) and quartile 4 at 50y (OR 1.6).	Adjusted for age and BMI at age 25y Not controlled for other risk factors, mainly occupational work load and past history of hip injuries.	Exposure to exercise obtained retrospectively Exposure to physical activity was too general (no details on sports exposure known). Subjects exposed to different sports at various intensities.	Recreational physical activities before menopause may increase the risk of radiographic and clinical hip OA.
McAlindon et al., 1999	Cohort study, Level II evidence	Framingham study cohort: 473 participants without knee OA in whom risk factors for developing the disease were studied: mean age 70y (SD 4.5), 62% women. Clinical and radiological knee OA	Not reported Sports probably mixed & not reported	Exposure to sports not reported. Level of physical activity: heavy (lifting weights, gardening with heavy tools, digging, sports, etc.), moderate (lifting light weights, brisk walking, sweeping, etc.), light (leisure walk, standing, etc.)	Knee	Adjusted risk of radiographic knee OA: only increased in heavy physical activity if 1, 3 or >4h of exposure per day (OR 2.2 (1.2-4.2, OR 2.9 (1.2-6.9), OR 7.2 (2.5-21), respectively). Sex-adjusted risk of radiographic knee OA: increased only in heavy physical activity: men if >4h of exposure per day (OR 7 (1.7-29)) and women for 1 and >4h of exposure per day (OR 2.6 (1.3-5.3), OR 9 (1.7-48), respectively). Adjusted risk of clinical knee OA: only increased in heavy physical activity if >3h of exposure per day OR 5.3 (1.2-24).	Adjusted for age, sex, BMI, weight, smoking, knee injuries, health status, and total calorie intake, simultaneously in the same analysis Occupational work load not isolated and mixed in the physical activity exposure.	Grade I radiographic OA not considered knee OA at baseline Subjects developing grade I in the follow-up not considered incident cases Not aimed to assess long-term effects of specific sports on knee OA	Heavy general physical activity is an important risk factor for the development of clinical and radiological knee OA
Sandmark and Vingard, 1999	Case-control, Level III evidence	625 cases with and 548 controls without knee prosthesis Cases: men 52%, women 48%; Controls: men 48%, women 52%	Soccer, cross-country ski, track and filed, ice hockey, many others	Total number of self-reported hours in all sports reported	Knee	21% women and 57% men had participated in regular sports activity Risk of knee OA in exposed to sports compared to not or low exposure:<65y 2.9 (1.3-6.5), >65y 1.1 (0.7-1.7); men soccer OR 2 (1.4-2.8), track and field OR 1.6 (1-2.7), cross-country OR <65y 2.5 (1.3-5.1), >65y 0.9 (0.6-1.4), Ice hockey OR 1.9 (1.2-1.9); women all sports OR 0.9 (0.6-1.6)	Subjects with prior injury excluded Age, weight, smoking, hormone therapy, and occupation controlled	Exposure to sports heterogeneous Exposure to sports not much detailed Women were active in sports to a limited extend	Cross-country ski, soccer, and ice hockey increases OA in men; Moderate daily activity not related to OA

Author	Type of study	Study / Patient characteristics	Exercise	Exposure to sport	Joints	Results	Confounding factors considered	Observations	Conclusions
Cooper et al., 2000	Cohort study, Level II evidence	Baseline data collection was obtained from a cohort and after mean 5y of follow-up, 354 (99 men, 255 women) were included, mean age 75y. Radiographic knee OA.	Not reported	Not reported.	Knee	Incident radiographic knee OA: K-L grade 1: regular sports participation had an OR 3.2 (1.1-9.1); K-L grade 2 OR for sports participation of 1 (0.5-2.1). Progression radiographic knee OA: K-L grade 1: regular sports participation had an OR 0.7 (0.4-1.6); K-L grade 2 OR for sports participation of 0.9 (0.3-2.5).	Information on smoking, alcohol, family history, knee injuries obtained. Analysis for sports adjusted for age, sex, BMI, knee pain, Heberden's node. Occupational load not controlled.	Participation 60%. Subjects exposed to different types of sports. Details on sports exposure and level not provided.	Sports increase the incidence, but not progression of radiographic knee OA
Kettunen et al., 2000	Case series, Level IV evidence	Ex-elite athletes from 1920-1965; 28 runners mean age 59y (range 51-67y) (long-distance), 31 soccer mean age 56y (45-67y), 29 weight lifters (WL) mean age 59y (46-66y), 29 shooters mean age 61y (50-687) Hip pain, disability, occupation and athletic loading	Running, Soccer, WL, Shooters	Soccer: median lifetime endurance training (h): 1530 (range 0-9936); team sport training 8240 (3864-18514); power training 0 (0-1600) WL: median lifetime endurance training (h): 1520 (range 0-8483); team sport training 1150 (0-4888); power training 9460 (284-16752)	Hip	Hip OA: runners 12%, soccer 12%, WL 20%, Shooters 24%; Hip pain: runners 21%, soccer 13%, WL 7%, Shooters 17%; Hip disability: runners 7%, soccer 3%, WL 3%, Shooters 3% In hip OA, more disability but not necessarily more pain	Age- and occupation-adjusted History of hip injury not reported Interviews, physical exam and radiography by independent investigator	No control group Small sample Only includes worst grades of hip OA Study not targeted towards hip OA; Statistics for between-groups differences in hip OA not reported Runners also exposed to other types of exercise	Sports had no influence on hip OA
Lau et al., 2000	Case-control, Level III evidence	138 subjects with hip OA and 414 controls. 658 subjects with knee OA, 658 controls. Clinical and radiological hip and knee OA	Running, badminton, soccer, gymnastics, kung fu	Not detailed	Hip Knee	Hip OA: Low number of cases in all sports, except gymnastics in women; Knee OA: Low number of cases except running, soccer in men, and running, gymnastics, kung-fu in women. Hip OA: men: running OR 0.7 (0.2-2.3), soccer 1.3 (0.3-5.4), gymnastics 1.2 (0.2-6.9), kung-fu 0.8 (0.08-6.7); women: running 0.9 (0.2-3.3), badminton 1 (0.2-5), gymnastics 6 (2.1-17.6). Knee OA: men: running OR 0.6 (0.3-1.4), soccer 1.3 (0.6-2.8), gymnastics 2 (0.8-5.3), kung-fu 1.4 (0.4-4.4); women: running 1.4 (0.7-2.8), badminton 0.5 (0.1-2.7), gymnastics 7.2 (3.1-16.8), kung-fu 20 (2.7-149).	Age-, sex-, weight-, occupation-, hip/knee injuries-controlled, but analysis only differentiating for sex.	Only includes worst grades of OA Too high risk of type II error in sports with low number of cases. No data on number of injuries in each group or sport.	Gymnastics increase the risk of hip and knee OA in women Kung-fu increases the risk of knee OA in women

Author	Type of study	Study / Patient characteristics	Exercise	Exposure to sport	Joints	Results	Confounding factors considered	Observations	Conclusions
Turner et al., 2000	Case series (soccer players), cross-sectional, Level IV evidence	284 ex-professional soccer players, mean age 56y, mean age at retirement 32y Diagnosis, treatments, disability and HRQOL in former players	Soccer	Exposure of mean 13.5y (SD 5.3); 60% played > 450 matches	Not joint-specific	49% (138 players) had OA, mean age 40.4y (SD 12.5y): Frequency: 1) knee; 2) ankle; 3) spine; 4) hip. OA patients had worst scores of HRQOL, more surgeries, medications, & other treatments	Not controlled for other risk factors	Response rate 55% No control group Low causal-effect relationship for OA	Professional soccer causes health problems later in life
Sandmark 2000	Case-control, Level III evidence	416 physical education teachers graduated between 1957-1965 median age 57y (range 53-65), and 512 age-matched controls General health, musculoskeletal dysfunction, including OA	Soccer, cross-country ski, downhill ski, jogging, swimming, gymnastics	Sports at elite level: men cases 73%, women cases 40%, men controls 17%, women controls 3% 63% men, 47% women exercised 4 times/week for at least 30 years, vs 13% and 5% in controls, respectively	Knee	Cases more knee, but not hip, injuries than controls Men and women cases more symptomatic knee OA after adjusting for age, BMI, sports compared to controls, but not more OA if knee injury excluded (PR 2.1 (0.5-8.5) men, 2 (0.6-6.7). Men cases not more hip OA compared to controls; Women cases more hip OA than controls after adjusting for age, BMI and sports (PR 3 (1.1-8.1), 3.2 (1.1-9), 5.5 (1.2-25.2, respectively).	Age, BMI, sports, injury adjusted for OA Exposure to each sport not detailed; OA can not be related to any sport	Controls had participated in sports Radiographic OA not known	OA can not be attributed to any sport General sports exposure: not increases risk of hip OA, knee OA not increased if controlled by knee injury
Kettunen et al., 2001	Case-control, Level III evidence	Initial sample: 2448 male ex-elite athletes representing Finland in sport events from 1920-1965 vs 1712 healthy age-matched controls at age 20y; Follow-up in 1995: 1321 athletes available, 814 in controls. Hip and knee OA in <45y / >45y Study through questionnaires Athletes of endurance, track and field, mixed and power sport Mean age: endurance 68y, track and field 64y, team sports 61, Power sport 64y, Shooters 70y, controls 62y	Endurance: Running Cross-country ski; Track & field; Mixed sports: Soccer, hockey Basketball Power: Boxing Wrestling Weight lifting Throwing; Shooters	Not reported; Former athletes at an elite level: Olympic games, World championships, European championships	Hip Knee	For age, weight, occupation-adjusted analysis (only significant results showed): -Hip disability: endurance OR 0.35 (0.14-0-85), Track and field OR 0.3 (0.12-0.73), All sports OR 0.54 (0.36-0.82) -Knee disability: Team sport OR 1.76 (1.03-3) -Hip OA: no differences. -Knee OA: Team sport OR 2.04 (1.35-3.07) -Hip pain: Endurance OR 0.32 (0.17-0.61), Shooting OR 0.32 (0.12-0.87), all sports OR 0.66 (0.5-0.88) -Knee pain: Team sports OR 1.56 (1.07-2.28)	Adjusted for age, weight and occupation History of joint injury not excluded from the analysis of OA	Exposure not quantified Likely influence of injury on hip and knee pain, disability, and OA	Sports protective against hip pain and disability Team sports risk for knee pain, disability, and OA

Author	Type of study	Study / Patient characteristics	Exercise	Exposure to sport	Joints	Results	Confounding factors considered	Observations	Conclusions
Sutton et al., 2001	Case-control, Level III evidence	216 cases (66 men, 150 women) mean age 57y (range 40-96) and 864 age, and sex-matched controls. Sports: Vigorous (team sports, boxing, weight lift, skiing, running, martial arts, racquet sports, etc.), moderate (swimming, cricket, gymnastics, aerobics, sailing, horse riding, etc.), gentle (shooting, golf, yoga, motor sports, fishing, etc.).	Many sports, grades as vigorous, moderate, and gentle activities	Exposure detailed, but reported as number of activities instead of details on training parameters. Exposure to sports considered for 2 time periods: 5-14y before, and 15-24y before the age of diagnosis.	Knee	Neither activity level in any of the 2 periods elicited a significant increased risk of knee OA. Walking for both time periods had a risk of knee OA: OR 1.7 (1.1-2.4) and OR 2.1 (1.5-3), respectively. Performing lot of exercise increased the risk of knee OA OR 1.8 (1-3) for exposure 15-24y. Being physically active did not increase the risk of knee OA in either period.	Analysis adjusted for knee injuries and BMI. Use of age-, and sex-matched controls. Occupational load not assessed.	Subjects participated in more than 1 sport. Controls exposed to same sports. Specific sport exposure not provided Knee OA was self-reported; knee replacement cases not collected. No details in average time spent in sports per week/month.	Increased levels of regular physical activity throughout life did not increase the risk of knee OA.
Drawer and Fuller, 2001	Case series (soccer players), cross-sectional, Level IV evidence	185 ex-professional soccer players, mean age 47y (range 20-84y); Players became professional mean 18y (16-27), retired from soccer 32y (17-42) Assessment of diagnosed lower limb OA through questionnaires	Soccer	Professional level for mean 4.1y (SD 2) Mean hours/week: Schoolboy stage soccer specific 4.8 (SD 4.9), endurance 1.6 (3), power 0.3 (0.8); Professional soccer specific 8.1 (4), endurance 3.3 (2.6) power 1.5 (1.2); Retired: soccer specific 3.5 (2.1), endurance 1.1 (1.6), power 0.8 (1.5)	Hip Knee Ankle	Injuries: Hip acute 0%, chronic 9%; knee acute 46%, chronic 37%; ankle acute 21%, chronic 7% OA at least in 1 location in 32%. OA in players retired because of injury 51% vs 25% in retired for other reasons. More knee OA than hip and ankles ($p<0.001$) OA: 20-29y 0%, 30-39y 36%, 40-49y 35%, 50-59y 32%, 60-69 42%, >70y 50% ($p>0.05$)	47% retired because of injury Significant differences in level of soccer between included subjects OA not evaluated adjusting for joint injury	Low response rate (37%) Rates of OA likely affected by joint injury Direct causal-effect relationship between soccer itself and OA can not be established	Soccer at professional increases the risk of lower limb OA

Author	Type of study	Study / Patient characteristics	Exercise	Exposure to sport	Joints	Results	Confounding factors considered	Observations	Conclusions
Manninen et al., 2001	Case-control, Level III evidence	281 cases undergoing TKR for knee OA (men 55, women 226, mean age 28y) and 524 age-, sex-matched controls	Running, cross-country skiing, biking, track and field, volleyball, tennis, baseball, walking, swimming, motor sports, gymnastics	Only few at competitive level. Exposure: hours per week, month per year, total years, cumulative hours of physical exercise. High exposure: >8654h in men, >6862h in women. Low exposure lower than these values.	Knee	Men with high cumulative exercise were protected against knee OA compared to low exposure OR 0.28 (0.08-0.96) for all ages. Women with high exposure were protected against knee OA in age ranges 30-49y, and >49y compared to low exposure OR 0.51 (0.23-1.15) and 0.59 (0.3-1.16), respectively. Women participating in cross-country skiing, walking, and swimming were protected against knee OA: OR 0.59 (0.37-0.94), 0.32 (0.16-0.65), and 0.64 (0.43-0.96), respectively; not for other sports in women, and for any sport in men.	Analysis adjusted for age, BMI, physical work stress, knee injury, and smoking.	Participation 70% Subjects participated in more than 1 sport. Controls exposed to same sports. Specific sport exposure not provided.	Moderate recreational exercise (especially cross-country skiing, walking and swimming) is associated with decreased risk of knee OA
Schmitt et al., 2001	Case series, Level IV evidence	21 ex-élite javelin throwers at an average of 19y after retirement, mean age at examination 50y (range 35-60). Clinical and radiological shoulder and elbow OA.	Javelin throwers	Details provided: number of years at élite level: mean 13y (range 4-23y); mean training hours per week 14h (5-25); mean hours of strength training per week 5 (1-12); javelin throws per week mean 190 (60-500); ball and shot throws per week mean 422 (120-1200)	Shoulder Elbow	Shoulder: Major injuries 19%, pain 24% (dominant), lack of internal 67% and external rotation 19%, cranialisation of humeral head 65%, labrum injury 65%. Positive association between duration of elite participation and degenerative changes in glenoid. Training with weights >3kg led to higher risk of shoulder OA. No correlation with other parameters. Elbow: No intraarticular injuries. Pain in 14%. Osteophytes and sclerosis 100%, joint space narrowing 38%, cysts and calcifications 67%. Joint space narrowing more frequent in athletes who trained with weights >3kg (p=0.07).	Main risk factors not controlled and likely influencing OA rates.	No control group. Definition and report of radiological changes not much detailed. Most radiological changes alone have poor direct relationship with actual OA.	Javelin throws were not associated with increased risk of shoulder and elbow OA, but weight train may be related to shoulder OA.
Rogers et al., 2002	Case-control, Level III evidence	415 cases (men 306, women 109) with diagnosis of hip/knee OA at follow-up compared to 1995 controls (men 1521, women 474).	Walking, treadmill, cycling, swimming, aerobic, weight train, running, racquet sports, soccer, basketball	Not detailed. Sports categorized in low and moderate/high joint stress	Hip Knee	Activities associated with moderate/high joint stress were associated with the lowest risk of hip/knee OA in both men and women: men OR 0.62 (0.43-0.89); women OR 0.24 (0.11-0.52).	Analysis adjusted for age, BMI, history of knee or hip injury, and years of follow-up.	Minimum follow-up of only 2 years. Minimum exposure to sports of only 3 months. Controls not exposed to sports Combination of moderate and high joint stress activities. Hip/knee OA not disclosed	Physical activity in terms of sports may reduce the risk of hip/knee OA, especially in women.

Author	Type of study	Study / Patient characteristics	Exercise	Exposure to sport	Joints	Results	Confounding factors considered	Observations	Conclusions
Schmitt et al., 2003	Case-control, Cross-sectional study, Level III evidence	40 men ex-élite high jumpers retired at least 10 years earlier, mean age 42 (SD 5.4), BMI 23 (2.4), years of retirement 16 (5), and 40 age-, sex-, and BMI-matched controls. Clinical and radiological ankle OA	High jumpers	Duration of career mean 10y (SD 3), training 18h/week (8), strength training 5h/week (2), jumps per week 716 (317), sports after retirement 4h/week (3)	Ankle	Worst functional scores for athletes performing a higher number of jumps. The more jumps during active phase, the worse radiological scores (r=0.4; p=0.01). No differences in radiological ankle OA between athletes and control. No radiological differences between takeoff and swinging leg. No correlations of outcomes with training history	Main risk factors not controlled Probable influence of ankle injury on risk of OA.	Participation 81% Subjects may have participated in other sports after retirement Statistics for radiology not reported because of small sample size	Ankles of former elite jumpers have not increased risk of clinical and radiological OA.
Schmitt et al., 2004	Case-control, Level III evidence	19 male ex-élite javelin throwers (mean age 52y, range 40-59) and 22 male ex-élite high jumpers (47y, range 42-57) compared to correspondent age, sex, and BMI-matched controls. Follow-up mean 19y (range 10-28) after retirement from competitive sports. Duration of sports career: javelin 13y (4-23); Jumpers 11y (5-17).	Javelin throwers, high jumpers	Training (h/week): javelin 14 (5-25), jumpers 17 (8-28). Strength train (h/week): javelin 5 (1-12), jumpers 5 (2-10). Sports activity (h/week): javelin 5 (2-12), jumpers 5 (1-15)	Hip	Javelin throwers: hip OA was 3 times greater compared to age-, and BMI-matched controls: OR 6.1 (2.1-17). High jumpers: hip OA was 2.5 times greater than age-, and BMI-matched controls: OR 3.3 (1.1-9.5). OR of pooled sample 4.4 (2.1-9.1).	None of athletes had heavy labor, were regular smokers or had chronic disease. Analysis not adjusted for occupational exposure and joint injury.	Controls have also participated in sports, although to a lesser degree and not at competitive level. Athletes have participated in other sports after retirement.	Javelin throwers and high jumpers have an increased risk of hip OA.
Shepard et al., 2003	Cross-sectional, Level III evidence	68 ex-elite soccer players mean age 44y (range 32-59) and 136 age-, sex-matched controls	Soccer	Playing career mean 16y (range 5-25); Number of matches 474 (range 1-850)	Hip	13% soccer players had hip OA (none reported to have hip injury during career) vs 1.5% hip OA in controls (p<0.001); OR 10.2 (2.1-48.8)	Age-, sex-, injury-adjusted analysis BMI not controlled Occupation not controlled (assumed subjects fully dedicated to soccer)	Cross-sectional: hip OA in controls in the subsequent years unknown	Elite soccer increases the risk of hip OA
Szoeke et al., 2006	Cohort study, Level II evidence	224 women assessed for hand and knee OA 11y after inclusion in a prospective study. Radiological OA.	General physical activity	Not detailed. Baseline: 25% daily physical activity, 20 no physical activity; Follow-up: 40% daily physical activity, 13% no physical activity	Knee hand	Overall OA 56%: 21% knee OA, 44% hand OA. Physical activity not associated with hand OA. Physical activity at ages 20-29y associated with higher risk of knee OA (p=0.03): daily exercise 10 times greater (0.3-13.1), exercise 2-6 times a week 8 times greater (0.3-13.1), once a week 7 times greater (0.1-7.3), and few times per month 1.8 times greater (0.04-4).	Controlled for age, BMI, hormone use and smoking. Occupational load and joint injuries not controlled.	Participation 51% Subjects exposed to many sports. Intensity not reported Sports not reported. Sports involving hand use not known.	High physical activity was associated with knee, but not hand, OA.

Author	Type of study	Study / Patient characteristics	Exercise	Exposure to sport	Joints	Results	Confounding factors considered	Observations	Conclusions
Thelin et al., 2006	Case-control, Level III evidence	778 cases with knee OA and 695 controls; mean age 62.6y (range 51-70)	Soccer, Track & field, cross-country ski, ice hockey, tennis, orientation	Not reported; Most recreational level Cases 9% competition level; controls 6%	Knee	Knee OA only associated to soccer (OR 1.56 (1.12-2.17)), ice hockey (OR 1.89 (1.17-3.04)), and tennis (OR 2.01 (1.07-3.77)) in men. After adjusting for smoking, BMI, occupation, heredity and injuries, no sports increased the risk of knee OA compared to controls, even further adjusting for sports at competition level	Age, sex, smoking, BMI, occupation, injuries controlled	Larger non-response rate in controls 15.7% vs cases 5.7% Low number of subjects at competition level	Sports-related knee OA is explained by knee injuries rather than exposition to sports itself
Elleuch et al., 2008	Cross-sectional, Level III evidence	50 ex-elite male soccer players mean age 49.2y (range 45-55); 50 male controls mean 47.8y (45-58) Clinical and radiographic knee OA	Soccer	Mean 14h (range 9-18) training/week élite Mean participation soccer 17y (range 14-24); in élite 10y (5-15)	Knee	Overweight 80% soccer / 64% controls (n.s.) Axis deviation 58% soccer / 50% controls (n.s.) Radiographic OA 80% soccer / 68% controls (n.s.); Soccer had worst K-L OA (p=0.05) Knee pain 15% soccer / 50% controls (p=0.004) Functional impairment greater in controls p<0.05	Age, sex, BMI, controlled Knee injuries excluded History of occupation not reported; 46% of ex-soccer players were sports-related teachers	Small sample OA in soccer is influenced by other risk factors (although similarly distributed in controls)	Soccer similar risk of knee OA compared to controls Controls worst function if OA
Frobell et al., 2008	Case series (soccer players), cross-sectional, Level IV evidence	188 active amateur soccer players (123 men, 65 women) mean age 21.6y (SD 3.7) Clinical knee OA (KOOS questionnaire)	Soccer	Not reported; soccer at amateur level Tegner Activity Scale score 9	Knee	Age, sex, BMI had no influence on KOOS Injury significantly associated with worst KOOS Lower divisions higher scores for symptoms Mean (SD) score pain 93.5 (10), symptoms 88 (13), ADL 96 (8), Sports 88 (16), QOL 88 (17)	43% had minor and/or severe knee injuries. Within the group of soccer, controlled by age, sex, BMI, and injuries; not controlled by occupation	No control group 80% response rate Radiographic OA, and OA later in life unknown	Young active players have high scores in KOOS, but worst if injured
Dahaghin et al., 2009	Case-control, Level III evidence	480 cases with knee OA (mean age 57y SD 12y) vs 490 controls without knee OA (mean age 46y SD15y) (p<0.00001); 70% women in cases, 65% in controls; BMI 30 cases, 27 controls (p<0.00001)	Running, Body-building, Soccer, Volleyball, Others	Not reported	Knee	Participation in sports: 32% cases, 40% controls After adjusting for age, sex, BMI, sports did not increase risk of OA: running OR 1 (0.63), Body-building OR 0.97 (0.93-1.48), Soccer/volleyball OR 0.97 (0.67-1.39), Others OR 1.09 (0.7-1.7). Cycling more risk in men only OR 2.6 (1.4-4.7)	Age, sex, and BMI-adjusted History of knee injuries not reported	Subjects exposed to different sports Minimum exposure to sports = 6 months Low participation in sports in both groups	Sports participation does not increase the risk of knee OA

Author	Type of study	Study / Patient characteristics	Exercise	Exposure to sport	Joints	Results	Confounding factors considered	Observations	Conclusions
Juhakoski et al., 2009	Cohort study, Level II evidence	840 subjects with no hip OA at baseline (mean age 42y, range 30-72), evaluated 22 years later. Clinical hip OA.	Many not detailed physical activities and sports	Not detailed.	Hip	At 22 years, hip OA 4.9% men, 5.1% women. Adjusted risk of hip OA from physical activity: irregular exercise OR 1.2 (0.5-2.9), regular exercise OR 1.1 (0.4-2.8).	Adjusted for age, sex, BMI, education, occupational load, smoking, alcohol, and hip injury	Participation 63% Small number of patients with hip OA. No radiographs used Subjects exposed to different sports Sports not specified	Leisure time physical activity did not increase the risk of hip OA.
Verweij et al., 2009	Cohort study, Level II evidence	1678 subjects with no knee OA at baseline (mean age 68y, SD 8), evaluated 12 years later. Clinical knee OA.	General physical activity	Not reported. Physical activity reported in terms of muscle strength, intensity (low, medium, high), mechanical strain, turning actions	Knee	Knee OA 28%. Subjects with more current physical activity (minute/day) = more knee OA. High mechanical load and low muscle strength associated with higher knee OA: HR 1.43 (1.15-1.77) and 1.3 (1.01-1.68).	Adjusted for age, sex, region of living, education, lifetime physical work, BMI, depression, and physical activity. Knee injuries not controlled.	Radiographs not performed. Excluded patients were older, less active, more men, with lower education, more depressed than those included. Questionnaires only asked for 2 sports. Physical activity assessed at 12y, but not throughout the period. Sports not detailed.	Older adults performing activities with low muscle strength and high mechanical strains had an increased risk of knee OA.
Vrezas et al., 2010	Case-control, Level III evidence	295 male cases with knee OA and 327 male controls, aged 25-70y Radiographic knee OA	Running, cycling, swimming, soccer, ball games, gymnastics, weight lifting, body building	Cumulative hours in each sport Level of sport not reported	Knee	Running, swimming, body-building, weight lifting: not increase risk of knee OA Cycling: increases risk with more cumulative hours of exposure: OR 3.7 (1.7-7.8) if >7000h Soccer: if 1660-4000h of exposure, OR 2 (1-3.8); if 4000-7800h of exposure OR 2.2 (1-5). Ball games (hand, volley, basketball: >2100h OR 4 (1.8-8.9) Gymnastics: 400-2200h OR 3.2 (1-9.8)	Age, sex, BMI, occupation, running-adjusted History of joint injury not reported	61% cases and 55% controls participated Mild OA not included Participation in only one sport by same subject not known Effects of joint injury on knee OA not known	High exposure to cycling, soccer, and ball games increases the risk of knee OA
Krajnc et al., 2010	Case series, Level IV evidence	40 ex-professional soccer players mean age 49y, BMI 26 Radiographic knee OA	Soccer	Mean duration of soccer career 18.9y (SD 3.8); duration of professional career 11.3 (SD 4.2)	Knee	Knee injuries: 60% retired because of injuries, 35% being knee injuries; mean 1.95 acute (moderate/severe) knee injury; 28% no injuries Knee OA: 57.5% non-dominant leg, 42.5% dominant leg	Age, sex, BMI, occupation and injuries not controlled because was not the purpose of the study	87% participation No control group Excludes initial stages of knee OA	Approximately half of ex-élite soccer players had knee OA

Author	Type of study	Study / Patient characteristics	Exercise	Exposure to sport	Joints	Results	Confounding factors considered	Observations	Conclusions
Ratzlaff et al., 2011	Cohort study, Level II evidence	2918 subjects with no hip OA at baseline (mean age 61y, SD 7, mean BMI 27) evaluated for lifetime hip joint force. Self-reported physician-diagnosed hip OA	Many sports and physical activities; not detailed	Details on exposure collected but not reported in a disclosed way; use of cumulative peak force index (new tool)	Hip	Hip OA in 6% of subjects. Highest quintile of lifetime cumulative physical activity (HR 2.32 (1.31-4.12)) and high hip forces from 35-49y associated with hip OA. Sports participation were not associated with hip OA.	Controlled for age, sex, weight, height, ethnicity, hip injury, occupational physical load, education. Hip injury in 3.1%.	Participation 76% Only 2 years of follow-up Lifetime exercise assessed retrospectively	Lifetime physical activity was not associated with hip OA.
Wang et al., 2011	Cohort study, Level II evidence	39023 participants evaluated for hip and knee OA at baseline and physical activity exposure (mean age 58y Hip and knee OA with need of joint replacement.	Many sports and physical activities; not detailed	Details not reported; classified as vigorous, less vigorous, and walking, each for none, 1-2 times/week, and >3 times/week. Also total activity	Hip Knee	Knee replacement 1.4%, Hip replacement 1.2% Knee: Total activity level high HR 1.47 (1.09-1.96), vigorous activity HR 1.44 (1.02-2.04), less vigorous and walking HR not significant Hip: Risk of OA requiring joint replacement not increased in any parameter.	Adjusted for age, sex, BMI, country of birth, occupational physical activity, education, alcohol, and smoking (occupational load collected with not many details) Joint injuries not controlled.	Exposure to physical activity obtained at a single point in time and only for last 6mo No differentiation between different types of exercises	Increasing levels of physical activity may increase the risk of knee, but not hip OA

y, years; OA, osteoarthritis; PF, patellofemoral; LCL, lateral collateral ligament; kg, kilograms; n.s., non-significant; 1MTTP, first metatarsophalangeal joint; TF, tibiofemoral; THR, total hip replacement; BMI, body mass index; OR, odds ration reported as mean (95% confidence interval); vs, versus; RR, relative risk; WL, weight lifters; h, hours; PR, prevalence ratio reported as mean (95% confidence interval); SD, standard deviation; ROM, range of motion; K-L, Kellgren-Lawrence radiological classification of osteoarthritis; HRQOL, health-related quality of life; TKR, total knee replacement; KOOS, knee injury and osteoarthritis outcome score; ADL, activities of daily living; QOL, quality of life; HR, hazards ratio.

Table 2. Summary of studies evaluating the risk of osteoarthritis after exposure to sports.

Prevention of osteoarthritis may be categorized as primary, when measures aimed to avoid the onset of osteoarthritis are applied, or secondary, when measures aimed to avoid the progression of existing osteoarthritis are applied (Neogi T & Zhang Y, 2011). Increasing age, female sex, obesity, and prior knee injury are the risk factors with clearer relation with the incidence of osteoarthritis (Neogi T & Zhang Y, 2011).

Obesity is one of the most important modifiable risk factors. It is essential to prevent weight gain at young ages, as it was found that obesity in young individuals would evoke a greater risk of developing osteoarthritis in the future than becoming obese later in life (Gelber AC et al., 1999; Kohatsu ND & Schurman DJ, 1990). Weight reduction may decrease the risk of acquiring osteoarthritis (Felson DT et al., 1992). Felson and colleagues found that a decrease in body mass index of 2 units or more (weight loss of approximately 5,1 kg) over the 10 years before their current examination decreased the odds for developing osteoarthritis by over 50% (odds ratio, 0.46; 95% confidence interval 0.24-0.86; $P = 0.02$). Among women with a high risk for osteoarthritis due to elevated baseline body mass index (greater than or equal to 25), weight loss also decreased the risk (for 2 units of body mass index, odds ratio, 0.41; $P = 0.02$). Weight gain was associated with a slightly increased risk, which was not statistically significant (Felson DT et al., 1992). Once weight loss is achieved, maintaining a body mass index about 25 kg/m^2 or below would reduce osteoarthritis of the population by 27% to 53% (Felson DT, 1998; Helminen HJ, 2009). In obese patients, the principle of training referred to progression takes special relevance. If an obese patient wished to decrease weight, a rapid increase in physical activity would likely result in joint damage. It is recommended to begin with important diet modifications along with non weight-bearing exercises, until weight is decreased and the musculoskeletal system is adequately prepared. This may be accomplished by performing activities such as swimming or stationary cycling without resistance. After some weeks with non weight-bearing exercise and weight reduction through diet, a slow progression to weight-bearing activities may be initiated, but again, with caution. It would be recommended to begin with activities such as fast walking or slow jogging instead of playing tennis or volleyball. Failing to apply these principles may in turn induce a further damage to the articular cartilage.

One of the most important aspects to prevent osteoporosis is adequate lifestyle during childhood (Mark S & Link H, 1999; Nikander R et al., 2010). Bone strength at loaded sites can be increased in children but not in adults (Nikander R et al., 2010). Therefore, it is essential to promote healthy lifestyle in young subjects, based on adequate weight-bearing exercise combined with needed supplements of calcium, vitamin D, and sun, if possible.

Occupational physical loading may be sometimes preventable. Felson estimated that eliminating squatting, kneeling positions, and carrying heavy loads during work would reduce 15% to 30% the prevalence of osteoarthritis in men (Felson DT, 1998). This is sometimes difficult because of job demands. However, it should be understood that failure to take preventive measures at work will result in lower worker musculoskeletal health. In addition to creating a personal impairment, the company will have high economic costs when health problems develop in their employees. Measures as simple as offering easy prevention programs for those positions at risk, using adequate shoes, changing positions in the company for those jobs with higher physical demands, or increase routine physician's examination to detect preventable risk factors may in turn improve employees' health, reduce sick leaves, and prevent long-term consequences on both the company and the employee.

The risk of developing osteoarthritis in a subject with prior knee injury is increased 4-fold (Blagojevic M et al., 2010). This is, with obesity, one of the most important modifiable risk factors. History of joint injury may have primary and secondary preventive measures. In patients willing to participate in sports, it is essential to first provide the subject with adequate musculoskeletal health. The individual must understand that to do sports one must be in shape, and not use sports to get in shape. It is first crucial to offer adequate preventive programs based on muscle strengthening, aerobics (to decrease weight or prevent its increase), and plyometric (exercise through stretch-shortening cycles) and neuromuscular training aimed to improve proprioception and, in general, afferent somatosensory system (Alentorn-Geli E et al., 2009a; 2009b; Griffin LY et al., 2006; Myer GD et al., 2005; 2006; 2008; Roos EM et al., 2011). A clear example of potential preventive strategies for knee osteoarthritis would be the prevention of anterior cruciate ligament tears (Alentorn-Geli E et al., 2009a; 2009b; Griffin LY et al., 2000; 2006; Molloy MG & Molloy CB, 2011). Preventing joint injuries would additionally reduce the prevalence of osteoarthritis by approximately 14% to 25% (Felson DT, 1998; Helminen HJ, 2009). Based on the presented literature, the prevalence of osteoarthritis in middle-aged, obese individuals with prior knee injury is as high as 41% to 78%, demonstrating the relevance of preventive measures.

Whether or not a consequence of joint injury, muscle weakness and disorders of the neuromuscular system may have implications in osteoarthritis. Segal and colleagues assessed whether knee extensor strength or hamstring:quadriceps ratio predicted the risk for incident radiographic tibiofemoral and incident symptomatic whole knee osteoarthritis in adults aged 50 to 79 years (Segal NA et al., 2009). This longitudinal cohort of over 2000 individuals and demonstrated that subjects with greater knee extensor strength were protected against the development of incident symptomatic whole knee osteoarthritis in both sexes, with an adjusted odds ratio of 0.5 to 0.6. Hamstring:quadriceps ratio was not predictive of incident symptomatic knee osteoarthritis in either sex. Neither knee extensor strength nor the hamstring:quadriceps ratio was predictive of incident radiographic knee osteoarthritis (Segal NA et al., 2009). Therefore, providing the patient with adequate muscle strength and adequate neuromuscular control may prevent the development of symptoms of knee osteoarthritis.

Overall, exercise and sports participation do not place the subject at greater risk of osteoarthritis, except in those subjects with other risk factors who participate in sports with high impact and torsional loads (Buckwalter JA & Martin JA, 2004). Sports participation increases the risk of suffering from any ligament, cartilage or menisci injury that would induce osteoarthritis. Therefore, preventive programs are more needed to decrease the risk of injury in people participating in sports than for the participation in sports itself. In fact, it was shown that running protected against osteoarthritis (Lane NE et al., 1987; Wijayaratne SP et al., 2008; Willick SE & Hansen PA, 2010), although this finding was not consistent in all studies perhaps because of the influence of other risk factors poorly controlled. Of notice, sports and exercise can really change the properties of articular cartilage in children and adolescents by increasing its volume (Jones G et al., 2003). Thus, the prevention of osteoarthritis begins in children, as for osteoporosis. It was hypothesized that sports and exercise in children not only increase the volume of articular cartilage, but also its strength and resistance (Helminen HJ et al., 2000). This would be accomplished by strengthening the collagen network of cartilage that would prevent osteoarthritis later in life (Helminen HJ et al., 2000). Of special interest is the case-control study reported by Manninen and colleagues

(Manninen P et al., 2001). They demonstrated that some types of exercise (e.g., cross-country, skiing, walking and swimming) were associated with a decreased risk of knee osteoarthritis requiring knee arthroplasty in women but not men. Rogers and colleagues also found a protective effect of exercise on the development of hip and knee osteoarthritis, especially among women (Rogers LQ et al., 2002).

Investigation of potential preventive strategies to decrease the risk of osteoarthritis needs further development. There is a clear lack of studies dealing with long-term consequences of preventive programs on the incidence and progression of osteoarthritis. The incidence and prevalence of osteoarthritis is rising instead of decreasing (Zhang W, 2010). Therefore, further studies are warranted.

7. Discussion

The disease known as osteoarthritis is the most common form of arthritis (Lawrence RC et al., 2008). It has been estimated that 27 million United States adults aged 25 years or more have clinical osteoarthritis of either the hand, knee, or hip joint in 2008 (around 8.6%), an increase from 21 million in 1995 (Lawrence RC et al., 2008). Such a high prevalence and increase in the incidence of osteoarthritis may be likely related to aging of the population and rising prevalence of obesity (Neogi T & Zhang Y, 2011). This suggests how important the prevention of osteoarthritis is. Knowledge of the risk factors for osteoarthritis is of great relevance to implement adequate preventive strategies for a highly debilitating disease with a clear impact on the patient's quality of life (Guccione AA et al., 1994). This chapter has reviewed the principal risk factors for osteoarthritis. It has been described that older age, female sex, obesity, osteoporosis, occupation, sports activities, previous trauma, muscle weakness or dysfunction, proprioceptive deficit, lower limb malalignment, leg-length inequality, and genetic factors may increase the risk of osteoarthritis (Bosomworth NJ, 2009; Felson DT et al., 2000; Hunter DJ & Sambrook PN, 2002; Neogi T & Zhang Y, 2011). Age, sex, and genetic factors are non-modifiable, whereas the others may be modified by an appropriate intervention. The strongest risk factors are older age, obesity, and history of joint injury. The strongest modifiable risk factors are obesity, history of joint injury, and occupational physical load (Felson DT, 1998; 2000; Hunter DJ & Sambrook PN, 2002). The risk of osteoarthritis in obese subjects and individuals with history of joint injury would be 6-to-8-fold and 4-to-5-fold, respectively (Blagojevic M et al., 2010; Gelber AC et al., 2000; Hart DJ & Spector TD, 1993; Hunter DJ & Sambrook PN, 2002). The estimated decrease of the incidence of knee osteoarthritis by decreasing weight, preventing joint injury, and avoiding occupational risk factors was 27% to 52%, 25%, and 15% to 30% in men, respectively (Felson DT, 1998). In women, by decreasing weight and preventing joint injury, the incidence of knee osteoarthritis was reduced 27% to 52% and 14%, respectively (Felson DT, 1998). Additionally, the reduction of weight would decrease the incidence of hip osteoarthritis around 26% in both males and females (Felson DT, 1998).

Combination of risk factors multiplies the risk of osteoarthritis, thus increasing even more the relevance of preventive strategies. The fact that individuals will have their specific risk factors highlights the need for individualized preventive programs, where each factor is treated in accordance with the subject's characteristics and the type of physical activity that he/she wishes to practice. In patients with older age or increased weight who wish to participate in sports, it would be desirable to first lose weight and undergo a conditioning phase where non-impact exercise or sports are played (flat cycling, fast walking, and swimming) (Bliddal H & Christensen R, 2009). Once weight is decreased (in combination with diet) or after some weeks of a conditioning phase (in old non-obese patients), the subject may be better prepared to participate in more intense sports. Failing to do this progression may increase the risk of joint damage. In athletes, preventive strategies are very important to prevent long-term disability due to osteoarthritis because this population has a high risk of joint injury.

This chapter was focused on the review of the exposure to sports and exercise as potential risk factors for osteoarthritis. Overall, sports and exercise participation may not be considered an independent risk factor, but instead, would increase the risk of osteoarthritis if accompanied by other risk factors. There is a popular belief that participation in sports is good for health, and this is generally true. However, there are some exceptions. Running would not increase the risk of osteoarthritis in healthy joints. In fact, it has been demonstrated by some authors that running may be protective (Lane NE et al., 1987; Manninen P et al., 2001). High impact and torsional loads coming from the participation of many sports may increase the risk of osteoarthritis, whether or not associated with previous joint injuries. In general, running would be more protective against osteoarthritis than sports participation with more actions than just straight-ahead running. It was found that adult human articular cartilage had a potential to adapt to loading changes by increasing the glycosaminoglycan content (Roos EM & Dahlberg LE, 2005; Tiderius CJ et al., 2004), but may be damaged at high impact loads (Wilson W et al., 2006). Patients with existing osteoarthritis should be encouraged to attain a minimum individualized physical activity and keep as active as possible to delay the progression of degeneration and improve pain, disability and quality of life (Bosomworth NJ, 2009; Dunlop DD et al., 2011). It is likely that exercise interventions are underused in the management of established knee osteoarthritis symptoms (Bosomworth NJ, 2009).

A pooled analysis of all studies reviewed in Tables 1 and 2 is very complex. There are considerable variations in the results of these publications. This may be explained by differences in the outcomes, assessment methods, length of follow-up, exposure to risk factors, influence of confounding factors, demographic characteristics of the sample, or whether clinical or radiographic osteoarthritis was considered. The existing literature is very heterogeneous and this may difficult the elaboration of conclusions. In addition, many of the reviewed studies have reservations regarding the employed methodology. In fact, studies included in the systematic review performed by Lievense were scored in average only a 44.6% (range 0% to 77%), with 0% being worst quality and 100% highest quality (Lievense AM et al., 2003). The authors claimed for more prospective cohort investigations (Lievense AM et al., 2003). The presence of a control group is also crucial to prevent the influence of other risk factors, most importantly, ageing. Most adequate control subjects would be those completely comparable to athletes except for their absolute sedentary lifestyle. This would ensure that differences in osteoarthritis are explained by the exposure to exercise. However, finding completely sedentary controls is very difficult because almost all humans have been relatively active at some point in their life. Also, an investigator can not place a subject to a group that has to be sedentary because of ethical reasons. Most studies presented in this chapter are case-control or cross-sectional (Level III-evidence). It should be recognized that performing adequate at least Level II-evidence studies would be more appropriate to investigate causal-effect relationships and would lower risk of bias. However, prospective longitudinal cohort studies are much more expensive and time consuming than case-control or cross-sectional, especially if we consider that follow-up should be long to know the real effects of risk factors on articular cartilage. The use of retrospective studies may evoke in recall bias when self-assessed questionnaires are administered to subjects to assess past exposure to exercise and sports. The obtained information is usually pretty exact in professional athletes, but this is not the case for most individuals who were involved in the presented articles. In addition, self-assessments may depend on the level of education, which was not reported in many of the studies.

A major concern regarding many of the reviewed studies is the nature of sports pursued. It was suggested that the risk of osteoarthritis in sports and exercise in subjects without other risk factors may depend on the type of physical activity (Buckwalter JA, 2003; 2004). Sports with high impact and torsional loads would have a risk not comparable to other physical activities such as running or swimming. Many studies included subjects involved in different types of physical activity, thus preventing the elaboration of reliable recommendations for each one. In other words, if a group of patients exercised through different activities (jogging, tennis, cycling or soccer) and the risk of osteoarthritis is increased, that does not mean that running or cycling would be related to an increase in the risk of osteoarthritis. Moreover, many studies have not even detailed the physical activities in which the subjects were involved. In addition, volume, frequency, intensity and duration of training are not commonly reported in most of the studies. With the exception of some studies related to running (in which exact information on the exposure was provided), most of the studies in sports do not report the different parameters of training. For example, exposure to soccer may substantially differ between subjects performing 2 training sessions per week and subjects performing 5 sessions per week, and the same applies for intensity, duration and volume. It should be noticed that reporting the parameters of training would be very difficult if prospective studies are not conducted, as most subjects would not exactly know the above mentioned parameters. In contrast, a strong point of most of the presented publications is the fact that long-term follow-up was reported. Also, efforts to control potential confounding factors were made by the authors in most of the publications. Any study aimed to investigate the influence of sports and exercise in osteoarthritis may have a bias if the presence of other risk factors is not avoided.

Further studies are clearly needed to understand the genetic predisposition to osteoarthritis, the interaction between genetics and environmental factors, and the exact characterization of the risk of osteoarthritis depending on volume (in each session, season, and the whole life), frequency (number of sessions per week), intensity (in terms of velocity of running, percentage of strength with respect to the maximal repetition, etc…) and duration of training (of each session, and the total number of years exposed to training). A promising area would be investigation of the role of hormones, and their genetic regulations, on the development of osteoarthritis. As most studies deal with lower extremity, sports with predominance for upper extremity and their risk of osteoarthritis of the involved joints needs to be further investigated. Considering that osteoarthritis has a high personal and economic cost, and that the prevalence is not decreasing but increasing (Zhang W, 2010), it is crucial to investigate on preventive measures, either as primary, secondary, or even tertiary.

8. Conclusions

- The principal risk factors for osteoarthritis include: older age, female sex, obesity, osteoporosis, occupation, sports activities, previous trauma, muscle weakness or dysfunction, proprioceptive deficit, lower limb malalignment, leg-length inequality, and genetic factors.

- The strongest modifiable risk factors for osteoarthritis are obesity, occupational physical load, and history of joint injury.
- Participation in running and sports with minimal impact and torsional loads may not be independent risk factors for osteoarthritis; that is, may not cause osteoarthritis in the absence of other risk factors.
- Participation in sport with high impact and torsional loads increases the risk of osteoarthritis, especially in subjects with prior joint injury.
- Presence of a combination of risk factors multiples the risk of osteoarthritis.
- Subjects at higher risk of osteoarthritis are overweight women with prior joint injury who wish to participate in sports with high impact and torsional loads, and non professional athletes of these kind of sports with prior joint injury who additionally work on physically heavy jobs.
- Preventive strategies for osteoarthritis should be based on weight loss, neuromuscular training, occupational modifications, and regular exercise.
- Avoiding sports with high impact and torsional loads and perform other types of exercise may better prevent osteoarthritis and may also be useful to treat already existing osteoarthritis.

9. References

Adams JE. (1965). Injury to the throwing arm: a study of traumatic changes in the elbow joints of boy baseball players. *Calif Med*, 102, pp. 127-129.

Ageberg E, Pettersson A, & Friden T. (2007). 15-year follow-up of neuromuscular function in patients with unilateral nonreconstructed anterior cruciate ligament injury initially treated with rehabilitation and activity modification: a longitudinal prospective study. *Am J Sports Med*, 35, pp. 2109-2117.

Ahmed AM & Burke DL. (1983). In vitro measurement of static pressure distribution in synovial joints. Part I: tibial surface of the knee. *J Biomech Eng*, 105, pp. 216-225.

Alentorn-Geli E, Myer GD, Silvers HJ, Samitier G, Romero D, Lázaro-Haro C, & Cugat R. (2009a). Prevention of non-contact anterior cruciate ligament injuries in soccer players. Part 1: Mechanisms of injury and underlying risk factors. *Knee Surg Sports Traum Arthrosc*, 17, pp. 705-729.

Alentorn-Geli E, Myer GD, Silvers HJ, Samitier G, Romero D, Lazaro-Haro C, & Cugat R. (2009b). Prevention of non-contact anterior cruciate ligament injuries in soccer players. Part 2: a review of prevention programs aimed to modify risk factors and to reduce injury rates. *Knee Surg Sports Traum Arthrosc*, 17, pp. 859-879.

Aluoch MA & Wao HO. (2009). Risk factors for occupational osteoarthritis. A literature review. *AAOHN Journal*, 57, pp. 283-290.

Amin S, Baker K, Niu J, Clancy M, Goggins J, Guermazi A, Grigoryan M, Hunter DJ, & Felson DT. (2009). Quadriceps strength and the risk of cartilage loss and symptom progression in knee osteoarthritis. *Arthritis Rheum*, 60, pp. 189-198.

Anderson JJ & Felson DT. (1988). Factors associated with osteoarthritis of the knee in the first national Health and Nutrition Examination Survey (HANES I). Evidence for an association with overweight, race, and physical demands of work. *Am J Epidemiol*, 128, pp. 179-189.

Andersson S, Nilsson B, Hessel T, Saraste M, Noren A, Stevens-Andersson A, & Rydholm D. (1989). Degenerative joint disease in ballet dancers. *Clin Orthop Relat Res*, 238, pp. 233-236.

Astephen Wilson JL, Deluzio KJ, Dunbar MJ, Caldwell GE, & Hubley-Kozey CL. (2011). The association between knee joint biomechanics and neuromuscular control and moderate knee osteoarthritis radiographic and pain severity. *Osteoarthritis Cartilage*, 19, pp. 186-193.

Baratz M, Fu F, & Mengato R. (1986). Meniscal tears: the effect of meniscectomy and of repair on intra-articular contact areas and stress in the human knee: a preliminary report. *Am J Sports Med*, 14, pp. 270-275.

Berchuck M, Andriacchi TP, Bach BR, & Reider B. (1990). Gait adaptations by patients who have a deficient anterior cruciate ligament. *J Bone Joint Surg Am*, 72, pp. 871-877.

Blagojevic M, Jinks C, Jeffery A, & Jordan KP. (2010). Risk factors for onset of osteoarthritis of the knee in older adults: a systematic review and meta-analysis. *Osteoarthritis Cartilage*, 18, pp. 24-33.

Bliddal H & Christensen R. (2009). The treatment and prevention of knee osteoarthritis: a tool for clinical decision-making. *Expert Opin Pharmacother*, 10, pp. 1793-1804.

Bosomworth NJ. (2009). Exercise and knee osteoarthritis: benefit or hazard? *Can Fam Physician*, 55, pp. 871-878.

Brandt KD. (1997). Putting some muscle into osteoarthritis. *Ann Intern Med*, 127, pp. 154-156.

Brodelius A. (1961). Osteoarthrosis of the talar joints in footballers and ballet dancers. *Acta Orthop Scand*, 30, pp. 309-314.

Brouwer GM, van Tol AW, Bergink AP, Belo JN, Bernsen RM, Reijman M, Pols HA, & Bierma-Zeinstra SM. (2007). Association between valgus and varus alignment and the development and progression of radiographic osteoarthritis of the knee. *Arthritis Rheum*, 56, pp. 1204-1211.

Buckwalter JA. (2003). Sports, joint injury, and posttraumatic osteoarthritis. *J Orthop Sports Phys Ther*, 33, pp. 578-588.

Buckwalter JA & Martin JA. (2004). Sports and osteoarthritis. *Curr Opin Rheumatol*, 16, pp. 634-639.

Burke DL, Ahmed AH, & Miller J. (1978). A biomechanical study of partial and total medial meniscectomy of the knee. *Trans Orthop Res Soc*, 3:91.

Chaganti RK, Lane NE. (2011). Risk factors for incident osteoarthritis of the hip and knee. *Curr Rev Musculoskelet Med*, Aug 2 .[Epub ahead of print].

Chakravarty EF, Hubert HB, Lingala VB, Zatarain E, & Fries JF. (2008). Long distance running and knee osteoarthritis. A prospective study. *Am J Prev Med*, 35, pp. 133-138.

Chantraine A. (1985). Knee joint in soccer players: osteoarthritis and axis deviation. *Med Sci Sports Exerc*, 17, pp. 434-439.

Cheng Y, Macera CA, Davis DR, Ainsworth BE, Troped PJ, & Blair SN. (2000). Physical activity and self-reported, physician-diagnosed osteoarthritis: is physical activity a risk factor? *J Clin Epidemiol*, 53, pp. 315-322.

Christoforakis J, Pradhan R, Sanchez-Ballester J, Hunt N, & Strachan RK. (2005). Is there an association between articular cartilage changes and degenerative meniscus tears? *Arthroscopy*, 21, pp. 1366-1369.

Cooper C, Inskip H, Croft P, Campbell L, Smith G, McLaren M, & Coggon D. (1998). Individual risk factors for hip osteoarthritis: obesity, hip injury, and physical activity. *Am J Epidemiol*, 147, pp. 516-522.

Cooper C, McAlindon T, Snow S, Vines K, Young P, Kirwan J, & Dieppe P. (1994). Mechanical and constitutional risk factors for symptomatic knee osteoarthritis: differences between medial tibiofemoral and patellofemoral disease. *J Rheumatol*, 21, pp. 307-313.

Cooper C, Snow S, McAlindon TE, Kellingray S, Stuart B, Coggon D, & Dieppe PA. (2000). Risk factors for the incidence and progression of radiographic knee osteoarthritis. *Arthritis Rheum*, 43, pp. 995-1000.

Dahaghin S, Tehrani-Banihashemi SA, Faezi ST, Jamshidi AR, & Davatchi F. (2009). Squatting, sitting on the floor, or cycling: are life-long daily activities risk factors for clinical knee osteoarthritis? Stage III results of a community-based study. *Arthritis Rheum*, 61, pp. 1337-1342.

Darling EM & Athanasiou KA. (2003). Articular cartilage bioreactors and bioprocesses. *Tissue Eng*, 9, pp. 9-26.

Davis MA, Ettinger WH, Neuhaus JM, & Hauck WW. (1988). Sex differences in osteoarthritis of the knee. The role of obesity. *Am J Epidemiol*, 127, pp. 1019-1030.

de Klerk BM, Schiphof D, Groeneveld FP, Koes BW, van Osch GJ, van Meurs JB, & Bierna-Zeinstra SM. (2009). Limited evidence for a protective effect of unopposed oestrogen therapy for osteoarthritis of the hip: a systematic review. *Rheumatology (Oxford)*, 48, pp. 104-112.

Deacon A, Bennell K, Kiss ZS, Crossley K, & Brukner P. (1997). Osteoarthritis of the knee in retired, elite Australian Rules footballers. *Med J Aust*, 166, pp. 187-190.

Drawer S & Fuller CW. (2001). Propensity for osteoarthritis and lower limb joint pain in retired professional soccer players. *Br J Sports Med*, 35, pp. 402-408.

Dunlop DD, Song J, Semanik PA, Sharma L, & Chang RW. (2011). Physical activity levels and functional performance in the osteoarthritis initiative: a graded relationship. *Arthritis Rheum*, 63, pp. 127-136.

Eastmond CJ, Hudson A, & Wright V. (1979). A radiological survey of the hips and knees in female specialist teachers of physical education. *Scand J Rheumatol*, 8, pp. 264-268.

Eckstein F, Lemberger B, Gratzke C, Hudelmaier M, Glaser C, Englmeier KH, & Reiser M. (2005). In vivo cartilage deformation after different types of activity and its dependence on physical training status. *Ann Rheum Dis*, 64, pp. 291-295.

Elleuch MH, Guermazi M, Mezghanni M, Ghroubi S, Fki H, Mefteh S, Baklouti S, & Sellami S. (2008). Knee osteoarthritis in 50 former top-level footballers: a comparative (control group) study. *Ann Readapt Med Phys*, 51, pp. 174-178.

Englund M, Guermazi A, Gale D, Hunter DJ, Aliabadi P, Clancy M, & Felson DT. (2008). Incidental meniscal findings on knee MRI in middle-aged and elderly persons. *N Engl J Med*, 359, pp. 1108-1115.

Englund M & Lohmander LS. (2004). Risk factors for symptomatic knee osteoarthritis fifteen to twenty-two years after meniscectomy. *Arthritis Rheum*, 50, pp. 2811-2819.

Englund M, Roos EM, & Lohmander LS. (2003). Impact of type of meniscal tear on radiographic and symptomatic knee osteoarthritis: a sixteen-year follow-up of meniscectomy with matched controls. *Arthritis Rheum*, 48, pp. 2178-2187.

Englund M, Roos EM, & Lohmander LS. (2004). Radiographic hand osteoarthritis is associated with radiographic knee osteoarthritis after meniscectomy. *Arthritis Rheum*, 50, pp. 469-475.

Englund M, Roos EM, Roos HP, & Lohmander LS. (2001). Patient-relevant outcomes fourteen years after meniscectomy: influence of type of meniscal tear and size of resection. *Rheumatology*, 40, pp. 631-639.

Fairbank TJ. (1948). Knee joint changes after meniscectomy. *J Bone Joint Surg Br*, 30, pp. 664-670.

Felson DT. (1998). Preventing knee and hip osteoarthritis. *Bull Rheum Dis*, 47, pp. 1-4.

Felson DT, Gross KD, Nevitt MC, Yang M, Lane NE, Torner JC, Lewis CE, & Hurley MV. (2009). The effects of impaired joint position sense on the development and progression of pain and structural damage in knee osteoarthritis. *Arthritis Rheum*, 61, pp. 1070-1076.

Felson DT, Lawrence RC, Dieppe PA, Hirsch R, Helmick CG, Jordan JM, Kington RS, Lane NE, Nevitt MC, Zhang Y, Sowers M, McAlindon T, Spector TD, Poole AR, Yanovski SZ, Ateshian G, Sharma L, Buckwalter JA, Brandt KD, & Fries JF. (2000). Osteoarthritis: New insights. Part 1. The disease and its risk factors. *Ann Intern Med*, 133, pp. 635-646.

Felson DT, Niu J, Clancy M, Sack B, Aliabadi P, & Zhang Y. (2007). Effect of recreational physical activities on the development of knee osteoarthritis in older adults of different weights: the Framingham Study. *Arthritis Rheum*, 57, pp. 6-12.

Felson DT, Zhang Y, Anthony JM, Naimark A, & Anderson JJ. (1992). Weight loss reduces the risk of symptomatic knee osteoarthritis in women: The Framingham Study. *Ann Intern Med*, 116, pp. 535-539.

Felson DT, Zhang Y, Hannan MT, Naimark A, Weissman BN, Aliabadi P, & Levy D. (1995). The incidence and natural history of knee osteoarthritis in the elderly. The Framingham Osteoarthritis Study. *Arthritis Rheum*, 38, pp. 1500-1505.

Felson DT, Zhang Y, Hannan MT, Naimark A, Weissman BN, Aliabadi P, & Levy D. (1997). Risk factors for incident radiographic knee osteoarthritis in the elderly: the Framingham Study. *Arthritis Rheum*, 40, pp. 728-733.

Fries JF, Singh G, Morfeld D, Hubert HB, Lane NE, & Brown BW. (1994). Running and the development of disability with age. *Ann Intern Med*, 121, pp. 502-509.

Frobell RB, Svensson E, Gothrick M, & Roos EM. (2008). Self-reported activity level and knee function in amateur football players: the influence of age, gender, history of knee injury and level of competition. *Knee Surg Sports Traum Arthrosc*, 16, pp. 713-719.

Fukubayashi TK & Kurosawa H. (1980). The contact area and pressure distribution pattern of the knee. *Acta Orthop Scand*, 51, pp. 871-879.

Gelber AC, Hochberg MC, Mead LA, Wang NY, Wigley FM, & Klag MJ. (1999). Body mass index in young men and the risk of subsequent knee and hip osteoarthritis. *Am J Med*, 107, pp. 542-548.

Gelber AC, Hochberg MC, Mead LA, Wang NY, Wigley FM, & Klag MJ. (2000). Joint injury in young adults and risk for subsequent knee and hip osteoarthritis. *Ann Intern Med*, 133, pp. 321-328.

Gillquist J & Messner K. (1999). Anterior cruciate ligament reconstruction and the long-term incidence of gonarthrosis. *Sports Med*, 27, pp. 143-156.

Golightly YM, Allen KD, Helmick CG, Schwartz TA, Renner JB, & Jordan JM. (2010). Hazard of incident and progression knee and hip radiographic osteoarthritis and chronic joint symptoms in individuals with and without limb length inequality. *J Rheumatol*, 37, pp. 2133-2140.

Golightly YM, Allen KD, Renner JB, Helmick CG, Salazar A, & Jordan JM. (2007). Relationship of limb length inequality with radiographic knee and hip osteoarthritis. *Osteoarthritis Cartilage*, 15, pp. 824-829.

Griffin LY, Agel J, Albohm MJ, Arendt EA, Dick RW, Garrett WE, Garrick JG, Hewett TE, Huston LJ, Ireland ML, Johnson RJ, & Kibler WB. (2000). Non-contact anterior cruciate ligament injuries: risk factors and prevention strategies. *J Am Acad Orthop Surg*, 8, pp. 141-150.

Griffin LY, Albohm MJ, Arendt EA, Bahr R, Beynnon BD, DeMaio M, Dick RW, Engebretsen L, Garrett WE, Hannafin JA, Hewett TE, & Huston LJ. (2006). Understanding and preventing non-contact anterior cruciate ligament injuries. A review of the Hunt Valley II Meeting, January 2005. *Am J Sports Med*, 34, pp. 1512-1532.

Grotle M, Hagen KB, Natvig B, Dahl FA, & Kvien TK. (2008). Obesity and osteoarthritis in knee, hip and/or hand: an epidemiological study in the general population with 10 years follow-up. *BMC Musculoskeletal Disord*, 9:132.

Guccione AA, Felson DT, Anderson JJ, Anthony JM, Zhang Y, & Wilson PW. (1994). The effects of specific medical conditions on the functional limitations of elders in the Framingham Study. *Am J Public Health*, 84, pp. 351-358.

Hannan MT, Anderson JJ, Zhang Y, Levy D, & Felson DT. (1993). Bone mineral density and knee osteoarthritis in elderly men and women: The Framingham Study. *Arthritis Rheum*, 36, pp. 1671-1680.

Hardingham T & Bayliss M. (1990). Proteoglycans of articular cartilage: changes in aging and in joint disease. *Semin Arthritis Rheum*, 20, pp. 12-33.

Hart DJ, Doyle DV, & Spector TD. (1999). Incidence and risk factors for radiographic knee osteoarthritis in middle-aged women: the Chingford study. *Arthritis Rheum*, 42, pp. 17-24.

Hart DJ & Spector TD. (1993). The relationship of obesity, fat distribution and osteoarthritis in women in the general population: The Chingford Study. *J Rheumatol*, 20, pp. 331-335.

Harvey WF, Yang M, Cooke TD, Segal NA, Lane N, Lewis CE, & Felson DT. (2010). Association of leg-length inequality with knee osteoarthritis: a cohort study. *Ann Intern Med*, 152, pp. 287-295.

Helminen HJ. (2009). Sports, loading of cartilage, osteoarthritis and its prevention. *Scand J Med Sci Sports*, 19, pp. 143-145.

Helminen HJ, Hyttinen MM, Lammi MJ, Arokoski JP, Lapveteläinen T, Jurvelin J, Kiviranta I, & Tammi MI. (2000). Regular joint loading in youth assists in the establishment and strengthening of the collagen network of articular cartilage and contributes to the prevention of osteoarthrosis later in life: a hypothesis. *J Bone Miner Metab*, 18, pp. 245-257.

Herzog W & Longino D. (2007). The role of muscles in joint degeneration and osteoarthritis. *J Biomech*, 40, pp. S54-S63.

Hinman RS, Hunt MA, Creaby MW, Wrigley TV, McManus FJ, & Bennell KL. (2010). Hip muscle weakness in individuals with medial knee osteoarthritis. *Arthritis Care Res (Hoboken)*, 62, pp. 1190-1193.

Hootman JM, Macera CA, Helmick CG, & Blair SN. (2003). Influence of physical activity-related joint stress on the risk of self-reported hip/knee osteoarthritis: a new method to quantify physical activity. *Prev Med*, 36, pp. 636-644.

Horton WE, Bennion P, & Yang L. (2006). Cellular, molecular, and matrix changes in cartilage during aging and osteoarthritis. *J Musculoskeletal Neuronal Interact*, 6, pp. 379-381.

Hoser C, Fink C, Brown C, Reichkendler M, Hackl W, & Bartlett J. (2001). Long-term results of arthroscopic partial lateral meniscectomy in knees without associated damage. *J Bone Joint Surg Br*, 83, pp. 513-516.

Hunt A. (2003). Musculoskeletal fitness: the keystone in overall well-being and injury prevention. *Clin Orthop*, 409, pp. 96-105.

Hunter DJ & Eckstein F. (2009). Exercise and osteoarthritis. *J Anat*, 214, pp. 197-207.

Hunter DJ, Niu J, Felson DT, Harvey WF, Gross KD, McCree P, Aliabadi P, Sack B, & Zhang Y. (2007). Knee alignment does not predict incident osteoarthritis: the Framingham Osteoarthritis Study. *Arthritis Rheum*, 56, pp. 1212-1218.

Hunter DJ & Sambrook PN. (2002). Knee osteoarthritis: the influence of environmental factors. *Clin Exp Rheumatol*, 20, pp. 93-100.

Hunter DJ, Zhang YQ, Niu JB, Tu X, Amin S, Clancy M, Guermazi A, Grigorian M, Gale D, & Felson DT. (2006). The association of meniscal pathologic changes with cartilage loss loss in symptomatic knee osteoarthritis. *Arthritis Rheum*, 54, pp. 795-801.

Hurley MV, Rees J, & Newham DJ. (1998). Quadriceps function, proprioceptive acuity and functional performance in healthy young, middle-aged and elderly subjects. *Age Ageing*, 27, pp. 55-62.

Ichiba A & Kishimoto I. (2009). Effects of articular cartilage and meniscus injuries at the time of surgery on osteoarthritic changes after anterior cruciate ligament reconstruction in patients under 40 years old. *Arch Orthop Trauma Surg*, 129, pp. 409-415.

Imeokparia RL, Barrett JP, Arrieta MI, Leaverton PE, Wilson AA, Hall BJ, & Marlowe SM. (1994). Physical activity as a risk factor for osteoarthritis of the knee. *Ann Epidemiol*, 4, pp. 221-230.

Jones G, Bennell K, & Cicuttini FM. (2003). Effect of physical activity on cartilage development in healthy kids. *Br J Sports Med*, 37, pp. 382-383.

Jordan JM, Luta G, Renner JB, Linder GF, Dragomir A, Hochberg MC, & Fryer JG. (1996). Self-reported functional status in osteoarthritis of the knee in a sural southern community: the role of sociodemographic factors, obesity, and knee pain. *Arthritis Care Res*, 9, pp. 273-278.

Jorgensen U, Sonne-Holm U, Lauridsen F, & Rosenklint A. (1987). A long-term follow-up of meniscectomy in athletes. *J Bone Joint Surg Br*, 69, pp. 80-83.

Juhakoski R, Heliövaara M, Impivaara O, Kröger H, Knekt P, Lauren H, & Arokoski JP. (2009). Risk factors for the development of hip osteoarthritis: a population-based prospective study. *Rheumatology (Oxford)*, 48, pp. 83-87.

Keays SL, Newcombe PA, Bullock-Saxton JE, Bullock MI, & Keays AC. (2010). Factors involved in the development of osteoarthritis after anterior cruciate ligament surgery. *Am J Sports Med*, 38, pp. 455-463.

Kettunen JA, Kujala UM, Kaprio J, Koskenvuo M, & Sarna S. (2001). Lower-limb function among former elite male athletes. *Am J Sports Med*, 29, pp. 2-8.

Kettunen JA, Kujala UM, Räty H, Videman T, Sarna S, Impivaara O, & Koskinen S. (2000). Factors associated with hip joint rotation in former elite athletes. *Br J Sports Med*, 34, pp. 44-48.

King D. (1936). The function of semilunar cartilages. *J Bone Joint Surg Am*, 18, pp. 1069-1076.

Klunder KB, Rud B, & Hansen J. (1980). Osteoarthritis of the hip and knee joint in retired football players. *Acta Orthop Scand*, 51, pp. 925-927.

Kohatsu ND & Schurman DJ. (1990). Risk factors for the development of osteoarthritis of the knee. *Clin Orthop Relat Res*, 261, pp. 242-246.

Konradsen L, Hansen EM, & Songard L. (1990). Long distance running and osteoarthritis. *Am J Sports Med*, 18, pp. 379-381.

Koralewicz LM & Engh GA. (2000). Comparison of proprioception in arthritic and age-matched normal knees. *J Bone Joint Surg Am*, 82, pp. 1582-1588.

Krajnc Z, Vogrin M, Recnik G, Crnjac A, Drobnic M, & Antolic V. (2010). Increased risk of knee injuries and osteoarthritis in the non-dominant leg of former professional football players. *Wien Klin Wochenschr*, 122 Suppl 2, pp. 40-43.

Krampla WW, Newrkla SP, Kroener AH, & Hruby WF. (2008). Changes on magnetic resonance tomography in the knee joints of marathon runners: a 10-year longitudinal study. *Skeletal Radiol*, 37, pp. 619-626.

Kujala UM, Kaprio J, & Sarna S. (1994). Osteoarthritis of weight bearing joints of lower limbs in former elite male athletes. *BMJ*, 308, pp. 231-234.

Kujala UM, Kettunen J, Paananen H, Aalto T, Battié MC, Impivaara O, Videman T, & Sarna S. (1995). Knee osteoarthritis in former runners, soccer players, weight lifters, and shooters. *Arthritis Rheum*, 38, pp. 539-546.

Kujala UM, Marti P, Kaprio J, Hernelahti M, Tikkanen H, & Sarna S. (2003). Occurrence of chronic disease in former top-level athletes. Predominance of benefits, risks or selection effects? *Sports Med*, 33, pp. 553-561.

Kujala UM, Sarna S, Kaprio J, Koskenvuo M, & Karjalainen J. (1999). Heart attacks and lower-limb function in master endurance athletes. *Med Sci Sports Exerc*, 31, pp. 1041-1046.

Lane NE, Bloch DA, Hubert HB, Jones H, Simpson U, & Fries JF. (1990). Running, osteoarthritis, and bone density: initial 2-year longitudinal study. *Am J Med*, 88, pp. 452-459.

Lane NE, Bloch DA, Jones HH, Marshall WH, Wood PD, & Fries JF. (1986). Long-distance running, bone density, and osteoarthritis. *JAMA*, 255, pp. 1147-1151.

Lane NE, Bloch DA, Wood PD, & Fries JF. (1987). Aging, long-distance running, and the development of musculoskeletal disability. A controlled study. *Am J Med*, 82, pp. 772-780.

Lane NE, Hochberg MC, Pressman A, Scott JC, & Nevitt MC. (1999). Recreational physical activity and the risk of osteoarthritis of the hip in elderly women. *J Rheumatol*, 26, pp. 849-854.

Lane NE, Michel B, Bjorkengren A, Oehlert J, Shi H, Bloch DA, & Fries JF. (1993). The risk of osteoarthritis with running and aging: a five year longitudinal study. *J Rheumatol*, 20, pp. 461-468.

Lane NE, Oehlert JW, Bloch DA, & Fries JF. (1998). The relationship of running to osteoarthritis of the knee and hip and bone mineral density of the lumbar spine: a 9 year longitudinal study. *J Rheumatol*, 25, pp. 334-341.

Lau EC, Cooper C, Lam D, Chan VN, Tsang KK, & Sham A. (2000). Factors associated with osteoarthritis of the hip and knee in Hong Kong Chinese: obesity, joint injury, and occupational activities. *Am J Epidemiol*, 152, pp. 855-862.

Lawrence RC, Felson DT, Helmick CG, Arnold LM, Choi HS, Deyo RA, Gabriel S, Hirsch R, Hochberg MC, Hunder GG, Jordan JM, Katz JN, Kremers HM, & Wolfe F. (2008). Estimates of the prevalence of arthritis and other rheumatic conditions in the United States. Part II. *Arthritis Rheum*, 58, pp. 26-35.

Lidén M, Sernert N, Rostgard-Christensen L, Kartus C, & Ejerhed L. (2008). Osteoarthritic changes after anterior cruciate ligament reconstruction using bone-patellar tendon-bone or hamstring tendon autografts: a retrospective, 7-year radiographic and clinical follow-up study. *Arthroscopy*, 24, pp. 899-908.

Lievense AM, Bierma-Zeinstra SM, Verhagen AP, Bernsen RM, Verhaar JA, & Koes BW. (2003). Influence of sporting activities on the development of osteoarthritis of the hip: a systematic review. *Arthritis Rheum*, 49, pp. 228-236.

Lindberg H, Roos H, & Gardsell P. (1993). Prevalence of coxarthrosis in former soccer players. 286 players compared with matched controls. *Acta Orthop Scand*, 64, pp. 165-167.

Lohmander LS, Englund PM, Dahl LL, & Roos EM. (2007). The long-term consequence of anterior cruciate ligament and meniscus injuries: osteoarthritis. *Am J Sports Med*, 35, pp. 1756-1769.

Lohmander LS, Ostenberg A, Englund M, & Roos H. (2004). High prevalence of knee osteoarthritis, pain, and functional limitations in female soccer players twelve years after anterior cruciate ligament injury. *Arthritis Rheum*, 50, pp. 3145-3152.

Lohmander LS & Roos H. (1994). Knee ligament injury, surgery and osteoarthrosis: truth or consequences? *Acta Orthop Scand*, 65, pp. 605-609.

Longino D, Frank c, & Herzog W. (2005). Acute botulinum toxin-induced muscle weakness in the anterior cruciate ligament-deficient rabbit. *J Orthop Res*, 23, pp. 1404-1410.

Loughlin J. (2011). Genetics of osteoarthritis. *Curr Opin Rheumatol*, 23, pp. 479-483.

Maetzel A, Makela M, Hawker G, & Bombardier C. (1997). Osteoarthritis of the hip and knee and mechanical occupational exposure. A systematic overview of the evidence. *J Rheumatol*, 24, pp. 1599-1607.

Maffulli N, Binfield PM, & King JB. (2003). Articular cartilage lesions in the symptomatic anterior cruciate ligament-deficient knee. *Arthroscopy*, 19, pp. 685-690.

Maffulli N, Longo UG, Spiezia F, & Denaro V. (2011). Aetiology and prevention of injuries in elite young athletes. *Med Sport Sci*, 56, pp. 187-200.

Magnussen RA, Mansour AA, Carey JL, & Spindler KP. (2009). Meniscus status at anterior cruciate ligament reconstruction associated with radiographic signs of osteoarthritis at 5- to 10-year follow-up: a systematic review. *J Knee Surg*, 22, pp. 347-357.

Manninen P, Riihimäki H, Heliövaara M, & Suomalainen O. (2001). Physical exercise and risk of severe knee osteoarthritis requiring arthroplasty. *Rheumatology*, 41, pp. 432-437.

Mark S & Link H. (1999). Reducing osteoporosis: prevention during childhood and adolescence. *Bull World Health Organ, 77*, pp. 423-424.

Marti B, Knobloch M, Tschopp A, Jucker A, & Howald H. (1989). Is excessive running predictive of degenerative hip disease? Controlled study of former elite athletes. *BMJ*, 299, pp. 91-93.

McAlindon TE, Felson DT, Zhang Y, Hannan MT, Aliabadi P, Weissman BN, Rush D, Wilson PW, & Jacques P. (1996). Relation of dietary intake and serum levels of vitamin D to progression of osteoarthritis of the knee among participants in the Framingham Study. *Ann Intern Med*, 125, pp. 353-359.

McAlindon TE, Wilson PW, Aliabadi P, Weissman BN, & Felson DT. (1999). Level of physical activity and the risk of radiographic and symptomatic knee osteoarthritis in the elderly: The Framingham Study. *Am J Med*, 106, pp. 151-157.

McDermott M & Freyne P. (1983). Osteoarthritis in runners with knee pain. *Br J Sports Med*, 17, pp. 84-87.

Meulenbelt I, Kraus VB, Sandell LJ, & Loughlin J. (2011). Summary of the OA biomarkers workshop 2010 - genetics and genomics: new targets in OA. *Osteoarthritis Cartilage*, 19, pp. 1091-1094.

Mikesky AE, Meyer A, & Thompson KL. (2000). Relationship between quadriceps strength and rate of loading during gait in women. *J Orthop Res*, 18, pp. 171-175.

Molloy MG & Molloy CB. (2011). Contact sport and osteoarthritis. *Br J Sports Med*, 45, pp. 275-277.

Myer GD, Ford KR, McLean SG, & Hewett TE. (2006). The effects of plyometric versus dynamic stabilization and balance training on lower extremity biomechanics. *Am J Sports Med*, 34, pp. 445-455.

Myer GD, Ford KR, Palumbo JP, & Hewett TE. (2005). Neuromuscular training improves performance and lower extremity biomechanics in female athletes. *J Strength Cond Res*, 19, pp. 51-60.

Myer GD, Paterno MV, Ford KR, & Hewett TE. (2008). Neuromuscular training techniques to target deficits before return to sport after anterior cruciate ligament reconstruction. *J Strength Cond Res*, 22, pp. 987-1014.

Neogi T & Zhang Y. (2011). Osteoarthritis prevention. *Curr Opin Rheumatol*, 23, pp. 185-191.

Neuman P, Englund M, Kostogiannis I, Fridén T, Roos H, & Dahlberg LE. (2008). Prevalence of tibiofemoral osteoarthritis 15 years after nonoperative treatment of anterior cruciate ligament injury: a prospective cohort study. *Am J Sports Med*, 36, pp. 1717-1725.

Nevitt MC, Lane NE, Scott JC, Hochberg MC, Pressman AR, Genant HK, & Cummings SR. (1995). Radiographic osteoarthritis of the hip and bone mineral density. The Study of Osteoporotic Fractures Research Group. *Arthritis Rheum*, 38, pp. 907-916.

Nikander R, Sievänen H, Heinonen A, Daly RM, Uusi-Rasi K, & Kannus P. (2010). Targeted exercise against osteoporosis: a systematic review and meta-analysis for optimising bone strength throughout life. *BMC Med*, 21, pp. 8-47.

Nüesch E, Dieppe P, Reichenbach S, Williams S, Iff S, & Jüni P. (2011). All cause and disease specific mortality in patients with knee or hip osteoarthritis: population based cohort study. *BMJ*, Mar 8;342:d1165.

Oiestad BE, Holm I, Aune AK, Gunderson R, Myklebust G, Engebretsen L, Fosdahl MA, & Risberg MA. (2010a). Knee function and prevalence of knee osteoarthritis after anterior cruciate ligament reconstruction: a prospective study with 10 to 15 years of follow-up. *Am J Sports Med*, 38, pp. 2201-2210.

Oiestad BE, Holm I, Gunderson R, Myklebust G, & Risberg MA. (2010b). Quadriceps muscle weakness after anterior cruciate ligament reconstruction: a risk factor for knee osteoarthritis? *Arthritis Care Res (Hoboken)*, 62, pp. 1706-1714.

Oliveria SA, Felson DT, Reed JI, Cirillo PA, & Walker AM. (1995). Incidence of symptomatic hand, hip, and knee osteoarthritis among patients in a health maintenance organization. *Arthritis Rheum*, 38, pp. 1134-1141.

Pai YC, Rymer WZ, Chang RW, & Sharma L. (1997). Effect of age and osteoarthritis on knee proprioception. *Arthritis Rheum*, 40, pp. 2260-2265.

Pallu S, Francin PJ, Guillaume C, Gegout-Pottie P, Netter P, Mainard D, Terlain B, & Presle N. (2010). Obesity affects the chondrocyte responsiveness to leptin in patients with osteoarthritis. *Arthritis Res Ther*, 12:R112.

Palmieri-Smith RM & Thomas AC. (2009). A neuromuscular mechanism of posttraumatic osteoarthritis associated with ACL injury. *Exerc Sport Sci Rev*, 37, pp. 147-153.

Panush RS, Hanson C, Caldwell J, Longley S, Stork J, & Thoburn R. (1995). Is running associated with osteoarthritis? An eight year follow-up study. *J Clin Rheumatol*, 1, pp. 35-39.

Panush RS, Schmidt C, Caldwell JR, Edwards NL, Longley S, Yonker R, Webster E, Nauman J, Stork J, & Pettersson H. (1986). Is running associated with degenerative joint disease? *JAMA*, 255, pp. 1152-1154.

Pietrosimone BG, Hertel J, Ingersoll CD, Hart JM, & Saliba SA. (2011). Voluntary quadriceps activation deficits in patients with tibiofemoral osteoarthritis: a meta-analysis. *PM R*, 3, pp. 153-162.

Puranen J, Ala-Ketola L, Peltokallio P, & Saarela J. (1975). Running and primary osteoarthritis of the hip. *BMJ*, 2, pp. 424-425.

Raty HP, Battie MC, Videman T, & Sarna S. (1997). Lumbar mobility in former élite male weight-lifters, soccer players, long-distance runners and shooters. *Clin Biomech*, 12, pp. 325-330.

Ratzlaff CR, Steininger G, Doerfling P, Koehoorn M, Cibere J, Liang MH, Wilson DR, Esdaile JM, & Kopec JA. (2011). Influence of lifetime hip joint force on the risk of self-reported hip osteoarthritis: a community-based cohort study. *Osteoarthritis Cartilage*, 19, pp. 389-398.

Raynauld JP, Martel-Pelletier J, Berthiaume MJ, Beaudoin G, Choquette D, Haraoui B, Tannenbaum H, Meyer JM, Beary JF, Cline GA, & Pelletier JP. (2006). Long term evaluation of disease progression through the quantitative magnetic resonance imaging of symptomatic knee osteoarthritis patients: correlation with clinical symptoms and radiographic changes. *Arthritis Res Ther*, 8:R21.

Riancho JA, García-Ibarbia C, Gravani A, Raine EV, Rodriguez-Fontenla C, Soto-Hermida A, Rego-Perez I, Dodd AW, Gómez-Reino JJ, Zarrabeitia MT, Garcés CM, Carr A, Blanco F, González A, & Loughlin J. (2010). Common variations in estrogen-related genes are associated with severe large-joint osteoarthritis: a multicenter genetic and functional study. *Osteoarthritis Cartilage*, 18, pp. 927-933.

Riddle DL, Kong X, & Jiranek WA. (2011). Factors associated with rapid progression of knee arthroplasty: complete analysis of three-year data from the osteoarthritis initiative. *Joint Bone Spine*, July 2 [Epub ahed of print].

Rogers LQ, Macera CA, Hootman JM, Ainsworth BE, & Blairi SN. (2002). The association between joint stress from physical activity and self-reported osteoarthritis: an analysis of the Cooper Clinic data. *Osteoarthritis Cartilage*, 10, pp. 617-622.

Roos EM & Dahlberg LE. (2005). Positive effects of moderate exercise on glycosaminoglycan content in knee cartilage: a four-month, randomized, controlled trial in patients at risk of osteoarthritis. *Arthritis Rheum*, 52, pp. 3507-3514.

Roos EM, Herzog W, Block JA, & Bennell KL. (2011). Muscle weakness, afferent sensory dysfunction and exercise in knee osteoarthritis. *Nat Rev Rheumatol*, 7, pp. 57-63.

Roos H, Lauren M, Adalberth T, Roos E, Jonsson K, & Lohmander L. (1998). Knee osteoarthritis after meniscectomy: prevalence of radiographic changes after twenty-one years, compared to matched controls. *Arthritis Rheum*, 41, pp. 687-693.

Roos H, Lindberg H, Gärdsell P, Lohmander LS, & Wingstrand H. (1994). The prevalence of gonarthrosis and its relation to meniscectomy in former soccer players. *Am J Sports Med*, 22, pp. 219-222.

Rosner IA, Goldberg VM, & Moskowitz RW. (1986). Estrogens and osteoarthritis. *Clin Orthop*, 213, pp. 77-83.

Sandmark H. (2000). Musculoskeletal dysfunction in physical education teachers. *Occup Environ Med*, 57, pp. 673-677.

Sandmark H & Vingärd E. (1999). Sports and risk for severe osteoarthrosis of the knee. *Scand J Med Sci Sports*, 9, pp. 279-284.

Schmitt H, Brocai DR, & Lukoschek M. (2004). High prevalence of hip arthrosis in former elite javelin throwers and high jumpers: 41 athletes examined more than 10 years after retirement from competitive sports. *Acta Orthop Scand*, 75, pp. 34-39.

Schmitt H, Hansmann HJ, Brocai DR, & Loew M. (2001). Long term changes of the throwing arm of former elite javelin throwers. *Int J Sports Med*, 22, pp. 275-279.

Schmitt H, Lemke JM, Brocai DR, & Parsch D. (2003). Degenerative changes in the ankle in former elite high jumpers. *Clin J Sport Med*, 13, pp. 6-10.

Seedhom BB & Hargreaves DJ. (1979). Transmission of load in the knee joint with special reference to the role of the menisci: part II: experimental results, discussions, and conclusions. *Eng Med Biol*, 8, pp. 220-228.

Segal NA, Glass NA, Felson DT, Hurley M, Yang M, Nevitt M, Lewis CE, & Torner JC. (2010). Effect of quadriceps strength and proprioception on risk for knee osteoarthritis. *Med Sci Sports Exerc*, 42, pp. 2081-2088.

Segal NA, Torner JC, Felson DT, Niu J, Sharma L, Lewis CE, & Nevitt M. (2009). Effect of thigh strength on incident radiographic and symptomatic knee osteoarthritis in a longitudinal cohort. *Arthritis Rheum*, 15, pp. 1210-1217.

Sharma L. (1999). Proprioceptive impairment in knee osteoarthritis. *Rheum Dis Clin North Am*, 25, pp. 299-314.

Sharma L & Pai YC. (1997). Impaired proprioception and osteoarthritis. *Curr Opin Rheumatol*, 9, pp. 253-258.

Sharma L, Song J, Dunlop D, Felson D, Lewis CE, Segal N, Torner J, Cooke TD, Hietpas J, Lynch J, & Nevitt M. (2010). Varus and valgus alignment and incident and progressive knee osteoarthritis. *Ann Rheum Dis*, 69, pp. 1940-1945.

Shepard GJ, Banks AJ, & Ryan WG. (2003). Ex-professional association footballers have an increased prevalence of osteoarthritis of the hip compared with age matched controls despite not having sustained notable hip injuries. *Br J Sports Med*, 37, pp. 80-81.

Slemenda C, Brandt KD, Heilman DK, Mazzuca S, Braunstein EM, Katz BP, & Wolinsky FD. (1997). Quadriceps weakness and osteoarthritis of the knee. *Ann Intern Med*, 127, pp. 97-104.

Slemenda C, Heilman DK, Brandt KD, Katz BP, Mazzuca S, Braunstein EM, & Byrd D. (1998). Reduced quadriceps strength relative to body weight: a risk factor for knee osteoarthritis in women? *Arthritis Rheum*, 41, pp. 1951-1959.

Snyder-Mackler L, Binder-Macleod SA, & Williams PR. (1993). Fatigability of human quadriceps femoris muscle following anterior cruciate ligament reconstruction. *Med Sci Sports Exerc*, 25, pp. 783-789.

Sohn RS & Micheli LJ. (1985). The effect of running on the pathogenesis of osteoarthritis of the hips and knees. *Clin Orthop Relat Res*, 198, pp. 106-109.

Solonen KA. (1966). The joints of the lower extremities of football players. *Ann Chir Gynecol Fen*, 55, pp. 176-180.

Sortland O, Tysvaer AT, & Storli OV. (1982). Changes in the cervical spine in association football players. *Br J Sports Med*, 16, pp. 80-84.

Spector TD, Cicuttini F, Baker J, Loughlin J, & Hart D. (1996a). Genetic influences on osteoarthritis in women: a twin study. *BMJ*, 312, pp. 940-943.

Spector TD, Harris PA, Hart DJ, Cicuttini FM, Nandra D, Etherington J, Wolman RL, & Doyle DV. (1996b). Risk of osteoarthritis associated with long-term weight-bearing sports: a radiographic survey of the hips and knees in female ex-athletes and population controls. *Arthritis Rheum*, 39, pp. 988-995.

Spector TD, Nandra D, Hart DJ, & Doyle DV. (1997). Is hormone replacement therapy protective for hand and knee osteoarthritis in women? The Chingford Study. *Ann Rheum Dis*, 56, pp. 432-434.

Stevens-Lapsley JE & Kohrt WM. (2010). Osteoarthritis in women: effects of estrogen, obesity, and physical activity. *Womens Health (Lond Engl)*, 6, pp. 601-615.

Suter E & Herzog W. (2000). Does muscle inhibition after knee injury increase the risk of osteoarthritis? *Exerc Sport Sci Rev*, 28, pp. 15-18.

Sutton AJ, Muir KR, Mockett S, & Fentem P. (2001). A case-control study to investigate the relationship between low and moderate levels of physical activity and osteoarthritis of the knee using data collected as part of the Allied Dunbar National Fitness Survey. *Ann Rheum Dis*, 60, pp. 756-764.

Szoeke CE, Cicuttini FM, Guthrie JR, Clark MS, & Dennerstein L. (2006). Factors affecting the prevalence of osteoarthritis in healthy middle-aged women: data from the longitudinal Melbourne Women's Midlife Health Project. *Bone*, 39, pp. 1149-1155.

Thelin N, Holmberg S, & Thelin A. (2006). Knee injuries account for the sports-related increased risk of knee osteoarthritis. *Scand J Med Sci Sports*, 16, pp. 329-333.

Tiderius CJ, Svensson J, Leander P, Ola T, & Dahlberg LE. (2004). dGEMRIC (delayed gadolinium-enhanced MRI of cartilage) indicates adaptive capacity of human knee cartilage. *Magn Reson Med*, 51, pp. 286-290.

Turner AP, Barlow JH, & Heathcote-Elliott C. (2000). Long term health impact of playing professional football in the United Kingdom. *Br J Sports Med*, 34, pp. 332-337.

Vairo GL, McBrier NM, Miller SJ, & Buckley WE. (2010). Premature knee osteoarthritis after anterior cruciate ligament reconstruction dependent on autograft. *J Sport Rehabil,* 19, pp. 86-97.

Van Dijk CN, Lim LS, Poortman A, Strubbe EH, & Marti RK. (1995). Degenerative joint disease in female ballet dancers. *Am J Sports Med,* 23, pp. 295-300.

Vanwanseele B, Eckstein F, Knecht H, Stussi E, & Spaepen A. (2002). Knee cartilage of spinal cord-injured patients displays progressive thinning in the absence of normal joint loading and movement. *Arthritis Rheum,* 46, pp. 2073-2078.

Verweij LM, van Schoor NM, Deeg DJ, Dekker J, & Visser M. (2009). Physical activity and incident clinical knee osteoarthritis in older adults. *Arthritis Rheum,* 61, pp. 152-157.

Vingard E. (1991). Overweight predisposes to coxarthrosis: body-mass index studied in 239 males with hip arthroplasty. *Acta Orthop Scand,* 62, pp. 106-109.

Vingard E, Alfredsson L, Goldie I, & Hogstedt C. (1993). Sports and osteoarthritis of the hip. An epidemiologic study. *Am J Sports Med,* 1993, pp. 195.

Vingard E, Alfredsson L, & Malchau H. (1998). Osteoarthrosis of the hip in women and its relationship to physical load from sports activities. *Am J Sports Med,* 26, pp. 78-84.

Vingard E, Sandmark H, & Alfredsson L. (1995). Musculoskeletal disorders in former athletes: a cohort study in 114 track and field champions. *Acta Orthop Scand,* 66, pp. 289-291.

von Porat A, Roos EM, & Roos H. (2004). High prevalence of osteoarthritis 14 years after an anterior cruciate ligament tear in male soccer players: a study of radiographic and patient-relevant outcomes. *Ann Rheum Dis,* 63, pp. 269-273.

Vrezas I, Elsner G, Bolm-Audorff U, Abolmaali N, & Seidler A. (2010). Case-control study of knee osteoarthritis and lifestyle factors considering their interaction with physical workload. *Int Arch Occup Environ Health,* 83, pp. 291-300.

Wang BW, Ramey DR, Schettler JD, Hubert HB, & Fries JF. (2002). Postponed development of disability in elderly runners: a 13-year longitudinal study. *Arch Intern Med,* 162, pp. 2285-2294.

Wang Y, Simpson JA, Wluka AE, Teichtahl AJ, English DR, Giles GG, Graves S, & Cicuttini FM. (2011). Is physical activity a risk factor for primary knee or hip replacement due to osteoarthritis? A prospective cohort study. *J Rheumatol,* 38, pp. 350-357.

Ward MM, Hubert HB, Shi H, & Bloch DA. (1995). Physical disability in older runners: prevalence, risk factors, and progression with age. *J Gerontol A Biol Sci Med Sci,* 50, pp. M70-M77.

White JA, Wright V, & Hudson AM. (1993). Relationships between habitual physical activity and osteoarthrosis in ageing women. *Public Health,* 107, pp. 459-470.

Wijayaratne SP, Teichtahl AJ, Wluka AE, Hanna F, Bell R, Davis SR, Adams J, & Cicuttini FM. (2008). The determinants of change in patella cartilage volume. A cohort study of healthy middle-aged women. *Rheumatology (Oxford),* 47, pp. 1426-1429.

Willick SE & Hansen PA. (2010). Running and osteoarthritis. *Clin Sports Med,* 29, pp. 417-428.

Wilson W, van Burken C, van Donkelaar C, Buma P, van Rietbergen B, & Huiskes R. (2006). Causes of mechanically induced collagen damage in articular cartilage. *J Orthop Res,* 24, pp. 220-228.

Wolf BR & Amendola A. (2005). Impact of osteoarthritis on sports carers. *Clin Sports Med,* 24, pp. 187-198.

Yelin E & Callahan LF. (1995). The economic cost and social and psychological impact of musculoskeletal conditions. National Arthritis Data Work Groups. *Arthritis Rheum,* 38, pp. 1351-1362.

Zhang W. (2010). Risk factors of knee osteoarthritis. Excellent evidence but little has been done. *Osteoarthritis Cartilage,* 18, pp. 1-2.

Zhang Y, Hannan MT, Chaisson CE, McAlindon TE, Evans SR, Aliabadi P, Levy D, & Felson DT. (2000). Bone mineral density and risk of incident and progressive radiographic knee osteoarthritis in women: the Framingham Study. *J Rheumatol,* 27, pp. 1032-1037.

Zhang Y & Jordan JM. (2010). Epidemiology of osteoarthritis. *Clin Geriatr Med,* 26, pp. 355-369.

10

Post-Traumatic Osteoarthritis: Biologic Approaches to Treatment

Sukhwinderjit Lidder[1] and Susan Chubinskaya[1,2,3]
[1]*Department of Biochemistry, Rush University Medical Center, Chicago, IL*
[2]*Section of Rheumatology, Department of Internal Medicine*
[3]*Department of Orthopedic Surgery, Rush University Medical Center, Chicago, IL, USA*

1. Introduction

Joint injuries are becoming increasingly common, with young adults between the ages of 18-44 seeking medical attention for joint sprains, dislocation, fractures, anterior cruciate ligament (ACL) and meniscal tears, and others. The cascade of events that follow these joint injuries have been shown to increase the risk of post-traumatic osteoarthritis (PTOA) by 20-50% (Anderson et al,2011). Therefore, understanding biological responses that predispose to PTOA should help in determining treatment strategies to delay and/or prevent the progression of the disease. Ex vivo and in vivo studies (Anderson et al,2011;Buckwalter et al,2004;Furman et al, 2007; Guilak et al,2004; Hurtig et al, 2009) have provided evidence that the force and severity of the impact applied to the joint are among the risk factors involved in the development of PTOA. Recent research on the events that follow joint trauma have shown chondrocyte death and apoptosis, inflammation (elevation of caspases, selected pro-inflammatory cytokines, matrix fragments, nitric oxide, reactive oxygen species [ROS], etc.) and matrix damage/fragmentation to be early phase responses to injury. Together they lead to the development of OA-like focal cartilage lesions characterized by the loss of matrix constituents, surface fibrillation, and fissures that if untreated have a tendency to expand and progress to fully-blown disease.

Currently, the only treatments available for joint trauma are surgical interventions, such as microfracture, articular chondrocyte transplantation, autografting, allografting, debridement and lavage. There are also some experimental approaches that involve engineering of cartilage with the use of juvenile cartilage, scaffolds and various polymeric matrices, but those are still in development. To the best of our knowledge none of them could regenerate normal adult hyaline cartilage that is able to perform required functions, sustain the load and integrate with the host tissue. Furthermore, newly repaired tissue, due to its imperfect structural organization, may also be more susceptible to re-injury, an important aspect that often remains forgotten. Therefore, there is an unmet need in the development of novel therapeutic approaches based on the mechanisms that drive the onset and progression of PTOA in order to stimulate biologic repair, delay or prevent the need of surgery, or when used together, improve the outcome of surgical interventions if biologics are applied prior, during, or soon after surgery. Based on our current understanding of the molecular and cellular manifestations of injury the following therapeutic options could be considered for PTOA: chondroprotection, anti-inflammatory, matrix protection, and stimulation of matrix remodeling with pro-anabolic factors. These and other approaches will be discussed in details in the current book chapter.

2. Joint injuries and the risk of post-traumatic osteoarthritis (PTOA)

Although joint injuries are not as life threatening as myocardial infarctions and strokes, they are similarly life changing. They are progressive and debilitating, with progression often leading to OA. Traumatic insult to a joint, as a precursor to OA, has been studied since it was first described by Hunter in 1743 (Key,1933). It was reported that 13 to 18% of total hip or knee patients had an identifiable acute trauma to the joint (Kern et al,1988). Further evidence of joint injury being a major factor in the development and progression of PTOA came from the work of Roos, in which it was shown that early onset of OA can occur within 10 years after injury (Roos et al,1995). With increased social and sport-related activities of today's society there are more and more younger people (18-44 years) who present with the evidence of post-traumatic focal cartilage lesions and OA- like changes occurred as a result of joint injury. This is in comparison to idiopathic OA, where its prevalence is increased with ageing and is more evident after the age of 50 (Anderson et al,2011;Brown et al,2006;Dirschl et al,2004;Gelber et al,2000). Approximately 12% of the overall prevalence of severe OA is attributable to post-traumatic hip, knee and ankle OA which corresponds to about 5.6 million people in the US suffering from PTOA (Brown et al,2006). With such a high prevalence of a lifelong nonfatal disability, there is enormous annual socioeconomic burden on the health system estimated to be $3.06 billion (Brown et al,2006). These numbers may be underestimated because they were based on patients presenting with severe OA that required total joint replacement and did not include patients with early or less advanced OA. A more recent study in 2008 (Murphy et al,2008) revealed that a history of knee injury carried a 56.8% lifetime risk of symptomatic knee OA.

3. Pathogenesis of PTOA

The pathogenesis of PTOA is not fully understood, in part due to the lack of correlation between the disease progression and the symptoms; therefore, it is difficult to estimate the number of individuals suffering from PTOA. Diagnosis is usually based on parameters used to diagnose idiopathic OA such as joint pain, visible signs of joint deformity, radiographic changes and biochemical tests that detect inflammation. However, many of these may not be presented at early stages after joint injury (Brown et al,2006). PTOA is not a unifactorial disease and there are a number of factors that could contribute to the onset and progression of PTOA: lost structural integrity of menisci and ACL, joint incongruence, lost muscle strength, continued physical activity, excessive biomechanical overload of the joint, intra-articular inflammation, and others (Furman et al,2006). The key difference between the two types of OA is the presence of precipitating insult to the joint in patients that suffer from PTOA versus idiopathic OA associated with ageing, genetics, obesity, occupation, bone density, metabolic disease, inflammation and abnormal biomechanics. Since it takes years and decades for the development of PTOA after injury, aforementioned factors known to contribute to the idiopathic OA may also play a role in the progression of PTOA. Regardless what causes PTOA it develops as a result of poor intrinsic regenerative ability of hyaline articular cartilage

(Anderson et al,2011;Pelletier et al,1998;Sandell et al,2001). In clinical setting, patients with signs of PTOA usually present with an advanced form of the disease in which the meniscus, ACL and the cartilage have eroded. As a result, there is a reduction in cartilage thickness with areas of complete loss and formation of fibrocartilagenous repair tissue. Biomechanically these patients have a decreased tensile strength and compressive stiffness (Furman et al,2006).
The extent of cartilage damage depends on the intensity and force of the impact (Anderson et al,2011;Butler et al,2008; Furman et al,2006). The type of damage can be categorized as: a) cartilage only disruption characterized by changes in structural components of the matrix and chondrocyte death. These may progress to focal lesions. b) Fracturing along the tidemark, in which the cartilage tissue above the calcified zone can exhibit blistering and full thickness cartilage loss can be seen. c) Fracturing through the calcified cartilage into the subchondral plate that can in most severe cases form osteochondral fragments (Anderson et al,2011).

4. Current clinical treatments for PTOA

Joint injuries have a high prevalence especially in young individuals and unfortunately, predominantly surgical interventions are currently available for their treatment:

a. Arthroscopic lavaging and debridement (Avouac et al,2010;Reichenbach et al,2010), which wash and remove pieces of degenerative cartilage, fibrous tissue and synovial fluid full of catabolic mediators that may cause joint inflammation, swelling and destruction. The removal of loose debris, cartilage flaps, torn meniscal fragments and synovial fluid may provide a temporary relief but does not prevent the generation of more fragments and more inflammation. Hence, this method has shown little to no evidence of significant improvement in pain relief or restoration of joint function (Avouac et al,2010;Reichenbach et al,2010). The arthroscopic nature of this method limits its use to patients with small cartilage defects.
b. Viscosupplementation with hyaluronic acid via intra-articular injections into the knee joint potentially improves joint lubrication and may help to restore cartilage. It also provides some relief of pain not seen with other analgesics such as ibuprofen or nonsteroidal anti-inflammatory drugs (NSAIDs) (Iannitti et al,2011;Kappler et al,2010;Migliore et al,2011). This approach has been only effective in mild to moderate OA.
c. Recently, the usage of autologous blood products became a potential breakthrough in augmenting joint tissue healing (Anitua et al,2004,2006;Sanchez et al,2009). This new method provides cellular and humeral mediators which have been greatly beneficial in regenerative processes of cartilage and other connective tissues. Autologous blood products are heavily populated with platelets, which have the capacity to release growth factors from their α-granules (chemokines and newly synthesised metabolites) and thus positively influence the tissues with low healing potential. Intra-articular injection of platelet concentrate may represent an innovative treatment to improve cartilage remodelling. More studies are indicated to understand the mechanism of action and to optimize, standardize, and widely implement into the clinic this new technology.
d. Osteochondral grafting makes up about 10% of surgical procedures available up to date to repair cartilage lesions (Cole et al,2009). Unlike procedures that target repair or regeneration, osteochondral grafting has garnered significant attention because of its ability to replace the lesion with true hyaline cartilage and allow for a relatively short recovery period (Convery et al,1972;Horas et al,2003;Nam et al,2004;Shasha et al,2003). Osteochondral grafting involves harvesting a cylindrical donor plug of cartilage attached

to underlying subchondral bone and implanting the graft into the recipient site covering the cartilage lesion. This procedure has a lot of potential for the treatment of isolated cartilage defects in young, active patients; however, graft survival is still limited with survival rates under 50% after 15 years (Shasha et al,2003). Other problems with grafting are the integration with the host cartilage and reduced viability and metabolism of residing chondrocytes in case of prolong stored allograft tissue (Kirk et al,2011).

e. Microfracture and bone marrow stimulation. These surgical options are employed when cartilage damage is confined to small focal areas. The damaged cartilage is removed to expose and perforate the subchondral bone. This can stimulate new cartilage growth in the subchondrol defect through the generation of a fibrin clot and recruitment of bone marrow mesenchymal stem cells. The fibrocartilage that covers the full thickness chondral lesion does not have the biomechanical strength and resilience of the native cartilage. Although this fibrocartilage has been shown to provide relief from the symptoms for several years (Miller et al,2004), it does not alter the progression of PTOA as patients present with OA symptoms 5 years after microfracture surgery (Miller et al,2004). In a majority of the patients, the size of the cartilage defect increases after microfracture (Von Keudell et al,2011). The implantation of collagen membranes over the microfracture in a technique referred to as Autologous matrix induced chondrogenesis (AMIC) have been used to improve the chondrogenic differentiation of the mesenchymal stem cells (Behrens et al,2006) into more hyaline like cartilage. In other efforts to improve cartilage regeneration after microfracture, Saw et al (Saw et al,2009) have developed an *in vivo* method in goats that used intra-articular injections of autologous peripheral blood progenitor cells and hyaluronic acid. The results have been promising and a clinical pilot study has shown regeneration of articular hyaline cartilage (Saw et al,2011).

f. Autologous chondrocyte implantation (ACI) was first described by Brittberg *et al* (Brittberg et al,1994). Although cartilage regeneration of the defect was observed, several serious problems have been associated with this method. 1) It is a two-step procedure. 2) The need to create additional defects within the normal and un-affected joint for the extraction of autologous chondrocytes. 3) The need for a two-week in vitro cell expansion to obtain a sufficient number of chondrocyte to cover and fill the original defect. 4) Reduced viability and altered phenotype of autologous cells; and finally, the quality and properties of regenerated fibrocartilage (Horas et al,2003).

g. Articular cartilage regeneration with stem cells is another cell-based cartilage repair procedure. Similar in concept to ACI, autologous mesenchymal stem cells have been used to decrease knee pain (Kuroda et al,2007). However, for the most part all listed methods generate fibrocartilage or a mixture of hyaline-like and fibrocartilage (Kuroda et al,2007).

h. Knee replacement surgery with a metal shell is often used to treat advanced PTOA in patients that show severe destruction of the joint and exhibit increasing joint stiffness and pain. However, the knee replacement itself has been associated with chronic pain, joint stiffness, post-operative inflammation, and prolong recovery (Gonzalez et al,2004).

Current surgical approaches are mainly utilized to treat the developed disease, while the whole idea of biologic treatment is based on the premise to arrest and/or prevent the onset and progression of the disease. Ideally, biologic interventions should be applied immediately or soon after the trauma incident. But, in reality patients present with moderate to severe PTOA when meniscus and cartilage erosion has already advanced. The lack of satisfactory surgical and other therapeutic approaches to successfully restore cartilage structure and function still remains a challenge in current orthopedics. Only few clinical trials have been conducted to investigate the efficacy of various classes of therapeutics in PTOA. Therefore, advances in our understanding of the mechanisms that govern the development of the disease come primarily from in vitro or in vivo animal models of the PTOA.

5. *In vivo* and *in vitro* approaches to study PTOA

Animal models that resemble human OA pathology have been difficult to develop and generally require some surgical insult. In Table 1 we summarized the majority of *in vivo* and *in vitro* studies that focused on joint trauma and the fate of cartilage after chondral or osteochondral damage (Borrelli et al,2003;Clements et al,2004;Green et al,2006a,2006b;Lewis et al,2003;Newberry et al,1998;Vener et al,1992). As outlined, this literature consistently points to three overlapping phases after acute cartilage injury that include a death/apoptosis phase, an inflammatory phase, and a limited repair phase. Studying cellular responses initiated by acute injury we identified and characterized a sequence of biologic events (both catabolic and anabolic) that cause the progressive joint degeneration leading to PTOA (Anderson et al,2011;Bajaj et al,2010;Hurtig et al,2009;Pascual Garrido et al,2009).

Target	Therapeutic Agent	Reference
Chondroprotection	PI88	(Martin et al, 2009); (Phillips&Haut, 2004); (Pascual Garrido et al, 2009); (Bajaj et al, 2010)
	Caspase Inhibitors (Z-VAD-FMK; Q-VD-Oph; Caspase-3; Caspase-9)	(Martin et al, 2009); (Pascual Garrido et al, 2009); (D'Lima et al, 2006); (D'Lima et al, 2001); (Huser & Davies 2006) (Lotz, 2010)
		(Kurz et al, 2004)
	Anti-oxidants iNOS inhibitors (L-NAME; L-NIL)	(Marsh et al, 2002); (Pelletier et al, 1998, 1999, 2000)
	Rotenone	(Goodwin et al, 2010)
	N-acetylcysteine	(Martin et al, 2009); (Martin et al, 2009)
Anti-inflammatory	IRAP/IL-1Ra	(Fox & Stephens, 2010); (Frisbie et al, 2002); (Evans et al, 2004); (Meijer et al, 2003)
	Anti-TNFα, PEGylated soluble TNFα	(Zafarullah et al, 2003), (Martel-Pelletier, 1999); (Furman et al, 2006); (Fukui et al, 2001); (Evans et al, 2004); (Elsaid et al, 2009)
Matrix protection	MMP inhibitors/ TIMPs	(Jarvinen et al, 1995); (Murrell et al, 1995) (Chockalingam et al, 2011)
	ADAMTS inhibitors (AGG-523)	(Glasson et al, 2005); (Chockalingam et al, 2011)
Pro-anabolic, inducers of repair	BMPs (BMP-2; BMP-7)	(Hunter et al, 2010); (Hayashi et al, 2008, 2010); (Hurtig et al, 2009); (Chubinskaya et al, 2007); (Cook et al, 2003); (Badlani et al, 2008)
	IGF-1	(Chubinskaya et al, 2011); (Fortier et al, 2002); (Im et al, 2003)
	FGF-18	(Moore et al, 2005); (Lotz & Kraus, 2010); (Ellsworth et al, 2002)

Table 1. Potential targets and therapeutic interventions for post-traumatic osteoarthritis. iNOS, inducible Nitric oxide synthase; IRAP, interleukin receptor antagonist protein; Anti-TNF-α, tumor necrosis factor (TNF)-α soluble receptor; MMP, matrix metalloproteinases; TIMPs, tissue inhibitors of matrix metalloproteinases; ADAMTS, A Disintegrin And Metalloproteinase with ThromboSpondin-like repeats; BMPs,Bone Morphogenetic Proteins; IGF-1, Insulin-like Growth Factor-1; FGF-18, fibroblast growth factor-18; L-NAME, N-Nitro-L-arginine methyl ester; L-NIL, N-iminoethyl-L-Lysine; Z-VAD-FMK, benzyloxycarbonyl-Val-Ala-Asp(OMe) fluoromethylketone; AGG-523, Aggrecanase inhibitor.

Cartilage impact models can be divided into two types: impaction to the closed joint, which maintains normal joint biology; and open impaction applied directly to the open joint or to the surface of articular cartilage explants. Closed impactions have been studied primarily in canine, Flemish giant rabbit or mice (Ewers et al,2002,2000b;Newberry et al,1997;Oegema et al,1993;Thompson et al,1991). In the canine model, cell death and fractures in the subchondral bone and calcified cartilage were observed without full-thickness cracks in the cartilage. OA-like degenerative changes were reported at 6 months, but these had stabilized by 12 months (Thompson et al,1991). In the rabbit model, the effect of trauma depended on the level of stress and varied from cartilage softening with no thickening of subchondral bone to cartilage softening accompanied by subchondral bone thickening/remodeling at 4.5 and 12 months post-trauma. It is not clear whether the damage seen in either of these models would progress to OA if sufficient time was given for end-stage OA to become apparent.

Open impact models. In open *in vitro* and *in vivo* impact models, the outcome depends on the impact forces. Forces above 500 N created more damage in the medial femoral condyle of the New Zealand white rabbits than forces below 500 N (Zhang et al,1999). The subchondral bone remained intact with only superficial fibrillation; although micro-structural injuries may have been present. When an impact was applied on an unconstrained plug of cartilage attached to subchondral bone, a stress of 25MPa at 25% strain disrupted chondrocytes and the cartilage matrix (Ewers et al,2001). Since chondrocyte death would eventually lead to matrix loss (Simon et al,1976), cell death has become the focus of cartilage trauma research and has been primarily studied *in vitro* in the open impact models (Ewers et al,2001;Jeffrey et al,1995;Repo et al,1977;Silyn-Roberts et al,1990;Torzilli et al,1999). Cell death was observed around cracks (Repo et al,1977) and there was a linear relationship between cell death and impact energy with stress levels up to 200 MPa (Jeffrey et al,1995). Cell death was already observed in the surface layer at 15-20 MPa, while extensive cell death in the deep layer was evident at higher levels (Torzilli et al,1999). In an open joint impact model with the impaction level of 25 MPa it has been shown (Hurtig et al,2009)that, if untreated, impact injuries progress to OA-like lesions radially from the center of impaction and present the loss of cartilage matrix components, surface fibrillation and fissures typical for OA-like pathology.

6. Immediate cellular responses to acute trauma and intervention strategies

The immediate responses that occur after joint trauma involve cell death by necrosis and apoptosis, activation of various catabolic events (inflammation, release of free radicals, nitric oxide [NO], proteinases, etc) and mechanical and enzymatic matrix disruption characterized by collagen fragmentation, loss of major matrix components (proteoglycan, hyaluronan, and other), and matrix structural disorganization. Often joint trauma is also accompanied by intra-articular bleeding. All these events identify **intervention strategies** that are based on specific molecular and metabolic pathways. Strategies that prevent post-traumatic cartilage degeneration and loss of cartilage and joint homeostasis would be valuable; and there is considerable experimental evidence that this goal may be attainable (Boileau et al,2002;El Hajjaji et al,2004;Ewers et al,2000a;Jovanovic et al,2001;Myers et al,1999;Pelletier et al,2000b;Phillips et al,2004;Smith et al,1999). The ideal therapy must be multi-varied and include anabolic effects on chondrocyte metabolism and stimulation of intrinsic repair while protecting integrity of cell membrane and inhibiting catabolic pathways that lead to chondrocyte death and matrix loss. In other words, the following are the key mechanisms that should be considered while developing biologic intervention therapies: 1) Chondroprotection; 2) Anti-inflammatory; 3) Matrix protection; and 4) Pro-anabolic, inducers of repair (Table 1). They are discussed below in more details.

7. Chondrocyte death

It has been well documented that cell death is the first response in all injuries that involve blunt trauma or direct insult (impaction, injurious compression, wound creation, etc) to cartilage surface or the entire joint. The role of cell death in PTOA has been widely studied using *in vivo* animal models, *ex vivo* animal and human models and *in vitro* culture approaches with cartilage from different species including humans (Table 2). Chondrocyte death in response to a single impact was first reported in the 1970's (Finlay et al,1978;Repo et al,1977) and was extensively studied in the last few decades. It was shown that controlled single impacts of 15-21 MPa on bovine cartilage explants resulted in chondrocyte death within 24 hours after the injury (Oegema et al,1993; Torzilli et al,1999).

This phenomena has been confirmed in multiple studies using cartilage from different species and applying various forces (15-53MPa) (Newberry et al,1998; Thompson,1975; Lewis et al,2003;Oegema et al, 1993; D'Lima et al,2001b;Ewers et al,2000b,2001,2002; Jeffrey et al,1995; Bolam et al,2006; Hurtig et al,2009; Beecher et al,2007; Pascual Garrido et al,2009; Bajaj et al,2010; Huser et al,2006a). The level of cell death and the depth of damage were proportional to the energy of the impact (Huser et al,2006a; Bolam et al,2006). These observations of the impact induced chondrocyte death in bovine, rabbit, canine, equine, and human cartilage point towards a general mechanism of trauma-mediated effects suggesting that cellular responses to injury could be studied in species that are readily available as models of PTOA. In the PTOA models chondrocytes could die by two mechanisms, necrosis and apoptosis. Necrosis occurs as a direct effect of impact/injury on the cell resulting in the disruption of the cellular membrane and loss of its integrity as well as the damage of the intracellular organelles. This type of death occurs immediately after the insult and is difficult to prevent in the PTOA models. Necrotic cell death also leads to the release of calcium, free radicals, nitric oxide, and the activation of intracellular catabolic mediators, including caspases, interleukins, proteinases, etc. All of them are capable of triggering the process called "apoptosis" leading to the programmed cell death. This second type of death could be prevented and arrested by using targeted therapeutics. For the most part, in the studies on PTOA types of death are not distinguished. Good examples that address both mechanisms are *in vitro* and *in vivo* studies with canine, sheep, or human cartilages (Chen et al,2001; Bajaj et al,2010;Hurtig et al,2009;Pascual Garrido et al,2009). Importantly, necrosis and apoptosis are usually spaced out in time, as it was reported for canine cartilage (Chen et al,2001), where a cyclic impaction induced necrosis during the first 4 hours after the impact, while apoptosis was seen 48 hours after the impact. As was already stated, the level of cell death depends upon the energy of the impact, but cell death is always observed at the surface and in the superficial cartilage zone; it is less pronounced in the middle and deep layers of cartilage (Beecher et al,2007;Pascual Garrido et al,2009).

Species	Model	Impact	Follow-up	Major parameters	Ref
	In Vitro Models				
Human cart /bone	in vitro impact	drop-tower device up to 25N		Cell survival	(Repo & Finkay, 1977)
	in vitro impact	25 MPa		Cell death	(Silyn-Roberts & Broom, 1990)
Canine	in vitro injury	1-2.4 kN	Immediate	Gross evaluation, histology, EM	(Vener et al, 1992)
Bovine cart w/o bone	impact load in vitro	100g-1kg/5-50cm height	3-15 days culture	Cell survival, Matrix integrity, EM	(Jeffrey et al, 1995)
Bovine cart/bone	In vitro impact	50-75 MPa		force displacement curves, histology, Water content, EM	(Borrelli et al, 1997)
Rabbit	In vitro impact	low and high intensity impact	immediate	Indentation, histology	(Newberry et al, 1998)
Bovine	in vitro impact	15-20 MPa		Cell viability, water content	(Torzilli et al, 1999)
Rabbit	impact load		96 hr	apoptosis, GAG release	(D'Lima et al, 2001a)
Human	in vitro impact	14 MPa	0-7, 24,48, 96 hrs	apoptosis, GAG release	(D'Lima et al, 2001b)
Porcine patella's/bone	blunt low impact	0.06, 0.1, 0.2 J	Immediate	Cell death, EM	(Duda et al, 2001)
Bovine patella	acute impact in vitro	53 MPa	18hr-5 days	Cell viability	(Lewis et al, 2003)
Canine	cyclic impacts		21 days	apoptosis, GAG and NO release	(Clements et al, 2004)
Bovine cart w/o bone	single impact	100g/10cm high drop tower	3 min, 20 min	Cell viability, LDH levels	(Bush et al, 2005)
Canine	impact ex vivo	20-25 MPa	7 days	Cell viability, NO, ICAM-1	(Green et al, 2006)
Equine cart w/o bone	single-impact load	130 MPa	48 hr	cell death, apoptosis, GAGs	(Huser et al, 2006)
Porcine	single impact	2, 8, 14 MPa	0,3,7, 14 days	Cell viability, Histology, Immunohistochem	(Otsuki et al, 2008)
Bovine	cyclic impacts	25 MPa	7, 14, 21 days	PG synthesis, cell viability	(Wei et al, 2008)
Porcine	cyclic impacts	5, 30-40MPa	4,24hr	Viability, lactate assay, PG synthesis, gene expression of MMP3,AGG	(Ramakrishnan et al, 2009)
Human	Single impact	600N	0,2,7,14 days	Viability, apoptosis, histology	(Pascual-Garrido et al, 2009)
Bovine	single impact	7J/cm2,14J/cm^2	48hr	Viability,GAG content	(Martin et al, 2009)
Bovine	single impact	14J/cm^2	20min, 1,3,6,12,24,48hr,	Histology,viability,PG synthesis, confocal	(Ding et al, 2010)
Human	single impact	1Ns	20min, 1,24hr	Western blots for ERK, Jun, JNK,P38, Stat3, GSK3	(Bajaj et al, 2010)
Bovine	single impact	20MPa	10,20,30,40,50mins, 1,3,6,24,48hr	Histology, viability,SOD production	(Goodwin et al, 2010)
Bovine	single impact	0, 0.35,0.71, 1.07, 1.43 J	1, 4 days	Viability	(Szczodry et al, 2011)
	In Vitro Compression Model				
Bovine	unconfined compression	17MPa	over night	Histology	(Kurz et al 2004)
Bovine cart w/o bone	unconfined compression	40-900 MPa/s	4 days	Cell death, GAGs	(Ewers et al, 2001)
Bovine, Human cart w/o bone	mechanical load			apoptosis, GAG release	(D'Lima et al, 2001a)
Rabbits	acute Osteochondral injury	2 mm drill	4 days	Apoptosis	(Costouros et al, 2003)
Bovine	mechanical load in vitro		Immediate or 7 day culture	PCR:18S,b-actin,b-2-Microglobulin	(Lee et al, 2005)
Calves	mechanical load	50% Strain	4-16 days	Aggrecanase immunohistochem, AGG western, NITEGE, anti-G1	(Lee et al, 2006)
Bovine	mechanical load	35MPa	0,24,48,72, 96, 120 hrs	cell proliferation, PG synthesis, ERK expression	(Ryan et al, 2009)
	Ex Vivo Models				
Canine	in vivo surgically-created OA	ex vivo	12 wks post op	viability, effect of caspase, COX and iNOS inhibitors	(Pelletier et al, 2001)
	In Vivo Models				
Canine	in vivo surgically-created trauma		1-110 wks post-op	acid hydrolase	(Thompson, 1975)
Canine	closed-joint impact in vivo	2000 N	2,12,24,52 wks	Histology, Immunohistochemistry Fibronectin, 3-B-3, IL-1b, TNF-a	(Pickvance et al, 1993)
Canine	transarticular load in vivo	2000 N	2,8,16, 36, 52 wks	Scanning EM, histology, MRI	(Thompson et al 1993)
Canine	closed impact		2wks, 3 mo	IL-1, TNF, GAG	(Oegema et al, 1993)
Canine	impact in vivo		6,12mo	Cell viability	(Thompson et al 1991)
Rabbit	Impact in vivo		up to 12 mo	Biomechanics, histology	(Newberry et al, 1997)
Rabbit	impact	120N	Immediate	structural changes	(Borrelli et al, 1997)
Canine	in vivo surgically-created OA		10wks post op	Histology, MMP activity, IL-1β PGE, NO assay	(Pelletier JP et al, 1998)
Canine	in vivo surgically-created OA		12wks post op	Gross evaluation, histology	(Pelletier et al, 1999)
Rabbit	closed impact	10KHz	0,4.5,12 mo post-op	stress , histology	(Ewers et al, 2000)
Rabbit	closed impact	5ms/peak or 50 ms/peak		histology, bone softening	(Ewers et al, 2002)
Equine	in vivo surgically-created trauma		48 hr, 7, 14,21,28,35 and 70 day post op	Histology, GAG content, IL-1Ra, PGE	(Frisbie et al, 2002)
Rabbit	impact in vivo	Low and high impact	Immediate	Apoptosis, EM, light microscopy	(Borrelli et al, 2003)
Canine	impact in vivo	18-25 MPa	1,2,4,8,12,116,20,24 wks	TNF, blood, NO, MMPs, GAG	(Green et al, 2006)
Rabbit	in vivo surgically-created OA		9 wks post op	Histology, immunohistochemistry	(D'Lima et al, 2006)
Mouse	closed fracture		2,4,8,50wks	Histology, Micro CT	(Furman et al, 2007)
Rabbit	in vivo surgically-created trauma		4,8,12 wks post op	Histology, immunohistochemistry, micro CT Effects of intra articular BMP7 injections	(Hayashi et al, 2008)
Goat	in vivo surgically-created defects	Full thickness chondral defects	42 wks post op	Histology, immunhistochemistry	(Saw KY et al, 2009)
Goat	open joint impact	25-MPa	90, 118, and 187 days	Histology, apoptosis, GAG, leucocytes	(Hurtig et al, 2009)
Rabbit	open joint single impact	4350g(low); 4900g(high)	0,1,6 mo	Histology, Immunohistochemistry, Viability	(Borrelli et al, 2009)
Mouse	in vivo surgically-created trauma		4 -8wks post-op	Aggrecan, histology	(Little et al, 2009)
Rabbit	open joint Single impact	3.76MPa	4 day post op	Gross evaluation, viability	(Isaac et al, 2010)
Sheep	partial thickness articular cartilage lesion		12wks	Histology, GAG content, Collagen II, NO, IL-1β	(Kaplan et al. 2011)
Rat	in vivo surgically-created OA		4day, 1,2,3,5,8 wks	Aggrecan,	(Chockalingam et al, 2011)

Table 2. *In vivo*, *ex vivo*, and *in vitro* modeling of PTOA. GAG, glycosaminoglycan; PGE2, prostaglandin E2; EM, extracellular matrix; NO, nitric oxide; PG, proteoglycan; TNF-α, tumor necrosis factor (TNF)-α; MMP, matrix metalloproteinases; ADAMTS, A Disintegrin And Metalloproteinase with ThromboSpondin-like repeats; BMPs,Bone morphogenetic proteins; IGF-1, Insulin-like Growth Factor-1; IL, Interleukin; Micro CT, micro computed tomography.

Every model has its advantages and limitations, but each provides important information adding to our understanding of the PTOA. Studying the cartilage explants out of their joint environment eliminates the external influences that cartilage would experience in its natural environment. Factors such as weight bearing, vascularization, fluid dynamics of the joint and the biomechanics of the supporting tissue cannot be controlled in the *in vitro* system, but it provides an opportunity to distinguish truly cartilage responses to trauma without other contributing mechanisms. On the flip side, it makes interpretation of results and extrapolation to actual clinical situations more challenging. Investigating cellular events using humans is almost impossible due to the nature of experimental approaches and end measures. Furthermore, patients come to see the doctor only when pain and signs of degenerative changes have been already developed, which eliminates the option of studying early cellular responses to trauma. In order to overcome some of these limitations *in vivo* animal models have been employed. Unfortunately, many PTOA studies are conducted on rodents or rabbits (Beecher et al,2007;D'Lima et al,2001c;Guilak et al,2004;Isaac et al,2010), the animals that either have a tendency to self-repair or are far from resembling human joint structure and biomechanics. In all these models cell death by necrosis and apoptosis was the most prominent feature, though the degree of death varied between the models and the energy of the impact (Beecher et al,2007;D'Lima et al,2001c;Milentijevic et al,2005). Chondrocyte death and superficial matrix damage were always observed immediately after impaction. The changes that were reported 3 to 52 weeks post impactions were those typically seen in early and late stage osteoarthritis, such as matrix damage, chondrocytes death and proteoglycan loss (Milentijevic et al,2005;Rundell et al,2005), and at later stages, characteristic cartilage fibrillation, clone formation, matrix disorganization, and joint space narrowing (Hurtig et al,2009). All these models indicate that even smaller forces could be sufficient to initiate cell necrosis and higher forces may be needed to initiate massive apoptosis (D'Lima et al,2001b;Milentijevic et al,2005;Rundell et al,2005). The majority of studies used a drop-tower device in an open joint injury models. Borrelli et al (Borrelli et al,2003) used a pendulum type apparatus to apply a rapid impact to the articular surface of the femoral condyle. We used a pneumatically controlled impactor in our studies to generate cartilage damage (Bajaj et al,2010;Pascual Garrido et al,2009; Hurtig et al,2009). Common injuries, such as sports or vehicular, are usually attained in a closed system. Hence, studying open joint impaction may not necessarily reflect real clinical scenario. Therefore, investigating chondrocyte responses that occur in a closed fracturing system could become more relevant, especially since Gaber et al (Gaber et al,2009) also observed significant chondrocyte death after a mid- diaphyseal closed fracture of the tibia.

In summary, in all PTOA models significant chondrocyte death occurs as earlier as 4 hours after the impact and persists for up to 48 hours. If left untreated, it leads to another mechanism of cell death, apoptosis and, eventually with time the cartilage develops OA-like changes. Consequently, therapeutic strategies aimed at minimizing the results of mechanical stress during the early stages post injury may help to preserve structural integrity of cartilage and slow or prevent the development of PTOA.

8. Chondroprotection as an early stage therapy

Since cell death is the first response in all injuries, the most obvious approach is to protect the cells and promote their survival and viability. Chondroprotection could be achieved via targeting different mechanisms: cell membrane protection, anti-oxidant therapy, mitochondria protection, inhibition of NO release, inhibition of apoptosis through the inhibition of caspase signaling, inhibition of calcium quenching, etc. These approaches are addressed below.

As mentioned above, there are two major mechanisms of cell death: necrosis, in which fluid uptake increases causing the cell to swell and rupture resulting in the release of the intracellular contents that incites an inflammatory cascade; and apoptosis, in which there is a chromatin condensation, DNA fragmentation, cell shrinkage, membrane blebbing that cause the cell to self-destruct. Two cellular pathways have been identified in the apoptotic signaling, the extrinsic pathway that involves the Fas receptor pathway and the intrinsic pathway that involves the mitochondrial pathway (Borrelli,2006). Oxygen and reactive oxygen species (ROS) have a role in cartilage homeostasis and are involved in chondrocyte activation, proliferation and matrix remodeling (Henrotin et al,2003). In excess amounts, they induce chondrocyte death and matrix degradation. Mechanical injury has been associated with an increase in production of ROS (Henrotin et al,2003) and decreased antioxidant capacity (Martin et al,2004), which becomes insufficient once structural and functional cartilage damage occurred. The use of exogenous antioxidants, such as vitamin E, N-acetyl-L-cysteine (NAC) and superoxide dismutase have the potential to protect the chondrocytes from the elevated oxidants. Beecher et al (Beecher et al,2007) have shown that pre-treatment with antioxidants can significantly increase chondrocyte survival up to 40-80% in the superficial zone and up to 53-80% in the middle zone. In their study, cartilage explants from non-osteoarthritic human cadaver ankle were pre-treated with NAC, superoxide dismutase or vitamin E before cyclic impaction of either 2MPa or 5MPa was applied. Pre-treatments with NAC and superoxide dismutase were the most effective at preventing chondrocyte death, when forces of 5MPa were applied. Although these finding are promising in showing that human chondrocyte survival can be attained by the treatment with antioxidants, the timing of the antioxidant treatment is not practical, because most joint injuries occur without advance warning. This approach may be valuable when antioxidants are either injected intra-articularly or applied during surgery, when the joint area that undergoes surgical intervention is pretreated with the antioxidants. By the time of surgery, which usually takes place much after the injury, the window of opportunity for antioxidant therapy could have been missed. In a similar study by Martin et al (Martin et al,2009) bovine osteochondral explants subjected to a single blunt end impact were treated with NAC, vitamin E, poloxamer 188 (P188) or Z-VAD-FMK after impaction. The agents were administered either immediately after injury or were delayed by 4 hours. Immediate treatment with NAC improved chondrocyte viability by up to 74%, while delayed treatment also promoted cell survival, but to a lesser extent, 59%, though still being relatively high. Z-VAD-FMK, a caspase inhibitor and anti-apoptotic agent, improved chondrocyte survival to the level of delayed NAC treatment. Vitamin E and P188 did not significantly increase cell survival. In our studies with the human cartilage *ex vivo* injury model, NAC was effective only while it was present in culture media (first 48 hours). It promoted cell survival and inhibited apoptosis in the superficial layer, which was two times lower in the NAC treated explants than in the untreated control. However, after NAC removal, apoptosis returned to the levels of untreated impacted control. Similar observations were found for PG synthesis, which was elevated by two-fold at day 2 under the NAC treatment, but declined to the untreated controls levels as the agent was removed. Adjacent, not impacted areas remained protected by NAC treatment and cell viability was comparable to that of the non-impacted controls. Though in our experiments NAC was effective in protecting the cells, it was ineffective in providing the protection for cartilage matrix integrity. Similarly to Beecher et al, Kurz et al compared the pre-treatment option versus post-injury treatment to see whether pre-treatment with antioxidants could enhance chondrocyte viability (Kurz et al,2004), though clinical relevance of this approach remains to be justified. Superoxide dismutase reduced apoptosis in a dose dependent manner with complete inhibition of apoptosis when the highest dose of 2.5μM was used, while vitamin E had no effect. Despite the efforts, a consensus cannot be achieved on whether the treatment with antioxidants prior to or after the injury has a beneficial effect in enhancing cell survival (Beecher et al,2007;Kurz et al,2004;Martin et al,2009). 1) Different time points and different methods were used to assess cell viability; 2) no distinction was made between necrosis and apoptosis; 3) different species were often used; and 4) distinct responses to the same agent were observed. Differences in responses can be attributed to species- and model-specific distinctions. It has been suggested that blunt versus cyclic impaction model may trigger distinct cellular responses and induce, for example, lipid peroxidation that has a damaging effect on plasma membrane (Beecher et al,2007). Therefore, accumulation of Vitamin E in the plasma membrane could have a protective effect (Claassen et al,2005). This is also supported by the fact that Vitamin E was the most active within the first 4 hours. Together these data indicate an anti-necrotic mechanism of Vitamin E activity. Despite the differences, above referenced studies generate one important message: a window of opportunity for treatment does exist and mechanism-based timely delivery of biologics could provide necessary protection in post-traumatic degenerative events.

The beneficial effects of ROS scavenger NAC (a powerful hydroxyl and hypochlorous radical scavenger) and superoxide dismutase on chondrocyte survival implicate chondrocyte death by apoptosis being secondary to the production of ROS, although the source of ROS excess remains unclear. Chondrocyte survival experiments with superoxide dismutase suggest a role for the mitochondria in early cellular responses to injury. Rotenone, an agent that suppresses the release of superoxide from the mitochondria, has been tested to confirm the role of the mitochondrial electron transport chain in the production of ROS (Goodwin et al,2010). Although rotenone significantly reduced chondrocyte death by more than 40% when administered 2 hours post injury (Goodwin et al,2010), it is unsuitable for an *in vivo* use due to its high cellular toxicity. Accepting the importance of the mitochondria in ROS release, factors that control mitochondrial depolarization have to be considered. Furthermore, it has been shown that injury increases intracellular cytoplasmic calcium due to its release by the endoplasmic reticulum. This leads to depolarization of the mitochondrial membrane, which is associated with the release of cytochrome C, caspase dependent apoptosis and Bcl-2 degradation (Huser et al,2007). Altered intracellular calcium homeostasis has been implied in chondrocyte death (Browning et al,2004;Ohashi et al,2006) and studies with calcium chelating agents have shown significant reduction in chondrocyte death (Huser et al,2007). Thus, calcium quenching inhibitors may have therapeutic value, although the mechanism between the mechanical impact and the cytoplasmic calcium increase remains to be understood.

NO and superoxide anion are the two main ROS produced by the chondrocyte (Hiran et al,1997;Moulton et al,1997). NO in the chondrocyte is synthesized by endothelial nitric oxide synthase (eNOS) or inducible nitric oxide synthase (iNOS) (Henrotin et al,2003) that are reportedly regulated by growth factors, cytokines and endotoxins (Henrotin et al,2003).

Factors such as Tumor Necrosis Factor (TNF)-α, Interleukin (IL)-β, Interferon (INF)-γ and Lipopolysaccharides (LPS) stimulate NO production and Transforming Growth Factor (TGF)-β, IL-4, IL-10 and IL-13 inhibit NO production (Henrotin et al,2003). NO has been shown to be up-regulated after trauma and to possess cartilage degradative properties, which suggests a potential role for iNOS inhibitors in matrix protection. Evidence for chondroprotective effect of NO inhibition comes from studies by Beecher et al (Beecher et al,2007), where human cartilage explants, were pre-treated with the nitric oxide synthase inhibitor N-Nitro-L-arginine methyl ester (L-NAME) before cyclic impaction loads. In treated explants cell survival was considerably higher (82-90%) in the superficial and middle layers compared to the 40-53% in the same areas of the untreated explants. The mechanism, through which L-NAME exhibited its anti-apoptotic effect, is thought to be via interference with the IL-1β pathway (Marsh et al,2002;Pelletier et al,1999,1998). In an *in vivo* canine OA model, Pelletier et al (Pelletier et al,1999,2000a) tested the effect of two concentrations of another iNOS inhibitor, N-iminoethyl-L-Lysine (L-NIL). The dogs that received the higher dose of L-NIL (10mg/kg/day) showed marked decrease in Tunel-positive chondrocytes and macroscopically and histologically their cartilage lesions were less severely affected by the OA-like changes than the placebo treated dogs. In addition, a reduced level of caspase 3 and MMP activity was found in the L-NIL treated dogs (Pelletier et al,1998,2000a). These data suggest that iNOS inhibitors reduce the progression of PTOA through the caspase 3 mediated inhibition of apoptosis that results in the diminished MMP activity (Pelletier et al,1998,2000a).

Apoptosis is one of the main causes of chondrocyte death after mechanical injury (Chen et al,2001;D'Lima et al,2001a; Borrelli,2006), which is mediated by a complex proteolytic system known as the cysteinyl aspartate-specific proteases (caspases). D'Lima et al have successfully demonstrated that caspase inhibitors reduce the severity of cartilage lesion in an *in vivo* rabbit OA model. Using intra-articular injections of the pan caspase inhibitor Z-VAD-FMK (benzyloxycarbonyl-Val-Ala-Asp(OMe) fluoromethylketone), a cell permeable fluoromethylketone, the authors demonstrated reduced cartilage degradation, reduced activity of caspase 3 and reduced p85 fragment suggesting that this broad spectrum caspase inhibitor prevents apoptosis and slows the disease progression. The effect of Z-VAD-FMK has also been studied in full thickness human cartilage explants subjected to single impacts of relatively low stress, 14MPa (D'Lima et al,2001a). These results were reliably reproduced in several other types of injury (static compression and blunt impact) applied to cartilage from different species (bovine, rabbit, equine and human) (Huser et al,2006a;Huser et al,2006b). However, in our studies with human cartilage impact induced by a higher stress, 25-30MPa, the effect of caspase inhibitors (inhibitors of caspase 3 & 9;(Pascual Garrido et al,2009) or pan-caspase inhibitors (Z -VAD-FMK or Q -VD-OPh)), was not as pronounced. In a 14-day follow-up study we found that caspase 3 inhibitor temporarily halted cartilage degenerative changes, while caspase 9 inhibitor was ineffective. Pan caspase inhibitors, contrary to studies of others (D'Lima et al,2001c;Huser et al,2006a;Huser et al,2006b), in our acute injury model on human explants, were not able to inhibit apoptosis. Yet the cells that survived impaction showed elevated PG synthesis after a treatment with caspase inhibitors. This resulted in preservation of matrix integrity (low Mankin score) especially in the areas adjacent to the impact. Both pan-caspase inhibitors demonstrated similar efficacy.

Despite a wide range of effects, evidence suggests that caspase inhibitors could be and should be considered for targeted therapeutic intervention in PTOA, if they are utilized immediately or soon after joint injury before the fully-blown apoptotic cascade takes place.

Another way to fight cell death is physical protection of cell membrane integrity (Duke et al,1996). Therefore, a number of laboratories (including ours) focused on the use of poloxamer 188 (P188), a nontoxic nonionic surfactant that has a hydrophilic and a hydrophobic center, similar to the lipid bilayer composition (Bajaj et al,2010;Isaac et al,2010;Martin et al,2009;Pascual Garrido et al,2009;Phillips et al,2004). It has been suggested that surfactant molecules, (i.e. P188), insert into the membrane to restore the cell membrane integrity post injury, protecting the cell form subsequent catabolic activation.

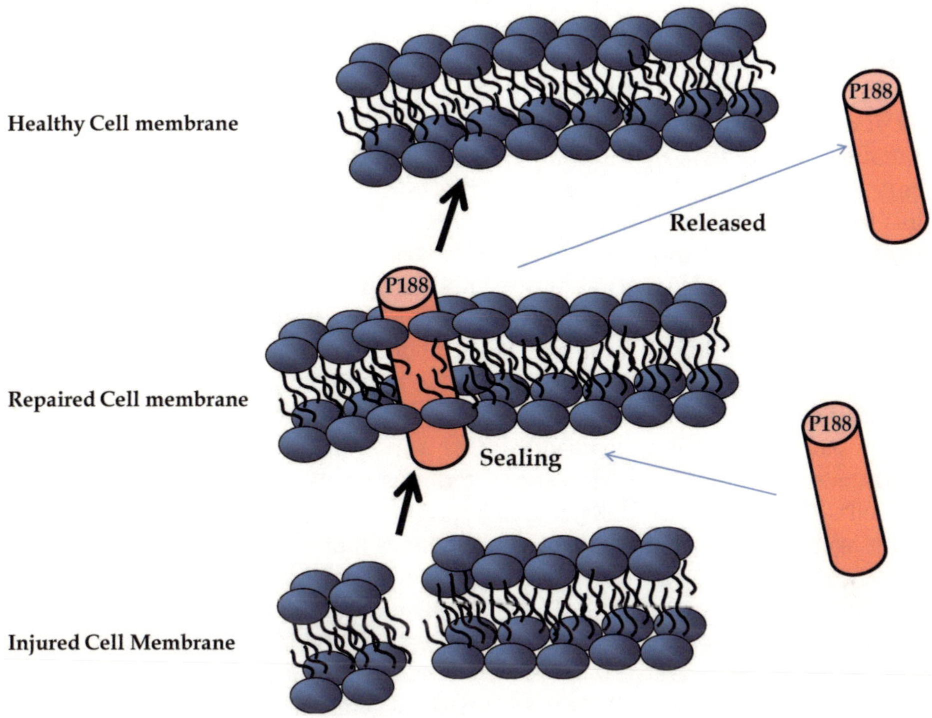

Fig. 1. Diagrammatic representation of P188 surfactant restoring membrane integrity

The role of P188 in bovine chondroprotection was first discovered by the group of Haut (Phillips et al,2004) who showed that P188 statistically reduced the level of apoptosis in the *ex vivo* blunt impaction model. In follow-up studies, an increase in chondrocyte viability with early P188 treatment in short- and long-term has been also documented *in vivo* in rabbits (Isaac et al,2010). We undertook a more comprehensive approach in an attempt to understand the mechanism of P188 action. We demonstrated that P188 was superior to inhibitors of caspase 3 and 9 in promoting cell survival after acute injury (Pascual Garrido et al, 2009). We also found that a single treatment with P188 (8mg/ml; added immediately after injury) was able to inhibit cell death by necrosis and apoptosis and, more importantly, was able to prevent horizontal and longitudinal spread of cell death to the areas that were not directly affected by the impaction. Though P188 was present in the explant culture only for 48 hours, the effect was sustainable for 7 of 14 days. Furthermore, we identified the mechanisms through which P188 exhibited its effect (Bajaj et al,2010). Earlier, the role for mitogen-activated protein kinases (MAPKs), c-Jun-N-terminal kinase and p38, in P188 mediated effects was implied in neural tissue (Serbest et al,2006). We found that among the mechanisms, through which the surfactant directly or indirectly inhibited cell death by apoptosis and prevented its expansion, was the inhibition of the IL-6 signaling pathway. Specifically, phosphorylation of key mediators of the IL-6 pathway, Stat1, Stat3, and p38, was significantly inhibited or prevented. Furthermore, glycogen synthase kinase 3 (GSK3) signaling involved in apoptosis was also inhibited. Our data, both biochemical and histological, suggest that p38 kinase may act up-stream of Stats signaling; activation of p38 kinase as a result of injury, may be partially responsible for initiation of IL-6/Stats mediated catabolic events. A single treatment with P188 blocked phosphorylation of Stats as well as their translocation in to the nucleus, thus potentially preventing transcription of catabolic genes. Furthermore, the role of p38 in injury-induced catabolic responses was further verified by the application of specific synthetic p38 inhibitor confirming previous data (Serbest et al,2006). Treatment with p38 inhibitor not only inhibited the IL-6 pathway, but also promoted cell survival by reducing apoptotic cell death. In addition, we observed an inhibitory effect of P188 on Vascular Endothelial Growth Factor and Monocyte Chemotactic Protein-1 and a stimulatory effect on IL-7 and especially IL-12, effects that remain to be explained. Stimulation of IL-12 may indicate another anabolic response that has not been widely explored in cartilage; IL-12 is an important regulatory cytokine that functions centrally in the initiation and regulation of cellular immune responses. Because a single treatment with P188 lasted only for the first 7 days, we explored multiple applications, adding fresh agent to the culture every 48 hours to sustain its presence for the duration of the experiments. Multiple treatments with P188 were not superior to its single application, suggesting that the primary mechanism of P188 activity is sealing the cellular membrane, which prevents trauma-induced cell necrosis and thus the release of catabolic mediators by necrotic cells. Treatment with P188 prior to impaction was also ineffective, pointing to the role of this agent in repair/restoration of the membrane that was damaged.

In summary, chondroprotective therapy should be seen as the earliest possible approach to treat cartilage tissue post-injury. Chondroprotection has a high potential in the development of targeted biologic interventions in PTOA, because when chondrocyte death is reduced and cartilage cellularity is preserved, there are more chances for the remaining cells to initiate anabolic responses to prevent the expansion of degenerative changes and to remodel damaged matrix.

9. Inhibition of pro-inflammatory mediators as early biologic treatment in PTOA

There are three major anti-catabolic interventions that could be considered at the present time: NAC as an antioxidant (described in details above), interleukin-1 receptor antagonist (IRAP), and TNF-α antagonist. NAC inhibits activation of c-Jun N-terminal kinase, p38 MAP kinase, redox-sensitive activating protein-1 and NF-κB transcription factor activities regulating expression of numerous genes. NAC can also prevent apoptosis and promote cell survival by activating extracellular signal-regulated kinase pathway (Zafarullah et al,2003). Interleukin-1 (IL-1) and tumor necrosis factor (TNF)-α are the most studied cytokines in post-traumatic OA (Evans et al,2004;Fukui et al,2001;Furman et al,2006;Guilak et al,2004). Both are potent activators of cartilage degradation (Martel-Pelletier,1999) and their activity has been significantly increased after acute injury. The levels of these mediators are shown to correlate with the disease severity (Lotz et al,2010;Marks et al,2005). Studies have also reported that IL-6, IL-8 and IL-10 (Bajaj et al,2010; Irie et al,2003;Perl et al,2003) play a role in cartilage loss and the progression of PTOA (Furman et al,2006).The increased expression of these cytokines is attributed to the stressed chondrocytes, synoviocytes and infiltrating inflammatory cells. We documented an elevation of IL-6, TNF-α, basic fibroblast growth factor, and other cytokines as early cellular responses to injury (Anderson et al,2011;Bajaj et al,2010).

Currently, the most effective approaches to inhibit activity of catabolic cytokines are the ones that could interfere with their signaling: receptor blockers, neutralizing monoclonal antibodies, soluble receptors, receptor antagonists, extracellular and intracellular binding proteins, as well as various intracellular repressors and cofactors that prevent the transcription of catabolic genes. IL-1 activity is mediated by its binding to specific IL-1 receptor (IL-1R). Therefore, the antagonist of the IL-1 receptor called interleukin receptor antagonist protein (IRAP) or IL-RA competes for binding to IL-1 and thus prevents the activation of IL-1 signaling. IRAP has been studied in the *in vivo* OA equine model (Frisbie et al,2002), where Ad-EqIL-1Ra was injected intra-articularly. Clinical observation based on pain (lameness) and radiographic examination showed significant improvement in treated horses compared to the untreated horses. Histological examination revealed significant reduction in subintimal edema, joint fibrillation, and chondrocyte necrosis in horses treated with IL-1Ra. Significant, improvement with IL-1Ra treatment seen in the equine model strongly supports its potential use in clinics. Methods have been developed to generate autologous conditioned serum with enriched endogenous IL-1Ra (Orthokine) (Meijer et al,2003) that could be injected into the joint. Preliminary clinical data have shown that intra-articular injections of Orthokine can improve the clinical signs and symptoms of OA such as a reduction in pain and increase in joint function (Fox et al,2010). Whether these methods are chondroprotective or alter the progression of disease is still being investigated. Recombinant IL-1Ra has been used in clinical trials in rheumatoid arthritis, sepsis and graft versus host disease (Evans et al,2004). We investigated whether recombinant IL-RA could inhibit cell death and thus affect cartilage metabolism in the ankle cartilage *ex vivo* acute injury model. 100ng/ml IL-RA increased the percentage of live cells by two-fold in the superficial layer of the impacted tissue compared with the untreated control; while a low dose of IL-RA (20ng/ml) was ineffective. The effect on apoptosis of both concentrations was negligible. Although ineffective in promoting cell survival, a lower concentration of IL-RA stimulated PG synthesis by three-fold. Normal histological pattern of IL-RA treated samples was observed only while the agent was present in culture. As IL-RA was removed, loss of Safranin O staining and depletion of proteoglycan became apparent.

Another cytokine involved in cartilage loss of PTOA is tumor necrosis factor (TNF)-α (Sandell et al,2001). Antagonists of IL-1 and TNF-α, namely, IRAP and the PEGylated soluble TNF-α receptor I, alone and/or in combination, down-regulated MMP-1, MMP-3, and MMP-13 expression and promoted cartilage preservation. Early inhibition of TNF-α can provide chondroprotection and cartilage preservation by decreasing release of glycosaminoglycans and increasing lubricin production in the post traumatic arthritis rat model (Elsaid et al,2009). These results suggest that the inhibition of either or both of these cytokines may offer a useful therapeutic approach to the management of PTOA by reducing gene expression of MMPs involved in cartilage matrix degradation and favoring its repair.

10. Matrix protection

Matrix protection could be achieved by either direct inhibition of matrix proteinases or by affecting the factors responsible for their activation, such as ROS, NO, inflammatory cytokines, etc. NO has been long implicated in cartilage degradation, noting that arthritic patients showed elevated levels of nitrites (Spreng et al,2001) and lipid peroxidation products (Situnayake et al,1991a,1991b) in their biological fluids. The increased NO production has been reported to inhibit aggrecan synthesis (Evans et al,1995), increase iNOS activity, reduce proteoglycan synthesis (Jarvinen et al,1995) and increase MMP activity (Murrell et al,1995). Use of the iNOS inhibitor L-NIL has slowed the progression of PTOA in an experimental OA model in dogs (Pelletier et al,1999). It is plausible to explore iNOS inhibitors therapeutically for matrix protection in addition to chondroprotection.

As a result of cartilage damage, there is a marked increase in the release of matrix components and their fragments, such as proteoglycans, aggrecan cleavage products, collagen, fibronectin, and hyaluronan fragments (Otsuki et al,2008; Ryan et al,2009; Wei et al,2009). Determining a profile of the released metabolites during disease progression may be beneficial in the development of treatment strategy and targeted therapeutic interventions. Specific effective inhibitors of the MMPs could also protect the matrix and in turn halt the disease progression. The role of MMPs has been primarily addressed in various OA models or in patients with signs of arthritis. In PTOA, there is very little, if any, available information. Selective inhibitors are not widely available and the majority of studies have utilized broad spectrum MMP inhibitors, which in addition to a direct effect on MMPs, have been also associated with adverse musculoskeletal effects such as muscle stiffness, bursitis and fibrosis (Pelletier et al,2007). Studies with MMP-13 knockout mice (Little et al,2009) showed cartilage protection when OA was surgically induced, suggesting a crucial role of MMP-13 in cartilage degradation. Oral dosing of the MMP-13 inhibitor in a rabbit OA model has shown cartilage protection without the musculoskeletal adverse effects (Johnson et al,2007). These very promising but preliminary data may have potential in PTOA therapy, although clinical trials with several MMP inhibitors in patients with established OA have failed due to side effects and lack of efficacy. ADAMTS's have also been implicated in the pathogenesis of OA. The use of ADAM-TS5 knockout mice have shown that these mice do not develop OA (Glasson et al,2005), but display some side effects, such as fibrosis. Inhibitors of aggrecanases with higher specificity and lower toxicity are among future therapeutic agents for the treatment of PTOA.

11. Matrix remodeling with anabolic growth factors

One of the very important directions in the development of pharmacological interventions in PTOA is the ability to stimulate production of new cartilage extracellular matrix. The best candidates are growth factors including members of the TGF-β superfamily, FGFs, Insulin-like Growth Factor (IGF)-1. Bone Morphogenetic Proteins (BMPs) belong to the TGF-β superfamily and are important stimuli of mesenchymal cell differentiation and extracellular matrix formation. BMP-2 and BMP-7 appear to be extremely potent in cartilage and bone repair. The most studied BMP for cartilage repair is BMP-7, also known as osteogenic protein-1 (OP-1). It has been studied most extensively *in vitro* in our laboratory on human cartilage (reviewed in (Chubinskaya et al,2007,2011) as well as in OA and PTOA animal models (Badlani et al,2008;Cook et al,2003;Hayashi et al,2008,2010;Hurtig et al,2009). The results suggest that BMP-7 may be the best candidate for a disease-modifying OA drug and also for PTOA. Unlike TGF-β and other BMPs, BMP-7 up-regulates chondrocyte metabolism and protein synthesis without creating uncontrolled cell proliferation and formation of osteophytes. BMP-7 prevents chondrocyte catabolism induced by IL-1 or fragments of matrix components. It has synergistic anabolic effects with other growth factors such as IGF-1, in addition to its anabolic effect acts as a cell survival factor (reviewed in Chubinskaya et al,2007). BMP-7 restores the responsiveness of human chondrocytes to IGF-1 lost with ageing through the regulation of IGF-1 and its signaling pathway (Chubinskaya et al,2011; Im et al,2003). IGF-1 has chondroprotective activity in various animal models (Fortier et al,2002). In our most recent studies in the acute *ex vivo* cartilage trauma model, BMP-7 stimulated PG synthesis and preserved matrix integrity. Treatment with BMP-7 also significantly promoted cell survival in the impacted region (two-fold difference) and prevented expansion of cell death and matrix degeneration into the adjacent, but not impacted regions. BMP-7 has been also used in various PTOA animal models in dogs (Cook et al,2003), sheep (Hurtig et al,2009), goats (Louwerse et al,2000) and rabbits (Badlani et al,2008;Hayashi et al,2008,2010). In all these PTOA models (ACL transaction, osteochondral defect, and impaction), BMP-7 regenerated articular cartilage, increased repair tissue formation and improved integrative repair between new cartilage and the surrounding articular surface. In the impaction model (Hurtig et al,2009), a window of opportunity for the treatment with BMP-7 has been identified. It was found that therapeutic application of BMP-7 was most effective in arresting progression of cartilage degeneration if administered twice at weekly intervals either immediately after trauma or delayed by three weeks. If delayed by three months, the treatment was ineffective, suggesting that the development and progression of PTOA could be arrested and maybe even prevented if the right treatment is administered at the right time. Phase I clinical study produced very encouraging results by showing tolerability to the treatment, absence of toxic response, and a greater symptomatic improvement in patients that received a single injection of BMP-7 (Hunter et al,2010). Clinical efficacy of the BMP-7 treatment is currently being tested in a phase II clinical OA study.

Other growth factors from the fibroblast growth factor family have been also tested as potential DMOADs in PTOA. FGFs are important regulators of cartilage development and homeostasis (Ellman et al,2008). FGF-2 can stimulate cartilage repair responses (Henson et al,2005), but its potent mitogenic effects may lead to chondrocyte cluster formation and poor extracellular matrix due to a relatively low level of type II collagen (Ellman et al,2008). FGF-2 has been also shown to induce pro-catabolic and pro-inflammatory responses (Ellman et al,2008). In a rabbit ACL transection model, sustained release formulations of FGF-2 reduced OA severity (reviewed in Lotz et al, 2010). Another member of the same family, FGF-18, has been shown to induce anabolic effects in chondrocytes and chondroprogenitor cells and to stimulate cell proliferation and type II collagen production (Ellsworth et al,2002). In a rat meniscal tear model of OA, intra-articular FGF-18 injections induced remarkable formation of new cartilage and reduced the severity of experimental lesions (Moore et al,2005). Thus far, only two anabolic factors, FGF-18 and BMP-7, are currently being tested in clinical studies in patients with established OA. At this stage of our cumulative knowledge, BMP-7 appears to be one of the best candidate therapeutic agents for cartilage treatment after injury, since it affects multiple catabolic and anabolic pathways.

12. Conclusion

One of the unanswered PTOA questions is when and which therapies that have been developed as disease-modifying OA drugs are indicated for patients with post-traumatic OA and whether a different set of treatments and molecular targets has to be considered. Through basic and clinical research an impressive progress has been made towards elucidation of pathogenesis of PTOA and understanding the mechanisms that govern immediate cellular responses to injury. However, this still requires further validation in a large cohort of patients with various types of joint injuries. The ideal therapy to arrest and prevent the development and progression of PTOA must be multi-varied and include anabolic effects on chondrocyte metabolism characterized by elevated intrinsic repair, while protecting integrity of cell membrane and inhibiting catabolic pathways that lead to chondrocyte death and matrix loss (Lotz et al,2010). The following are the key mechanisms that should constitute the basis for the design of intervention therapies: 1) Chondroprotection; 2) Anti-inflammatory; 3) Matrix protection; and 4) Pro-anabolic, stimuli of cartilage remodeling and regeneration. The most beneficial agents are those that target multiple pathways and mechanisms. A number of molecular targets have been identified (Table 1) and many of the existing therapeutic agents have been already tested *in vitro* and *in vivo*. The biggest remaining challenge is the translation of this knowledge into the clinic and the development of appropriate effective therapy/therapies administered within the window of opportunity. Currently, the most suitable route for administering such therapy appears to be intra-articular injections that allow accumulation of critical doses of the drug within the damaged area and also reduce the risk of systemic side effects. To monitor the efficacy of the PTOA therapy, an appropriate set of bio- and imaging markers is needed that could predict and correlate with the progression of the disease, since it takes years and decades for the disease to develop.

13. Acknowledgements

This work was supported by the National Football League Charity Foundation, Ciba-Geigy Endowed Chair and Department of Biochemistry, Rush University Medical Center. The authors would like to acknowledge Drs. Markus A. Wimmer, Theodore R Oegema, and Jeffrey A. Borgia for their important contributions to this work. The authors would like to acknowledge Dr. Arkady Margulis for tissue procurement and Dr. Lev Rappoport and Mrs. Arnavaz Hakimiyan for their technical assistance. The authors also would like to acknowledge the Gift of Hope Organ & Tissue Donor Network and donor's families.

14. References

Anderson, DD; Chubinskaya, S; Guilak, F; Martin, JA; Oegema, TR; Olson, SA and Buckwalter, JA. (2011). Post-traumatic osteoarthritis: improved understanding and opportunities for early intervention. *J Orthop Res*, 29(6):802-9.

Anitua, E; Andia, I; Ardanza, B; Nurden, P and Nurden, AT. (2004). Autologous platelets as a source of proteins for healing and tissue regeneration. *Thromb Haemost*, 91(1):4-15.

Anitua, E; Sanchez, M; Nurden, AT; Zalduendo, M; de la Fuente, M; Orive, G; Azofra, J and Andia, I. (2006). Autologous fibrin matrices: a potential source of biological mediators that modulate tendon cell activities. *J Biomed Mater Res A*, 77(2):285-93.

Avouac, J; Vicaut, E; Bardin, T and Richette, P. (2010). Efficacy of joint lavage in knee osteoarthritis: meta-analysis of randomized controlled studies. *Rheumatology (Oxford)*, 49(2):334-40.

Badlani, N; Inoue, A; Healey, R; Coutts, R and Amiel, D. (2008). The protective effect of OP-1 on articular cartilage in the development of osteoarthritis. *Osteoarthritis Cartilage*, 16(5):600-6.

Bajaj, S; Shoemaker, T; Hakimiyan, AA; Rappoport, L; Pascual-Garrido, C; Oegema, TR; Wimmer, MA and Chubinskaya, S. (2010). Protective effect of P188 in the model of acute trauma to human ankle cartilage: the mechanism of action. *J Orthop Trauma*, 24(9):571-6.

Beecher, BR; Martin, JA; Pedersen, DR; Heiner, AD and Buckwalter, JA. (2007). Antioxidants block cyclic loading induced chondrocyte death. *Iowa Orthop J*, 27(1-8.

Behrens, P; Bitter, T; Kurz, B and Russlies, M. (2006). Matrix-associated autologous chondrocyte transplantation/implantation (MACT/MACI)--5-year follow-up. *Knee*, 13(3):194-202.

Boileau, C; Martel-Pelletier, J; Jouzeau, JY; Netter, P; Moldovan, F; Laufer, S; Tries, S and Pelletier, JP. (2002). Licofelone (ML-3000), a dual inhibitor of 5-lipoxygenase and cyclooxygenase, reduces the level of cartilage chondrocyte death in vivo in experimental dog osteoarthritis: inhibition of pro-apoptotic factors. *J Rheumatol*, 29(7):1446-53.

Bolam, CJ; Hurtig, MB; Cruz, A and McEwen, BJ. (2006). Characterization of experimentally induced post-traumatic osteoarthritis in the medial femorotibial joint of horses. *Am J Vet Res*, 67(3):433-47.

Borrelli, J, Jr. (2006). Chondrocyte apoptosis and posttraumatic arthrosis. *J Orthop Trauma*, 20(10):726-31.

Borrelli, J, Jr.; Tinsley, K; Ricci, WM; Burns, M; Karl, IE and Hotchkiss, R. (2003). Induction of chondrocyte apoptosis following impact load. *J Orthop Trauma*, 17(9):635-41.

Brittberg, M; Lindahl, A; Nilsson, A; Ohlsson, C; Isaksson, O and Peterson, L. (1994). Treatment of deep cartilage defects in the knee with autologous chondrocyte transplantation. *N Engl J Med*, 331(14):889-95.

Brown, TD; Johnston, RC; Saltzman, CL; Marsh, JL and Buckwalter, JA. (2006). Posttraumatic osteoarthritis: a first estimate of incidence, prevalence, and burden of disease. *J Orthop Trauma*, 20(10):739-44.

Browning, JA; Saunders, K; Urban, JP and Wilkins, RJ. (2004). The influence and interactions of hydrostatic and osmotic pressures on the intracellular milieu of chondrocytes. *Biorheology*, 41(3-4):299-308.

Buckwalter, JA and Brown, TD. (2004). Joint injury, repair, and remodeling: roles in post-traumatic osteoarthritis. *Clin Orthop Relat Res*, 423):7-16.

Butler, DL; Juncosa-Melvin, N; Boivin, GP; Galloway, MT; Shearn, JT; Gooch, C and Awad, H. (2008). Functional tissue engineering for tendon repair: A multidisciplinary strategy using mesenchymal stem cells, bioscaffolds, and mechanical stimulation. *J Orthop Res*, 26(1):1-9.

Chen, CT; Burton-Wurster, N; Borden, C; Hueffer, K; Bloom, SE and Lust, G. (2001). Chondrocyte necrosis and apoptosis in impact damaged articular cartilage. *J Orthop Res*, 19(4):703-11.

Chubinskaya, S; Hurtig, M and Rueger, DC. (2007). OP-1/BMP-7 in cartilage repair. *Int Orthop*, 31(6):773-81.

Chubinskaya, S; Otten, L; Soeder, S; Borgia, JA; Aigner, T; Rueger, DC and Loeser, RF. (2011). Regulation of chondrocyte gene expression by osteogenic protein-1. *Arthritis Res Ther*, 13(2):R55.

Claassen, H; Schunke, M and Kurz, B. (2005). Estradiol protects cultured articular chondrocytes from oxygen-radical-induced damage. *Cell Tissue Res*, 319(3):439-45.

Clements, KM; Burton-Wurster, N and Lust, G. (2004). The spread of cell death from impact damaged cartilage: lack of evidence for the role of nitric oxide and caspases. *Osteoarthritis Cartilage*, 12(7):577-85.

Cole, BJ; Pascual-Garrido, C and Grumet, RC. (2009). Surgical management of articular cartilage defects in the knee. *J Bone Joint Surg Am*, 91(7):1778-90.

Convery, FR; Akeson, WH and Keown, GH. (1972). The repair of large osteochondral defects. An experimental study in horses. *Clin Orthop Relat Res*, 82(253-62.

Cook, SD; Patron, LP; Salkeld, SL and Rueger, DC. (2003). Repair of articular cartilage defects with osteogenic protein-1 (BMP-7) in dogs. *J Bone Joint Surg Am*, 85-A Suppl 3(116-23.

D'Lima, D; Hermida, J; Hashimoto, S; Colwell, C and Lotz, M. (2006). Caspase inhibitors reduce severity of cartilage lesions in experimental osteoarthritis. *Arthritis Rheum*, 54(6):1814-21.

D'Lima, DD; Hashimoto, S; Chen, PC; Colwell, CW, Jr. and Lotz, MK. (2001a). Human chondrocyte apoptosis in response to mechanical injury. *Osteoarthritis Cartilage*, 9(8):712-9.

D'Lima, DD; Hashimoto, S; Chen, PC; Colwell, CW, Jr. and Lotz, MK. (2001b). Impact of mechanical trauma on matrix and cells. *Clin Orthop Relat Res*, 391 Suppl):S90-9.

D'Lima, DD; Hashimoto, S; Chen, PC; Lotz, MK and Colwell, CW, Jr. (2001c). In vitro and in vivo models of cartilage injury. *J Bone Joint Surg Am*, 83-A Suppl 2(Pt 1):22-4.

Dirschl, DR; Marsh, JL; Buckwalter, JA; Gelberman, R; Olson, SA; Brown, TD and Llinias, A. (2004). Articular fractures. *J Am Acad Orthop Surg*, 12(6):416-23.

Duke, RC; Ojcius, DM and Young, JD. (1996). Cell suicide in health and disease. *Sci Am*, 275(6):80-7.

El Hajjaji, H; Williams, JM; Devogelaer, JP; Lenz, ME; Thonar, EJ and Manicourt, DH. (2004). Treatment with calcitonin prevents the net loss of collagen, hyaluronan and proteoglycan aggregates from cartilage in the early stages of canine experimental osteoarthritis. *Osteoarthritis Cartilage*, 12(11):904-11.

Ellman, MB; An, HS; Muddasani, P and Im, HJ. (2008). Biological impact of the fibroblast growth factor family on articular cartilage and intervertebral disc homeostasis. *Gene*, 420(1):82-9.

Ellsworth, JL; Berry, J; Bukowski, T; Claus, J; Feldhaus, A; Holderman, S; Holdren, MS; Lum, KD; Moore, EE; Raymond, F; Ren, H; Shea, P; Sprecher, C; Storey, H; Thompson, DL; Waggie, K; Yao, L; Fernandes, RJ; Eyre, DR and Hughes, SD. (2002). Fibroblast growth factor-18 is a trophic factor for mature chondrocytes and their progenitors. *Osteoarthritis Cartilage*, 10(4):308-20.

Elsaid, KA; Machan, JT; Waller, K; Fleming, BC and Jay, GD. (2009). The impact of anterior cruciate ligament injury on lubricin metabolism and the effect of inhibiting tumor necrosis factor alpha on chondroprotection in an animal model. *Arthritis Rheum*, 60(10):2997-3006.

Evans, CH; Gouze, JN; Gouze, E; Robbins, PD and Ghivizzani, SC. (2004). Osteoarthritis gene therapy. *Gene Ther*, 11(4):379-89.

Evans, CH; Stefanovic-Racic, M and Lancaster, J. (1995). Nitric oxide and its role in orthopaedic disease. *Clin Orthop Relat Res*, 312):275-94.

Ewers, BJ; Dvoracek-Driksna, D; Orth, MW and Haut, RC. (2001). The extent of matrix damage and chondrocyte death in mechanically traumatized articular cartilage explants depends on rate of loading. *J Orthop Res*, 19(5):779-84.

Ewers, BJ and Haut, RC. (2000a). Polysulphated glycosaminoglycan treatments can mitigate decreases in stiffness of articular cartilage in a traumatized animal joint. *J Orthop Res*, 18(5):756-61.

Ewers, BJ; Jayaraman, VM; Banglmaier, RF and Haut, RC. (2002). Rate of blunt impact loading affects changes in retropatellar cartilage and underlying bone in the rabbit patella. *J Biomech*, 35(6):747-55.

Ewers, BJ; Newberry, WN and Haut, RC. (2000b). Chronic softening of cartilage without thickening of underlying bone in a joint trauma model. *J Biomech*, 33(12):1689-94.

Finlay, JB and Repo, RU. (1978). Instrumentation and procedure for the controlled impact of articular cartilage. *IEEE Trans Biomed Eng*, 25(1):34-9.

Fortier, LA; Mohammed, HO; Lust, G and Nixon, AJ. (2002). Insulin-like growth factor-I enhances cell-based repair of articular cartilage. *J Bone Joint Surg Br*, 84(2):276-88.

Fox, BA and Stephens, MM. (2010). Treatment of knee osteoarthritis with Orthokine-derived autologous conditioned serum. *Expert Rev Clin Immunol*, 6(3):335-45.

Frisbie, DD; Ghivizzani, SC; Robbins, PD; Evans, CH and McIlwraith, CW. (2002). Treatment of experimental equine osteoarthritis by in vivo delivery of the equine interleukin-1 receptor antagonist gene. *Gene Ther*, 9(1):12-20.

Fukui, N; Purple, CR and Sandell, LJ. (2001). Cell biology of osteoarthritis: the chondrocyte's response to injury. *Curr Rheumatol Rep*, 3(6):496-505.

Furman, BD; Olson, SA and Guilak, F. (2006). The development of posttraumatic arthritis after articular fracture. *J Orthop Trauma*, 20(10):719-25.

Furman, BD; Strand, J; Hembree, WC; Ward, BD; Guilak, F and Olson, SA. (2007). Joint degeneration following closed intraarticular fracture in the mouse knee: a model of posttraumatic arthritis. *J Orthop Res*, 25(5):578-92.

Gaber, S; Fischerauer, EE; Frohlich, E; Janezic, G; Amerstorfer, F and Weinberg, AM. (2009). Chondrocyte apoptosis enhanced at the growth plate: a physeal response to a diaphyseal fracture. *Cell Tissue Res*, 335(3):539-49.

Gelber, AC; Hochberg, MC; Mead, LA; Wang, NY; Wigley, FM and Klag, MJ. (2000). Joint injury in young adults and risk for subsequent knee and hip osteoarthritis. *Ann Intern Med*, 133(5):321-8.

Glasson, SS; Askew, R; Sheppard, B; Carito, B; Blanchet, T; Ma, HL; Flannery, CR; Peluso, D; Kanki, K; Yang, Z; Majumdar, MK and Morris, EA. (2005). Deletion of active ADAMTS5 prevents cartilage degradation in a murine model of osteoarthritis. *Nature*, 434(7033):644-8.

Gonzalez, MH and Mekhail, AO. (2004). The failed total knee arthroplasty: evaluation and etiology. *J Am Acad Orthop Surg*, 12(6):436-46.

Goodwin, W; McCabe, D; Sauter, E; Reese, E; Walter, M; Buckwalter, JA and Martin, JA. (2010). Rotenone prevents impact-induced chondrocyte death. *J Orthop Res*, 28(8):1057-63.

Green, DM; Noble, PC; Ahuero, JS and Birdsall, HH. (2006a). Cellular events leading to chondrocyte death after cartilage impact injury. *Arthritis Rheum*, 54(5):1509-17.

Green, DM; Noble, PC; Bocell, JR, Jr.; Ahuero, JS; Poteet, BA and Birdsall, HH. (2006b). Effect of early full weight-bearing after joint injury on inflammation and cartilage degradation. *J Bone Joint Surg Am*, 88(10):2201-9.

Guilak, F; Fermor, B; Keefe, FJ; Kraus, VB; Olson, SA; Pisetsky, DS; Setton, LA and Weinberg, JB. (2004). The role of biomechanics and inflammation in cartilage injury and repair. *Clin Orthop Relat Res*, 423):17-26.

Hayashi, M; Muneta, T; Ju, YJ; Mochizuki, T and Sekiya, I. (2008). Weekly intra-articular injections of bone morphogenetic protein-7 inhibits osteoarthritis progression. *Arthritis Res Ther*, 10(5):R118.

Hayashi, M; Muneta, T; Takahashi, T; Ju, YJ; Tsuji, K and Sekiya, I. (2010). Intra-articular injections of bone morphogenetic protein-7 retard progression of existing cartilage degeneration. *J Orthop Res*, 28(11):1502-6.

Henrotin, YE; Bruckner, P and Pujol, JP. (2003). The role of reactive oxygen species in homeostasis and degradation of cartilage. *Osteoarthritis Cartilage*, 11(10):747-55.

Henson, FM; Bowe, EA and Davies, ME. (2005). Promotion of the intrinsic damage-repair response in articular cartilage by fibroblastic growth factor-2. *Osteoarthritis Cartilage*, 13(6):537-44.

Hiran, TS; Moulton, PJ and Hancock, JT. (1997). Detection of superoxide and NADPH oxidase in porcine articular chondrocytes. *Free Radic Biol Med*, 23(5):736-43.

Horas, U; Pelinkovic, D; Herr, G; Aigner, T and Schnettler, R. (2003). Autologous chondrocyte implantation and osteochondral cylinder transplantation in cartilage repair of the knee joint. A prospective, comparative trial. *J Bone Joint Surg Am*, 85-A(2):185-92.

Hunter, DJ; Pike, MC; Jonas, BL; Kissin, E; Krop, J and McAlindon, T. (2010). Phase 1 safety and tolerability study of BMP-7 in symptomatic knee osteoarthritis. *BMC Musculoskelet Disord*, 11(232.

Hurtig, M; Chubinskaya, S; Dickey, J and Rueger, D. (2009). BMP-7 protects against progression of cartilage degeneration after impact injury. *J Orthop Res*, 27(5):602-11.

Huser, CA and Davies, ME. (2006a). Validation of an in vitro single-impact load model of the initiation of osteoarthritis-like changes in articular cartilage. *J Orthop Res*, 24(4):725-32.

Huser, CA and Davies, ME. (2007). Calcium signaling leads to mitochondrial depolarization in impact-induced chondrocyte death in equine articular cartilage explants. *Arthritis Rheum*, 56(7):2322-34.

Huser, CA; Peacock, M and Davies, ME. (2006b). Inhibition of caspase-9 reduces chondrocyte apoptosis and proteoglycan loss following mechanical trauma. *Osteoarthritis Cartilage*, 14(10):1002-10.

Iannitti, T; Lodi, D and Palmieri, B. (2011). Intra-articular injections for the treatment of osteoarthritis: focus on the clinical use of hyaluronic Acid. *Drugs R D*, 11(1):13-27.

Im, HJ; Pacione, C; Chubinskaya, S; Van Wijnen, AJ; Sun, Y and Loeser, RF. (2003). Inhibitory effects of insulin-like growth factor-1 and osteogenic protein-1 on fibronectin fragment- and interleukin-1beta-stimulated matrix metalloproteinase-13 expression in human chondrocytes. *J Biol Chem*, 278(28):25386-94.

Irie, K; Uchiyama, E and Iwaso, H. (2003). Intraarticular inflammatory cytokines in acute anterior cruciate ligament injured knee. *Knee*, 10(1):93-6.

Isaac, DI; Golenberg, N and Haut, RC. (2010). Acute repair of chondrocytes in the rabbit tibiofemoral joint following blunt impact using P188 surfactant and a preliminary investigation of its long-term efficacy. *J Orthop Res*, 28(4):553-8.

Jarvinen, TA; Moilanen, T; Jarvinen, TL and Moilanen, E. (1995). Nitric oxide mediates interleukin-1 induced inhibition of glycosaminoglycan synthesis in rat articular cartilage. *Mediators Inflamm*, 4(2):107-11.

Jeffrey, JE; Gregory, DW and Aspden, RM. (1995). Matrix damage and chondrocyte viability following a single impact load on articular cartilage. *Arch Biochem Biophys*, 322(1):87-96.

Johnson, AR; Pavlovsky, AG; Ortwine, DF; Prior, F; Man, CF; Bornemeier, DA; Banotai, CA; Mueller, WT; McConnell, P; Yan, C; Baragi, V; Lesch, C; Roark, WH; Wilson, M; Datta, K; Guzman, R; Han, HK and Dyer, RD. (2007). Discovery and characterization of a novel inhibitor of matrix metalloprotease-13 that reduces cartilage damage in vivo without joint fibroplasia side effects. *J Biol Chem*, 282(38):27781-91.

Jovanovic, DV; Fernandes, JC; Martel-Pelletier, J; Jolicoeur, FC; Reboul, P; Laufer, S; Tries, S and Pelletier, JP. (2001). In vivo dual inhibition of cyclooxygenase and lipoxygenase by ML-3000 reduces the progression of experimental osteoarthritis: suppression of collagenase 1 and interleukin-1beta synthesis. *Arthritis Rheum*, 44(10):2320-30.

Kappler, J; Kaminski, TP; Gieselmann, V; Kubitscheck, U and Jerosch, J. (2010). Single-molecule imaging of hyaluronan in human synovial fluid. *J Biomed Opt*, 15(6):060504.

Kern, D; Zlatkin, MB and Dalinka, MK. (1988). Occupational and post-traumatic arthritis. *Radiol Clin North Am*, 26(6):1349-58.

Key JA (1933) Experimental arthritis, Chronic and Atrophic. *Med. J and Rec* 138:369-372.

Kirk, S; Gitelis, S; Ruta, D; Filardo, G; Hakimiyan, AA; Rappoport, L; Cole, BJ; Chubinskaya, S. (2011). New Insight into Allograft Cartilage: Lessons to be considered. ORS meeting, Long Beach, CA, Jan 13-16 2011. Trans ORS, 36: Poster#1975

Kuroda, R; Ishida, K; Matsumoto, T; Akisue, T; Fujioka, H; Mizuno, K; Ohgushi, H; Wakitani, S and Kurosaka, M. (2007). Treatment of a full-thickness articular cartilage defect in the femoral condyle of an athlete with autologous bone-marrow stromal cells. *Osteoarthritis Cartilage*, 15(2):226-31.

Kurz, B; Lemke, A; Kehn, M; Domm, C; Patwari, P; Frank, EH; Grodzinsky, AJ and Schunke, M. (2004). Influence of tissue maturation and antioxidants on the apoptotic response of articular cartilage after injurious compression. *Arthritis Rheum*, 50(1):123-30.

Lewis, JL; Deloria, LB; Oyen-Tiesma, M; Thompson, RC, Jr.; Ericson, M and Oegema, TR, Jr. (2003). Cell death after cartilage impact occurs around matrix cracks. *J Orthop Res*, 21(5):881-7.

Little, CB; Barai, A; Burkhardt, D; Smith, SM; Fosang, AJ; Werb, Z; Shah, M and Thompson, EW. (2009). Matrix metalloproteinase 13-deficient mice are resistant to osteoarthritic cartilage erosion but not chondrocyte hypertrophy or osteophyte development. *Arthritis Rheum*, 60(12):3723-33.

Lotz, MK and Kraus, VB. (2010). New developments in osteoarthritis. Posttraumatic osteoarthritis: pathogenesis and pharmacological treatment options. *Arthritis Res Ther*, 12(3):211.

Louwerse, RT; Heyligers, IC; Klein-Nulend, J; Sugihara, S; van Kampen, GP; Semeins, CM; Goei, SW; de Koning, MH; Wuisman, PI and Burger, EH. (2000). Use of recombinant human osteogenic protein-1 for the repair of subchondral defects in articular cartilage in goats. *J Biomed Mater Res*, 49(4):506-16.

Marks, PH and Donaldson, ML. (2005). Inflammatory cytokine profiles associated with chondral damage in the anterior cruciate ligament-deficient knee. *Arthroscopy*, 21(11):1342-7.

Marsh, JL; Buckwalter, J; Gelberman, R; Dirschl, D; Olson, S; Brown, T and Llinias, A. (2002). Articular fractures: does an anatomic reduction really change the result? *J Bone Joint Surg Am*, 84-A(7):1259-71.

Martel-Pelletier, J. (1999). Proinflammatory mediators and osteoarthritis. *Osteoarthritis Cartilage*, 7(3):315-6.

Martin, JA; Brown, T; Heiner, A and Buckwalter, JA. (2004). Post-traumatic osteoarthritis: the role of accelerated chondrocyte senescence. *Biorheology*, 41(3-4):479-91.

Martin, JA; McCabe, D; Walter, M; Buckwalter, JA and McKinley, TO. (2009). N-acetylcysteine inhibits post-impact chondrocyte death in osteochondral explants. *J Bone Joint Surg Am*, 91(8):1890-7.

Meijer, H; Reinecke, J; Becker, C; Tholen, G and Wehling, P. (2003). The production of anti-inflammatory cytokines in whole blood by physico-chemical induction. *Inflamm Res*, 52(10):404-7.

Migliore, A; Giovannangeli, F; Bizzi, E; Massafra, U; Alimonti, A; Lagana, B; Diamanti Picchianti, A; Germano, V; Granata, M and Piscitelli, P. (2011). Viscosupplementation in the management of ankle osteoarthritis: a review. *Arch Orthop Trauma Surg*, 131(1):139-47.

Milentijevic, D; Rubel, IF; Liew, AS; Helfet, DL and Torzilli, PA. (2005). An in vivo rabbit model for cartilage trauma: a preliminary study of the influence of impact stress magnitude on chondrocyte death and matrix damage. *J Orthop Trauma*, 19(7):466-73.

Miller, BS; Steadman, JR; Briggs, KK; Rodrigo, JJ and Rodkey, WG. (2004). Patient satisfaction and outcome after microfracture of the degenerative knee. *J Knee Surg*, 17(1):13-7.

Moore, EE; Bendele, AM; Thompson, DL; Littau, A; Waggie, KS; Reardon, B and Ellsworth, JL. (2005). Fibroblast growth factor-18 stimulates chondrogenesis and cartilage repair in a rat model of injury-induced osteoarthritis. *Osteoarthritis Cartilage*, 13(7):623-31.

Moulton, PJ; Hiran, TS; Goldring, MB and Hancock, JT. (1997). Detection of protein and mRNA of various components of the NADPH oxidase complex in an immortalized human chondrocyte line. *Br J Rheumatol*, 36(5):522-9.

Murphy, L; Schwartz, TA; Helmick, CG; Renner, JB; Tudor, G; Koch, G; Dragomir, A; Kalsbeek, WD; Luta, G and Jordan, JM. (2008). Lifetime risk of symptomatic knee osteoarthritis. *Arthritis Rheum*, 59(9):1207-13.

Murrell, GA; Jang, D and Williams, RJ. (1995). Nitric oxide activates metalloprotease enzymes in articular cartilage. *Biochem Biophys Res Commun*, 206(1):15-21.

Myers, SL; Brandt, KD; Burr, DB; O'Connor, BL and Albrecht, M. (1999). Effects of a bisphosphonate on bone histomorphometry and dynamics in the canine cruciate deficiency model of osteoarthritis. *J Rheumatol*, 26(12):2645-53.

Nam, EK; Makhsous, M; Koh, J; Bowen, M; Nuber, G and Zhang, LQ. (2004). Biomechanical and histological evaluation of osteochondral transplantation in a rabbit model. *Am J Sports Med*, 32(2):308-16.

Newberry, WN; Garcia, JJ; Mackenzie, CD; Decamp, CE and Haut, RC. (1998). Analysis of acute mechanical insult in an animal model of post-traumatic osteoarthrosis. *J Biomech Eng*, 120(6):704-9.

Newberry, WN; Zukosky, DK and Haut, RC. (1997). Subfracture insult to a knee joint causes alterations in the bone and in the functional stiffness of overlying cartilage. *J Orthop Res*, 15(3):450-5.

Oegema, TR, Jr.; Lewis, JL and Thompson, RC, Jr. (1993). Role of acute trauma in development of osteoarthritis. *Agents Actions*, 40(3-4):220-3.

Ohashi, T; Hagiwara, M; Bader, DL and Knight, MM. (2006). Intracellular mechanics and mechanotransduction associated with chondrocyte deformation during pipette aspiration. *Biorheology*, 43(3-4):201-14.

Otsuki, S; Brinson, DC; Creighton, L; Kinoshita, M; Sah, RL; D'Lima, D and Lotz, M. (2008). The effect of glycosaminoglycan loss on chondrocyte viability: a study on porcine cartilage explants. *Arthritis Rheum*, 58(4):1076-85.

Pascual Garrido, C; Hakimiyan, AA; Rappoport, L; Oegema, TR; Wimmer, MA and Chubinskaya, S. (2009). Anti-apoptotic treatments prevent cartilage degradation after acute trauma to human ankle cartilage. *Osteoarthritis Cartilage*, 17(9):1244-51.

Pelletier, J; Jovanovic, D; Fernandes, JC; Manning, P; Connor, JR; Currie, MG and Martel-Pelletier, J. (1999). Reduction in the structural changes of experimental osteoarthritis by a nitric oxide inhibitor. *Osteoarthritis Cartilage*, 7(4):416-8.

Pelletier, JP; Jovanovic, D; Fernandes, JC; Manning, P; Connor, JR; Currie, MG; Di Battista, JA and Martel-Pelletier, J. (1998). Reduced progression of experimental osteoarthritis in vivo by selective inhibition of inducible nitric oxide synthase. *Arthritis Rheum*, 41(7):1275-86.

Pelletier, JP; Jovanovic, DV; Lascau-Coman, V; Fernandes, JC; Manning, PT; Connor, JR; Currie, MG and Martel-Pelletier, J. (2000a). Selective inhibition of inducible nitric oxide synthase reduces progression of experimental osteoarthritis in vivo: possible link with the reduction in chondrocyte apoptosis and caspase 3 level. *Arthritis Rheum*, 43(6):1290-9.

Pelletier, JP; Lajeunesse, D; Jovanovic, DV; Lascau-Coman, V; Jolicoeur, FC; Hilal, G; Fernandes, JC and Martel-Pelletier, J. (2000b). Carprofen simultaneously reduces progression of morphological changes in cartilage and subchondral bone in experimental dog osteoarthritis. *J Rheumatol*, 27(12):2893-902.

Pelletier, JP and Martel-Pelletier, J. (2007). DMOAD developments: present and future. *Bull NYU Hosp Jt Dis*, 65(3):242-8.

Perl, M; Gebhard, F; Knoferl, MW; Bachem, M; Gross, HJ; Kinzl, L and Strecker, W. (2003). The pattern of preformed cytokines in tissues frequently affected by blunt trauma. *Shock*, 19(4):299-304.

Phillips, DM and Haut, RC. (2004). The use of a non-ionic surfactant (P188) to save chondrocytes from necrosis following impact loading of chondral explants. *J Orthop Res*, 22(5):1135-42.

Reichenbach, S; Rutjes, AW; Nuesch, E; Trelle, S and Juni, P. (2010). Joint lavage for osteoarthritis of the knee. *Cochrane Database Syst Rev*, 12(5):CD007320.

Repo, RU and Finlay, JB. (1977). Survival of articular cartilage after controlled impact. *J Bone Joint Surg Am*, 59(8):1068-76.

Roos, H; Adalberth, T; Dahlberg, L and Lohmander, LS. (1995). Osteoarthritis of the knee after injury to the anterior cruciate ligament or meniscus: the influence of time and age. *Osteoarthritis Cartilage*, 3(4):261-7.

Rundell, SA; Baars, DC; Phillips, DM and Haut, RC. (2005). The limitation of acute necrosis in retro-patellar cartilage after a severe blunt impact to the in vivo rabbit patello-femoral joint. *J Orthop Res*, 23(6):1363-9.

Ryan, JA; Eisner, EA; DuRaine, G; You, Z and Reddi, AH. (2009). Mechanical compression of articular cartilage induces chondrocyte proliferation and inhibits proteoglycan synthesis by activation of the ERK pathway: implications for tissue engineering and regenerative medicine. *J Tissue Eng Regen Med*, 3(2):107-16.

Sanchez, M; Anitua, E; Orive, G; Mujika, I and Andia, I. (2009). Platelet-rich therapies in the treatment of orthopaedic sport injuries. *Sports Med*, 39(5):345-54.

Sandell, LJ and Aigner, T. (2001). Articular cartilage and changes in arthritis. An introduction: cell biology of osteoarthritis. *Arthritis Res*, 3(2):107-13.

Saw, KY; Anz, A; Merican, S; Tay, YG; Ragavanaidu, K; Jee, CS and McGuire, DA. (2011). Articular cartilage regeneration with autologous peripheral blood progenitor cells and hyaluronic acid after arthroscopic subchondral drilling: a report of 5 cases with histology. *Arthroscopy*, 27(4):493-506.

Saw, KY; Hussin, P; Loke, SC; Azam, M; Chen, HC; Tay, YG; Low, S; Wallin, KL and Ragavanaidu, K. (2009). Articular cartilage regeneration with autologous marrow aspirate and hyaluronic Acid: an experimental study in a goat model. *Arthroscopy*, 25(12):1391-400.

Serbest, G; Horwitz, J; Jost, M and Barbee, K. (2006). Mechanisms of cell death and neuroprotection by poloxamer 188 after mechanical trauma. *FASEB J*, 20(2):308-10.

Shasha, N; Krywulak, S; Backstein, D; Pressman, A and Gross, AE. (2003). Long-term follow-up of fresh tibial osteochondral allografts for failed tibial plateau fractures. *J Bone Joint Surg Am*, 85-A Suppl 2(33-9.

Silyn-Roberts, H and Broom, ND. (1990). Fracture behavior of cartilage-on-bone in response to repeated impact loading. *Connect Tissue Res*, 24(2):143-56.

Simon, WH; Richardson, S; Herman, W; Parsons, JR and Lane, J. (1976). Long-term effects of chondrocyte death on rabbit articular cartilage in vivo. *J Bone Joint Surg Am*, 58(4):517-26.

Situnayake, RD; Crump, BJ; Thurnham, DI and Taylor, CM. (1991a). Further evidence of lipid peroxidation in post-enteropathic haemolytic-uraemic syndrome. *Pediatr Nephrol*, 5(4):387-92.

Situnayake, RD; Thurnham, DI; Kootathep, S; Chirico, S; Lunec, J; Davis, M and McConkey, B. (1991b). Chain breaking antioxidant status in rheumatoid arthritis: clinical and laboratory correlates. *Ann Rheum Dis*, 50(2):81-6.

Smith, GN, Jr.; Myers, SL; Brandt, KD; Mickler, EA and Albrecht, ME. (1999). Diacerhein treatment reduces the severity of osteoarthritis in the canine cruciate-deficiency model of osteoarthritis. *Arthritis Rheum*, 42(3):545-54.

Spreng, D; Sigrist, N; Schweighauser, A; Busato, A and Schawalder, P. (2001). Endogenous nitric oxide production in canine osteoarthritis: Detection in urine, serum, and synovial fluid specimens. *Vet Surg*, 30(2):191-9.

Thompson, RC, Jr. (1975). An experimental study of surface injury to articular cartilage and enzyme responses within the joint. *Clin Orthop Relat Res*, 107):239-48.

Thompson, RC, Jr.; Oegema, TR, Jr.; Lewis, JL and Wallace, L. (1991). Osteoarthrotic changes after acute transarticular load. An animal model. *J Bone Joint Surg Am*, 73(7):990-1001.

Torzilli, PA; Grigiene, R; Borrelli, J, Jr. and Helfet, DL. (1999). Effect of impact load on articular cartilage: cell metabolism and viability, and matrix water content. *J Biomech Eng*, 121(5):433-41.

Vener, MJ; Thompson, RC, Jr.; Lewis, JL and Oegema, TR, Jr. (1992). Subchondral damage after acute transarticular loading: an in vitro model of joint injury. *J Orthop Res*, 10(6):759-65.

Von Keudell, A; Atzwanger, J; Forstner, R; Resch, H; Hoffelner, T and Mayer, M. (2011). Radiological evaluation of cartilage after microfracture treatment: A long-term follow-up study. *Eur J Radiol*,

Wei, F and Haut, RC. (2009). High levels of glucosamine-chondroitin sulfate can alter the cyclic preload and acute overload responses of chondral explants. *J Orthop Res*, 27(3):353-9.

Zafarullah, M; Li, WQ; Sylvester, J and Ahmad, M. (2003). Molecular mechanisms of N-acetylcysteine actions. *Cell Mol Life Sci*, 60(1):6-20.

Zhang, H; Vrahas, MS; Baratta, RV and Rosler, DM. (1999). Damage to rabbit femoral articular cartilage following direct impacts of uniform stresses: an in vitro study. *Clin Biomech (Bristol, Avon)*, 14(8):543-8.

Part 4

Genetics

11

The Genetics of Osteoarthritis

Antonio Miranda-Duarte
Genetics Department, National Rehabilitation Institute, Mexico City, Mexico

1. Introduction

Complex or common diseases are those which are common in the population-at-large, are responsible for the majority of morbidity and mortality, and substantially affect individuals and society health-care costs. As such, they are responsible for the greatest burden to society and to the population. It is widely accepted that all complex diseases possess a genetic component that, in addition, plays a role in their pathogenesis. Therefore, clarification of their genetic determinants will lead to a better understanding of the causes and it will be possible to develop tools to identify persons who are at risk in families and in the population in general (Schork, 1997).

Osteoarthritis (OA) is a complex disease with multiple environmental and genetic factors contributing to its pathogenesis (Felson, 2004; Peach et al., 2005). It is strongly age-related, rare prior to the age of 40 years, but importantly increasing in frequency later; in fact, it is estimated that approximately up to 80% of people aged > 65 years exhibit radiographic evidence of OA (Oddis, 1996). OA has been classified into two classes: primary OA, which is the late-onset form and that has no obvious causes, and secondary OA, which has a clearly identifiable cause comprising a developmental abnormality or a major environmental effect (Altman, 1995). It has long been suggested that OA is inherited. The clinical studies by Stecher (1941) on Heberden's nodes, a common manifestation of OA and by Kellgren et al. (1963) on generalized OA suggested that specific forms of common OA clusters in families.

Due to its nature, primary OA is the target of studies on the genetic factors associated with its development and, as in other complex diseases, different strategies have been employed to investigate this genetic contribution. This chapter will be centered on familial aggregation studies, twin studies, and association studies on candidate genes. Other strategies, such as linkage analysis and Genome-wide association studies (GWAS), will be contemplated elsewhere.

2. Familial aggregation

2.1 Sibling risk studies

A genetic component for a disease may be suspected if there is clustering in families. Sibling risk studies may be useful to clarify this search if the frequency of disease in the siblings of affected probands is higher than that in general population; if so, the disease probably has a genetic component and the susceptibility genes probably are segregated in the proband's family. Nevertheless, the disease may afflict several family members because several predisposing environmental factors also share a greater frequency in the proband's family and this could also result in higher disease concordance. To limit this possibility, researchers are required to match population controls to proband siblings as closely as possible. From sibling risk studies, a risk of recurrence to a relative of an affected individual, given that these share a particular allele compared with the general population, can be calculated through a measurement termed lambda sib (λs) (Guo, 2002; Rich & Sellers, 2002).

In OA, sibling studies have been conducted that principally identify subjects who have undergone total joint replacement due to primary OA. In a study in the U.K., the prevalence of OA in siblings of probands who had undergone primary OA-related Total hip (THR) or Total knee replacement (TKR) surgery was compared with the prevalence in a control group consisting of siblings' spouses; the latter were selected because they share a common environment to sibling group but they differ from these regarding possible genetic determinants and are representative of general population in terms of their disease susceptibility. The frequency of OA in siblings was higher compared with controls; hence, an increased risk to siblings to undergo THR (λs = 1.8), TKR (λs = 4.8), or both (combined λs = 1.98) for idiopathic end-stage OA was determined (Chitnavis et al., 1997). A similar study also carried out in the U.K. recruited probands who had experienced THR, compared the frequency of hip OA between their siblings to that of unrelated matched controls who had undergone intravenous urography and in whom a pelvic x-ray was obtained to document OA. As in the previous study, the frequency of hip OA was greater in siblings, indicating an increased risk for developing definite and severe hip OA (λs = 5.0 and 9.8, respectively). When stratification by gender was performed, the increased risk was maintained; however, this was greater for THR in males than in females (λs 14.4 and 7.7, respectively) (Lanyon et al., 2000). Another sibling study, conducted by the same research group, analized the genetic contribution to knee OA including siblings of probands with TKR. Siblings were assessed for radiographic knee OA of all knee compartments and were compared with subjects from the general population, finding an increasing risk for tibiofemoral and patellofemoral OA (λs = 2.9 and 1.7, respectively), which was maintained after stratification by gender (Neame et al., 2004).

As mentioned previously, sibling studies require a control group whose participants reflect as possible general population in order to compare disease frequencies and to deduce a Relative risk through λs. Another related design, denominated sib pair study, does not employ a control group and only siblings of probands are recruited and compared among themselves to determine whether siblings or other close relatives tend to express the same disease phenotype or similar values of a quantitative trait. From these studies, it is possible to estimate a risk calculated by means of Odds ratios (ORs), and heritability (h^2), which is the proportion of the population variance in the trait that is attributable to the segregation of a gene or genes and whose values are between 0 and 1; the greater the h^2, the more significant the genetic component. However, due to their methodological differences with those of sibling risk studies and that measurement of familial aggregation as ORs does not yield the risk of recurrence, these results are not comparable with those of sibling risk studies. They do, however, contribute substantially to the study of genetic determinants in OA.

The GARP study (Genetics, Arthrosis, and Progression) was conducted in The Netherlands and was designed to identify determinants of OA susceptibility and progression. For this, the study recruited Caucasian probands and their siblings of Dutch ancestry with symptomatic OA at multiple sites. To analyze whether there is some familial aggregation of OA at specific joint sites, such as hands, knees, and hips, and at combination of joint sites, the control population comprised probands and their siblings with OA but not at the specific disease site. ORs were calculated to estimate possible risks. After adjustment of ORs for age, gender, and Body mass index (BMI), siblings were affected in an increased manner at the same joint sites as the proband in OA of the hand (OR 4.4) and hip (OR 3.9); OA of the knee showed no increased risk (OR 1.0). When different joint-site combinations were analyzed, hand-hip demonstrated the most increased risk (OR 4.7) (Riyazi et al., 2008). Later, the same group analyzed familial aggregation of radiologic progression of OA at multiple joint sites in a longitudinal study from the GARP cohort. To assess radiologic progression, x-rays were graded on a scale of 0 - 3 for Joint space narrowing (JSN) and osteophytes including all hand, hip, and knee joints to obtain a total score. Radiologic progression of OA was defined as a 1-point score increase in total scores of JSN or osteophytes on x-rays obtained at baseline and after 2 years. ORs adjusted for age, gender, and the BMI, of a sibling having radiologic progression if the proband had progression were 3.0 for JSN progression and 1.5 for osteophyte progression. A dose-response relationship was found between the amount of increase in JSN total scores among probands and the progression of JSN in siblings (Botha-Scheepers et al., 2007).

Some other studies have analyzed the genetic contribution in characteristics associated with OA development through a sib pair design. In a sib pair study designed to assess whether the h^2 of knee structural components is independent of radiologic OA, 115 siblings of patients who had had a TKR were recruited. Muscle strength of lower limbs was measured, x-rays of the knees were obtained to assess JSN and osteophytes, and Magnetic resonance imaging (MRI) of the knee to determine cartilage volume was carried out. Lower limb muscle strength showed a high h^2 (42%); nonetheless, this was higher for medial tibial, for lateral tibial, and for patellar cartilage volume (h^2 = 65, 77, and 84%, respectively). For radiographic OA, h^2 was 61% for presence and 61% for severity (Zhai et al., 2004). Later, to search for longitudinal changes, this same sib pair cohort was followed for 2.4 years. Successful follow-up was achieved in 95 sibling pairs, and a higher h^2 was observed for changes in medial and lateral cartilage (73 and 43%, respectively), muscular strength (64%), and for progression of medial and lateral chondral defects, (90 and 80%, respectively) (Zahi et al., 2005).

2.2 Population-based family studies

Designs that involve family- and population-based sampling allow for the investigation of both genes and environment, separately or together, and permit valid inference to the population. These designs can be utilized for determining familial risks and to understand the nature of the transmittal of the OA genetic component better.

In an interesting study developed in Iceland to assess the genetic contribution to hip OA leading to THR, a population-wide study was conducted. The researchers used information obtained from a national registry of patients who underwent THR, as well as data from an Icelandic genealogy data base that includes the entire current population and the majority of their ancestors back to the IX century. With these resources, numerous large family clusters from 2,713 patients with THR for OA were identified. In order to assess whether these familial clusters were significantly different from what could be expected, matched control sets were generated utilizing the national genealogy database; subsequently, the following tests were performed to assess the genetic contribution: determination of the degree of familial clustering of OA in patients with THR; estimation of the minimum number of founders who could account for the genealogy of these patients and comparison of this with the average number of founders for their controls; determination of the overall degree of relatedness among Icelandic controls, and an estimate of RR. This analysis demonstrated that the cases were more related to each other than would be expected if no genetic component predisposing to OA were segregated in these, and supports the existence of a significant genetic component in familial aggregation of hip OA in Iceland. On the other hand, the siblings of these patients were found to be three times more likely to require THR than were controls. (Ingvarsson et al., 2000).

To evaluate whether OA is inherited and to investigate the most likely transmission pattern, a segregation analysis was performed taking data from the Framingham Study. This study was not designed to analyze OA, but rather to evaluate risk factors for heart disease; the study cohort was assembled in 1948 as a random sample of adults. Segregation analysis was performed in 337 families with radiographic OA on hand and knee and included both parents and at least one of their adult children. An OA count was generated, adding up the number of joints affected and creating standardized residuals that were used to obtain correlations in pairs drawn from each family. There was little correlation between pairs of spouses; however, correlations between parents and offspring (r = 0.115) or between siblings (r = 0.306) were higher. Remarkably, mother-daughter and mother-son correlations were 0.206 and 0.158, respectively, whereas father-daughter and father-son correlations were 0.084 and 0.007, respectively, suggesting that mothers are more likely to transmit OA to their offspring than are fathers. The analysis also revealed a significant genetic component of the disease and suggested that this component may involve a major recessive locus (Felson et al., 1998). These results showed a greater female h^2 for OA.

A cohort of families drawn from the Baltimore Longitudinal Study of Ageing was obtained to assess OA changes in order to determine the familial aggregation of OA; as in the previous study, this was not designed for analysis of OA. X-rays of hands and knees were obtained and identified 167 nuclear families with hand, 157 with knee, and 148 with hand and knee radiographic data. The outcome variable was OA defined as presence/absence of disease or as severity, taking into account the number of joints affected or the sum of all joints of a given site. When data were analyzed as presence or absence, no significant sib-sib correlations were observed; however, in terms of OA severity, significant correlations were found for Distal interphalangeal (DIP)- and Proximal phalangeal (PIP)-joint OA, and for OA affecting two or three hands sites (r = 0.81, 0.45, and 0.33, respectively). For OA of the knee, no significant correlation was found (r = 0.33); however, as the authors themselves stated, this finding could be due to underestimating of the number of cases of knee OA. The results from this cohort demonstrate familial aggregation of OA and suggest that genes could play a more significant role in severity than in occurrence (Hirsch et al., 1998). This, however, does not exclude a role for environmental influences because the authors did not look for putative environmental factors, as frequently occurs in large-scale studies in which control or ascertainment of all variables is difficult.

As part of the Rotterdam Study, which is a prospective population- based, follow-up study of the determinants and prognosis of chronic diseases in the elderly, a random sample of 1,583 individuals was calculated to estimate the genetic influence on the occurrence of radiographic OA in knees, hips, and hands. From the random sample, 118 probands with multiple-affected joint sites and their 257 siblings were identified, and OA frequency between these and the remainder of study participants was compared. Hand OA was found to be more common in proband siblings, knee OA was no more common in probands, and hip OA was even less common than that in the random sample. The h^2 for a score that summed the number of joints affected was 78%. For individual joint sites, the h^2 of OA of the hand was 56%; however, OA of the knee was not significantly correlated (h^2 = 7%). These data suggest that there is a strong genetic effect for hand, but not for knee or hip OA (Bijkerk et al., 1999). These findings do not support the results of other studies in which a greater contribution for hip and knee OA was demonstrated.

3. Twin studies

Familial aggregation does not result exclusively from genetic factors and may reflect an environmental exposure shared by family members. An alternative method for assessing the actual genetic contribution to a condition, in this case OA, is the use of classic twin studies, which enable researchers to quantify the environmental and genetic factors that contribute to a trait or disease. In these studies each member of a twin pair are evaluated with respect to the presence or absence of a disease or trait and the disease concordance rates are compared in Monozygotic (MZ) and Dizygotic (DZ) twin pairs. While higher concordance in MZ than in DZ twin pairs suggests that a significant part of familial aggregation is due to genetic factors and to equal rates of concordance or to the presence of an MZ twin concordance, <100% emphasizes the importance of environmental factors. From these concordance rates, it is possible to estimate the h^2 of the trait (Hawkes, 1997; Risch & Sellers, 2002).

The first large-scale OA twin study was published in 1996 on 130 MZ and 120 DZ female twin pairs in whom radiographic examination of hand and knee were carried out. MZ twins exhibited a higher intra-class correlation compared with DZ twins for several clinical and radiographic features of OA. The concordance rate in MZ twins was 64% compared with 38% in DZ pairs, and the h^2 ranged between 39 and 65%. Incomplete concordance in MZ pairs clearly showed an environmental component of disease expression; however, these authors demonstrate an important genetic contribution to primary OA (Spector et al., 1996). The same research group performed another twin study, but on this occasion they focused on radiographic hip OA. Concordance for JSN was higher in MZ than in DZ twin pairs (43 and 21%, respectively), as well as for other radiographic characteristics, and h^2 was ~60% (MacGregor et al., 2000). Later, this research group searched for genetic influences, but at different skeletal sites. They observed a strong genetic correlation in OA of the hand (h^2 = 53–68%) but not of hip or knee. This suggests that OA is unlikely to be explained by a single, common genetic mechanism, and it is possible that the genetic factors that contribute to OA are specific to individual joint sites (MacGregor, et al., 2009).

Different from these previously mentioned studies, a twin study from Finland included both genders with a large proportion of male pairs. This was a questionnaire-based twin study, and OA at any joint group was employed as the disease criterion. Concordance was higher in female MZ twin pairs compared with that of DZ female twin pairs, and an h^2 of 44% was obtained. However, in male twin pairs, concordance in MZ was of 34% and in DZ, this was 38%; therefore, no genetic component in the disease in males was detected. These results suggest that genes do not play a significant role in OA in males (Kaprio et al., 1996).

These twin studies have focused on hand, knee, and hip OA, each reporting a significant h^2 whose values vary among different joint groups; this could comprise evidence for differences in genetic susceptibilities at these sites; nevertheless, this remains unclear. On the other hand, it appears apparent that MZ twin concordance does not reach 100%, suggesting an important role for primary OA-associated environmental factors.

As in sibling studies, some twin studies have been employed to analyze disease progression and certain characteristics related with OA. To analyze genetic influences on OA progression, the T. Spector group designed a longitudinal twin study that included 114 MZ and 195 DZ female twin pairs in whom radiographic OA of the knees was documented during a 7.2-year follow-up time. Progression of osteophyte and JSN were assessed and the researchers observed that concordance for both radiographic characteristics were greater in MZ than in DZ pairs, with 69 and 38% for osteophyte, respectively, and 73 and 53% in JSN, respectively. The h^2 estimates were 69 and 80% for medial osteophyte and JSN, respectively, demonstrating a significant genetic influence in progression of OA of the knee (Zahi et al., 2007). To assess the genetic contribution of cartilage volume, 31 MZ and 37 DZ twin pairs, all females, were evaluated through MRI of the knees. Concordance was always higher in MZ than that of DZ twins, and estimated h^2 was 61 for femoral, 76 for tibial, for patella, 66, and total cartilage volume, 73% (Hunter et al., 2003). These results indicate the importance of genetic factors in determining cartilage volume.

4. Association studies

A case-control study is a useful method to determine whether there is an association between an exposure-of-interest, in this case, a candidate gene or a genetic marker, and a disease. Association tests determine whether a specific allele of a genetic marker is found with increased frequency in cases compared with the frequency of this marker in controls. If an association is found between the disease and the particular allele, this may suggest a causal relationship. Strength-of-association is quantified by the Odds ratio (OR); this signifies the odds of exposure to any given disease relative to the odds of exposure given to no disease. If a study yields an OR of 1.0, the odds of exposure are the same between cases and controls, implying no association. If the OR are >1, the event is more likely to happen than not, and if the OR is <1, the event is less likely to happen than not (Caporaso, 1999; Risch & Sellers, 2002).

The above mentioned segregation and twin pair studies have highlighted the fact that primary OA possesses a major genetic component. Association studies, through a case-control design, have been useful to investigate the relationship between candidate genes and OA. Even if, after a linkage analysis or a GWAS has encountered a probably relationship with a gene or a genetic marker, case-control studies are employed to replicate these findings. Several genes with different functions have been tested for an association, and Valdes & Spector (2009a) have categorized these genes in different molecular pathways or types of molecules as follows: inflammation; Extracellular matrix (ECM) molecules; Wnt signaling; Bone morphogenetic proteins (BMPs); proteases or their inhibitors, and genes related with modulation of osteocyte or chondrocyte differentiation (Table 1).

Gene	Name	Association Positive Trait	OR	Author	Negative Author
Inflammation					
CCL2	Chemokine (C-C motif) ligand 2	Knee	2,2	Park, 2007	
COX2 (PTGS2)	Cyclooxygenase 2 (Prostaglandin G/H Synthase2)	Knee	0,7	Valdes, 2004	Valdes, 2006
			1,5*	Valdes, 2006	
			1,5	Valdes, 2008	
			0,6	Schnider, 2010	
IL-1 gene cluster	Intrleukin 1-α, β, interleukin receptor antagonist (IL1RN)	Hand	1,6	Solovieva, 2009	Moxley, 2010
		Hip	2,4	Meulenbelt, 2004	Sezguin, 2007
			0,7	Jotanovic, 2011	
		Knee	0,1	Attur, 2010	
IL-6	Interleukin-6	Hand	4,7	Kämäräinen, 2008	Valdes, 2010
		Hip	0,4	Pola, 2005	
IL-10	Interleukin-10	Knee	4	Fytili, 2005a	Riyazi, 2005
HLA	Human leukocyte antigen system	Hand	2,4	Riyazi, 2003	Shi, 2010
		Knee	1,3	Nakajima, 2010	
		Knee/Hip	1,6	Moos, 2002	
Extracelular matrix molecules					
ASPN	Asporin	Knee/hip	2,4	Kizawa, 2005	Mustafa, 2005
			1,9	Jiang, 2006	Rodriguez-Lopez, 2006
			1,5	Nakamura, 2007	Kaliakatsos, 2006
COL2A1	Collagen type II α-1	Generalized	5,3	Meulenbelt, 1999	Baldwin, 2002
		Hand	1,6	Hämäläinen, 2008	Aersens, 1998
		Knee	2,1	Uitterlinden, 2000	
			4,1	Galves-Rosas, 2010	
		Knee/Hip	1,3	Ikeda, 2002	
COMP	Cartilage oligomeric matrix protein	Knee/Hip	1.5*	Valdes, 2007	Mabuchi, 2001
CILP	Cartilage intermediate layer protein	Knee	0.4*	Valdes, 2006	
MATN3	Matrilin-3	Hand	2,6	Steffanson, 2003	Pullig, 2007
			2	Min, 2006	
			4,3	Pullig, 2007	
Wnt signaling pathway					
CALM1	Calmodulin 1	Hip	2,4	Mototani, 2005	Shi, 2008b
				Mototani, 2010	Poulou, 2008
					Valdes, 2007
					Loughlin,2006
FRZB	Frizzled related protein 3	Generalized	1,4	Min, 2005	Kerkhof, 2008
		Knee	2,9	Valdes, 2007	Evangelou, 2009
			2	Ródriguez-López, 2007	
		Hip	4,1**	Loughlin, 2004	
			3,2	Lane, 2006	
LRP5	Low density lipoprotein receptor-related protein 5	Knee	1,6	Smith, 2005	Kerkhof, 2008

Gene	Name	Association Positive Trait	OR	Author	Negative Author
Bone morphogenetic proteins					
BMP2	Bone morphogenetic protein 2	Knee	1,7 1,3**	Valdes, 2004 Valdes 2006	
BMP5	Bone morphogenetic protein 5	Hip	0.007¤ 0.018	Southam, 2004 Wilkins, 2009	
GDF5	Growth differentiation factor 5	Hip Hip/Knee Knee Hand/Hip/Knee	1,8 1,3 1,2 1,3 1,1	Miyamoto, 2007 Southam, 2007 Chapman, 2008 Valdes, 2009b Evangelou, 2009	Tsezou, 2008
Protease/protease inhibitors					
AACT	Alpha-1-antichymotrypsin	Knee	0,7**	Valdes, 2006	
ADAM12	A desintegrin and metalloproteinase domain 12	Knee	7,1** 2,5* 1,9 3,5	Valdes, 2006 Valdes, 2004 Kerna, 2009	Limer, 2008 Rodriguez-Lopez 2009
ADAMTS14	ADAM with trombospondin motif	Knee	1,4**	Rodríguez-López 2009	
MMPs	Matrix metalloproteinase	Knee	0.001¤	Barlas, 2009	
TNA	Tetranectin	Knee	1,5** 1,4*	Valdes, 2006	
Modulation of osteocyte or chondrocyte differentiation					
ESR1	Estrogen receptor α	Knee Hip	1,4 1,03 3,6** 0,5 0,7 0,8** 1,3*	Jin, 2004 Fytili, 2005b Valdes, 2006 Borgonio-Cuadra, 2011 Lian, 2007 Riancho, 2010	Wise, 2009 Loughlin, 2000b
IL-4R	Interleukin -4 receptor	Hip	2,1	Forster, 2004	
OPG	Osteoprotegerin	Knee	0,5**	Valdes, 2006	
VDR	Vitamin D receptor	Hand Knee	1,9 2,3 2,8 1,9*	Solovieva, 2006 Uitterlinden, 1997 Ken, 1997 Valdes, 2006	Aerssens, 1998 Huang, 2000 Loughlin, 2000b Baldwin, 2002 Lee, 2009
Others					
CALCA	Calcitonin	Knee	0,4	Magaña, 2010	
DIO2	Iodothyronine deionidase enzyme type 2	Hip	1,8	Meulenbelt, 2008	

Gene	Name	Association Positive Trait	OR	Author	Negative Author
LRCH1	Leucine-rich repeats and calponin homology (CH) domain containing 1	Knee	1,5	Spector, 2006	Snelling, 2007
RHOB	Ras homolog gene family member B	Knee	0,3*	Shi, 2008a	Loughlin, 2007
TXNDC3	Thioredoxin domain containing 3	Knee	1,4	Shi, 2008a	Loughlin, 2007

* Males; ** Females; ¤ p value, OR not available.

Table 1. Association studies on candidate genes in osteoarthritis.

4.1 Inflammation

Classically, OA has been considered a degenerative joint disease; however, the role is currently recognized of an inflammatory process in its pathogenesis, which is reflected by several clinical signs and symptoms as swelling of affected joints and joint stiffness. Synovial membrane also exhibits inflammatory changes which in addition to cartilage damage could result in the release of antigenic determinants leading to the production of inflammatory cytokines, chemokines, and destructive enzymes, between other inflammatory components, increasing the inflammatory process and damage to the articular structure (Yuan et al., 2003). It is unclear if this is actually caused by OA or by associated/complicating crystalline (e.g., calcium pyrophosphate or hydroxapatite) arthritis.

Several kinds of interleukins have been associated with OA; however, the results have been inconclusive. Results concerning *IL1* are controversial because while some reports suggest an association, there are reports in which no association has been found (Jotanovic et al., 2011; Meulenbelt et al., 2004; Moxley et al., 2010; Sezguin, 2007; Solovieva et al., 2009). However, there is a report in which a very significant association of *IL1* with severity of OA of the knee was shown ($p < 0.0001$) (Attur et al., 2010). *IL-6* has been reported to be associated with OA (Kämäräinen et al., 2008; Pola et al., 2005); however, in a large-scale meta-analysis, there was no reproducibility of the results (Valdes et al., 2010)

Prostaglandins are well known modulators of the activities of bone cells and inflammation. The COX2 protein is encoded by the *PTGS2* gene and is expressed in meniscus, synovial membrane, and osteophyte fibrocartilage, particularly during early OA (Hardy, 2002). *PTGS2* gene polymorphisms have been associated significantly with OA of the knee (Schnider et al., 2010; Valdes et al., 2004, 2006). Interestingly, during the replication stage of a GWA, this association was confirmed, and through an expression-analysis study, the transcripts of two genes related with the synthesis of *PGE2* were abundantly expressed in chondrocytes of patients with OA, underlying its importance in the pathogenesis of the disease (Valdes et al., 2008).

The association with Human leukocyte antigen (HLA) has also been shown (Moos et al., 2002; Nakajima et al., 2010; Riyazi et al., 2003), and in a GWA, two markers mapped to DQB1 and to the butyrophilin-like 2 protein (BTNL2), which regulates T-cell activation (Nguyen et al., 2006). These findings demonstrate the importance of the HLA system in risks for OA.

4.2 Extracellular matrix molecules

The alterations in osteoarthritic cartilage are numerous and involve morphologic and metabolic changes in chondrocytes, as well as biochemical and structural alterations in ECM macromolecules. A hallmark of OA is the degradation of ECM (Malemud et al., 1987; Martel-Pelletier et al., 2008); therefore, genes encoding its molecules have become strong candidates for association studies.

Of the structural genes, *COL2A1* has received the most attention because it encodes type II collagen, which is the most abundant protein of articular cartilage and because has been implicated in several osteochondrodysplasias that develop early OA. Several studies have demonstrated an association of *COL2A1* gene polymorphisms (Galves-Rosas et al., 2010; Hämäläinen et al., 2008; Ikeda et al., 2002; Meulenbelt et al., 1999; Uitterlinden et al., 2000); however, some other studies have not found such an association (Aersens et al., 1998; Baldwin et al., 2002).

One gene that exhibited interesting results is Asporin (*ASPN*). Asporin is an ECM protein member of the small leucine-rich proteoglycan subfamily of proteins that binds to Transforming growth factor-β (TGF-β), a key growth factor in cartilage metabolism, and to collagen and agrecan. The *ASPN* gene contains a polymorphic aspartic acid (D) repeat in its N-terminal region, and its mRNA is expressed abundantly in osteoarthritic articular cartilage (Henry et al., 2001; Lorenzo et al., 2001, Lorenzo, 2004). Kizawa et al. (2005) observed that *ASPN* containing 14 aspartic acid repeats (D14) was significantly associated with OA of the knee. Other length variants were identified, the most common being D13 repeats. The authors generated cell lines from a murine chondrogenesis model expressing different *ASPN* alleles, and they found that cells containing the D14 allele result in greater inhibition of AGC1 and COL2A1 than cells containing other alleles. Additionally, *in vitro* binding assays showed a direct interaction between *ASPN* and TGF-β, concluding that their findings demonstrate a functional link among ECM proteins, TGF-beta activity, and disease. These results were interesting; however, subsequent association studies in Caucasian populations did not support the association of D14 with OA (Kaliakatsos et al., 2006; Mustafa et al., 2005; Rodríguez-López et al., 2006). A meta-analysis including data on Asian and Caucasian individuals demonstrated that combined D14 is associated with OA (p = 0.0030; OR, 1.46); however, in the stratification analysis, a positive association between knee OA and the D14 allele (p = 0.0000013; summary OR, 1.95) was found only in Asians, suggesting that the association of *ASPN* and OA of the knee has global relevance, but that its effect possesses ethnic differences (Nakamura et al., 2007).

4.3 Wnt signaling pathway

Wnts comprise a family of glycoproteins involved in developmental processes such as embryogenesis, organogenesis, and tumor formation, as well as in cartilage and bone development and degeneration. The Wnt1 class activates the canonical Wnt signaling pathway, which involves the formation of a complex among Wnt proteins, frizzled, and LRP5/6 receptors, promoting the inhibition of β-catenin degradation and its subsequent accumulation in the nucleus, which was suggested to contribute to cartilage loss. This pathway also plays a role in the endochondral ossification that causes osteophytes (Yavropoulou & Yovos, 2007; Yuasa et al., 2008).

The association of *FRZB* with OA was analyzed after a genome-wide linkage scan mapped a hip OA susceptibility locus to 2q (Loughlin et al., 2000a). In the subsequent association analysis, a Single nucleotide polymorphism (SNP) in *FRZB* resulting in an Arg324Gly substitution at the carboxyl terminus was associated with hip OA in female probands (p = 0.04), and this was confirmed in an independent cohort of cases involved female hip OA (p = 0.04). Additionally, haplotype coding for substitutions of two highly conserved arginine residues (Arg200Trp and Arg324Gly) in *FRZB* was a strong risk factor for primary hip OA, with an OR of 4.1 (p = 0.004) (Loughlin et al., 2004). Several replication studies (Min et al., 2005; Lane et al., 2006; Rodríguez-López et al., 2007; Valdes et al., 2007) confirmed the association; however, others that were sufficiently powered failed to find any association. In a large meta-analysis, a weak association in a SNP to hip OA was found (OR = 1.12; p <0.016), but not with other OA sites (Evangelou et al., 2009).

Another gene of the Wnt signaling pathway, *LRP5*, has also been associated with OA (Smith et al., 2005), although the results were unable to be replicated in a large population-based study (Kerkhof et al., 2008).

4.4 Modulation of osteocyte or chondrocyte differentiation

Bone mass and probably rate of change in bone density are controlled to a great extent by genetic factors, and a range of regulatory and structural genes has been proposed as being involved, including Collagen 1α1 (*COL1A1*), the Estrogen receptor (*ER*), and the Vitamin D receptor (*VDR*). These genes have been studied in OA, but *VDR* has received the most attention, and first reports have shown significant associations with an increased risk in the presence of different polymorphisms (Ken et al., 1997; Uitterlinden et al., 1997; Solovieva et al., 2006; Valdes et al., 2006); however, this has not always been confirmed (Aerssens et al., 1998; Baldwin et al., 2002; Huang et al., 2000; Loughlin et al., 2000b). A meta-analysis on the most frequently studied *VDR* polymorphisms (TaqI, BsmI, and ApaI) in OA analyzed a total of 10 studies of persons of Asian or European origin involving a total of 1,591 patients with OA and 1,781 controls. Nine studies were performed on *VDR* TaqI polymorphisms, six on *VDR* BsmI polymorphisms, and 5 on *VDR* ApaI polymorphisms. The results showed no association between OA and the *VDR* TaqI T allele among all study subjects (OR, 0.841; p = 0.15). Stratification by ethnicity yielded no association between the *VDR* TaqI T allele and OA in Europeans or Asians. Moreover, no association was found between OA and *VDR* TaqI polymorphisms by meta-analysis of recessive and dominant models, and contrasts of homozygotes. And finally, no association was found between OA and *VDR* polymorphisms with respect to BsmI and ApaI polymorphisms by meta-analysis. Therefore, the authors concluded that there is no association between *VDR* gene polymorphisms and OA (Lee et al., 2009)

Several studies have tested for an association between *ESR1* gene polymorphisms and the risk of OA. Some studies reported an association for either increased or decreased risk (Borgonio-Cuadra et al, 2011; Fytili et al., 2005b; Jin et al., 2004; Lian et al., 2007; Valdes et al., 2006). A large study exploring the association of two common polymorphisms within the *ESR1* and aromatase (*CYP19A1*) genes polymorphism with severe OA included 2,176 patients with hip OA, 971 patients with knee OA, and 2,381 controls who were recruited at three centers in Spain and one in the U.K. The rs2234693 (*ESR1*) and rs1062033 (*CYP19A1*) single nucleotide polymorphisms were genotyped, and in the global analysis, both were associated with OA, but there was significant gender interaction. The GG genotype at rs1062033 was associated with an increased risk of knee OA in women (OR, 1.23; p = 0.04). The CC genotype at rs2234693 tended to be associated with reduced OA risk in women (OR,

0.76; $p = 0.028$ for knee OA and OR, 0.84; $p = 0.076$ for hip OA), but with an increased risk of hip OA in men (OR, 1.28; $p = 0.029$). The rs1062033 genotype associated with higher OA risk was also associated with reduced expression of the aromatase gene in bone. These results are consistent with the hypothesis that estrogen activity may influence the development of large-joint OA (Riancho et al., 2010).

4.5 Bone morphogenetic proteins

Bone morphogenetic proteins (BMPs) are multi-functional growth factors that belong to the TGF-β superfamily and they were first identified by their ability to induce the formation of bone and cartilage. They function as regulators of bone induction, maintenance, and repair and are critical determinants of the embryological development of mammalian organisms (van der Kraan et al., 2010).

BMP2 has been associated with OA of the knee ($p = 0.007$), particularly with JSN (Valdes et al., 2004). BMP5 was detected after a linkage analysis study; the linkage encompassed two strong candidate genes: *BMP5*, and *COL9A1*. When each marker was tested for association with a marker within intron 1 of *BMP5* was associated ($p < 0.05$) (Southam et al., 2004; Wilkins et al., 2009).

GDF5 is required for formation of bones and joints in the limbs, skull, and axial skeleton (Settle et al., 2003). This gene was shown to associate with hip OA in an Asian study, including Japanese and Chinese patients. An SNP, the rs143383, showed the strongest association ($p = 1.8 \times 10^{-13}$) (Miyamoto 2007). This SNP is located in the *GDF5* core promoter and exerts allelic differences on transcriptional activity in chondrogenic cells, with the susceptibility allele exhibiting reduced activity. These findings implicate *GDF5* as a susceptibility gene for OA and suggest that decreased *GDF5* expression is involved in its pathogenesis (Myamoto et al., 2007). This association was confirmed by other studies, and a meta-analysis employing a larger collection of European as well as Asian studies validated the association with OA. The combined association for both ethnic groups is highly significant for the allele frequency model (OR, 1.21; $p = 0.0004$). These findings represent the first highly significant evidence for a risk factor for the development of OA that affects two highly diverse ethnic groups (Chapman et al., 2008).

4.6 Proteases and their inhibitors

Increased proteolytic activity leads to degradation of ECM components such as agrecan and COL2A1, resulting in cartilage degradation. The Matrix metalloproteinases (MMPs) have been considered the main enzymes responsible for this degradation. Members of this MMP family include ADAM and ADAMTS (Nagase & Kashiwagi, 2002). A haplotype of the *ADAM12* gene polymorphism has been significantly associated with knee osteoarthritis demonstrating differences between genders, conferring a risk of up to 7-fold in women ($p < 1 \times 10^{-6}$) and 2-fold in men ($p < 0.014$) (Valdes et al., 2006). On the other hand, an *ADAM12* gene polymorphism has been associated with progression in OA of the knee, particularly with changes in Kellgren-Lawrence and osteophyte grades ($p < 0.07$ and 0.004, respectively) (Valdes et al., 2004).

4.7 Other genes

There are other genes that have shown susceptibility to OA. The *DIO2* gene encodes an intracellular enzyme in the thyroid pathway that converts thyroxin (T4) into an active thyroid hormone (T3), which in the growth plate specifically stimulates chondrocyte differentiation and induces hypertrophy of the chondrocytes, initiating terminal differentiation and formation of bone. As in other OA susceptibility genes, *DIO2* was identified by a genome-wide linkage scan, and during replication in UK, Dutch, and Japanese, an association of a common *DIO2* haplotype, exclusively containing the minor allele of rs225014 and common allele of rs12885300, was observed with a combined recessive OR of 1.79 ($p = 2.02 \times 10^{-5}$) in cases of females with advanced/symptomatic hip osteoarthritis, indicating *DIO2* as a new susceptibility gene that confers risk for osteoarthritis (Meulenbelt 2008).

5. Conclusions

The existence is clear of genetic determinants related with OA, as has been demonstrated in sibling studies, familial aggregation, and twin pair studies; however, it appears that there are differences in genetic susceptibility according to affected sites, gender, and disease stage. Association studies also show differences in site, gender, and ethnicity. To date, one of the most consistent associations is that of *GDF5;* however, it is clear that there are other genes implicated, not only with the disease prevalence, but also with disease progression. It is important to continue the search for genes implicated in development of OA in order to acquire a better understanding of its pathogenic mechanisms in order to plan prevention strategies in populations-at-risk and to design different therapeutic interventions.

6. References

Aerssens, J.; Dequeker, J.; Peeters, J.; Breemans, S. & Boonen, S. (1998). Lack of association between osteoarthritis of the hip and gene polymorphisms of VDR, COL1A1, and COL2A1 in postmenopausal women. *Arthritis Rheum*, 41, 11, 1946-1950

Altman, R.D. (1995). The classification of osteoarthritis. *J Rheumatol*, 22, (Suppl 43), 42-43

Attur, M.; Wang, H.Y.; Byers, K. V.; Bukowski, J.F.; Aziz, N.; Krasnokutsky, S.; Samuels, J.; Greenberg, J.; McDaniel, G.; Abramson, S.B.& Kornman, K.S. (2010). Radiographic severity of knee osteoarthritis is conditional on interleukin-1 receptor antagonist gene variations. *Ann Rheum Dis*, 69, 5, 856-861

Baldwin, C.T.; Cupples, L.A.; Joost, O.; Demissie, S.; Chaisson, C.; McAlindon, T.; Myers, R.H. & Felson, D. (2002). Absence of linkage or association for osteoarthritis with the vitamin D receptor/type II collagen locus: the Framingham Osteoarthritis Study. *J Rheumatol*, 29, 1, 161-165

Barlas, I.O.; Sezgin, M.; Erdal, M.E.; Sahin, G.; Ankarali, H.C.; Altintas, Z.M. & Türkmen, E (2009). Association of (-1,607) 1G/2G polymorphism of matrix metalloproteinase-1 gene with knee osteoarthritis in the Turkish population (knee osteoarthritis and MMPs gene polymorphisms). *Rheumatol Int*, 29, 4, 383-388

Bijkerk, C.; Houwing-Duistermaat, J.J.; Valkenburg, H.A.; Meulenbelt, I.; Hofman, A.; Breedveld, F.C,; Pols, H.A.; van Duijn, C.M. & Slagboom P.E. (1999). Heritabilities of radiologic osteoarthritis in peripheral joints and of disc degeneration of the spine. *Arthritis Rheum*, 42, 8, 1729-1735

Borgonio-Cuadra, V.M.; González-Huerta, C.; Duarte-Salazár, C.; Soria-Bastida M.; Cortés-González, S. & Miranda-Duarte A. (2011). Analysis of estrogen receptor alpha gene haplotype in Mexican mestizo patients with primary osteoarthritis of the knee. *Rheumatol Int*, Mar 29. [Epub ahead of print]

Botha-Scheepers, S.A.; Watt, I.; Slagboom, E.; Meulenbelt, I.; Rosendaal, F.R.; Breedveld, F.C. & Kloppenburg, M. (2007). Influence of familial factors on radiologic disease progression over two years in siblings with osteoarthritis at multiple sites: a prospective longitudinal cohort study. *Arthritis Rheum*, 57, 4, 626-632

Caporaso, N.; Rothman, N. & Wacholder, S. (1999).Case-control studies of common alleles and environmental factors. *J Natl Cancer Inst Monogr*, 26, 25-30

Chapman, K.; Takahashi, A.; Meulenbelt, I.; Watson, C.; Rodriguez-Lopez, J.; Egli, R.; Tsezou, A.; Malizos, K.N.; Kloppenburg, M.; Shi, D.; Southam, L.; van der Breggen, R.; Donn, R.; Qin, J.; Doherty, M.; Slagboom, P.E.; Wallis, G; Kamatani, N.; Jiang, Q.; Gonzalez, A.; Loughlin, J. & Ikegawa, S. (2008). A meta-analysis of European and Asian cohorts reveals a global role of a functional SNP in the 5' UTR of GDF5 with osteoarthritis susceptibility. *Hum Mol Genet*, 17, 10, 1497-1504

Chitnavis, J. ; Sinsheimer, J.S.; Clipsham, K.; Loughlin, J.; Sykes, B.; Burge, P.D. & Carr A.J. (1997). Genetic influences in end-stage osteoarthritis. Sibling risks of hip and knee replacement for idiopathic osteoarthritis. *J Bone Joint Surg Br*, 79, 4, 660-664

Evangelou, E.; Chapman, K.; Meulenbelt, I.; Karassa, F.B.; Loughlin, J.; Carr, A; Doherty, M.; Doherty, S.; Gómez-Reino, J.J.; Gonzalez, A.; Halldorsson, B.V.; Hauksson, V.B.; Hofman, A.; Hart, D.J.; Ikegawa, S.; Ingvarsson, T.; Jiang, Q.; Jonsdottir, I.; Jonsson, H.; Kerkhof, H.J.; Kloppenburg, M.; Lane, N.E.; Li, J.; Lories, R.J.; van Meurs, J.B.; Näkki, A.; Nevitt, M.C.; Rodriguez-Lopez, J.; Shi, D.; Slagboom, P.E.; Stefansson, K.; Tsezou, A.; Wallis, G.A.; Watson, C.M.; Spector, T.D.; Uitterlinden, A.G.; Valdes, A.M. & Ioannidis JP. (2009). Large-scale analysis of association between GDF5 and FRZB variants and osteoarthritis of the hip, knee, and hand. *Arthritis Rheum*, 60, 6, 1710-1721

Felson, D.T.; Couropmitree, N.N.; Chaisson, C.E.; Hannan, M.T.; Zhang, Y.; Mcalindon, T.E; LaValley, M.; Levy, D. & Myers, R.H. (1998). Evidence for a Mendelian gene in a segregation analysis of generalized radiographic osteoarthritis. *Arthritis Rheum*, 41, 6, 1064-1071

Felson, D.T. (2004). An update on the pathogenesis and epidemiology of osteoarthritis. *Radiol Clin North Am*. 42, 1, 1-9

Forster, T.; Chapman, K. & Loughlin J. (2004). Common variants within the interleukin 4 receptor alpha gene (IL4R) are associated with susceptibility to osteoarthritis. *Hum Genet*, 114, 4, 391–395

Fytili P.; Giannatou E.; Karachalios T; Malizos, K. & Tsezou, A. (2005a). Interleukin-10G and interleukin-10R microsatellite polymorphisms and osteoarthritis of the knee. *Clin Exp Rheumatol*, 23, 5, 621–627

Fytili, P.; Giannatou, E.; Papanikolaou, V.; Stripeli, F.; Karachalios, T.; Malizos, K. & Tsezou, A. (2005b). Association of repeat polymorphisms in the estrogen receptors alpha, beta, and androgen receptor genes with knee osteoarthritis. *Clin Genet*, 68, 3, 268–277

Gálvez-Rosas, A.; González-Huerta, C.; Borgonio-Cuadra, V.M.; Duarte-Salazár, C.; Lara-Alvarado, L.; de los Angeles Soria-Bastida, M.; Cortés-González, S.; Ramón-Gallegos, E. & Miranda-Duarte A (2010). A COL2A1 gene polymorphism is related with advanced stages of osteoarthritis of the knee in Mexican Mestizo population. *Rheumatol Int*, 30, 8, 1035-1039

Guo, S-W. (2002).Sibling recurrence risk ratio as a measure of genetic effect: caveat emptor! *Am J Hum Genet* .70(3):818–9.

Hämäläinen, S.; Solovieva, S.; Hirvonen, A.; Vehmas, T.; Takala, E.P.; Riihimäki, H. & Leino-Arjas P. (2009). COL2A1 gene polymorphisms and susceptibility to osteoarthritis of the hand in Finnish women. *Ann Rheum Dis,* 68, 10, 1633-1637

Hardy.; M.M.; Seibert.; K.; Manning.; P.T.; Currie.; M.G.; Woerner, B.M.; Edwards, D.; Koki, A. & Tripp. (2002). Cyclooxygenase 2-dependent prostaglandin E2 modulates cartilage proteoglycan degradation in human osteoarthritis explants. *Arthritis Rheum,* 46, 7, 1789–1803

Hawkes, C.H. (1997). Twin studies in medicine--what do they tell us? *QJM,* 90, 5, 311-321.

Henry, S.P.; Takanosu, M.; Boyd, T.C.; Mayne, P.M.; Eberspaecher, H.; Zhou, W.; de Crombrugghe, B.; Hook, M. & Mayne, R. (2001). Expression pattern and gene characterization of asporin: a newly discovered member of the leucine-rich repeat protein family. *J. Biol. Chem,* 276, 15, 12212-12221

Hirsch, R.; Lethbridge-Cejku, M.; Hanson, R.; Scott, W.W. Jr.; Reichle, R.; Plato, C.C.; Tobin, J.D. & Hochberg, M.C. (1998). Familial aggregation of osteoarthritis: data from the Baltimore longitudinal study on aging. *Arthritis Rheum,* 41, 7, 1227-1232

Huang, J.; Ushiyama, T.; Inoue, K.; Kawasaki, T. & Hukuda, S. (2000). Vitamin D receptor gene polymorphisms and osteoarthritis of the hand, hip, and knee: a case-control study in Japan. *Rheumatology,* 39, 1, 79-84

Hunter, D.J.; Snieder, H.; March, L. & Sambrook, P.N. (2003). Genetic Contribution to cartilage volume in women: a classical twin study. *Rheumatology (Oxford),* 42, 12, 1495-1500

Ikeda, T.; Mabuchi, A.; Fukuda, A.; Kawakami, A.; Ryo, Y.; Yamamoto, S.; Miyoshi, K.; Haga, N.; Hiraoka, H.; Takatori, Y.; Kawaguchi, H.; Nakamura, K. & Ikegawa, S. (2002). Association analysis of single nucleotide polymorphisms in cartilage-specific collagen genes with knee and hip osteoarthritis in the Japanese population. *J Bone Miner Res,* 17, 7, 1290–1296

Ingvarsson, T.; Stefánsson, S.E.; Hallgrímsdóttir, I.B.; Frigge, M.L.; Jónsson, H. Jr.; Gulcher, J.; Jónsson, H.; Ragnarsson, J.I.; Lohmander, L.S. & Stefánsson, K. (2000).The inheritance of hip osteoarthritis in Iceland. *Arthritis Rheum,* 43, 12, 2785-2792

Jiang, Q.; Shi, D.; Yi, L.; Ikegawa, S.; Wang, Y.; Nakamura, T.; Qiao, D.; Liu, C. & Dai, J. (2006). Replication of the association of the aspartic acid repeat polymorphism in the asporin gene with kneeosteoarthritis susceptibility in Han Chinese. *J Hum Genet,* 51, 12, 1068-1072

Jin SY.; Hong SJ.; Yang HI.; Park, S.D.; Yoo, M.C.; Lee, H.J.; Hong, M.S.; Park, H.J.; Yoon, S.H.; Kim, B.S.; Yim, S.V.; Park, H.K. & Chung, J.H. (2004). Estrogen receptor-alpha gene haplotype is associated with primary knee osteoarthritis in Korean population. *Arthritis Res Ther,* 6, 5, R415–421

Jotanovic, Z.; Etokebe, G.E.; Mihelic, R.; Heiland Kårvatn, M.; Mulac-Jericevic, B.; Tijanic, T.; Balen, S.; Sestan, B. & Dembic, Z. (2011). Hip osteoarthritis susceptibility is associated with IL1B -511(G>A) and IL1 RN (VNTR) genotypic polymorphisms in Croatian caucasian population. *J Orthop Res,* 29, 8, 1137-1144

Kaliakatsos, M.; Tzetis, M.; Kanavakis, E,: Fytili, P.; Chouliaras, G.; Karachalios, T; Malizos, K. & Tsezou, A. (2006). Asporin and knee osteoarthritis in patients of Greek origin. *Osteoarthritis Cartilage,* 14, 6, 609–611.

Kämäräinen, O.P.; Solovieva. S.; Vehmas. T.; Luoma. K.; Riihimaki. H.; Ala-Kokko. L.; Männikkö, M. & Leino-Arjas, P. (2008). Common interleukin-6 promoter variants associate with the more severe forms of distal interphalangeal osteoarthritis. *Arthritis Res Ther,* 10, 1, R21

Kaprio, J.; Kujala, U.M.; Peltonen, L. & Koskenvuo, M. (1996). Genetic liability to osteoarthritis may be greater in women than men. *BMJ,* 313, 7050, 232

Keen, R.W.; Hart, D.J.; Lanchbury, J.S. & Spector, T.D. (1997). Association of early osteoarthritis of the knee with a Taq I polymorphism of the vitamin D receptor gene. *Arthritis Rheum,* 40, 8, 1444-1449

Kellgren, J.H.; Lawrence, R.S. & Bier, F. (1963). Genetic factors in generalized osteoarthritis. *Ann Rheum Dis.* 22, 237-255.

Kerkhof, J.M.; Uitterlinden, A.G.; Valdes, A.M.; Hart, D.J.; Rivadeneira, F.; Jhamai, M.; Hofman, A.; Pols, H.A.; Bierma-Zeinstra, S.M.; Spector, T.D. & van Meurs, J.B. (2008). Radiographic osteoarthritis at three joint sites and FRZB, LRP5, and LRP6 polymorphisms in two population-based cohorts. *Osteoarthr Cartilage,* 16, 10, 1141-1149

Kerna, I.; Kisand, K.; Tamm, A.E.; Lintrop, M.; Veske, K. & Tamm, A.O. (2009). Missense single nucleotide polymorphism of the ADAM12 gene is associated with radiographic knee osteoarthritis in middle-aged Estonian cohort. *Osteoarthritis Cartilage,* 17, 8, 1093-1098

Kizawa, H.; Kou, I.; Iida, A.; Sudo, A; Miyamoto, Y.; Fukuda, A.; Mabuchi, A; Kotani, A.; Kawakami, A.; Yamamoto, S; Uchida, A.; Nakamura, K.; Notoya, K.; Nakamura, Y. & Ikegawa, S. (2005) An aspartic acid repeat polymorphism in asporin inhibits chondrogenesis and increases susceptibility to osteoarthritis. *Nat Genet,*37, 2, 138–144

Lane, N.E.; Lian. K.; Nevitt. M.C.; Zmuda, J.M; Lui, L.; Li, J.; Wang, J.; Fontecha, M.; Umblas, N.; Rosenbach, M.; de Leon, P. & Corr, M. (2006). Frizzled-related protein variants are risk factors for hip osteoarthritis. *Arthritis Rheum,* 54, 4, 1246–1254

Lanyon, P.; Muir, K.; Doherty, S. & Doherty, M. (2000). Assessment of a genetic contribution to osteoarthritis of the hip: sibling study. *BMJ,* 321, 7270, 1179–1183

Lee, Y.H.; Woo, J.H.; Choi, S.J.; Ji, J.D. & Song, G.G. (2010) Vitamin D receptor TaqI, BsmI and ApaI polymorphisms and osteoarthritis susceptibility: A meta-analysis. *Joint Bone Spine,* 76, 2, 156-161

Lian, K.; Lui, L.; Zmuda, J.M.; Nevitt, M.C.; Hochberg, M.C.; Lee, J,M.; Li, J. & Lane, N.E. (2007). Estrogen receptor alpha genotype is associated with a reduced prevalence of radiographic hip osteoarthritis in elderly Caucasian women. *Osteoarthritis Cartilage,* 15, 8, 972-978

Limer, K.L.; Tosh, K.; Bujac, S.R.; McConnell, R.; Doherty, S.; Nyberg, F.; Zhang, W.; Doherty, M.; Muir, K.R. & Maciewicz, R.A. (2008). Attempt to replicate published genetic associations in a large, well-defined osteoarthritis case-control population (the GOAL study). *Osteoarthritis Cartilage,* 17, 6, 782-789

Lorenzo, P.; Bayliss, M.T. & Heinegård, D. (2004). Altered patterns and synthesis of extracellular matrix macromolecules in early osteoarthritis. *Matrix Biol,* 23, 6, 381-391

Lorenzo, P.; Aspberg, A.; Onnerfjord, P.; Bayliss, M.T.; Neame, P.J. & Heinegard, D. (2001). Identification and characterization of asporin: a novel member of the leucine-rich repeat protein family closely related to decorin and biglycan. *J Biol Chem,* 276, 15, 12201-12211

Loughlin, J.; Dowling, B.; Chapman, K.; Marcelline, L; Mustafa, Z.; Southam, L; Ferreira, A; Ciesielski, C.; Carson, D.A. & Corr, M. (2004). Functional variants within the secreted frizzledrelated protein 3 gene are associated with hip osteoarthritis in females. *Proc Natl Acad Sci USA,* 101, 26, 9757–9762

Loughlin, J.; Meulenbelt, I.; Min, J.; Mustafa, Z; Sinsheimer, J.S.; Carr, A. & Slagboom, P.E. (2007). Genetic association analysis of RHOB and TXNDC3 in osteoarthritis. *Am J Hum Genet,* 80, 2, 383–386

Loughlin, J.; Mustafa, Z.; Smith, A.; Irven, C.; Carr, A.J.; Clipsham, K.; Chitnavis, J.; Bloomfield, V.A.; McCartney, M.; Cox, O.; Sinsheimer, J.S.; Sykes, B. & Chapman, K.E. (2000a). Linkage analysis of chromosome 2q in osteoarthritis. *Rheumatology,* 39, 4, 377-381

Loughlin, J.; Sinsheimer, J.S.; Carr, A. & Chapman, K. (2006). The CALM1 core promoter polymorphism is not associated with hip osteoarthritis in a United Kingdom Caucasian population. *Osteoarthritis Cartilage,* 14, 3, 295–298

Loughlin, J.; Sinsheimer, J.S.; Mustafa, Z.; Carr, A.J.; Clipsham, K.; Bloomfield, V.A.; Chitnavis, J.; Bailey, A.; Sykes, B. & Chapman K. (2000b). Association analysis of the vitamin D receptor gene, the type I collagen gene COL1A1, and the estrogen receptor gene in idiopathic osteoarthritis. *J Rheumatol,* 27, 3, 779-784

Mabuchi, A.; Ikeda, T.; Fukuda, A.; Koshizuka, Y.; Hiraoka, H.; Miyoshi, K.; Haga, N.; Kawaguchi, H.; Kawakami, A.; Yamamoto, S.; Takatori, Y.; Nakamura, K. & Ikegawa, S. (2001) .Identification of sequence polymorphisms of the COMP (cartilage oligomeric matrix protein) gene and association study in osteoarthrosis of the knee and hip joints. *J Hum Genet,* 46, 8, 456-462

MacGregor, A.J.; Antoniades, L.; Matson, M.; Andrew, T. & Spector, T.D. (2000). The genetic contribution to radiographic hip osteoarthritis in women. Results of a Classic Twin Study. *Arthritis Rheum,* 43, 11, 2410-2416

MacGregor, A.J.; Li, Q.; Spector, T.D. & Williams, F.M. (2009). The genetic influence on radiographic osteoarthritis is site specific at the hand, hip and knee. *Rheumatology (Oxford),* 48, 3, 277-280

Magaña, J.J.; Gálvez-Rosas, A.; González-Huerta, C.; Duarte-Salazár, C.; Lara-Alvarado, L.; Soria-Bastida, M.A.; Cortés-González, S. & Miranda-Duarte, A. (2010). Association of the calcitonin gene (CA) polymorphism with osteoarthritis of the knee in a Mexican mestizo population. *Knee,* 17, 2, 157-160

Malemud, C.J.; Martel-Pelletier, J. & Pelletier, J.P. (1987). Degradation of extracellular matrix in osteoarthritis: 4 fundamental questions. *J Rheumatol,* 14, Spec No, 20-22

Martel-Pelletier, J.; Boileau, C.; Pelletier, J.P. & Roughley, P.J. (2008). Cartilage in normal and osteoarthritis conditions. *Best Pract Res Clin Rheumatol,* 22, 2, 351-384.

Meulenbelt, I.; Bijkek, C.; De Wildt, S.C.; Miedema, H.S.; Breedveld, F.C.; Pols, H.A.; Hofman, A; Van Duijn, C.M. & Slagboom, P.E. (1999). Haplotype analysis of three polymorphisms of the COL2A1 gene and associations with generalised radiological osteoarthritis. *Ann Hum Genet,* 63, (Pt 5), 393-400

Meulenbelt, I.; Min, J.L.; Bos, S.; Riyazi, N; Houwing-Duistermaat, J.J.; van der Wijk, H.J.; Kroon, H.M.; Nakajima, M.; Ikegawa, S.; Uitterlinden, A.G.; van Meurs, J.B.; van der Deure, W.M.; Visser, T.J.; Seymour, A.B.; Lakenberg, N.; van der Breggen, R.;

Kremer, D.; van Duijn, C.M.; Kloppenburg, M.; Loughlin, J. & Slagboom, P.E. (2008). Identification of DIO2 as new susceptibility locus for symptomatic osteoarthritis. *Hum Mol Genet*, 17, 12, 1867-1875

Meulenbelt, I.; Seymour, A.B.; Nieuwland, M.; Huizinga, T.W.; van Duijn, C.M. & Slagboom, P.E. (2004). Association of the interleukin-1 gene cluster with radiographic signs of osteoarthritis of the hip. *Arthritis Rheum*, 50, 4, 1179–1186

Min, J.L.; Meulenbelt, I.; Riyazi, N.; Kloppenburg, M.; Houwing-Duistermaat, J.J.; Seymour, A.B.; Pols, H.A.; van Duijn, C.M. & Slagboom, P.E. (2005). Association of the frizzled-related protein gene with symptomatic osteoarthritis at multiple sites. *Arthritis Rheum*, 52, 4, 1077–1080

Min, J.L.; Meulenbelt, I.; Riyazi, N.; Kloppenburg, M; Houwing-Duistermaat, J.J.; Seymour, A.B.; van Duijn, C.M. & Slagboom, P.E. (2006). Association of matrilin-3 polymorphisms with spinal disc degeneration and osteoarthritis of the first carpometacarpal joint of the hand. *Ann Rheum Dis*, 65, 8, 1060–1066

Miyamoto, Y.; Mabuchi, A.; Shi, D.; Kubo, T.; Takatori, Y.; Saito, S.; Fujioka, M.; Sudo, A.; Uchida, A.; Yamamoto, S.; Ozaki, K.; Takigawa, M.; Tanaka, T.; Nakamura, Y.; Jiang, Q. & Ikegawa S. (2007). A functional polymorphism in the 5′-UTR of GDF5 is associated with susceptibility to osteoarthritis. *Nat Genet*, 39, 4, 529–533

Moos, V.; Menard, J.; Sieper, J.; Sparmann, M. & Müller, B. (2002). Association of HLA-DRB1*02 with osteoarthritis in a cohort of 106 patients. *Rheumatology (Oxford)*, 41, 6, 666–669

Mototani, H.; Iida, A.; Nakamura, Y. & Ikegawa, S. (2010). Identification of sequence polymorphisms in CALM2 and analysis of association with hip osteoarthritis in a Japanese population. *J Bone Miner Metab*, 28, 5, 547-553

Mototani, H.; Mabuchi, A.; Saito, S.; Fujioka, M.; Iida, A.; Takatori, Y.; Kotani, A.; Kubo, T.; Nakamura, K.; Sekine, A.; Murakami, Y.; Tsunoda, T.; Notoya, K.; Nakamura, Y. & Ikegawa, S. (2005). A functional single nucleotide polymorphism in the core promoter region of CALM1 is associated with hip osteoarthritis in Japanese. *Hum Mol Genet*, 14, 8, 1009–1017

Moxley, G.; Meulenbelt, I.; Chapman, K.; van Diujn, C.M.; Eline Slagboom, P.; Neale, M.C.; Smith, A.J.; Carr, A.J. & Loughlin, J. (2010). Interleukin-1 region meta-analysis with osteoarthritis phenotypes. *Osteoarthritis Cartilage*, 18, 2, 200-207

Mustafa, Z.; Dowling, B.; Chapman, K.; Sinsheimer, J.S.; Carr, A. & Loughlin, J. (2005). Investigating the aspartic acid (D) repeat of asporin as a risk factor for osteoarthritis in a UK Caucasian population. *Arthritis Rheum*, 52, 11, 3502–3506

Nagase, H. & Kashiwagi, M. (2003). Aggrecanases and cartilage matrix degradation. *Arthritis Res Ther*, 5, 2,94-103

Nakajima, M.; Takahashi, A.; Kou, I.; Rodriguez-Fontenla, C.; Gomez-Reino, J.J.; Furuichi, T.; Dai, J.; Sudo, A.; Uchida, A.; Fukui, N.; Kubo, M.; Kamatani, N.; Tsunoda, T.; Malizos, K.N.; Tsezou, A.; Gonzalez, A.; Nakamura, Y. & Ikegawa, S. (2010). New sequence variants in HLA class II/III region associated with susceptibility to knee osteoarthritis identified by genome-wide association study. *PLoS One*, 5, 3, e9723

Nakamura, T.; Shi D.; Tzetis M.; Rodriguez-Lopez J.; Miyamoto Y.; Tsezou, A.; Gonzalez, A.; Jiang, Q.; Kamatani, N.; Loughlin, J. & Ikegawa S. (2007). Meta-analysis of association between the ASPN D-repeat and osteoarthritis. *Hum Mol Genet*, 16, 14, 1676-1681

Neame, R.L.; Muir, K.; Doherty, S. & Doherty, M. (2004). Genetic risk of knee osteoarthritis: a sibling study. *Ann Rheum Dis,* 63, 9, 1022-1027

Nguyen, T.; Liu, X.K.; Zhang, Y. & Dong, C. (2006). BTNL2, a butyrophilin-like molecule that functions to inhibit T cell activation. *J Immun,* 176, 12, 7354-7360

Oddis, C.V. (1996). New perspectives on osteoarthritis. *Am J Med,* 26, 100, 10S-15S

Park, H.J.; Yoon, S.H.; Zheng, L.T.; Lee, K.H; Kim, J.W.; Chung, J.H.; Lee, Y.A. & Hong, S.J. (2007). Association of the -2510A/G chemokine (C-C motif) ligand 2 polymorphism with knee osteoarthritis in a Korean population. *Scand J Rheumatol,* 36, 4, 299-306

Peach, C.A.; Carr, A.J. & Loughlin, J. (2005). Recent advances in the genetic investigation of osteoarthritis. *Trends Mol Med,* 11, 4, 186-191

Pola, E.; Papaleo, P.; Pola, R.; Gaetani, E; Tamburelli, F.C.; Aulisa, L. & Logroscino, C.A. (2005). Interleukin-6 gene polymorphism and risk of osteoarthritis of the hip: a case-control study. *Osteoarthritis Cartilage,* 13, 11, 1025–1028

Poulou, M.; Kaliakatsos, M.; Tsezou, A.; Kanavakis, E.; Malizos, K.N. & Tzetis, M. (2008). Association of the CALM1 core promoter polymorphism with knee osteoarthritis in patients of Greek origin. *Genet Test,* 12, 2, 263-265

Pullig, O.; Tagariello, A.; Schweizer, A.; Swoboda, B.; Schaller, P. & Winterpacht, A. (2007). MATN3 (matrilin-3) sequence variation (pT303M) is a risk factor for osteoarthritis of the CMC1 joint of the hand, but not for knee osteoarthritis. *Ann Rheum Dis,* 66, 2, 279-80

Riancho, J.A.; García-Ibarbia, C.; Gravani, A.; Raine, E.V.; Rodríguez-Fontenla, C.; Soto-Hermida, A.; Rego-Perez, I.; Dodd, A.W.; Gómez-Reino, J.J.; Zarrabeitia, M.T.; Garcés, C.M.; Carr, A.; Blanco, F.; González, A. & Loughlin, J. (2010) Common variations in estrogen-related genes are associated with severe large-joint osteoarthritis: a multicenter genetic and functional study. *Osteoarthritis Cartilage,* 18, 7, :927-933

Rich, S.S. & Sellers, T.A. (2002) Genetic epidemiology methods, In: *Genetic basis of common diseases 2nd ed,* King, R.A., Rotter J.I., Motulsky, A.G., 39-49, Oxford University Press, ISBN 0-19-512582-7, New York.

Riyazi, N.; Kurreeman, F.A.; Huizinga, T.W.; Dekker, F.W.; Stoeken-Rijsbergen, G. & Kloppenburg, M. (2005). The role of interleukin 10 promoter polymorphisms in the susceptibility of distal interphalangeal osteoarthritis. *J Rheumatol,* .32, 8, 1571–1575

Riyazi, N.; Rosendaal, F.R.; Slagboom, E.; Kroon, H.M.; Breedveld, F.C. & Kloppenburg, M. (2008). Risk factors in familial osteoarthritis: the GARP sibling study. *Osteoarthritis Cartilage,* 16, 6, 654-659

Riyazi, N.; Spee, J.; Huizinga, T.W.; Schreuder, G.M.; de Vries, R.R.; Dekker, F.W. & Kloppenburg, M. (2003).HLA class II is associated with distal interphalangeal osteoarthritis. *Ann Rheum Dis,* 62, 3, 227–230

Rodriguez-Lopez J.; Pombo-Suarez M.; Liz M.; Gomez-Reino, J.J. & Gonzalez, A. (2007). Further evidence of the role of frizzledrelated protein gene polymorphisms in osteoarthritis. *Ann Rheum Dis,* 66, 8, 1052–1055

Rodriguez-Lopez, J.; Pombo-Suarez, M.; Liz, M.; Gomez-Reino, J.J. & Gonzalez, A. (2006). Lack of association of a variable number of aspartic acid residues in the asporin gene with osteoarthritis susceptibility: casecontrol studies in Spanish Caucasians. *Arthritis Res Ther,* 8, 3, R55

Rodriguez-Lopez, J.; Pombo-Suarez, M.; Loughlin, J.; Tsezou, A.; Blanco F.J.; Meulenbelt, I.; Slagboom, P.E.; Valdes, A.M.; Spector, T.D.; Gomez-Reino, J.J. & Gonzalez A. (2009). Association of a nsSNP in ADAMTS14 to some osteoarthritis phenotypes. *Osteoarthritis Cartilage*, 17, 3, 321-327

Schneider, E.M.; Du, W.; Fiedler, J.; Hogel, J.; Gunther, K.P.; Brenner, H. & Brenner, R.E. (2011). The (-765 G->C) promoter variant of the COX-2/PTGS2 gene is associated with a lower risk for end-stage hip and knee osteoarthritis. *Ann Rheum Dis*, 70, 8, 1458-60

Schork, N.J. (1997). Genetics of complex disease: approaches, problems, and solutions. *Am J Respir Crit Care Med*. 156, 4 Pt 2, 103-109.

Settle, S.H. Jr.; Rountree, R. B.; Sinha, A.; Thacker, A.; Higgins, K. & Kingsley, D.M. (2003). Multiple joint and skeletal patterning defects caused by single and double mutations in the mouse Gdf6 and Gdf5 genes. *Dev Biol*, 254, 1, 116-130

Sezgin, M.; Erdal, M.E.; Altintas, Z.M.; Ankarali, H.C.; Barlas, I.O.; Turkmen, E. & Sahin, G. (2007). Lack of association polymorphisms of the IL1RN, IL1A, and IL1B genes with knee osteoarthritis in Turkish patients. *Clin Invest Med*, 30, 2, 86-92

Shi, D.; Nakamura, T.; Nakajima, M.; Dai, J.; Qin, J.; Ni, H.; Xu, Y.; Yao, C.; Wei, J.; Liu, B.; Ikegawa, S. & Jiang, Q. (2008a). Association of single-nucleotide polymorphisms in RHOB and TXNDC3 with knee osteoarthritis susceptibility: two case-control studies in East Asian populations and a meta-analysis. *Arthritis Res Ther*, 10, 3, R54

Shi, D.; Ni, H.; Dai, J.; Qin, J.; Xu, Y.; Zhu, L.; Yao, C.; Shao, Z.; Chen, D.; Xu, Z.; Yi, L.; Ikegawa, S. & Jiang, Q. (2008b). Lack of association between the CALM1 core promoter polymorphism (-16C/T) and susceptibility to knee osteoarthritis in a Chinese Han population. *BMC Med Genet*, 22, 9, 91

Shi, D.; Zheng, Q.; Chen, D.; Zhu, L.; Qin, A.; Fan, J.; Liao, J.; Xu, Z.; Lin, Z.; Norman, P.; Xu, J.; Nakamura, T.; Dai, K.; Zheng, M. & Jiang, Q. (2010). Association of single-nucleotide polymorphisms in HLA class II/III region with knee osteoarthritis. *Osteoarthritis Cartilage*, 18, 11, 1454-1457

Smith, A.J.; Gidley, J.; Sandy, J.R.; Perry, M.J.; Elson, C.J.; Kirwan, J.R.; Spector, T.D.; Doherty, M.; Bidwell, J.L. & Mansell, J.P. (2005). Haplotypes of the low-density lipoprotein receptorrelated protein 5 (LRP5) gene: are they a risk factor in osteoarthritis? *Osteoarthritis Cartilage*, 13, 7, 608–613

Snelling, S.; Sinsheimer, J.S.; Carr, A. & Loughlin, J. (2007). Genetic association analysis of LRCH1 as an osteoarthritis susceptibility locus. *Rheumatology*, 46, 2, 250-252

Solovieva, S.; Hirvonen, A.; Siivola, P.; Vehmas, T.; Luoma, K.; Riihimaki, H. & Leino-Arjas, P. (2006). Vitamin D receptor gene polymorphisms and susceptibility of hand osteoarthritis in Finnish women. *Arthritis Res Ther*, 8, R20

Solovieva, S.; Kämäräinen, O.P.; Hirvonen, A.; Hämäläinen, S.; Laitala, M. Vehmas, T.; Luoma, K.; Näkki, A.; Riihimäki, H.; Ala-Kokko, L.; Männikkö, M. & Leino-Arjas P. (2009). Association between interleukin 1 gene cluster polymorphisms and bilateral distal interphalangeal osteoarthritis. *J Rheumatol*, 36, 9, 1977-1986

Southam, L.; Dowling, B.; Ferreira, A.; Marcelline, L.; Mustafa, Z.; Chapman, K.; Bentham, G.; Carr, A. & Loughlin, J. (2004). Microsatellite association mapping of a primary osteoarthritis susceptibility locus on chromosome 6p12.3-q13. *Arthritis Rheum*, 50, 12, 3910–3914

Southam, L.; Rodriguez-Lopez, J.; Wilkins, J.M.; Pombo-Suarez, M.; Snelling, S.; Gomez-Reino, J.J.; Chapman, K.; Gonzalez, A. & Loughlin J. (2007). An SNP in the 5'-UTR of GDF5 is associated with osteoarthritis susceptibility in Europeans and with in vivo differences in allelic expression in articular cartilage. *Hum Mol Genet,* 16, 18, 2226–2232

Spector, T.D.; Cicuttini, F.; Baker, J.; Loughlin, J. & Hart, D. (1996). Genetic influences on osteoarthritis in women: a twin study. *British Medical Journal*, 312, 7036, 940-943

Spector, T.D.; Reneland, R.H.; Mah, S.; Valdes, A.M.; Hart, D.J.; Kammerer, S.; Langdown, M.; Hoyal, C.R.; Atienza, J.; Doherty, M.; Rahman, P.; Nelson, M.R. & Braun, A. (2006). Association between a variation in LRCH1 and knee osteoarthritis: a genome-wide single-nucleotide polymorphism association study using DNA pooling. *Arthritis Rheum*, 54, 2, 524–532

Stecher, R.M. (1941). Heberdens´s nodes. Heredity in hypertrophic arthritis of finger joints. *Am J Med Sci*, 201, 6 ,801-809

Stefánsson, S.E.; Jónsson, H.; Ingvarsson, T.; Manolescu, I.; Jónsson, H.H.; Olafsdóttir, G.; Pálsdóttir, E.; Stefánsdóttir, G.; Sveinbjörnsdóttir, G.; Frigge, M.L.; Kong, A.; Gulcher, J.R. & Stefánsson, K. (2003). Genomewide scan for hand osteoarthritis: a novel mutation in matrilin-3. *Am J Hum Genet*, 72, 6, 1448-1459

Tsezou, A.; Satra, M.; Oikonomou, P.; Bargiotas, K. & Malizos, K.N. (2008). The growth differentiation factor 5 (GDF5) core promoter polymorphism is not associated with knee osteoarthritis in the Greek population. *J Orthop Res*, 26, 1, 136-140

Uitterlinden, A.G.; Burger, H.; Huang, Q.; Odding, E.; Duijn, C.M.; Hofman, A.; Birkenhäger, J.C.; van Leeuwen, J.P. & Pols, H.A. (1997). Vitamin D receptor genotype is associated with radiographic osteoarthritis at the knee. *J Clin Invest*, 100, 2, 259-263

Uitterlinden, A.G.; Burger, H.; van Duijn, C.M.; Huang, Q.; Hofman, A.; Birkenhager, J.C.; van Leeuwen, J.P. & Pols, H.A. (2000). Adjacent genes, for COL2A1 and the vitamin D receptor, are associated with separate features of radiographic osteoarthritis of the knee. *Arthritis Rheum*, 43, 7, 1456-1464

Valdes, A.M.; Arden, N.K.; Tamm, A.; Kisand, K.; Doherty, S.; Pola, E.; Cooper, C.; Tamm, A.; Muir, K.R.; Kerna, I.; Hart, D.; O'Neil, F.; Zhang, W.; Spector, T.D.; Maciewicz, R.A. & Doherty, M. (2010). A meta-analysis of interleukin-6 promoter polymorphisms on risk of hip and knee osteoarthritis. *Osteoarthritis Cartilage*, 18, 5, 699-704

Valdes, A.M.; Evangelou, E.; Kerkhof, H.J.; Tamm, A.; Doherty, S.A.; Kisand, K.; Tamm, A.; Kerna, I.; Uitterlinden, A.; Hofman, A.; Rivadeneira, F.; Cooper, C.; Dennison, E.M.; Zhang, W.; Muir, K.R.; Ioannidis, J.P.; Wheeler, M.; Maciewicz, R.A.; van Meurs, J.B.; Arden, N.K.; Spector, T.D. & Doherty, M. (2011). The GDF5 rs143383 polymorphism is associated with osteoarthritis of the knee with genome-wide statistical significance. *Ann Rheum Dis*, 70, 5, 873-875

Valdes, A.M.; Hart, D.J.; Jones, K.A.; Surdulescu, G.; Swarbrick, P.; Doyle, D.V.; Schafer, A.J. & Spector, T.D. (2004) Association study of candidate genes for the prevalence and progression of knee osteoarthritis. *Arthritis Rheum*, 50, 8, 2497–24507

Valdes, A.M.; Loughlin, J.; Oene, M.V.; Chapman, K.; Surdulescu, G.L.; Doherty, M. & Spector, T.D. (2007). Sex and ethnic differences in the association of ASPN, CALM1,

COL2A1, COMP, and FRZB with genetic susceptibility to osteoarthritis of the knee. *Arthritis Rheum*, 56, 1, 137–146.

Valdes, A.M.; Loughlin, J.; Timms, K.M.; van Meurs, J.J.; Southam, L.; Wilson, S.G.; Doherty, S.; Lories, R.J.; Luyten, F.P.; Gutin, A.; Abkevich, V.; Ge, D.; Hofman, A.; Uitterlinden, A.G.; Hart, D.J.; Zhang, F.; Zhai, G.; Egli, R.J.; Doherty, M.; Lanchbury, J. & Spector, T.D. (2008). Genome-wide association scan identifies a PTGS2 (prostaglandin-endoperoxide synthase 2) variant involved in risk of knee osteoarthritis. *Am J Hum Genet*, 82, 6, 1231–1240

Valdes, A.M. & Spector, T.D. (2009a). The contribution of genes to osteoarthritis. *Med Clin North Am*, 93, 1, 45-66

Valdes, A.M. & Spector, T.D.; Doherty, S.; Wheeler, M.; Hart, D.J. & Doherty, M. (2009b). Association of the DVWA and GDF5 polymorphisms with osteoarthritis in UK populations. *Ann Rheum Dis*. 68, 12, 1916-1920

Valdes, A.M.; Van Oene, M, Hart DJ, Surdulescu G.L.; Loughlin, J.; Doherty, M. & Spector, T.D. (2006). Reproducible genetic associations between candidate genes and clinical knee osteoarthritis in men and women. *Arthritis Rheum*, 54, 2, 533–539

van der Kraan, P.M.; Davidson, E.N. & van den Berg W.B. (2010). Bone morphogenetic proteins and articular cartilage: To serve and protect or a wolf in sheep clothing's? *Osteoarthritis Cartilage*, 18, 6, 735-741

Wilkins, J.M.; Southam, L.; Mustafa, Z.; Chapman, K. & Loughlin, J. (2009). Association of a functional microsatellite within intron 1 of the BMP5 gene with susceptibility to osteoarthritis. *BMC Med Genet*, 10:141

Wise, B. L.; Demissie, S.; Cupples, L. A. Felson, D.T.; Yang, M.; Shearman, A.M.; Aliabadi, P. & Hunter, D.J. (2009). The relationship of estrogen receptor-alpha and -beta genes with osteoarthritis of the hand. *J Rheumatol*, 36, 12, 2772-2779

Yavropoulou, M.P. & Yovos, J. G. (2007). The role of the Wnt signaling pathway in osteoblast commitment and differentiation. *Hormones*, 6, 4, 279-294

Yuan, G.H.; Masuko-Hongo, K.; Kato, T. & Nishioka K. (2003). Immunologic intervention in the pathogenesis of osteoarthritis. *Arthritis Rheum*, 48, 3, 602-611

Yuasa, T.; Otani, T.; Koike, T.; Iwamoto, M. & Enomoto-Iwamoto M. (2008). Wnt/beta-catenin signaling stimulates matrix catabolic genes and activity in articular chondrocytes: its possible role in joint degeneration. *Lab Invest*, 88, 3, 264-74

Zhai, G.; Ding, C; Stankovich, J.; Cicuttini, F. & Jones, G. (2005). The genetic contribution to longitudinal changes in knee structure and muscle strength: a sibpair study. *Arthritis Rheum*, 52, 9, 2830-2834

Zhai, G.; Hart, D. J.; Kato, B. S.; Macgregor, A. & Spector, T. D. (2007). Genetic influence on the progression of radiographic knee osteoarthritis: a longitudinal twin study. *Osteoarthritis Cartilage*, 15, 2, 222-225

Zhai, G.; Stankovich, J.; Ding, C.; Scott, F.; Cicuttini, F. & Jones, G. (2004). The genetic contribution to muscle strength, knee pain, cartilage volume, bone size, and radiographic osteoarthritis: a sibpair study. *Arthritis Rheum*, 50, 3, 805-810

12

Genetic Association and Linkage Studies in Osteoarthritis

Annu Näkki[1,2,3], Minna Männikkö[4] and Janna Saarela[1]
[1]*Institute for Molecular Medicine Finland (FIMM), University of Helsinki, Helsinki,*
[2]*Unit of Public Health Genomics, National Institute for Health and Welfare, Helsinki,*
[3]*Departments of Medical Genetics and Public Health, University of Helsinki, Helsinki,*
[4]*Oulu Center for cell-Matrix Research, Biocenter and Department of Medical Biochemistry and Molecular Biology, University of Oulu, Oulu,*
Finland

1. Introduction

Text Osteoarthritis (OA) is the most common musculoskeletal disease in developed countries. It is characterized by progressive degradation of articular cartilage that leads to joint space narrowing, subchondral sclerosis, osteophyte and cyst formation, and eventually loss of joint function. While OA can be secondary to various factors, the majority of cases are considered primary. Certain OA forms have long been known to have a genetic component. Based on twin studies the heritability of OA has been estimated to be around 50 %. Since the disease is complex, with environmental and genetic factors acting together, the knowledge of the etiology and development of preventive medication have been a challenge. A better understanding of the predisposing genes and biological mechanisms behind OA are essential for future drug development.

The current estimate of the number of genes in the human genome is 23 500 (Patterson 2011). Almost the entire genome of 3.2 x 10^9 base pairs is identical between any two individuals, excluding the 0.1 % that varies. A large fraction of the variation is common in the general population, i.e. the variant allele is seen as often or almost as often as the wild-type allele. However, some of the variation is rare, seen only in less than 1% of individuals or possibly even unique to one person. The early genetic studies were performed by selecting biologically interesting candidate genes and searching for sequence variants segregating with the disease in families with multiple affected individuals or variants identified from a small number of affected cases. Many of these studies concentrated on genes coding for the structural components of cartilage, like the collagens (for reviews, see (Kuivaniemi et al. 1997; Loughlin 2001)).

Next, genome-wide studies were launched to search for chromosomal regions co-segregating with a disease in families or in sibling pairs. The genome-wide linkage analyses utilized a set of variants throughout the genome without prior knowledge or hypothesis of the function of the genes. Initially a few hundred microsatellite markers, which were located on average 10 million base pairs apart, were selected throughout the human genome. The chromosomal regions identified by the linkage analysis were usually very large, containing hundreds of genes, and needed fine mapping with additional genetic markers to better locate the genome region of interest. The genome-wide linkage study approach has been very successful in locating disease-causing genes for monogenic diseases (for example (Kestilä et al. 1994; Mäkelä-Bengs et al. 1998; Nousiainen et al. 2008)). Genes causing rare, familial forms of OA have been identified by genetic linkage studies, which have also revealed novel insight on OA etiology, even though the identified variants have not been significant in predisposing to common forms of OA at the population level (Palotie et al. 1989; Ala-Kokko et al. 1990; Vikkula et al. 1993; Prockop et al. 1997; Jakkula et al. 2005).

In recent years, the knowledge of the human genome has grown substantially. The linkage disequilibrium (LD) structure of the human genome was studied in the international HapMap project, gaining understanding of genetic tag markers that are informative and can cover surrounding regions of the genome (Gibbs et al. 2003). That and the technological improvements in genotyping methods have decreased the cost of genotyping and thus enabled high throughput gene mapping studies with large numbers of informative variants in a large number samples (Craddock et al. 2010; Lango Allen et al. 2010). Genome-wide association studies use hundreds of thousands of tag markers throughout the genome and require no priori hypothesis on the disease etiology. The association is measured by a statistical test of the co-occurrence of an allele with a phenotype. The basic research frame in an association study is a case-control sample set of unrelated individuals. Genome-wide association analysis (GWAS) is usually performed with common single nucleotide polymorphism (SNP) markers. GWAS aiming to identify predisposing variants for common, multifactorial diseases require large sample sizes because the effect of a single variant is typically small. So far, GWAS studies of OA phenotypes have revealed few confirmed variants.

Many of the initial genetic associations have not been replicated in the follow-up studies. This may be due to many different factors such as a false positive original finding, a small sample size in the replication study, which does not have the power to detect a true association with a small effect size, or a difference in phenotypes between studies. An accurately defined phenotype should be reliably measurable and represent the biological phenomenon as closely as possible. Sometimes the optimal phenotyping method for a genetic study does not correspond with the diagnostic criteria used in patient care. For example, pain is an important symptom in evaluating the need for treatment in OA, but it is typically a poor phenotype for genetic studies since it can be caused by several factors and it is difficult to measure reliably.

Our aim is to review the studies aiming to identify disease-predisposing variants for different OA phenotypes. We will summarize different genome-wide linkage (GWL) and some of the earlier candidate gene studies performed in OA. Additionally we will present the novel findings in recent genome-wide association studies and discuss the challenges confronted in gene mapping studies of complex disease.

2. Heritability

Heritability is defined as the proportion of the total phenotypic variation that is caused by genetic factors. The heritability can vary between 1 - 100 % and it is dependent on the studied population. For example, the heritability of height is roughly 80 % (Silventoinen et al. 2003). Traditionally, twins have been used as study subjects for heritability estimates;

monozygotic twins share 100 % of their genome and dizygotic twins share on average 50 % of their genome. Since twins share their prenatal environment and often most of the environmental factors later in life, the higher concordance in the phenotype between monozygotic twins than between dizygotic twins is considered to be caused by genetic factors (Kempthorne et al. 1961).

In OA the heritability estimates have also varied between the study populations and different OA types, but can roughly be estimated to be between 50-60 %. Based on a twin study by Page et al. (2003), the heritability of hip OA was approximately more than half in males in the USA; the genetic effect on self-reported hip replacement surgery was 53 % and the effect for radiologically verified primary hip OA was 61%. Similar results were observed in a study by MacGregor et al. (2000) with a UK population-based cohort of women: Heritability of 58% was observed for radiographic hip OA and 64% for radiographic joint space narrowing. High heritability estimates were reported for radiological knee OA of medial osteophytes (69 %) and for joint space narrowing (80%) in a population-based study with twins from the UK (Zhai et al. 2007). The heritability of radiographic hand OA has been shown to vary between 47.6 % and 67.4 % in an UK population-based study sample of females. The lower value was for DIP OA based on joint space narrowing and osteophytes, and the upper value the total Kellgren and Lawrence value for all 30 hand joints (Livshits et al. 2007).

3. Genome-wide linkage studies

Similarly as in other complex diseases the early genetic studies in OA focused on rare families and genes known to have a biological role in the development and structure of cartilage (Palotie et al. 1989; Ala-Kokko et al. 1990; Vikkula et al. 1993; Jakkula et al. 2005). In the 1990s, the introduction of panels of highly informative microsatellite markers evenly covering the genome allowed hypothesis-free screening with no prior knowledge of the gene functions (Petrukhin et al. 1993; Straub et al. 1993).

The first genome-wide linkage studies in OA families were published over ten years ago (Leppävuori et al. 1999; Loughlin et al. 1999). They were followed by a number of twin, sib pair, and family-based studies and their meta-analysis, which together have identified at least fifteen OA loci with a genome-wide significant logarithm of odds score (LOD $\geq$ 3.3) (Leppävuori et al. 1999; Loughlin et al. 1999; Ingvarsson et al. 2001; Demissie et al. 2002; Loughlin et al. 2002b; Stefansson et al. 2003; Forster et al. 2004b; Hunter et al. 2004; Loughlin et al. 2004; Southam et al. 2004; Greig et al. 2006; Lee et al. 2006; Mabuchi et al. 2006; Meulenbelt et al. 2006; Livshits et al. 2007; Min et al. 2007; Meulenbelt et al. 2008). Of these, loci in 2p23-p24, 2q31-q33, 4q31-q32, 7q34-q36, and 19q13 have been implicated also in other independent studies. Table 1 lists loci identified with genome-wide significant evidence for linkage at least in one study and also additional studies showing suggestive evidence for linkage for these loci. However, since the identified linkage peaks have typically been wide and the marker maps quite sparse, it is challenging to evaluate the true overlap between the studies.

Although the linkage screens and their follow-up fine mapping studies have revealed several interesting OA candidate loci, very few, if any, OA predisposing variants that would explain the observed linkage have been identified within these loci. Loci with genome-wide significant evidence for linkage supported by at least one independent study, as well as some of the candidate genes within these regions, are shortly described below.

Chr	LOD	Phenotype	Country	n (individuals in screening/finemapping) n (families or sibpairs)**	Ref.
2p23.3–24.1	**4.4**	DIP/CMC1	Iceland	1143 cases + 939 relatives / 2162 cases + 873 controls 329 families (≥2 aff/fam)	(Stefansson et al. 2003)
2p23.3	2.2	JSN, hand	USA	1477 / - 296 families	(Demissie et al. 2002)
2p13.2–2p14 and **2p12–13.3**	2.9 and **4.0**	DIP and Tot-KL, hand	UK	1028 / - DZ twins	(Livshits et al. 2007)
2q12-2q21	2.3	DIP	Finland	54 27 sib pairs	(Leppävuori et al. 1999)
2q31.1	1.6	Thumb IP	USA	1214 / - 267 families	(Hunter et al. 2004)
2q24.3–31.1	1.6	Hip	UK	Finemapping > 962 / > 756 481 families (≥2 aff sib pair /fam) / 378 families (≥2 aff sib pair/fam)	(Loughlin et al. 2000) (Loughlin et al. 2002b)
2q32.1-2q34	p=0.03 meta	Knee, hip, hand	European + USA	3000 893 families	(Lee et al. 2006)
2q23	2.2	CMC1	Iceland	558 204 families	(Stefansson et al. 2003)
2q33.3	**6.1**	GOA	Netherlands	38 / 52+X 4/7 families 1228 assoc	(Meulenbelt et al. 2006)
4q12–21.2	3.1	Hip (women)	UK	178 female hip OA 85 families	(Loughlin et al. 1999)
4q13.1	2.7	PIIANP biomarker	Afr.Am/ Nat.Am.	350 1 extended family	(Chen et al. 2010) *
4q13.3	3.1	Hip (women)	UK	> 436 218 families (of which 146 THR)	(Forster et al. 2004b)
4q	2.3	DIP	Finland	54 27 sibpairs	(Leppävuori et al. 1999)
4q31.3	**3.3**	DIP	Iceland	1143 cases + 939 relatives / 2162 cases + 873 controls 329 families (≥2 aff/fam)	(Stefansson et al. 2003)
4q32.3	**3.8**	Tot-KL, hand	UK	1028 / - DZ twins	(Livshits et al. 2007)
6p21.1–q22.1	2.1	Hip	UK	416 194 families	(Loughlin et al. 1999)
6p21.1-q15	p=0.02 meta	Knee, hip, hand	European + USA	3000 893 families	(Lee et al. 2006) E

Chr	LOD	Phenotype	Country	n (individuals in screening/finemapping) n (families or sibpairs)**	Ref.
6p11.1	**4.8**	Hip (women)	UK	Finemapping > 292 146 families	(Southam et al. 2004)
6p12	**4.6**	THR, hip	UK	> 756 378 families (≥2 aff sib pair/fam)	(Loughlin et al. 2002c)
6q11.2–12	3.1	Tot-KL, hand	UK	1028 / - DZ twins	(Livshits et al. 2007)
7q34-36	p=0.004 meta	Knee, hip, hand	European + USA	3000 893 families	(Lee et al. 2006)
7q32	1.1	Knee, hip	UK	641 481 families	(Chapman et al. 1999)
7q35	3.1	DIP	USA	1214 / - 267 families	(Hunter et al. 2004)
8p23.2	**4.3**	PIIANP biomarker	Afr.Am/ Nat.Am..	350 1 extended family	(Chen et al. 2010)*
8p12	2.6	JSN, hand	UK	354 128 families	Greig et al. 2006
8q11	3.2	COMP biomarker	Afr.Am/ Nat.Am	350 1 extended family	(Chen et al. 2010)*
8q12–21	2.1	DIP	USA	1214 / - 267 families	(Hunter et al. 2004)
8q24.2	2.5	COMP	Afr.Am/ Nat.Am	350 1 extended family	(Chen et al. 2010)*
9q21.2	2.3	JSN, hand	USA	1477 / - 296 families	(Demissie et al. 2002)
9q34.2–34.3	**4.5**	DIP	UK	1028 / - DZ twins	(Livshits et al. 2007)
11p12–11q13.4	p=0.02 meta	Knee, hip, hand	European + USA	3000 893 families	(Lee et al. 2006)
11p11	1.32	Female knee, hip	UK	594 / 392 females 294 families / 192 pairs	(Chapman et al. 1999)
12q21.3–22	**3.9**	DIP	UK	1028 / - DZ twins	(Livshits et al. 2007)
12q24.3	1.7	JSN, hand	USA	1477 / - 296 families	(Demissie et al. 2002)
12q24.3	1.8	DIP	USA	1214 / - 267 families	(Hunter et al. 2004)
13q	2.3	First CMC	USA	1214 / - 267 families	(Hunter et al. 2004)

Chr	LOD	Phenotype	Country	n (individuals in screening/finemapping) n (families or sibpairs)**	Ref.
13q22.1	**3.6**	Hip associated with acetabular dysplasia	Japan	8 aff + 8 unaff 1 family	(Mabuchi et al. 2006)*
14q23-31	2.23	COMP, HA biomarkers	Afr.Am / Nat. Am	350 1 extended family	(Chen et al. 2010) *
14q32.11	3.0	GOA	Netherlands UK Japan	370 179 aff. siblings + 4 trios	(Meulenbelt et al. 2008)
15q21.3- 15q26.1	p=0.04 meta	Knee, hip, hand	European + USA	3000 893 families	(Lee et al. 2006)
15q25.3	**6.3**	First CMC	USA	1214 / - 267 families	(Hunter et al. 2004)
19q13.2 and 19q13.4	**4.3** and 4.0	Tot-KL, hand and DIP	UK	1028 / - DZ twins	(Livshits et al. 2007)
19q13.3	1.8	Tot-KL, hand	USA	1477 / - 296 families	(Demissie et al. 2002)
20p13	**3.7**	DIP (women)	USA	1214 / - 267 families	(Hunter et al. 2004)

*Only one family; DIP = distal interphalangeal; GOA = generalized OA; OST = osteophyte; PIP = proximal interphalangeal; JSN = joint space narrowing; Tot-KL = Kellgren Lawrence score sum for both hands; CMC1 = carpometacarpal; TIP = thumb interphalangeal; European background including the USA; In the study by Chen et al. (2010), the phenotype correlates with visually graded hand OA (Chen et al. 2008). Overlapping studies: Lee et al. (2006) meta-analysis includes Chapman et al. 1999, Stefansson et al. 2003, Hunter et al. 2004; Demissie et al. 2002, Hunter et al. 2004; Loughlin et al. 1999, Loughlin et al. 2000, Loughlin et al. 2002b, Chapman et al. 1999, Forster et al. 2004, Southam et al. 2004; Meulenbelt et al. 2006, Meulenbelt et al. 2008.

** the amount of individuals in screening / finemapping, and the amount of families or sibpairs used in the study;

Table 1. Results from OA linkage studies. Modified from Kämäräinen (2009).

The 2p23.3–24.1 region harboring the matrilin (*MATN3*) gene was shown to be significantly linked with hand OA (LOD = 4.4) in a study utilizing 1143 affected individuals and 939 relatives in 329 families (Stefansson et al. 2003). The same region had been previously implicated by Demissie et al. (2002) in 296 families, but without genome-wide significance (LOD=2.2). A possible disease-causing variant was pinpointed in the *MATN3* gene in the same study using 1312 cases and 873 controls, but the mutation was rare and did not fully explain the observed linkage.

A wide locus on 2q12-q34 has provided some evidence for linkage in four independent linkage studies: for DIP OA (Leppävuori et al. 1999), HIP OA (Loughlin et al. 2002a; Loughlin et al. 2002b), thumb IP (Hunter et al. 2004), and generalized OA (Meulenbelt et al. 2006). Only evidence for generalized OA peaking at 2q33.3 was statistically significant and was also supported by a meta-analysis combining three previously published screens (Chapman et al. 1999; Stefansson et al. 2003; Hunter et al. 2004; Lee et al. 2006). It is, however, unlikely that these linkage signals represent the same variant and none of the variants within this locus have yet provided convincing evidence for association, though several candidate genes with suggestive association have been reported: the neuropilin 2 gene (*NRP2*), $p = 0.02$; the "isocitrate dehydrogenase 1 (NADP+), soluble" gene (*IDH1*), $p = 0.03$ (Min et al. 2007); FRZB (Loughlin et al. 2004); and IL1R1 (Näkki et al. 2010).

The 6p12-p11 region has shown significant evidence for linkage with hip OA in two overlapping UK screens conducted in 375 (Loughlin et al. 2002c) and 146 families (Southam et al. 2004). No significant OA-associated variants have been identified, but interestingly a variant (rs987237, *TFAP2B*) previously shown to associate with BMI ($p = 2.90 \times 10^{-20}$, $n = 195{,}776$) maps within the linked region (Speliotes et al. 2010) - overweight being one of the known predisposing factors for OA.

The loci on 7q35 and 15q25 were identified in a linkage screen for hand OA ($n = 1216$ study subjects in a DIP OA study) (Hunter et al. 2004) and were further replicated in a meta-analysis extended with independent knee and hip OA families (in total $n = 3000$ knee, hip, and hand OA study subjects) (Chapman et al. 1999; Stefansson et al. 2003; Hunter et al. 2004; Lee et al. 2006). No OA predisposing variants have been identified.

A region on 4q31-q32 has provided significant evidence for linkage with DIP (Stefansson et al. 2003) and hand OA (Livshits et al. 2007). Further, the locus on 19q13 has shown significant evidence for linkage with hand and DIP OA (19q13.2 and 19q13.4, respectively, (Livshits et al. 2007) and this locus was also supported by a family based earlier linkage screen (Demissie et al. 2002). However to our knowledge, no significant OA predisposing variants have been identified within these loci.

4. Candidate gene studies

OA predisposing genes have been searched for through candidate gene studies, selecting genes based on their biological relevance or following a promising linkage study. Many of these genes participate in the cartilage extracellular matrix (ECM) composition/homeostasis by encoding structural proteins, matrix degrading enzymes, and different inflammatory mediator genes, as well as regulating signaling pathway genes. To date only a few of the putative positive findings in candidate gene association studies have been successfully replicated in an independent population, and the associated variants lack solid evidence for causality and functional differences between susceptibility alleles. For a review, see (Ikegawa 2007). In Table 2 we summarize those candidate genes that have shown the most suggestive evidence for association to OA. Replication of the initial finding in an independent study sample was used as a selection criterion. In addition, we will shortly describe genes with putative biological relevance to OA. They have shown suggestive association with OA in different candidate gene studies (for more details, see reviews by (Loughlin 2005; Bos et al. 2008; Ryder et al. 2008)), but have mostly not been confirmed.

Gene	Locus	Variation	OA*	Cases (n) / Controls (n)	OR	p-value	Population	Reference
ACAN	15q26	VNTR	Ha	43 / 50	3.23 (1.24-8.41)	<0.05	US	(Horton et al. 1998)
		VNTR/A27	Ha	112 / 153	0.46 (0.27-0.78)	0.012	Finnish	(Kämäräinen et al. 2006)
		VNTR/A27	Ha	tot. 134	na	0.04	Australian	(Kirk et al. 2003)
ASPN	9q22.31	Allele D14	K	137 / 234	2.63 (1.5–4.7)	0.00084	Japanese	(Kizawa et al. 2005)
		Allele D14	H	593 / 374	1.70 (1.1–2.5)	0.0078	Japanese	(Kizawa et al. 2005)
		Allele D14	H	364 / 356	1.48 (1.09-2.01)	0.016	British	(Mustafa et al. 2005)
		Allele D14	K	218 / 454	2.04 (1.32-3.15)	0.0013	Chinese	(Jiang et al. 2006)
		Allele D14	K	354 / -	na	0.004	Chinese	(Shi et al. 2007)
COL2A1	12q13.1	HT of HaeIII, HindIII	GOA	123 / 697	5.3 (2.2-12.7)	0.9983	Caucasian	(Meulenbelt et al. 1999)
		VNTR	K	183 / 668p	2.06 (1.27-3.34)	na	Caucasian	(Uitterlinden et al. 2000)
		HT of SNPs in exons 5, 32 and 51	K/H	417 / 280	1.30 (1.04-1.63)	0.024	Japanese	(Ikeda et al. 2002)
		rs2276455	H	160 / 383	1.58 (1.05-2.36)	0.005	Finnish	(Hämäläinen et al. 2009)
ESR1	6q25.1	PvuII, XbaI	GOA	65 / 318	1.86 (1.03-3.24)	0.039	Japanese	(Ushiyama et al. 1998)
		HT of PvuII, XbaI	K	316 / 1122p	1.3 (0.9-1.7)	<0.01	Caucasian	(Bergink et al. 2003)
FRZB	2q32.1	Arg324Gly	H	378 / 760	1.50 (1.1–2.1)	0.04	British	(Loughlin et al. 2004)
		Arg200Trp and Arg 324Gly	H	558 / 760	4.10 (1.6–10.7)	0.007	British	(Loughlin et al. 2004)
		Arg324Gly	G	545 / 1362	1.60 (1.1-2.3)	0.02	Dutch	(Min et al. 2005)
		Arg200Trp and Arg 324Gly	H	570 / 1317	1.90 (1.22–2.96)	0.1	US	(Lane et al. 2006)
		Arg200Trp and Arg 324Gly	K	603 / 599	2.87 (0.92–8.95)	0.04	UK	(Valdes et al. 2007)
GDF5	20q11.22	rs143383	K	718 / 861	1.30 (1.10–1.53)	0.0021	Japanese	(Miyamoto et al. 2007)
		rs143383	H	1000 / 981	1.79 (1.53–2.09)	$1.8x10^{-13}$	Japanese	(Miyamoto et al. 2007)
		rs143383	K	313 / 485	1.54 (1.22–1.95)	0.00028	Chinese	(Miyamoto et al. 2007)
		rs143383	K/H	2487 / 2018	1.28 (1.08–1.51)	0.004	Spanish UK	(Southam et al. 2007)
		rs143383	K/H	1842 / 1166	1.29 (1.14-1.47)	$8x10^{-5}$	UK	(Valdes et al. 2009b)
		rs143383	Ha	604 / 1102	0.68 (0.54-0.85)	$8x10^{-6}$	Dutch	(Vaes et al. 2009)
		rs143383	K	494 / 1174	0.68 (0.53-0.88)	0.003	Dutch	(Vaes et al. 2009)

Gene	Locus	Variation	OA*	Cases (n) / Controls (n)	OR	p-value	Population	Reference
		rs143383	H	5,789 / 7,850	1.16 (1.03-1.31)	0.016	Caucasian Japanese (8 cohorts)	(Evangelou et al. 2009) ***
		rs143383	K	5,085 / 8,135	1.15 (1.09-1.22)	9.4x 10^{-7}	Caucasian Japanese (10 cohorts)	(Evangelou et al. 2009) ***
		rs143383	Ha	4,040 / 4,792	1.08 (0.96-1.22)	0.19	Caucasian Japanese (6 cohorts)	(Evangelou et al. 2009) ***
IGF-1	12q22-24	CA-repeat	Ha/H K/S	615 /135p	1.9 (1.2-3.1)	0.02	Caucasian	(Meulenbelt et al. 1998)
		CA-repeat	Ha/H K/S	1355/191p	1.4 (1.0-1.8)	0.03	Caucasian	(Zhai et al. 2004)
IL1B	2q12-13	+3954C>T/TaqI	K/H	61 / 254	2.59 (1.4-4.7)	0.0096	Caucasian	(Moos et al. 2000)
		-511C>T/AvaI	H	70 / 816p	1.5 (0.8-2.9)	0.004	Caucasian	(Meulenbelt et al. 2004)
		+3954C>T/TaqI	H	70 / 816p	0.6 (0.4-1.2)	0.003	Caucasian	(Meulenbelt et al. 2004)
		5819G>A	Ha	68 / 51	3.82 (na)	0.021	US	(Stern et al. 2003)
		rs1143634	Ha	165 / 377p	1.6 (1.08-2.26)	0.001	Finnish	(Solovieva et al. 2009)
MATN3	2p24.1	Thr303Met	Ha	2162 / 873	2.12 (0.92-4.86)	na	Iceland	(Stefansson et al. 2003)
		Thr303Met	Ha	50 / 356	4.28 (1.18-14.8)	0.007	German	(Pullig et al. 2007)
ANP32A	15q23	rs7164503	H	1,288 / 1,741	0.67 (0.53-0.84)	3.8x10^{-4}	Caucasian (4 cohorts)	(Valdes et al. 2009a).
SMAD3	15q22	rs12901499	H	1,288 / 1,741	1.22 (1.12-1.34)	7.5x10^{-6}	Caucasian (5 cohorts)	(Valdes et al. 2010b)
		rs12901499	K	1,888 / 1,741	1.22 (1.09-1.36)	4.0x10^{-4}	Caucasian (5 cohorts)	(Valdes et al. 2010b)
DIO2	14q31	rs225014	H	1839 / 2687	1.79 (1.37-2.34)	2.02x10 -5	Caucasian Japanese (4 cohorts)	(Meulenbelt et al. 2008)
DIO3	14q32	rs945006	G	3,252 / 2,132	0.81 (0.70-0.93)	0.04**	Caucasian (4 cohorts)	(Meulenbelt et al. 2011)
VDR	12q12-14	I365I, TaqI	K	82 / 269p	2.60 (1.01-6.71)	<0.05	Caucasian	(Keen et al. 1997)
		HT of BsmI, ApaI, TaqI	K	179 / 667p	2.31 (1.48-3.59)	0.005	Caucasian	(Uitterlinden et al. 1997; Uitterlinden et al. 2000)

[a]Association for early onset OA; 3 Association for joint involvement and disease severity; *G = generalized; Ha = hand; K = knee; H = hip; na = not available; population based study; HT=haplotype, A27=27 repeats;** = permutation based; *** = including Vaes et al. 2008, Valdes et al. 2008, Southam et al. 2007, Miyamoto et al. 2007; bold font indicates region with linkage finding

Table 2. Candidate gene studies

The first structural genes analyzed were genes coding for major cartilage collagens II, IX, and XI, where mutations causing Stickler syndrome, a mild chondrodysplasia associated with OA, have been identified (for a review, see Robin et al. (2010)). Earlier reports suggested linkage between *COL2A1* and OA in two large families (Palotie et al. 1989; Vikkula et al. 1993), and a causal Arg519Cys mutation in the α1(II) chain was identified in OA families (Ala-Kokko et al. 1990; Fertala et al. 1997). In addition rare sequence variants in the genes for collagens II and XI have been associated with hip/knee OA (Jakkula et al. 2005). Several mutations have been identified in the collagen IX genes in patients with MED, a mild chondrodysplasia characterized by early-onset OA (Paassilta et al. 1999; Czarny-Ratajczak et al. 2001; Briggs et al. 2002). The roles of these genes are indisputable in mild chodrodysplasias, but so far only suggestive evidence for different common variants predisposing to OA have been reported (Ikeda et al. 2002; Hämäläinen et al. 2008; Näkki et al. 2011), none of which have yet been confirmed. Interestingly, mutations causing MED have also been identified in the vWF domain of the *MATN-3* gene (Chapman et al. 2001), which has been suggestively associated with OA later in a linkage and association study. The chromosomal region of 2p23.3–24.1 harboring the *MATN3* gene was shown to be significantly linked with hand OA (LOD = 4.4) in a study utilizing 1143 affected individuals and 939 relatives (Stefansson et al. 2003). A possible disease-causing variant was pinpointed in *MATN3.* Matrilins are ECM proteins expressed in the developing skeletal system. MATN3 is mostly restricted to developing cartilage, especially the epiphyseal cartilage (Stefansson et al. 2003). The expression of *MATN3* has been shown to be enhanced in OA cartilage of humans (Pullig et al. 2002).

Aggrecan (*AGC1, ACAN*) is the most abundant proteoglycan in cartilage and is an essential molecule for its osmotic properties (Roughley et al. 1994). Aggrecan gene transcription was shown to be elevated in early osteoarthritis in STR/ort mice (Gaffen et al. 1997). It contains a large polymorphic *VNTR* region that has been a target for several association studies, as it provides the attachment sites for numerous glycosaminoglycan side chains. Some level of association between *ACAN* and OA has been shown, but the results have been inconsistent (Horton et al. 1998; Kirk et al. 2003; Kämäräinen et al. 2006).

The transforming growth factor-β (TGF-β) signaling pathway has provided interesting candidate genes for OA, such as asporin (*ASPN*), which binds to TGF-β and suppresses the expression of both *ACAN* and *COL2A1* and reduces proteoglycan accumulation (Kizawa et al. 2005). Asporin is expressed in human osteoarthritic cartilage at high levels, but is barely detectable in cartilage of healthy individuals (Kizawa et al. 2005). The association between *ASPN* and knee/hip OA was first found in a Japanese population by Kizawa et al. (2005) and then replicated for knee OA by Nakamura et al. (2007) in a meta-analysis combining Europeans and Asians ($p = 0.003$, summary OR 1.46 with significant heterogeneity ($p=0.047$)). After stratification, association of the *ASPN* D14 allele with knee OA was seen only in the Asian populations. It is difficult to prove whether there is a true ethnical difference seen in the study, since there were also differences in the patient selection criteria between different ethnic populations.

Another member of the TGF-β superfamily is GDF5, growth and differentiation factor 5, which is closely related to the subfamily of bone- and cartilage-inducing molecules called the bone morphogenetic proteins (BMPs). GDF5 seems to induce cartilage and bone formation and stimulate de novo synthesis of proteoglycan ACAN (Erlacher et al. 1998). Mutations in this gene cause skeletal alterations both in humans (Thomas et al. 1996) and in mice (Storm et al. 1994). *GDF5* was first associated with hip and knee OA in Asian populations (1000 hip OA cases, 984 controls, $p = 1.8 \times 10^{-13}$) (Miyamoto et al. 2007), and the knee OA finding was replicated in a large meta-analysis (5085 knee OA cases and 8135 controls; OR 1.15, 95% CI 1.09-1.22, $p = 9.4\times10^{-7}$, Table 4) (Evangelou et al. 2009).

Participation of the TGF-β pathway was suggested also by a recent meta-analysis where the rs12901499 SNP in the *SMAD3* gene showed association with hip OA in a study utilizing five OA cohorts (1288 hip OA cases, 1741 controls; OR = 1.22, 95% CI 1.12-1.34, $p < 7.5 \times 10^{-6}$) and a similar trend was seen in knee OA (1888 knee OA cases, 3057 controls; OR = 1.22, 95% CI 1.09-1.36, $p < 4.0 \times 10^{-4}$) (Valdes et al. 2010b). SMAD3 has been suggested to act as an effector of the TGF-beta response (Zhang et al. 1996). *SMAD3* is located in chromosomal area 15q22.33 previously linked with OA: 15q21.3-15q26.1 with a p-value of 0.04 (Lee et al. 2006) and 15q25.3 with a LOD score of 6.3 (Hunter et al. 2004). In the same chromosomal region, *ANP32A* has been suggestively associated with hip OA in a study utilizing four patient cohorts (meta-analysis $p = 3.8\times10^{-4}$) and it was suggested to play a role in increased chondrocyte apoptosis (Valdes et al. 2009a). In mice, the over-expression of the Smurf2 gene seems to lead to dephosphorylation of Smad3 and cause the spontaneous OA phenotype (Wu et al. 2008).

The Wnt (wingless) signaling pathway that is involved in skeletal and joint patterning in embryogenesis has also raised interest in OA genetic studies. Previously, James et al. (2000) suggested that a member of this family, FrzB-2, may play a role in apoptosis and that the expression of this protein may be important in the pathogenesis of human OA. FRZB is a soluble antagonist of Wnt signalling and the gene showed some association with hip OA in a study by Loughlin et al. (2004) among others. However, the association could not be confirmed in a meta-analysis by Kerkhof et al. (2008) or in a large-scale association analysis of 5789 cases and 7859 controls with two *FRZB* variants (Evangelou et al. 2009), as the latter study revealed only a borderline association for hip OA ($p = 0.0199$).

The inflammatory cascade in OA cartilage is a widely studied topic in OA genetics. Interleukin 1 (IL-1) and tumor necrosis factor α (TNF-α) have been shown to inhibit collagen II production in chondrocytes by activating signaling pathways c-Jun N-terminal kinase (JNK), p38 mitogen-activated protein kinase (p38 MAPK), and nuclear factor kappa B (NF-κB) (Robbins et al. 2000; Seguin et al. 2003). Mechanical stress can also activate these pathways. The interleukin-1 gene family cluster is located on chromosome 2q12-13, and several association studies have shown a possible role for these genes in hip, knee, or hand OA (Moos et al. 2000; Loughlin et al. 2002a; Meulenbelt et al. 2004; Solovieva et al. 2009; Näkki et al. 2010). Individual associations have not been replicated, however. Kerkhof et al. (2011a) performed a meta-analysis to clarify the role of the common variants in the *IL1B* and *IL1RN* genes on the risk of knee and hip OA. No evidence of association was seen for individual variants ($p > 0.05$), but a suggestive association with reduced severity of knee OA was seen for a CTA-haplotype (rs419598, rs315952, and rs9005; OR 0.71, 95 % CI 0.56-0.91, $p = 0.006$).

Interleukin 6 (IL-6) is a pleiotropic proinflammatory cytokine that is markedly up-regulated in tissue inflammation. There is plenty of biological evidence of its role in OA pathogenesis. A significant rise in the level of IL-6 mRNA has been detected in OA-affected cartilage, and IL-6 levels in the serum and synovial fluid have been reported to be elevated among OA patients (Kaneko et al. 2000). Additionally, *IL-6* knockout mice develop more severe OA than wild-type animals (de Hooge et al. 2005). Genetic analyses have not been able to show compelling evidence for any of the common variants in *IL-6* with OA, however. *IL-6* promoter variant rs1800795 has been found to correlate for example with pain sensation in rheumatoid arthritis ($p = 0.014$) (Oen et al. 2005), and there is initial evidence for its association in a small set of symptomatic hand OA cases (OR 1.52, 95% CI 1.5-9.0, $p = 0.004$) (Kämäräinen et al. 2008). A recent meta-analysis of this SNP, however, (1101 hip OA patients, 1904 knee OA patients, and 2511 controls) showed no evidence for association with the risk of hip and knee osteoarthritis ($p = 0.95$ and $p = 0.30$, respectively) (Valdes et al. 2010a), although the study sample had 80 % power to observe association with the OR 1.12 for hip and OR 1.10 for knee OA with $p < 0.05$. IL-6 has been reported to contribute to the disease symptoms in rheumatoid arthritis and in OA ((Kaneko et al. 2000; Cronstein 2007), respectively), and as Valdes et al. (2010a) point out, confirming the lack of genetic association does not imply a lack of involvement in disease. In addition, IL4R has a known role in cartilage homeostasis by affecting inflammation due to mechanical stress. Common variants in this gene have shown suggestive evidence for association with OA (OR 2.1, 95 % CI 1.3-3.5, $p = 0.004$) (Forster et al. 2004a), but the associations have not been confirmed.

In OA, the degradation of cartilage ECM exceeds its synthesis and the primary cause has been suggested to be an increase in proteolytic enzyme activity, since aggrecan cleavage products accumulate in the synovial fluid of OA patients (Sandy et al. 1992). Two aggrecanases, *ADAMTS4* and *ADAMTS5*, are expressed in human OA cartilage and localize in the areas of aggrecan depletion, and have the highest specific activity for aggrecan cleavage *in vitro* (Tortorella et al. 2002). Suppression of both enzymes by siRNA reduces aggrecan degradation (Song et al. 2007). Tetlow et al. (2001) showed that several matrix metalloproteinases (MMPs 1, 3, 8, and 13), IL-1β, and TNF-α are present in the superficial zone of OA cartilage, where the chondrocyte clusters are located and where degenerative matrix changes appear. Matrix metalloproteinases break down collagens and MMP-13 is specialized in breaking the type II collagen.

In a study by Meulenbelt et al. (2008), a suggestive association between hip OA and variant rs225014 (Thr92Ala) in the iodothyronine-deiodinase enzyme type II gene (*DIO2*) was detected in 1839 hip OA cases and 2687 controls from Asia and Europe. The variant was located in close proximity to the linkage region on 14q32.11 (LOD 3.03). Some association was observed in four independent OA study samples of females with Caucasian and Asian background, and an OR = 1.79 (95% CI 1.37–2.34; $p = 2.02 \times 10^{-5}$) was obtained for rs225014 and rs12885300 haplotypes. The authors hypothesized that the link between this gene and OA is the role of *DIO2* in one of the following: endochondral ossification, OA progression, or inflammatory pathways including NFκB. The gene product of *DIO2* participates in the regulation of intracellular levels of active thyroid hormone (T3) in target tissues such as the growth plate. A meta-analysis of genes modulating intracellular T3 bioavailability has shown a role for another gene, deiodinase iodothyronine type III (*DIO3*), in OA (Meulenbelt et al. 2011). A total of 3252 hip/hand/knee cases and 2132 controls were studied and the suggestive association was seen with variant rs945006 for knee and/or hip OA (OR 0.81, 95 % CI 0.70-0.93, $p = 0.004$, permutation-based corrected $p = 0.039$).

Several studies have investigated the role of the vitamin D receptor gene (*VDR*) in OA. Restriction enzyme polymorphisms have been suggestively associated with knee and hand OA in limited sample sets (Keen et al. 1997; Uitterlinden et al. 1997; Uitterlinden et al. 2000;

Solovieva et al. 2006). However, a meta-analysis of ten studies on VDR polymorphisms and OA provided no evidence of association (Lee et al. 2009). The studies used in the meta-analysis differed in respect to the site of OA involvement, and heterogeneity in clinical features such as age and sex, which both affect the development of OA, and was recognized by the authors.

The role of variants in the estrogen receptor genes (*ESR1*, *ESR2*) has also been studied in OA. The role of estrogen may be important in OA since estrogen has been shown to be chondrodestructive via a receptor-mediated mechanism, and estrogen receptors are found in canine, rabbit, and human articular cartilage (Tsai et al. 1992). Suggestive association of restriction polymorphisms in *ESR1* has been detected in three studies (Ushiyama et al. 1998; Bergink et al. 2003; Jin et al. 2004). A meta-analysis of 2364 hip, 1983 knee, and 1431 hand OA cases and 6773, 4706, and 3883 controls, respectively, was performed for variants in *ESR2*. Variant rs1256031 showed some evidence for association with increased risk for hip OA in women (OR 1.36, 95 % CI 1.08-1.70, $p = 0.009$), but the combined analysis with knee and hand OA data did not show evidence for this variant (OR 1.06, 95 % CI 0.99-1.15, $p = 0.10$). The study had 80 % power to detect an OR of at least 1.14 for hip OA ($\alpha=0.05$).

5. Genome-wide association studies

Single nucleotide variants (SNPs) and information on the linkage disequilibrium (LD) structure between them identified by the HapMap and 1000 Genomes projects (Gibbs et al. 2003; Frazer et al. 2007; Durbin et al. 2011; Patterson 2011), as well as significant advancements in commercially available genotyping methods, have enabled development of genome-wide SNP arrays capable of genotyping a few hundred thousands to up to millions of evenly distributed variants within the genome at a reasonable cost in large amounts of samples. Genome-wide association studies (GWAS) have the advantage of not requiring knowledge and hypotheses on the gene functions beforehand, since the whole genome is under investigation in a systematic manner. GWAS analyses have proven a highly effective approach for identifying disease predisposing variants for common familial diseases (Wellcome Trust Case Control Consortium 2007).

The increased number of SNPs on arrays in recent years has improved the coverage of the common and especially the non-frequent variants; however, all common variations are still not fully covered. The increase in the number of SNPs represented on the arrays has also significantly increased the amount of association tests conducted in a project, thus making multiple testing correction and utilization of strict thresholds for statistically significant association very critical to avoid a multitude of false positive findings. The statistical significance threshold for the p-value suggested by the Wellcome Trust Case Control Consortium in 2007 was $p < 5x10^{-7}$ (2007), while the current broadly accepted threshold for genome-wide significance is $p < 5x10^{-8}$. The high quality genotype data produced from the commercially available arrays has also enabled the collection of sufficiently large data sets, which is a prerequisite for reliably identifying predisposing variants with low Odds Ratios (OR 1.1-1.5) typically seen in common, multi-factorial diseases (Manolio et al. 2009). Altogether four high density GWAS and one meta-analysis of GWAS have been conducted for OA phenotypes and the GWAS approach has proven to be a useful tool also in OA (Table 3). Three of the four genome-wide significant or highly probable OA predisposing variants have been identified by GWAS (Table 4).

Phenotype	Screening cases / controls, screening (population)*	Replication cases / controls, replication (population)**	Platform in screening phase	Ref
Hip: Radiological + clinical	93 / 631 (Japanese)	426 / 1006 (Japanese)	71,880 SNPs	(Mototani et al. 2005)
Knee: radiological, clinical	94 / 658 (Japanese)	1,399 / 2,141 (Japanese, Chinese)	99,295 SNPs The multiplex PCR-based Invader assay28 (Third Wave Technologies)	(Miyamoto et al. 2008)
Hand: radiological	1804 in total (UK, Dutch)	3266 in total (UK, Dutch, Caucasian from Russian Federation autonomous regions)	Illumina HumanHap 317 k Illumina HumanHap 550 k	(Zhai et al. 2009)
Hip: radiological or TJR Knee: radiological or TJR Hand: The American College of Rheumatology	hip + knee + hand: 248 + 515 + 578 / 1,411 + 1,047 + 1,038 (European ancestry: Dutch)	5,720 + 4,066 + 3,811/ 39,000 controls (European ancestry)	Illumina HumanHap 550v3 k Infinium HumanHap 300 k Affymetrix GeneChip Human Mapping	(Kerkhof et al. 2010)
Knee: radiological, clinical	906 / 3,396 (Japanese)	1,879 / 4,814 (Japanese, European ancestry)	Illumina HumanHap 550 k	(Nakajima et al. 2010)
Hip and knee: radiological, clinical	3177 / 4894 (UK)	~60.000 (European)	Illumina Human610 platform Illumina 1.2M Duo platform	(Panoutsopoulou et al. 2011)
Knee: radiological, clinical	2,371 / 35,909 (European ancestry: Icelandic, Dutch, UK, USA)	6,709 / 44.439 (European ancestry)	Illumina HumanHap 550v3 k Infinium HumanHap 300 k Affymetrix GeneChip Human Mapping	(Evangelou et al. 2011)

* In the screening phase, the nationality of the studied population is specified.

** Including the screening sample

Table 3. GWA studies performed in OA

Mototani and coworkers (2005) conducted a low density genome wide analysis by testing over 70,000 gene-based SNP markers for association with hip OA. The initial screening phase revealed a variant in the calmodulin 1 *CALM1* gene (rs3213718, IVS3 - 293C > T) on 14q24–q31 that showed some association in the small Japanese case-control set (OR=2.51, 95 % CI 1.40–4.50; p=0.0015). A replication in 334 individuals with hip OA and 375 control subjects provided a p-value of p=0.00065, (OR=2.40, 95 % CI 1.43–4.02) but when the reported genotype count data is combined into a meta-analysis, there is no genome wide significance (OR=1.35, 95 % CI 1.12-1.62; p = 0.0015, The Plink program (Purcell et al. 2007)).

The s3213718 SNP did not associate with knee OA in two low-powered Caucasian cohorts (298 male cases/300 male controls and 305 female cases, 299 female controls) (Valdes et al. 2007). Another SNP initially associating with hip OA in the Japanese study (rs12885713: 303 cases, 375 controls; OR = 2.56, 95 % CI 1.50–4.36, $p = 0.00036$) did not replicate in a study of 920 Caucasian hip OA cases and 752 controls, which had 97 % power to detect the original association (Loughlin et al. 2006). This might be due to a false positive original finding or due to substantial differences in the phenotypes, 40 % of the Japanese cases suffering from acetabular dysplasia (Hoaglund 2007).

Two GWA studies utilizing pooled knee OA and control DNA samples have been conducted. First, a low density genome-wide analysis of 25 494 SNPs located within gene regions utilizing pooled DNA samples of 335 female knee OA cases and 335 female controls was performed (Spector et al. 2006). The most significant SNPs were individually genotyped in the same samples and those with the most consistent difference were also genotyped in two replication sets of 1124 cases and 902 controls. One variant (rs912428a) in the *LRCH1* gene on chromosome 13 showed the most consistent difference in the replication samples, but the association was not significant after correcting for multiple testing (OR of 1.45, and a p-value $< 5 \times 10^{-4}$ in the analysis combining the screening and the replication sets).

A high-density GWAS was also conducted utilizing pooled samples. A three-phase study used a chip containing over 500 000 genome-wide variants to screen pools of 357 female knee OA cases and 285 female controls, replicated the most significant 28 variants in 871 knee OA cases and 1788 controls, and further validated seven variants in an additional 306 cases and 584 controls (Valdes et al. 2008). None of SNPs reached genome-wide significance in the screening phase, but one variant (rs4140564) located in an LD block containing the PTGS2 and PLA2G4A genes, which are involved in the prostaglandin E2 synthesis pathway, provided quite convincing evidence for association in the combined analysis of the screening and the replication samples (OR 1.55 (95% CI 1.30–1.85), $p = 6.9 \times 10^{-7}$).

A second low density genome-wide analysis utilizing individually genotyped cases and controls was conducted in a limited sample of 94 knee OA cases and 658 controls of Japanese origin using approximately 100 000 SNPs (Miyamoto et al. 2008). Fine-mapping of the initially identified susceptibility locus and further validation in independent OA cohorts revealed variants with genome-wide significant association to knee OA (a combined p-value of 7.3×10^{-11} with an OR of 1.43 (95% CI 1.28–1.59 for rs7639618). Re-sequencing of the novel *DVWA* gene identified three putatively functional SNPs: two missense SNPs, rs11718863 (encoding Y169N) and rs7639618 (encoding C260Y), and rs9864422 located in intron 1. The two coding variants were in almost complete LD and one of the four observed haplotypes (Tyr169-Cys260) was significantly overrepresented in osteoarthritis and was found to bind β-tubulin weaker than the other three isoforms in a *in vitro* functional assay. Later, Wagener and co-workers (Wagener et al. 2009) suggested that the *DVWA* might actually represent the COL6A4 gene, but according to current RefSeq annotation it is a transcribed pseudogene and represents the 5' end of a presumed ortholog to a mouse gene encoding a collagen VI alpha 4 chain protein (UCSC Genome Browser, GRCh37/hg19; http://genome.ucsc.edu/). Association of the variants in the *DVWA* gene was not replicated in a follow-up analysis of 1120 European knee OA cases and 2147 controls, which had approximately 96 % power to observe an association with an effect size (OR= 1.43) reported in the combined Japanese and Chinese population and an allele frequency of 0.14 in cases) (Meulenbelt et al. 2009). Whether the lack of association is due to a limited sample size and overestimation of the effect size in the original publication, difference in the phenotypes, heterogeneity in different populations, or a false positive initial finding, requires further analysis in a significantly large sample cohort.

A larger GWAS in a Japanese population genotyped over 500 000 SNPs in 906 knee OA cases and 3396 controls (Nakajima et al. 2010). Replication of the 15 SNPs with a p-value smaller than $1x10^{-5}$ in the initial screen in an independent Japanese cohort identified two SNPs (rs7775228 and rs10947262) showing genome-wide significant evidence for association in a combined analysis (p = $2.43x10^{-8}$, OR= 1.34; 95% CI = 1.21–1.49 and p = $6.73x10^{-8}$; OR= 1.32; 95% CI = 1.19–1.46, respectively). The two SNPs were in high LD with each other and were located within a 340-kb region within the HLA locus, including *BTNL2, HLA-DRA, HLA-DRB5, HLA-DRB1, HLA-DQA1,* and *HLA-DQB1.* Most of the genes within the associated region belong to the HLA class II molecules, which are expressed in antigen presenting cells and play a central role in the immune system by presenting peptides derived from extracellular proteins. The *BTNL2* gene encodes butyrophilin-like 2, which negatively regulates T-cell activation. The variant rs10947262 in the *BTNL2* gene showed nominal evidence for association also in a European cohort and provided a p-value of $5.10x10^{-9}$ in a meta-analysis combining the Japanese and European data. The authors did not report whether the previously identified variants in the *DVWA* gene (Miyamoto et al. 2008) were tagged by the SNPs in the array and showed no evidence for association in the screen.

Over 300 000 genome-wide variants were analyzed for association to hand OA in the TwinsUK cohort, which had radiographs of both hands available for 799 subjects (Zhai et al. 2009). None of the SNPs achieved significant evidence for association in the first screening phase, and the top 100 SNPs were selected for further analysis in a part of the Rotterdam cohort with both genotype and hand OA data available. Of the five SNPs nominally replicated in the second cohort, none were significantly associated with hand OA in the meta-analysis combining the two screening and four additional replication cohorts. The strongest evidence for association was observed with an SNP rs716508 located in the intron of the *A2BP1* gene (p = $4.75 x10^{-5}$), but did not reach genome-wide significance.

A high density GWAS of over 500 000 SNPs was aimed at identifying variants associated with a generalized OA (Kerkhof et al. 2010). In total, 1341 Dutch OA cases and 3496 Dutch controls were utilized in the screen, and SNPs associated with at least two OA phenotypes were analyzed in 12 additional cohorts including 14 938 independent OA cases and 39 000 controls in total. Of the twelve top hits analyzed in the replication cohorts, one variant (rs3815148) located in *COG5* on chromosome 7 was significantly associated with hand and/or knee OA in the meta-analysis combining screening and replication cohorts (p = $8x10^{-8}$, OR 1.14, 95% CI 1.09-1.19). Variants in the previously identified *GDF5* gene (Miyamoto et al. 2007) showed evidence for association to hand OA in the screening phase (p = $1x10^{-5}$), but the variant (rs6088813) provided only a p-value of 0.01 in the replication, although there were 8970 hand and/or knee of cases and almost 40 000 controls included in the analysis. None of the other previously identified OA variants were included in the replication effort. Although the authors monitored for their association in the screening cohort, it had only a limited power to observe the association. Variants rs225014 and 12885300 in the DIO2 gene were reported not to associate with hip OA in the Rotterdam Study, but they showed a trend towards the same direction observed in the original publication (Meulenbelt et al. 2008). The SNPs rs4140564 in *PTGS2* (Valdes et al. 2008) and rs7639618 in *DVWA* (Miyamoto et al. 2008) showed no evidence for association with knee OA in the to some extent undersized Rotterdam cohort.

Panoutsopoulou and co-workers (2011) conducted a GWAS of knee and hip OA with over 500 000 SNPs in 3,177 cases and 4,894 controls in the screening phase and almost 60,000 study subjects in the replication phase. Variant rs4512391 near the *TRIB1* gene showed the strongest association with combined hip and knee OA (OR=1.17, 95% CI 1.10-1.25; $p=1.8\times10^{-6}$) and with knee OA (OR = 1.23, 95% CI 1.13-1.33; $p = 1.1\times10^{-6}$) and rs4977469 in *FAM154A* with hip OA (OR = 1.30, 95% CI 1.17- 1.45; $p = 1.2\times10^{-6}$) in the initial screen. However, none of the SNPs included in the replication ($p<10^{-4}$) reached genome-wide significance in the analysis combining the screening and the replication data. The screening cohort had limited power to detect association with common variants with low Odds Ratios, thus the previously identified OA variants were not systematically followed-up. Yet, a few variants in biologically interesting genes providing suggestive evidence for association in the combined analysis (p-values between 1.2×10^{-6} and $7.59\text{x}10^{-5}$) were brought up in the discussion (rs13026243 in *NRP2,* rs7626795 in *IL1RAP,* rs2819358 in *ELF3,* rs2280465 in *ACAN,* rs2615977 in *COL11A1).*

The meta-analysis of GWAS for knee OA combined the data of the four previously published GWAS including in total 2371 knee OA cases and 35 909 controls of Caucasian origin in the screening phase (Evangelou et al. 2011). Altogether 11 SNPs (p-value < $5\text{x}10^{-5}$) in 10 different loci were replicated in 3326 cases and 7691 controls from eight European populations. Only two SNPs (rs4730250 and rs10953541), which are located in the previously identified 500 kb LD block on chromosome 7q22 containing six genes, replicated nominally in the combined analysis of the follow-up samples and showed genome-wide significant evidence for association with OA in the analysis combining the meta-analysis GWAS data and 10 replication cohorts of European origin ($p = 9.2\text{x}10^{-9}$, OR 1.17, 95% CI 1.11-1.24) for rs4730250. No evidence for either heterogeneity in the effect size between populations or gender-specific effects was observed. The association was not significantly replicated in an East-Asian cohort of 1183 knee OA cases and 1245 controls, which, however, had a limited power to observe an association of the effect size seen in the European populations (power of 6% when assuming MAF of 0.15 in controls based on HapMap). The meta-analysis combining the European and Asian samples yielded a global summary effect of 1.15 and showed no evidence of heterogeneity. The most significant variant rs4730250 is in high LD with rs10953541 (r2=0.63, D'=1 in HapMap-CEU) and with the previously identified variant rs3815148 (r2=0.77, D'=1 in HapMap CEU), and thus all three are likely to represent the same underlying association signal. None of the other previously confirmed OA variants yielded a p-value < $5\text{x}10^{-5}$, and were not followed up. This likely reflects the limited power of the meta-analysis, but may also indicate heterogeneity between the phenotypes or between European and Asian populations in at least some of the OA susceptibility variants.

As for the other confirmed OA loci, the predisposing gene/variant within the 7q22 locus remains yet to be defined. The associated 500 kb LD block contains six genes: *DUS4L, COG5, GPR22, BCAP29, PRKAR2B,* and *HPB1. DUS4L* encodes for a tRNA-dihydrouridine synthase 4-like. The protein encoded by *COG5* is one of eight proteins which form a Golgi-localized complex required for normal Golgi morphology and function (Ungar et al. 2002). Mutations in *COG5* have been shown to result in congenital disorder of glycosylation type 2I (Paesold-Burda et al. 2009). GPR22 encodes for a G protein-coupled receptor 22, which belongs to a family of the G-protein coupled receptors (O'Dowd et al. 1997). *BCAP29* encodes for a B-cell receptor-associated protein 29. The Bap29/31 complex has been shown to influence the intracellular traffic of MHC class I molecules (Paquet et al. 2004). *PRKAR2B* encodes for a cAMP-dependent protein kinase, which is a signaling molecule important for a variety of cellular functions. *HPB1* encodes for a HMG-box transcription factor 1, which is a transcriptional repressor regulating the cell cycle and of the Wnt pathway (Sampson et al. 2001).

Chr.	Variant	Putative gene	Predispo-sing allele /Freq	p	OR (95 % CI)	Study population: cases/controls	Ref
3p24	rs7639618	DVWA/ COL6A4P1 CAPN7	C / 0.64	$7.3x10^{-11}$	1.43 (1.28–1.60)	1,399 knee / 2,141 Asian	(Miyamoto et al. 2008)
6p21	rs10947262 (rs7775228)	BTNL2 HLA-DQB1 HLA-DRA HLA-DRB5 HLA-DRB1 HLA-DQA1 HLA-DQB1 HLA-DRB3 HLA-DRB4	C / 0.58	$5.1x10^{-9}$	1.31 (1.20–1.44)	1,879 knee / 4,814 Asian & European	(Nakajima et al. 2010)
7q22	rs4730250 (rs3815148) (rs10953541)	DUS4L COG5 GPR22 BCAP29 PRKAR2B HPB1	G / 0.17	$9.2x10^{-9}$	1.17 (1.11-1.24)	6,709 knee / 44.439 European	(Evangelou et al. 2011) (Kerkhof et al. 2010)
20q11	rs143383	GDF5 UQCC CEP250	T / 0.26	$1.8x10^{-13}$	1.79 (1.53–2.09)	998 hip / 983 Asian	(Miyamoto et al. 2007)

Chr = chromosome; variant= rs number of the most significant reported variant (other reported variants shown in the parenthesis), p-value = combined p-value of screening and replication; OR = odds ratio; Study population= number of cases/controls utilized in the analysis providing the most significant p-value, OA= generalized OA, knee= knee OA, hip= hip OA, All findings were identified by a GWAS approach, except rs143383 in GDF5, which was identified by a candidate gene study.

Table 4. Loci with genome-wide significant evidence for association ($p < 5x10^{-8}$) with OA.

6. Other approaches

There have not been sufficiently large, systematic genome-wide expression studies on human cartilage samples to undoubtedly confirm or exclude any expression patterns in OA cartilage. Some examples of alternative approaches are shortly described below.

Genome-wide expression profiling by Karlsson et al. (2010) of healthy (n = 5) and osteoarthritic cartilage (n = 5) revealed several genes up- or downregulated in OA cartilage. The study analyzing over 47 000 transcripts suggested changes for several gene families: cytokines, such as the tumor necrosis factors (TNF), chemokines like interleukin 8 (IL8), enzymes like matrix metalloproteinase (MMP), growth factors like insulin growth factor (IGF), matrix components like collagen I (COL1), and others such as HLA-DQA1.

In the first serum-based metabolomic study of osteoarthritis in humans, the ratio of two branched-chain amino acids, valine and combination of leusine and isoleucine, to histidine was significantly associated with the disease. The study was conducted in 123 + 76 knee OA cases and 299 + 100 controls by analyzing 163 serum metabolites (Zhai et al. 2010).

In a candidate biomarker study using blood samples (n = 287), hyaluronan (HA), cartilage oligomeric matrix protein (COMP) and collagen IIA N-propeptide (PIIANP), high sensitive C-reactive protein (hs-CRP), and glycated serum protein (GSP) showed an association ($p < 0.05$) with clinical phenotypes of hand OA or hand symptoms, of which PIIANP (0.57), HA (0.49), and COMP (0.43) showed some level of heritability (Chen et al. 2008). PIIANP is a marker of a fetal form of collagen II recapitulated in OA (Chen et al. 2008). The COMP molecule binds to the collagenous structure in cartilage and can initiate the alternative complement pathway (Happonen et al. 2010). HA has a role in cartilage structure as well.

7. Conclusions

Earlier studies have shown the importance of some structural genes in familial OA, but their role in predisposition to common forms of OA remains unclear. It is possible that there are rare mutations with high risk for OA affecting single families (or individuals), and perhaps there are more common alleles with smaller effects functioning at the population level. In population-based genome wide association studies utilizing common variants a handful of genes have been confirmed to affect OA (Table 4), however these studies have not revealed additional evidence that common variants in the earlier candidate genes associate with OA.

The few confirmed genome-wide significant gene variants in OA (Table 4) locate in or near genes that have a role in cell signaling and immunity. For practically all the recognized variants, the functional gene and the predisposing variant is still unknown due to the LD structure of the pinpointed area, thus the mechanism how these loci increase OA susceptibility is yet unknown. The causative gene might not be located in close proximity to the observed variant, but the variant might also affect the gene expression of genes further away in the genome.

As presented in the current review, false positive findings and limited power are issues in many genetic studies of common diseases. In general the power to detect predisposing variants depends on the effect size of the single variant to the disease. The smaller the effect of one variant to the disease the larger the study sample that is needed to observe the effect. Usually in complex diseases the effect size of any single variant is very small thus small effect variants will be missed and negative findings do not exclude the role of a variant to the studied trait (Purcell et al. 2003). A positive finding from an association study could mean that a disease-causing or predisposing variant has been found or a variant in high LD with the true disease-causing or predisposing variant has been identified. However, many aspects in gene mapping need to be taken into account when interpreting the results.

One of the challenges in genetic studies is population stratification, which occurs when the studied population contains genetically different subsets. Significant association might be due to the genetic difference between the case and control groups, which is unrelated to a given trait. In family-based analysis this is not an issue since the studied individuals share their genetic background, and in the GWAS studies it is possible to better control for the substructure by utilizing the genetic profiles of all the GWAS variants.

Type 1 error is unfortunately a common cause of positive findings. It arises from the fact that the more tests that are performed, the more positive findings that are seen by chance. Bonferroni correction and methods taking into account the LD structure of the genome are used to correct for multiple testing (Nyholt 2004; Li et al. 2005). To exclude the possibility of type 1 error, adequately stringent limit for p-value significance and replication of findings in independent study cohorts are needed. Many of the earlier suggestive candidate gene associations have not been followed-up in the recent GWAS projects leaving the significance of the many earlier findings still unconvincing. The lack of replication in the follow-up cohort may indicate false positive initial association, but might also be due to a limited size of the replication cohort not having enough statistical power to detect an association with a small effect size.

Differences in the phenotype definition may also be a cause for a seeming lack of replication (Kerkhof et al. 2011b). Very diverse diagnostic criteria have been used in different cohorts, which may have potentially enriched for specific subtypes of OA. However, in last few years there has also been successful attempts to harmonize the phenotype designation between cohorts (Evangelou et al. 2011). Further, the clinically used diagnostic criteria for OA are not always the optimal phenotypes in genetic studies. The clinical diagnosis has usually evolved historically on the basis of symptoms rather than the etiology of the disease (Plomin et al. 2009). Pain and disability caused by OA are likely affected by even a greater variety of genetic and environmental factors than the radiological findings of the joints, although they are naturally significant determinants in patient care.

According to current understanding OA is a multi-factorial disease, and several genetic and environmental factors are expected to affect the susceptibility. Although a few genetic predisposing variants have been identified, most of the disease heritability remains unsolved. It has been suggested that OA is a polygenic disease with hundreds or even thousands of predisposing variants, each having very small effect on the disease susceptibility (Evangelou et al. 2011). The challenge of missing heritability has been brought up in search for genes for other complex diseases, where significantly larger international collaborative efforts have already been made, and tens of confirmed and well-replicated disease variants have been identified (International Multiple Sclerosis Genetics Consortium and Wellcome Trust Case Control Consortium 2, 2011; De Jager et al. 2009; Lango Allen et al. 2010). In such cases GWAS conducted by large consortia have been able to identify disease variants that explain approximately 10-20% of the heritable component. Although recent international collaborative efforts have identified a few confirmed variants for OA, significantly larger efforts are needed to tackle the yet unidentified OA predisposing variants.

The methods in molecular genetics are developing rapidly, making it soon possible to sequence the entire human genome in a very reasonable time and cost, opening novel opportunities for genetic studies. Today we have plenty of suggestive evidence of the genes possibly involved in the etiology of OA, but what do we know for sure? We have rare mutations or variants in familial forms of OA, and a handful of confirmed genetic associations of common variants to continue in future studies on their biological function and role in the disease pathology. Significantly larger study cohorts with accurately defined phenotypes, as well as studies on transcriptomics, proteomics, and lipidomics are needed for complete understanding of the disease.

8. List of abbreviations

Osteoarthritis: OA; linkage disequilibrium: LD; logarithm of odds: LOD; Genome-wide association analysis: GWAS; single nucleotide polymorphism: SNP; genome-wide linkage: GWL; distal interphalangeal: DIP; generalized OA: GOA; osteophyte: OST; proximal interphalangeal: PIP; joint space narrowing JSN; Kellgren Lawrence score KL; carpometacarpal CMC1; thumb interphalangeal: TIP, thumb IP; matrilin: MATN3; interphalangeal: IP; neuropilin 2: NRP2; isocitrate dehydrogenase 1 (NADP+) soluble: IDH1; frizzled-related protein: FRZB; interleukin 1 receptor 1: IL1R1; transcription factor AP-2 beta (activating enhancer binding protein 2 beta): TFAP2B; body mass index: BMI; Aggrecan: AGC1, ACAN: Aspirin: ASPN; collagen, type II, alpha 1: COL2A1; estrogen receptor 1: ESR1; growth differentiation factor 5: GDF5; odds ratio: OR; confidence interval: CI; insulin-like growth factor 1: IGF-1; interleukin 1 beta: IL1B; matrilin 3: MATN3; acidic (leucine-rich) nuclear phosphoprotein 32 family, member A: ANP32A; SMAD family member 3: SMAD3; deiodinase, iodothyronine, type II: DIO2; deiodinase, iodothyronine, type III: DIO3; vitamin D (1,25- dihydroxyvitamin D3) receptor: VDR; multiple epiphyseal dysplasia: MED; arginine: Arg; cysteine: Cys; bone morphogenetic protein: BMP; SMAD specific E3 ubiquitin protein ligase 2: Smurf2; Wingless: Wnt; Interleukin: 1 IL-1; tumor necrosis factor α: TNF-α; c-Jun N-terminal kinase: JNK; p38 mitogen-activated protein kinase: p38 MAPK; nuclear factor kappa B: NF-κB; interleukin 1 receptor antagonist IL1RN; interleukin 6: IL-6; interleukin 4 receptor: IL4R; messenger RNA: mRNA; extracellular matrix: ECM; ADAM metallopeptidase with thrombospondin type 1 motif, 4: ADAMTS4; ADAM metallopeptidase with thrombospondin type 1 motif, 5: ADAMTS5; small interfering: siRNA; matrix metalloproteinase: MMP; interleukin 1 beta: IL-1β; estrogen receptor 2: ESR2; total joint replacement: TJR; calmodulin 1: CALM1; leucine-rich repeats and calponin homology (CH) domain containing 1: LRCH1; prostaglandin-endoperoxide synthase 2: PTGS2; phospholipase A2, group IVA (cytosolic, calcium-dependent): PLA2G4A; collagen, type VI, alpha 4 pseudogene 1: DVWA, COL6A4P1; butyrophilin-like 2 (MHC class II associated): BTNL2; major histocompatibility complex, class II, DR alpha: HLA-DRA; major histocompatibility complex, class II, DR beta 5: HLA-DRB5; major histocompatibility complex, class II, DR beta 1: HLA-DRB1; major histocompatibility complex, class II, DQ alpha 1: HLA-DQA1; major histocompatibility complex, class II, DQ beta 1: HLA-DQB1; RNA binding protein, fox-1 homolog (C. elegans) 1: A2BP1, RBFOX1; component of oligomeric golgi complex 5: COG5; tribbles homolog 1 (Drosophila): TRIB1; interleukin 1 receptor accessory protein: IL1RAP; E74-like factor 3 (ets domain transcription factor, epithelial-specific): ELF3; collagen, type XI, alpha 1: COL11A1; minor allele frequency: MAF; Utah residents with Northern and Western European ancestry from the CEPH collection: CEU; dihydrouridine synthase 4-like (S. cerevisiae): DUS4L; component of oligomeric golgi complex 5: COG5; G protein-coupled receptor 22: GPR22; B-cell receptor-associated protein 29: BCAP29; protein kinase, cAMP-dependent, regulatory, type II, beta: PRKAR2B; PBRM1 polybromo 1: HPB1, PBRM1; calpain 7: CAPN7; ubiquinol-cytochrome c reductase complex chaperone: UQCC; centrosomal protein 250kDa: CEP250; hyaluronan: HA; cartilage oligomeric matrix protein: COMP; collagen IIA N-propeptide: PIIANP; high sensitive C-reactive protein: hs-CRP; glycated serum protein: GSP.

9. References

Ala-Kokko, L., C. T. Baldwin, R. W. Moskowitz and D. J. Prockop, (1990). Single base mutation in the type II procollagen gene (COL2A1) as a cause of primary osteoarthritis associated with a mild chondrodysplasia, *Proc Natl Acad Sci U S A*. Vol 87, No. 17, pp. 6565-8. ISSN 0027-8424 (Print) 0027-8424 (Linking).

Bergink, A. P., J. B. van Meurs, J. Loughlin, P. P. Arp, Y. Fang, A. Hofman, J. P. van Leeuwen, C. M. van Duijn, A. G. Uitterlinden and H. A. Pols, (2003). Estrogen receptor alpha gene haplotype is associated with radiographic osteoarthritis of the knee in elderly men and women, *Arthritis Rheum*. Vol 48, No. 7, pp. 1913-22. ISSN 0004-3591 (Print) 0004-3591 (Linking).

Bos, S. D., P. E. Slagboom and I. Meulenbelt, (2008). New insights into osteoarthritis: early developmental features of an ageing-related disease, *Curr Opin Rheumatol*. Vol 20, No. 5, pp. 553-9. ISSN 1531-6963 (Electronic).

Briggs, M. D. and K. L. Chapman, (2002). Pseudoachondroplasia and multiple epiphyseal dysplasia: mutation review, molecular interactions, and genotype to phenotype correlations, *Hum Mutat*. Vol 19, No. 5, pp. 465-78. ISSN 1098-1004 (Electronic) 1059-7794 (Linking)

Chapman, K., Z. Mustafa, C. Irven, A. J. Carr, K. Clipsham, A. Smith, J. Chitnavis, J. S. Sinsheimer, V. A. Bloomfield, M. McCartney, O. Cox, L. R. Cardon, B. Sykes and J. Loughlin, (1999). Osteoarthritis-susceptibility locus on chromosome 11q, detected by linkage, *Am J Hum Genet*. Vol 65, No. 1, pp. 167-74. ISSN 0002-9297 (Print)0002-9297 (Linking).

Chapman, K. L., G. R. Mortier, K. Chapman, J. Loughlin, M. E. Grant and M. D. Briggs, (2001). Mutations in the region encoding the von Willebrand factor A domain of matrilin-3 are associated with multiple epiphyseal dysplasia, *Nat Genet*. Vol 28, No. 4, pp. 393-6. ISSN 1061-4036 (Print) 1061-4036 (Linking)

Chen, H. C., V. B. Kraus, Y. J. Li, S. Nelson, C. Haynes, J. Johnson, T. Stabler, E. R. Hauser, S. G. Gregory, W. E. Kraus and S. H. Shah, (2010). Genome-wide linkage analysis of quantitative biomarker traits of osteoarthritis in a large, multigenerational extended family, *Arthritis Rheum*. Vol 62, No. 3, pp. 781-90. ISSN 1529-0131 (Electronic) 0004-3591 (Linking).

Chen, H. C., S. Shah, T. V. Stabler, Y. J. Li and V. B. Kraus, (2008). Biomarkers associated with clinical phenotypes of hand osteoarthritis in a large multigenerational family: the CARRIAGE family study, *Osteoarthritis Cartilage*. Vol 16, No. 9, pp. 1054-9. ISSN 1522-9653 (Electronic) 1063-4584 (Linking).

Craddock, N., M. E. Hurles, N. Cardin, R. D. Pearson, V. Plagnol, S. Robson, D. Vukcevic, C. Barnes, D. F. Conrad, E. Giannoulatou, C. Holmes, J. L. Marchini, K. Stirrups, M. D. Tobin, L. V. Wain, C. Yau, J. Aerts, T. Ahmad, T. D. Andrews, H. Arbury, et al., (2010). Genome-wide association study of CNVs in 16,000 cases of eight common diseases and 3,000 shared controls, *Nature*. Vol 464, No. 7289, pp. 713-20. ISSN 0028-0836.

Cronstein, B. N., (2007). Interleukin-6--a key mediator of systemic and local symptoms in rheumatoid arthritis, *Bull NYU Hosp Jt Dis*. Vol 65 Suppl 1, No. pp. S11-5. ISSN 1936-9719 (Print) 1936-9719 (Linking).

Czarny-Ratajczak, M., J. Lohiniva, P. Rogala, K. Kozlowski, M. Perala, L. Carter, T. D. Spector, L. Kolodziej, U. Seppänen, R. Glazar, J. Krolewski, A. Latos-Bielenska and

L. Ala-Kokko, (2001). A mutation in COL9A1 causes multiple epiphyseal dysplasia: further evidence for locus heterogeneity, *Am J Hum Genet*. Vol 69, No. 5, pp. 969-80. ISSN 0002-9297 (Print) 0002-9297 (Linking).

de Hooge, A. S., F. A. van de Loo, M. B. Bennink, O. J. Arntz, P. de Hooge and W. B. van den Berg, (2005). Male IL-6 gene knock out mice developed more advanced osteoarthritis upon aging, *Osteoarthritis Cartilage*. Vol 13, No. 1, pp. 66-73. ISSN 1063-4584 (Print) 1063-4584 (Linking).

De Jager, P. L., X. Jia, J. Wang, P. I. de Bakker, L. Ottoboni, N. T. Aggarwal, L. Piccio, S. Raychaudhuri, D. Tran, C. Aubin, R. Briskin, S. Romano, S. E. Baranzini, J. L. McCauley, M. A. Pericak-Vance, J. L. Haines, R. A. Gibson, Y. Naeglin, B. Uitdehaag, P. M. Matthews, et al., (2009). Meta-analysis of genome scans and replication identify CD6, IRF8 and TNFRSF1A as new multiple sclerosis susceptibility loci, *Nat Genet*. Vol 41, No. 7, pp. 776-82. ISSN 1546-1718 (Electronic) 1061-4036 (Linking).

Demissie, S., L. A. Cupples, R. Myers, P. Aliabadi, D. Levy and D. T. Felson, (2002). Genome scan for quantity of hand osteoarthritis: the Framingham Study, *Arthritis Rheum*. Vol 46, No. 4, pp. 946-52. ISSN 0004-3591 (Print) 0004-3591 (Linking).

Durbin, R. M., G. R. Abecasis, D. L. Altshuler, A. Auton, L. D. Brooks, R. A. Gibbs, M. E. Hurles and G. A. McVean, (2011). A map of human genome variation from population-scale sequencing, *Nature*. Vol 467, No. 7319, pp. 1061-73. ISSN 1476-4687 (Electronic) 0028-0836 (Linking).

Erlacher, L., J. McCartney, E. Piek, P. ten Dijke, M. Yanagishita, H. Oppermann and F. P. Luyten, (1998). Cartilage-derived morphogenetic proteins and osteogenic protein-1 differentially regulate osteogenesis, *J Bone Miner Res*. Vol 13, No. 3, pp. 383-92. ISSN 0884-0431 (Print).

Evangelou, E., K. Chapman, I. Meulenbelt, F. B. Karassa, J. Loughlin, A. Carr, M. Doherty, S. Doherty, J. J. Gomez-Reino, A. Gonzalez, B. V. Halldorsson, V. B. Hauksson, A. Hofman, D. J. Hart, S. Ikegawa, T. Ingvarsson, Q. Jiang, I. Jonsdottir, H. Jonsson, H. J. Kerkhof, et al., (2009). Large-scale analysis of association between GDF5 and FRZB variants and osteoarthritis of the hip, knee, and hand, *Arthritis Rheum*. Vol 60, No. 6, pp. 1710-21. ISSN ISSN: 1529-0131 (Electronic).

Evangelou, E., A. M. Valdes, H. J. Kerkhof, U. Styrkarsdottir, Y. Zhu, I. Meulenbelt, R. J. Lories, F. B. Karassa, P. Tylzanowski, S. D. Bos, T. Akune, N. K. Arden, A. Carr, K. Chapman, L. A. Cupples, J. Dai, P. Deloukas, M. Doherty, S. Doherty, G. Engstrom, et al., (2011). Meta-analysis of genome-wide association studies confirms a susceptibility locus for knee osteoarthritis on chromosome 7q22, *Ann Rheum Dis*. Vol 70, No. 2, pp. 349-55. ISSN 1468-2060 (Electronic) 0003-4967 (Linking).

Fertala, A., L. Ala-Kokko, R. Wiaderkiewicz and D. J. Prockop, (1997). Collagen II containing a Cys substitution for arg-alpha1-519. Homotrimeric monomers containing the mutation do not assemble into fibrils but alter the self-assembly of the normal protein, *J Biol Chem*. Vol 272, No. 10, pp. 6457-64. ISSN 0021-9258 (Print) 0021-9258 (Linking).

Forster, T., K. Chapman and J. Loughlin, (2004a). Common variants within the interleukin 4 receptor alpha gene (IL4R) are associated with susceptibility to osteoarthritis, *Hum Genet*. Vol 114, No. 4, pp. 391-5. ISSN 0340-6717 (Print) 0340-6717 (Linking).

Forster, T., K. Chapman, L. Marcelline, Z. Mustafa, L. Southam and J. Loughlin, (2004b). Finer linkage mapping of primary osteoarthritis susceptibility loci on chromosomes 4 and 16 in families with affected women, *Arthritis Rheum*. Vol 50, No. 1, pp. 98-102. ISSN 0004-3591 (Print) 0004-3591 (Linking).

Frazer, K. A., D. G. Ballinger, D. R. Cox, D. A. Hinds, L. L. Stuve, R. A. Gibbs, J. W. Belmont, A. Boudreau, P. Hardenbol, S. M. Leal, S. Pasternak, D. A. Wheeler, T. D. Willis, F. Yu, H. Yang, C. Zeng, Y. Gao, H. Hu, W. Hu, C. Li, et al., (2007). A second generation human haplotype map of over 3.1 million SNPs, *Nature*. Vol 449, No. 7164, pp. 851-61. ISSN 0028-0836.

Gaffen, J. D., M. T. Bayliss and R. M. Mason, (1997). Elevated aggrecan mRNA in early murine osteoarthritis, *Osteoarthritis Cartilage*. Vol 5, No. 4, pp. 227-33. ISSN 1063-4584 (Print) 1063-4584 (Linking).

Gibbs, R. A., J. W. Belmont, P. Hardenbol, T. D. Willis, F. Yu, H. Yang, L. Ch'ang, W. Huang, B. Liu, Y. Shen, P. K. Tam, L. Tsui, M. M. Y. Waye and J. Tze-Fei, (2003). The International HapMap Project, *Nature*. Vol 426, No. 6968, pp. 789-96. ISSN 0028-0836.

Greig, C., K. Spreckley, R. Aspinwall, E. Gillaspy, M. Grant, W. Ollier, S. John, M. Doherty and G. Wallis, (2006). Linkage to nodal osteoarthritis: quantitative and qualitative analyses of data from a whole-genome screen identify trait-dependent susceptibility loci, *Ann Rheum Dis*. Vol 65, No. 9, pp. ISSN 1131-8. 0003-4967 (Print) 0003-4967 (Linking).

Hafler, D. A., A. Compston, S. Sawcer, E. S. Lander, M. J. Daly, P. L. De Jager, P. I. de Bakker, S. B. Gabriel, D. B. Mirel, A. J. Ivinson, M. A. Pericak-Vance, S. G. Gregory, J. D. Rioux, J. L. McCauley, J. L. Haines, L. F. Barcellos, B. Cree, J. R. Oksenberg and S. L. Hauser, (2007). Risk alleles for multiple sclerosis identified by a genomewide study, *N Engl J Med*. Vol 357, No. 9, pp. 851-62. ISSN 1533-4406 (Electronic) 0028-4793 (Linking).

Happonen, K. E., T. Saxne, A. Aspberg, M. Morgelin, D. Heinegard and A. M. Blom, (2010). Regulation of complement by cartilage oligomeric matrix protein allows for a novel molecular diagnostic principle in rheumatoid arthritis, *Arthritis Rheum*. Vol 62, No. 12, pp. ISSN 3574-83. 1529-0131 (Electronic) 0004-3591 (Linking).

Hoaglund, F. T., (2007). CALM1 promoter polymorphism gene and Japanese congenital hip disease, *Osteoarthritis Cartilage*. Vol 15, No. 5, pp. 593.

Horton, W. E., Jr., M. Lethbridge-Cejku, M. C. Hochberg, R. Balakir, P. Precht, C. C. Plato, J. D. Tobin, L. Meek and K. Doege, (1998). An association between an aggrecan polymorphic allele and bilateral hand osteoarthritis in elderly white men: data from the Baltimore Longitudinal Study of Aging (BLSA), *Osteoarthritis Cartilage*. Vol 6, No. 4, pp. 245-51. ISSN 1063-4584 (Print).

Hunter, D. J., S. Demissie, L. A. Cupples, P. Aliabadi and D. T. Felson, (2004). A genome scan for joint-specific hand osteoarthritis susceptibility: The Framingham Study, *Arthritis Rheum*. Vol 50, No. 8, pp. 2489-96. ISSN 0004-3591 (Print) 0004-3591 (Linking).

Hämäläinen, S., S. Solovieva, A. Hirvonen, T. Vehmas, E. P. Takala, H. Riihimäki and P. Leino-Arjas, (2009). COL2A1 gene polymorphisms and susceptibility to osteoarthritis of the hand in Finnish women, *Ann Rheum Dis*. Vol 68, No. 10, pp. 1633-7. ISSN 1468-2060 (Electronic) 0003-4967 (Linking).

Hämäläinen, S. H., S. Solovieva, A. Hirvonen, T. Vehmas, E. P. Takala, H. Riihimäki and P. Leino-Arjas, (2008). COL2A1 gene polymorphisms and susceptibility to hand osteoarthritis in Finnish women, *Ann Rheum Dis*. Vol, No. ISSN 1468-2060 (Electronic).

International Multiple Sclerosis Genetics Consortium; Wellcome Trust Case Control Consortium 2, Sawcer S, Hellenthal G, Pirinen M, Spencer CC, Patsopoulos NA, Moutsianas L, Dilthey A, Su Z, Freeman C, Hunt SE, Edkins S, Gray E, Booth DR, Potter SC, Goris A, Band G, Oturai AB, Strange A et al. (2011). Genetic risk and a primary role for cell-mediated immune mechanisms in multiple sclerosis. *Nature*. Vol 476, No. 7359, pp 214-9. ISSN 0028-0836.

Ikeda, T., A. Mabuchi, A. Fukuda, A. Kawakami, Y. Ryo, S. Yamamoto, K. Miyoshi, N. Haga, H. Hiraoka, Y. Takatori, H. Kawaguchi, K. Nakamura and S. Ikegawa, (2002). Association analysis of single nucleotide polymorphisms in cartilage-specific collagen genes with knee and hip osteoarthritis in the Japanese population, *J Bone Miner Res*. Vol 17, No. 7, pp. ISSN 1290-6. 0884-0431 (Print).

Ikegawa, S., (2007). New gene associations in osteoarthritis: what do they provide, and where are we going?, *Curr Opin Rheumatol*. Vol 19, No. 5, pp. 429-34. ISSN 1040-8711 (Print) 1040-8711 (Linking).

Ingvarsson, T., S. E. Stefansson, J. R. Gulcher, H. H. Jonsson, H. Jonsson, M. L. Frigge, E. Palsdottir, G. Olafsdottir, T. Jonsdottir, G. B. Walters, L. S. Lohmander and K. Stefansson, (2001). A large Icelandic family with early osteoarthritis of the hip associated with a susceptibility locus on chromosome 16p, *Arthritis Rheum*. Vol 44, No. 11, pp. 2548-55. ISSN 0004-3591 (Print) 0004-3591 (Linking).

Jakkula, E., M. Melkoniemi, I. Kiviranta, J. Lohiniva, S. S. Räinä, M. Perälä, M. L. Warman, K. Ahonen, H. Kröger, H. H. Göring, and L. Ala-Kokko, (2005). The role of sequence variations within the genes encoding collagen II, IX and XI in non-syndromic, early-onset osteoarthritis, *Osteoarthritis Cartilage*. Vol 13, No. 6, pp. 497-507. ISSN 1063-4584 (Print) 1063-4584 (Linking).

James, I. E., S. Kumar, M. R. Barnes, C. J. Gress, A. T. Hand, R. A. Dodds, J. R. Connor, B. R. Bradley, D. A. Campbell, S. E. Grabill, K. Williams, S. M. Blake, M. Gowen and M. W. Lark, (2000). FrzB-2: a human secreted frizzled-related protein with a potential role in chondrocyte apoptosis, *Osteoarthritis Cartilage*. Vol 8, No. 6, pp. 452-63. ISSN 1063-4584 (Print).

Jiang, Q., D. Shi, L. Yi, S. Ikegawa, Y. Wang, T. Nakamura, D. Qiao, C. Liu and J. Dai, (2006). Replication of the association of the aspartic acid repeat polymorphism in the asporin gene with knee-osteoarthritis susceptibility in Han Chinese, *J Hum Genet*. Vol 51, No. 12, pp. 1068-72. ISSN 1434-5161 (Print) 1434-5161 (Linking).

Jin, S. Y., S. J. Hong, H. I. Yang, S. D. Park, M. C. Yoo, H. J. Lee, M. S. Hong, H. J. Park, S. H. Yoon, B. S. Kim, S. V. Yim, H. K. Park and J. H. Chung, (2004). Estrogen receptor-alpha gene haplotype is associated with primary knee osteoarthritis in Korean population, *Arthritis Res Ther*. Vol 6, No. 5, pp. R415-21. ISSN 1478-6362 (Electronic) 1478-6354 (Linking).

Kaneko, S., T. Satoh, J. Chiba, C. Ju, K. Inoue and J. Kagawa, (2000). Interleukin-6 and interleukin-8 levels in serum and synovial fluid of patients with osteoarthritis, *Cytokines Cell Mol Ther*. Vol 6, No. 2, pp. 71-9. ISSN 1368-4736 (Print) 1368-4736 (Linking).

Karlsson, C., T. Dehne, A. Lindahl, M. Brittberg, A. Pruss, M. Sittinger and J. Ringe, (2010). Genome-wide expression profiling reveals new candidate genes associated with osteoarthritis, *Osteoarthritis Cartilage*. Vol 18, No. 4, pp. 581-92. ISSN 1522-9653 (Electronic) 1063-4584 (Linking).

Keen, R. W., D. J. Hart, J. S. Lanchbury and T. D. Spector, (1997). Association of early osteoarthritis of the knee with a Taq I polymorphism of the vitamin D receptor gene, *Arthritis Rheum*. Vol 40, No. 8, pp. 1444-9. ISSN 0004-3591 (Print) 0004-3591 (Linking).

Kempthorne, O. and R. H. Osborne, (1961). The interpretation of twin data, *Am J Hum Genet*. Vol 13, No. pp. 320-39.

Kerkhof, H. J., M. Doherty, N. K. Arden, S. B. Abramson, M. Attur, S. D. Bos, C. Cooper, E. M. Dennison, S. A. Doherty, E. Evangelou, D. J. Hart, A. Hofman, K. Javaid, I. Kerna, K. Kisand, M. Kloppenburg, S. Krasnokutsky, R. A. Maciewicz, I. Meulenbelt, K. R. Muir, et al., (2011a). Large-scale meta-analysis of interleukin-1 beta and interleukin-1 receptor antagonist polymorphisms on risk of radiographic hip and knee osteoarthritis and severity of knee osteoarthritis, *Osteoarthritis Cartilage*. Vol 19, No. 3, pp. 265-71. ISSN 1522-9653 (Electronic) 1063-4584 (Linking).

Kerkhof, H. J., R. J. Lories, I. Meulenbelt, I. Jonsdottir, A. M. Valdes, P. Arp, T. Ingvarsson, M. Jhamai, H. Jonsson, L. Stolk, G. Thorleifsson, G. Zhai, F. Zhang, Y. Zhu, R. van der Breggen, A. Carr, M. Doherty, S. Doherty, D. T. Felson, A. Gonzalez, et al., (2010). A genome-wide association study identifies an osteoarthritis susceptibility locus on chromosome 7q22, *Arthritis Rheum*. Vol 62, No. 2, pp. 499-510. ISSN 0004-3591 (Print) 0004-3591 (Linking).

Kerkhof, H. J., I. Meulenbelt, T. Akune, N. K. Arden, A. Aromaa, S. M. Bierma-Zeinstra, A. Carr, C. Cooper, J. Dai, M. Doherty, S. A. Doherty, D. Felson, A. Gonzalez, A. Gordon, A. Harilainen, D. J. Hart, V. B. Hauksson, M. Heliovaara, A. Hofman, S. Ikegawa, et al., (2011b). Recommendations for standardization and phenotype definitions in genetic studies of osteoarthritis: the TREAT-OA consortium, *Osteoarthritis Cartilage*. Vol 19, No. 3, pp. 254-64. ISSN 1522-9653 (Electronic) 1063-4584 (Linking).

Kerkhof, J. M., A. G. Uitterlinden, A. M. Valdes, D. J. Hart, F. Rivadeneira, M. Jhamai, A. Hofman, H. A. Pols, S. M. Bierma-Zeinstra, T. D. Spector and J. B. van Meurs, (2008). Radiographic osteoarthritis at three joint sites and FRZB, LRP5, and LRP6 polymorphisms in two population-based cohorts, *Osteoarthritis Cartilage*. Vol 16, No. 10, pp. 1141-9. ISSN 1522-9653 (Electronic) 1063-4584 (Linking).

Kestilä, M., M. Männikkö, C. Holmberg, G. Gyapay, J. Weissenbach, E. R. Savolainen, L. Peltonen and K. Tryggvason, (1994). Congenital nephrotic syndrome of the Finnish type maps to the long arm of chromosome 19, *Am J Hum Genet*. Vol 54, No. 5, pp. 757-64. ISSN 0002-9297 (Print) 0002-9297 (Linking).

Kirk, K. M., K. J. Doege, J. Hecht, N. Bellamy and N. G. Martin, (2003). Osteoarthritis of the hands, hips and knees in an Australian twin sample--evidence of association with the aggrecan VNTR polymorphism, *Twin Res*. Vol 6, No. 1, pp. 62-6. ISSN 1369-0523 (Print).

Kizawa, H., I. Kou, A. Iida, A. Sudo, Y. Miyamoto, A. Fukuda, A. Mabuchi, A. Kotani, A. Kawakami, S. Yamamoto, A. Uchida, K. Nakamura, K. Notoya, Y. Nakamura and S. Ikegawa, (2005). An aspartic acid repeat polymorphism in asporin inhibits chondrogenesis and increases susceptibility to osteoarthritis, *Nat Genet.* Vol 37, No. 2, pp. 138-44. ISSN 1061-4036 (Print).

Kuivaniemi, H., G. Tromp and D. J. Prockop, (1997). Mutations in fibrillar collagens (types I, II, III, and XI), fibril-associated collagen (type IX), and network-forming collagen (type X) cause a spectrum of diseases of bone, cartilage, and blood vessels, *Hum Mutat.* Vol 9, No. 4, pp. 300-15.

Kämäräinen, O. P. The search for susceptibility genes in osteoarthritis, PhD thesis. Faculty of Medicine, University of Oulu, Acta Univ. Oul. D 1018, Oulu, Finland (2009) 112 p.

Kämäräinen, O. P., S. Solovieva, T. Vehmas, K. Luoma, P. Leino-Arjas, H. Riihimäki, L. Ala-Kokko and M. Männikkö, (2006). Aggrecan core protein of a certain length is protective against hand osteoarthritis, *Osteoarthritis Cartilage.* Vol 14, No. 10, pp. 1075-80. ISSN 1063-4584 (Print) 1063-4584 (Linking).

Kämäräinen, O. P., S. Solovieva, T. Vehmas, K. Luoma, H. Riihimäki, L. Ala-Kokko, M. Männikkö and P. Leino-Arjas, (2008). Common interleukin-6 promoter variants associate with the more severe forms of distal interphalangeal osteoarthritis, *Arthritis Res Ther.* Vol 10, No. 1, pp. R21. ISSN 1478-6362 (Electronic) 1478-6354 (Linking).

Lane, N. E., K. Lian, M. C. Nevitt, J. M. Zmuda, L. Lui, J. Li, J. Wang, M. Fontecha, N. Umblas, M. Rosenbach, P. de Leon and M. Corr, (2006). Frizzled-related protein variants are risk factors for hip osteoarthritis, *Arthritis Rheum.* Vol 54, No. 4, pp. 1246-54. ISSN 0004-3591 (Print) 0004-3591 (Linking).

Lango Allen, H., K. Estrada, G. Lettre, S. I. Berndt, M. N. Weedon, F. Rivadeneira, C. J. Willer, A. U. Jackson, S. Vedantam, S. Raychaudhuri, T. Ferreira, A. R. Wood, R. J. Weyant, A. V. Segre, E. K. Speliotes, E. Wheeler, N. Soranzo, J. H. Park, J. Yang, D. Gudbjartsson, et al., (2010). Hundreds of variants clustered in genomic loci and biological pathways affect human height, *Nature.* Vol 467, No. 7317, pp. 832-8. ISSN 0028-0836.

Lee, Y. H., Y. H. Rho, S. J. Choi, J. D. Ji and G. G. Song, (2006). Osteoarthritis susceptibility loci defined by genome scan meta-analysis, *Rheumatol Int.* Vol 26, No. 11, pp. 959-63. ISSN 0172-8172 (Print) 0172-8172 (Linking).

Lee, Y. H., J. H. Woo, S. J. Choi, J. D. Ji and G. G. Song, (2009). Vitamin D receptor TaqI, BsmI and ApaI polymorphisms and osteoarthritis susceptibility: a meta-analysis, *Joint Bone Spine.* Vol 76, No. 2, pp. 156-61. ISSN 1778-7254 (Electronic) 1297-319X (Linking).

Leppävuori, J., U. Kujala, J. Kinnunen, J. Kaprio, M. Nissilä, M. Heliövaara, N. Klinger, J. Partanen, J. D. Terwilliger and L. Peltonen, (1999). Genome scan for predisposing loci for distal interphalangeal joint osteoarthritis: evidence for a locus on 2q, *Am J Hum Genet.* Vol 65, No. 4, pp. 1060-7. ISSN 0002-9297 (Print) 0002-9297 (Linking).

Li, J. and L. Ji, (2005). Adjusting multiple testing in multilocus analyses using the eigenvalues of a correlation matrix, *Heredity.* Vol 95, No. 3, pp. 221-227.

Livshits, G., B. S. Kato, G. Zhai, D. J. Hart, D. Hunter, A. J. MacGregor, F. M. Williams and T. D. Spector, (2007). Genomewide linkage scan of hand osteoarthritis in female twin pairs showing replication of quantitative trait loci on chromosomes 2 and 19, *Ann Rheum Dis.* Vol 66, No. 5, pp. 623-627. ISSN

Loughlin, J., (2001). Genetic epidemiology of primary osteoarthritis, *Curr Opin Rheumatol.* Vol 13, No. 2, pp. 111-6. ISSN

Loughlin, J., (2005). The genetic epidemiology of human primary osteoarthritis: current status, *Expert Rev Mol Med*. Vol 7, No. 9, pp. 1-12. ISSN 1462-3994 (Electronic)

Loughlin, J., B. Dowling, K. Chapman, L. Marcelline, Z. Mustafa, L. Southam, A. Ferreira, C. Ciesielski, D. A. Carson and M. Corr, (2004). Functional variants within the secreted frizzled-related protein 3 gene are associated with hip osteoarthritis in females, *Proc Natl Acad Sci U S A*. Vol 101, No. 26, pp. 9757-62. ISSN 0027-8424 (Print).

Loughlin, J., B. Dowling, Z. Mustafa and K. Chapman, (2002a). Association of the interleukin-1 gene cluster on chromosome 2q13 with knee osteoarthritis, *Arthritis Rheum*. Vol 46, No. 6, pp. 1519-1527. ISSN 0004-3591.

Loughlin, J., B. Dowling, Z. Mustafa, L. Southam and K. Chapman, (2002b). Refined linkage mapping of a hip osteoarthritis susceptibility locus on chromosome 2q, *Rheumatology (Oxford)*. Vol 41, No. 8, pp. 955-6. ISSN 1462-0324 (Print) 1462-0324 (Linking).

Loughlin, J., Z. Mustafa, B. Dowling, L. Southam, L. Marcelline, S. S. Raina, L. Ala-Kokko and K. Chapman, (2002c). Finer linkage mapping of a primary hip osteoarthritis susceptibility locus on chromosome 6, *Eur J Hum Genet*. Vol 10, No. 9, pp. 562-8. ISSN 1018-4813 (Print) 1018-4813 (Linking).

Loughlin, J., Z. Mustafa, C. Irven, A. Smith, A. J. Carr, B. Sykes and K. Chapman, (1999). Stratification analysis of an osteoarthritis genome screen-suggestive linkage to chromosomes 4, 6, and 16, *Am J Hum Genet*. Vol 65, No. 6, pp. 1795-8. ISSN 0002-9297 (Print) 0002-9297 (Linking).

Loughlin, J., Z. Mustafa, A. Smith, C. Irven, A. J. Carr, K. Clipsham, J. Chitnavis, V. A. Bloomfield, M. McCartney, O. Cox, J. S. Sinsheimer, B. Sykes and K. E. Chapman, (2000). Linkage analysis of chromosome 2q in osteoarthritis, *Rheumatology (Oxford)*. Vol 39, No. 4, pp. 377-381.

Loughlin, J., J. S. Sinsheimer, A. Carr and K. Chapman, (2006). The CALM1 core promoter polymorphism is not associated with hip osteoarthritis in a United Kingdom Caucasian population, *Osteoarthritis Cartilage*. Vol 14, No. 3, pp. 295-8.

Mabuchi, A., S. Nakamura, Y. Takatori and S. Ikegawa, (2006). Familial osteoarthritis of the hip joint associated with acetabular dysplasia maps to chromosome 13q, *Am J Hum Genet*. Vol 79, No. 1, pp. 163-8. ISSN 0002-9297 (Print) 0002-9297 (Linking).

MacGregor, A. J., L. Antoniades, M. Matson, T. Andrew and T. D. Spector, (2000). The genetic contribution to radiographic hip osteoarthritis in women: results of a classic twin study, *Arthritis Rheum*. Vol 43, No. 11, pp. 2410-6.

Manolio, T. A., F. S. Collins, N. J. Cox, D. B. Goldstein, L. A. Hindorff, D. J. Hunter, M. I. McCarthy, E. M. Ramos, L. R. Cardon, A. Chakravarti, J. H. Cho, A. E. Guttmacher, A. Kong, L. Kruglyak, E. Mardis, C. N. Rotimi, M. Slatkin, D. Valle, A. S. Whittemore, M. Boehnke, et al., (2009). Finding the missing heritability of complex diseases, *Nature*. Vol 461, No. 7265, pp. 747-53. ISSN 1476-4687 (Electronic) 0028-0836 (Linking).

Meulenbelt, I., C. Bijkerk, S. C. De Wildt, H. S. Miedema, F. C. Breedveld, H. A. Pols, A. Hofman, C. M. Van Duijn and P. E. Slagboom, (1999). Haplotype analysis of three polymorphisms of the COL2A1 gene and associations with generalised radiological osteoarthritis, *Ann Hum Genet*. Vol 63, No. Pt 5, pp. 393-400. ISSN 0003-4800 (Print) 0003-4800 (Linking).

Meulenbelt, I., C. Bijkerk, H. S. Miedema, F. C. Breedveld, A. Hofman, H. A. Valkenburg, H. A. Pols, P. E. Slagboom and C. M. van Duijn, (1998). A genetic association study of the IGF-1 gene and radiological osteoarthritis in a population-based cohort study (the Rotterdam Study), *Ann Rheum Dis.* Vol 57, No. 6, pp. 371-4. ISSN 0003-4967 (Print) 0003-4967 (Linking).

Meulenbelt, I., S. D. Bos, K. Chapman, R. van der Breggen, J. J. Houwing-Duistermaat, D. Kremer, M. Kloppenburg, A. Carr, A. Tsezou, A. Gonzalez, J. Loughlin and P. E. Slagboom, (2011). Meta-analyses of genes modulating intracellular T3 bio-availability reveal a possible role for the DIO3 gene in osteoarthritis susceptibility, *Ann Rheum Dis.* Vol 70, No. 1, pp. 164-7.

Meulenbelt, I., K. Chapman, R. Dieguez-Gonzalez, D. Shi, A. Tsezou, J. Dai, K. N. Malizos, M. Kloppenburg, A. Carr, M. Nakajima, R. van der Breggen, N. Lakenberg, J. J. Gomez-Reino, Q. Jiang, S. Ikegawa, A. Gonzalez, J. Loughlin and E. P. Slagboom, (2009). Large Replication Study and Meta-Analyses of Dvwa as an Osteoarthritis Susceptibility Locus in European and Asian Populations, *Hum Mol Genet.* Vol, No. ISSN 1460-2083 (Electronic).

Meulenbelt, I., J. L. Min, S. Bos, N. Riyazi, J. J. Houwing-Duistermaat, H. J. van der Wijk, H. M. Kroon, M. Nakajima, S. Ikegawa, A. G. Uitterlinden, J. B. van Meurs, W. M. van der Deure, T. J. Visser, A. B. Seymour, N. Lakenberg, R. van der Breggen, D. Kremer, C. M. van Duijn, M. Kloppenburg, J. Loughlin, et al., (2008). Identification of DIO2 as a new susceptibility locus for symptomatic osteoarthritis, *Hum Mol Genet.* Vol 17, No. 12, pp. 1867-75. ISSN 1460-2083 (Electronic).

Meulenbelt, I., J. L. Min, C. M. van Duijn, M. Kloppenburg, F. C. Breedveld and P. E. Slagboom, (2006). Strong linkage on 2q33.3 to familial early-onset generalized osteoarthritis and a consideration of two positional candidate genes, *Eur J Hum Genet.* Vol 14, No. 12, pp. 1280-7. ISSN 1018-4813 (Print) 1018-4813 (Linking).

Meulenbelt, I., A. B. Seymour, M. Nieuwland, T. W. Huizinga, C. M. van Duijn and P. E. Slagboom, (2004). Association of the interleukin-1 gene cluster with radiographic signs of osteoarthritis of the hip, *Arthritis Rheum.* Vol 50, No. 4, pp. 1179-1186. ISSN 0004-3591.

Min, J. L., I. Meulenbelt, M. Kloppenburg, C. M. van Duijn and P. E. Slagboom, (2007). Mutation analysis of candidate genes within the 2q33.3 linkage area for familial early-onset generalised osteoarthritis, *Eur J Hum Genet.* Vol 15, No. 7, pp. 791-9. 1018-4813 (Print) 1018-4813 (Linking).

Min, J. L., I. Meulenbelt, N. Riyazi, M. Kloppenburg, J. J. Houwing-Duistermaat, A. B. Seymour, H. A. Pols, C. M. van Duijn and P. E. Slagboom, (2005). Association of the Frizzled-related protein gene with symptomatic osteoarthritis at multiple sites, *Arthritis Rheum.* Vol 52, No. 4, pp. 1077-80. 0004-3591 (Print) 0004-3591 (Linking).

Miyamoto, Y., A. Mabuchi, D. Shi, T. Kubo, Y. Takatori, S. Saito, M. Fujioka, A. Sudo, A. Uchida, S. Yamamoto, K. Ozaki, M. Takigawa, T. Tanaka, Y. Nakamura, Q. Jiang and S. Ikegawa, (2007). A functional polymorphism in the 5' UTR of GDF5 is associated with susceptibility to osteoarthritis, *Nat Genet.* Vol 39, No. 4, pp. 529-33. 1061-4036 (Print).

Miyamoto, Y., D. Shi, M. Nakajima, K. Ozaki, A. Sudo, A. Kotani, A. Uchida, T. Tanaka, N. Fukui, T. Tsunoda, A. Takahashi, Y. Nakamura, Q. Jiang and S. Ikegawa, (2008). Common variants in DVWA on chromosome 3p24.3 are associated with susceptibility to knee osteoarthritis, *Nat Genet*. Vol 40, No. 8, pp. 994-8. 1546-1718 (Electronic).

Moos, V., M. Rudwaleit, V. Herzog, K. Hohlig, J. Sieper and B. Muller, (2000). Association of genotypes affecting the expression of interleukin-1beta or interleukin-1 receptor antagonist with osteoarthritis, *Arthritis Rheum*. Vol 43, No. 11, pp. 2417-2422. ISSN 0004-3591.

Mototani, H., A. Mabuchi, S. Saito, M. Fujioka, A. Iida, Y. Takatori, A. Kotani, T. Kubo, K. Nakamura, A. Sekine, Y. Murakami, T. Tsunoda, K. Notoya, Y. Nakamura and S. Ikegawa, (2005). A functional single nucleotide polymorphism in the core promoter region of CALM1 is associated with hip osteoarthritis in Japanese, *Hum Mol Genet*. Vol 14, No. 8, pp. 1009-17.

Mustafa, Z., B. Dowling, K. Chapman, J. S. Sinsheimer, A. Carr and J. Loughlin, (2005). Investigating the aspartic acid (D) repeat of asporin as a risk factor for osteoarthritis in a UK Caucasian population, *Arthritis Rheum*. Vol 52, No. 11, pp. 3502-6. 0004-3591 (Print) 0004-3591 (Linking).

Mäkelä-Bengs, P., N. Järvinen, K. Vuopala, A. Suomalainen, J. Ignatius, M. Sipilä, R. Herva, A. Palotie and L. Peltonen, (1998). Assignment of the disease locus for lethal congenital contracture syndrome to a restricted region of chromosome 9q34, by genome scan using five affected individuals, *Am J Hum Genet*. Vol 63, No. 2, pp. 506-16. 0002-9297 (Print) 0002-9297 (Linking).

Nakajima, M., A. Takahashi, I. Kou, C. Rodriguez-Fontenla, J. J. Gomez-Reino, T. Furuichi, J. Dai, A. Sudo, A. Uchida, N. Fukui, M. Kubo, N. Kamatani, T. Tsunoda, K. N. Malizos, A. Tsezou, A. Gonzalez, Y. Nakamura and S. Ikegawa, (2010). New sequence variants in HLA class II/III region associated with susceptibility to knee osteoarthritis identified by genome-wide association study, *PLoS One*. Vol 5, No. 3, pp. e9723. 1932-6203 (Electronic) 1932-6203 (Linking).

Nakamura, T., D. Shi, M. Tzetis, J. Rodriguez-Lopez, Y. Miyamoto, A. Tsezou, A. Gonzalez, Q. Jiang, N. Kamatani, J. Loughlin and S. Ikegawa, (2007). Meta-analysis of association between the ASPN D-repeat and osteoarthritis, *Hum Mol Genet*. Vol 16, No. 14, pp. 1676-81. 0964-6906 (Print).

Näkki, A., T. Videman, U. M. Kujala, M. Suhonen, M. Männikkö, L. Peltonen, M. C. Battie, J. Kaprio and J. Saarela, (2011). Candidate gene association study of magnetic resonance imaging-based hip osteoarthritis (OA): evidence for COL9A2 gene as a common predisposing factor for hip OA and lumbar disc degeneration, *J Rheumatol*. Vol 38, No. 4, pp. 747-52. 0315-162X (Print) 0315-162X (Linking).

Nousiainen, H. O., M. Kestilä, N. Pakkasjärvi H. Honkala, S. Kuure, J. Tallila, K. Vuopala, J. Ignatius, R. Herva and L. Peltonen, (2008). Mutations in mRNA export mediator GLE1 result in a fetal motoneuron disease, *Nat Genet*. Vol 40, No. 2, pp. 155-7. 1546-1718 (Electronic) 1061-4036 (Linking).

Nyholt, D. R., (2004). A simple correction for multiple testing for single-nucleotide polymorphisms in linkage disequilibrium with each other, *Am J Hum Genet*. Vol 74, No. 4, pp. 765-9.

Näkki, A., S. T. Kouhia, J. Saarela, A. Harilainen, K. Tallroth, T. Videman, M. C. Battie, J. Kaprio, L. Peltonen and U. M. Kujala, (2010). Allelic variants of IL1R1 gene associate with severe hand osteoarthritis, *BMC Med Genet*. Vol 11, No. 1, pp. 50. 1471-2350 (Electronic) 1471-2350 (Linking).

O'Dowd, B. F., T. Nguyen, B. P. Jung, A. Marchese, R. Cheng, H. H. Heng, L. F. Kolakowski, Jr., K. R. Lynch and S. R. George, (1997). Cloning and chromosomal mapping of four putative novel human G-protein-coupled receptor genes, *Gene*. Vol 187, No. 1, pp. 75-81. 0378-1119 (Print) 0378-1119 (Linking).

Oen, K., P. N. Malleson, D. A. Cabral, A. M. Rosenberg, R. E. Petty, P. Nickerson and M. Reed, (2005). Cytokine genotypes correlate with pain and radiologically defined joint damage in patients with juvenile rheumatoid arthritis, *Rheumatology (Oxford)*. Vol 44, No. 9, pp. 1115-21. 1462-0324 (Print) 1462-0324 (Linking).

Paassilta, P., J. Lohiniva, S. Annunen, J. Bonaventure, M. Le Merrer, L. Pai and L. Ala-Kokko, (1999). COL9A3: A third locus for multiple epiphyseal dysplasia, *Am J Hum Genet*. Vol 64, No. 4, pp. 1036-44. 0002-9297 (Print) 0002-9297 (Linking).

Paesold-Burda, P., C. Maag, H. Troxler, F. Foulquier, P. Kleinert, S. Schnabel, M. Baumgartner and T. Hennet, (2009). Deficiency in COG5 causes a moderate form of congenital disorders of glycosylation, *Hum Mol Genet*. Vol 18, No. 22, pp. 4350-6. 1460-2083 (Electronic) 0964-6906 (Linking).

Page, W. F., F. T. Hoaglund, L. S. Steinbach and A. C. Heath, (2003). Primary osteoarthritis of the hip in monozygotic and dizygotic male twins, *Twin Res*. Vol 6, No. 2, pp. 147-51.

Palotie, A., P. Väisänen, J. Ott, L. Ryhänen, K. Elima, M. Vikkula, K. Cheah, E. Vuorio and L. Peltonen, (1989). Predisposition to familial osteoarthrosis linked to type II collagen gene, *Lancet*. Vol 1, No. 8644, pp. 924-7. 0140-6736 (Print) 0140-6736 (Linking).

Panoutsopoulou, K., L. Southam, K. S. Elliott, N. Wrayner, G. Zhai, C. Beazley, G. Thorleifsson, N. K. Arden, A. Carr, K. Chapman, P. Deloukas, M. Doherty, A. McCaskie, W. E. Ollier, S. H. Ralston, T. D. Spector, A. M. Valdes, G. A. Wallis, J. M. Wilkinson, E. Arden, et al., (2011). Insights into the genetic architecture of osteoarthritis from stage 1 of the arcOGEN study, *Ann Rheum Dis*. Vol 70, No. 5, pp. 864-7.

Paquet, M. E., M. Cohen-Doyle, G. C. Shore and D. B. Williams, (2004). Bap29/31 influences the intracellular traffic of MHC class I molecules, *J Immunol*. Vol 172, No. 12, pp. 7548-55. 0022-1767 (Print) 0022-1767 (Linking).

Patterson, K., (2011). 1000 GENOMES: A World of Variation, *Circ Res*. Vol 108, No. 5, pp. 534-6. 1524-4571 (Electronic) 0009-7330 (Linking).

Petrukhin, K. E., M. C. Speer, E. Cayanis, M. F. Bonaldo, U. Tantravahi, M. B. Soares, S. G. Fischer, D. Warburton, T. C. Gilliam and J. Ott, (1993). A microsatellite genetic linkage map of human chromosome 13, *Genomics*. Vol 15, No. 1, pp. 76-85.

Plomin, R., C. M. Haworth and O. S. Davis, (2009). Common disorders are quantitative traits, *Nat Rev Genet*. Vol 10, No. 12, pp. 872-8. 1471-0064 (Electronic) 1471-0056 (Linking).

Prockop, D. J., L. Ala-Kokko, D. A. McLain and C. Williams, (1997). Can mutated genes cause common osteoarthritis?, *Br J Rheumatol*. Vol 36, No. 8, pp. 827-9. 0263-7103 (Print) 0263-7103 (Linking).

Pullig, O., G. Weseloh, A. R. Klatt, R. Wagener and B. Swoboda, (2002). Matrilin-3 in human articular cartilage: increased expression in osteoarthritis, *Osteoarthritis Cartilage*. Vol 10, No. 4, pp. 253-63. 1063-4584 (Print).

Pullig, O., A. Tagariello, A. Schweizer, B. Swoboda, P. Schaller and A. Winterpacht, (2007). MATN3 (matrilin-3) sequence variation (pT303M) is a risk factor for osteoarthritis of the CMC1 joint of the hand, but not for knee osteoarthritis, *Ann Rheum Dis*. Vol 66, No. 2, pp. 279-80. 1468-2060 (Electronic).

Purcell, S., S. S. Cherny and P. C. Sham, (2003). Genetic Power Calculator: design of linkage and association genetic mapping studies of complex traits, *Bioinformatics*. Vol 19, No. 1, pp. 149-50.

Purcell, S., B. Neale, K. Todd-Brown, L. Thomas, M. A. Ferreira, D. Bender, J. Maller, P. Sklar, P. I. de Bakker, M. J. Daly and P. C. Sham, (2007). PLINK: a tool set for whole-genome association and population-based linkage analyses, *Am J Hum Genet*. Vol 81, No. 3, pp. 559-75.

Robbins, J. R., B. Thomas, L. Tan, B. Choy, J. L. Arbiser, F. Berenbaum and M. B. Goldring, (2000). Immortalized human adult articular chondrocytes maintain cartilage-specific phenotype and responses to interleukin-1beta, *Arthritis Rheum*. Vol 43, No. 10, pp. 2189-201. 0004-3591 (Print).

Robin, N. H., R. T. Moran, M. Warman and L. Ala-Kokko, (2010). Stickler Syndrome. Vol, No.

Roughley, P. J. and E. R. Lee, (1994). Cartilage proteoglycans: structure and potential functions, *Microsc Res Tech*. Vol 28, No. 5, pp. 385-97. 1059-910X (Print) 1059-910X (Linking).

Ryder, J. J., K. Garrison, F. Song, L. Hooper, J. Skinner, Y. Loke, J. Loughlin, J. P. Higgins and A. J. MacGregor, (2008). Genetic associations in peripheral joint osteoarthritis and spinal degenerative disease: a systematic review, *Ann Rheum Dis*. Vol 67, No. 5, pp. 584-91. 1468-2060 (Electronic).

Sampson, E. M., Z. K. Haque, M. C. Ku, S. G. Tevosian, C. Albanese, R. G. Pestell, K. E. Paulson and A. S. Yee, (2001). Negative regulation of the Wnt-beta-catenin pathway by the transcriptional repressor HBP1, *EMBO J*. Vol 20, No. 16, pp. 4500-11. ISSN 0261-4189 (Print) 0261-4189 (Linking).

Sandy, J. D., C. R. Flannery, P. J. Neame and L. S. Lohmander, (1992). The structure of aggrecan fragments in human synovial fluid. Evidence for the involvement in osteoarthritis of a novel proteinase which cleaves the Glu 373-Ala 374 bond of the interglobular domain, *J Clin Invest*. Vol 89, No. 5, pp. 1512-6. ISSN 0021-9738 (Print) 0021-9738 (Linking).

Seguin, C. A. and S. M. Bernier, (2003). TNFalpha suppresses link protein and type II collagen expression in chondrocytes: Role of MEK1/2 and NF-kappaB signaling pathways, *J Cell Physiol*. Vol 197, No. 3, pp. 356-69. ISSN 0021-9541 (Print).

Shi, D., T. Nakamura, J. Dai, L. Yi, J. Qin, D. Chen, Z. Xu, Y. Wang, S. Ikegawa and Q. Jiang, (2007). Association of the aspartic acid-repeat polymorphism in the asporin gene with age at onset of knee osteoarthritis in Han Chinese population, *J Hum Genet*. Vol 52, No. 8, pp. 664-7. ISSN 1434-5161 (Print) 1434-5161 (Linking).

Silventoinen, K., S. Sammalisto, M. Perola, D. I. Boomsma, B. K. Cornes, C. Davis, L. Dunkel, M. De Lange, J. R. Harris, J. V. Hjelmborg, M. Luciano, N. G. Martin, J. Mortensen, L. Nistico, N. L. Pedersen, A. Skytthe, T. D. Spector, M. A. Stazi, G. Willemsen and J. Kaprio, (2003). Heritability of adult body height: a comparative study of twin cohorts in eight countries, *Twin Res*. Vol 6, No. 5, pp. 399-408.

Solovieva, S., A. Hirvonen, P. Siivola, T. Vehmas, K. Luoma, H. Riihimäki and P. Leino-Arjas, (2006). Vitamin D receptor gene polymorphisms and susceptibility of hand osteoarthritis in Finnish women, *Arthritis Res Ther*. Vol 8, No. 1, pp. R20. ISSN 1478-6362 (Electronic) 1478-6354 (Linking).

Solovieva, S., O.-P. Kämäräinen, A. Hirvonen, S. Hämäläinen, M. Laitala, T. Vehmas, K. Luoma, A. Näkki, H. Riihimäki, L. Ala-Kokko, M. Männikkö and P. Leino-Arjas, (2009). Association between interleukin 1 gene cluster polymorphisms and bilateral dip osteoarthritis, *The Journal of Rheumatology*. Vol 36, No. 9, pp. 1977-1986. ISSN

Song, R. H., M. D. Tortorella, A. M. Malfait, J. T. Alston, Z. Yang, E. C. Arner and D. W. Griggs, (2007). Aggrecan degradation in human articular cartilage explants is mediated by both ADAMTS-4 and ADAMTS-5, *Arthritis Rheum*. Vol 56, No. 2, pp. 575-85. ISSN 0004-3591 (Print) 0004-3591 (Linking).

Southam, L., B. Dowling, A. Ferreira, L. Marcelline, Z. Mustafa, K. Chapman, G. Bentham, A. Carr and J. Loughlin, (2004). Microsatellite association mapping of a primary osteoarthritis susceptibility locus on chromosome 6p12.3-q13, *Arthritis Rheum*. Vol 50, No. 12, pp. 3910-4. ISSN 0004-3591 (Print) 0004-3591 (Linking).

Southam, L., J. Rodriguez-Lopez, J. M. Wilkins, M. Pombo-Suarez, S. Snelling, J. J. Gomez-Reino, K. Chapman, A. Gonzalez and J. Loughlin, (2007). An SNP in the 5'-UTR of GDF5 is associated with osteoarthritis susceptibility in Europeans and with in vivo differences in allelic expression in articular cartilage, *Hum Mol Genet*. Vol 16, No. 18, pp. 2226-32. ISSN 0964-6906 (Print) 0964-6906 (Linking).

Spector, T. D., R. H. Reneland, S. Mah, A. M. Valdes, D. J. Hart, S. Kammerer, M. Langdown, C. R. Hoyal, J. Atienza, M. Doherty, P. Rahman, M. R. Nelson and A. Braun, (2006). Association between a variation in LRCH1 and knee osteoarthritis: a genome-wide single-nucleotide polymorphism association study using DNA pooling, *Arthritis Rheum*. Vol 54, No. 2, pp. 524-32. ISSN 0004-3591 (Print).

Speliotes, E. K., C. J. Willer, S. I. Berndt, K. L. Monda, G. Thorleifsson, A. U. Jackson, H. L. Allen, C. M. Lindgren, J. Luan, R. Magi, J. C. Randall, S. Vedantam, T. W. Winkler, L. Qi, T. Workalemahu, I. M. Heid, V. Steinthorsdottir, H. M. Stringham, M. N. Weedon, E. Wheeler, et al., (2010). Association analyses of 249,796 individuals reveal 18 new loci associated with body mass index, *Nat Genet*. Vol 42, No. 11, pp. 937-48. ISSN 1546-1718 (Electronic) 1061-4036 (Linking).

Stefansson, S. E., H. Jonsson, T. Ingvarsson, I. Manolescu, H. H. Jonsson, G. Olafsdottir, E. Palsdottir, G. Stefansdottir, G. Sveinbjornsdottir, M. L. Frigge, A. Kong, J. R. Gulcher and K. Stefansson, (2003). Genomewide scan for hand osteoarthritis: a novel mutation in matrilin-3, *Am J Hum Genet*. Vol 72, No. 6, pp. 1448-59. ISSN 0002-9297 (Print).

Stern, A. G., M. R. de Carvalho, G. A. Buck, R. A. Adler, T. P. Rao, D. Disler and G. Moxley, (2003). Association of erosive hand osteoarthritis with a single nucleotide polymorphism on the gene encoding interleukin-1 beta, *Osteoarthritis Cartilage*. Vol 11, No. 6, pp. 394-402. ISSN 1063-4584 (Print) 1063-4584 (Linking).

Storm, E. E., T. V. Huynh, N. G. Copeland, N. A. Jenkins, D. M. Kingsley and S. J. Lee, (1994). Limb alterations in brachypodism mice due to mutations in a new member of the TGF beta-superfamily, *Nature*. Vol 368, No. 6472, pp. 639-43. ISSN 0028-0836 (Print).

Straub, R. E., M. C. Speer, Y. Luo, K. Rojas, J. Overhauser, J. Ott and T. C. Gilliam, (1993). A microsatellite genetic linkage map of human chromosome 18, *Genomics*. Vol 15, No. 1, pp. 48-56.

Tetlow, L. C., D. J. Adlam and D. E. Woolley, (2001). Matrix metalloproteinase and proinflammatory cytokine production by chondrocytes of human osteoarthritic cartilage: associations with degenerative changes, *Arthritis Rheum*. Vol 44, No. 3, pp. 585-94. ISSN 0004-3591 (Print).

Thomas, J. T., K. Lin, M. Nandedkar, M. Camargo, J. Cervenka and F. P. Luyten, (1996). A human chondrodysplasia due to a mutation in a TGF-beta superfamily member, *Nat Genet*. Vol 12, No. 3, pp. 315-7. ISSN 1061-4036 (Print).

Tortorella, M. D., R. Q. Liu, T. Burn, R. C. Newton and E. Arner, (2002). Characterization of human aggrecanase 2 (ADAM-TS5): substrate specificity studies and comparison with aggrecanase 1 (ADAM-TS4), *Matrix Biol*. Vol 21, No. 6, pp. 499-511. ISSN 0945-053X (Print) 0945-053X (Linking).

Tsai, C. L. and T. K. Liu, (1992). Osteoarthritis in women: its relationship to estrogen and current trends, *Life Sci*. Vol 50, No. 23, pp. 1737-44. ISSN 0024-3205 (Print).

Uitterlinden, A. G., H. Burger, Q. Huang, E. Odding, C. M. Duijn, A. Hofman, J. C. Birkenhager, J. P. van Leeuwen and H. A. Pols, (1997). Vitamin D receptor genotype is associated with radiographic osteoarthritis at the knee, *J Clin Invest*. Vol 100, No. 2, pp. 259-63. ISSN 0021-9738 (Print) 0021-9738 (Linking).

Uitterlinden, A. G., H. Burger, C. M. van Duijn, Q. Huang, A. Hofman, J. C. Birkenhager, J. P. van Leeuwen and H. A. Pols, (2000). Adjacent genes, for COL2A1 and the vitamin D receptor, are associated with separate features of radiographic osteoarthritis of the knee, *Arthritis Rheum*. Vol 43, No. 7, pp. 1456-64. ISSN 0004-3591 (Print) 0004-3591 (Linking).

Ungar, D., T. Oka, E. E. Brittle, E. Vasile, V. V. Lupashin, J. E. Chatterton, J. E. Heuser, M. Krieger and M. G. Waters, (2002). Characterization of a mammalian Golgi-localized protein complex, COG, that is required for normal Golgi morphology and function, *J Cell Biol*. Vol 157, No. 3, pp. 405-15. ISSN 0021-9525 (Print) 0021-9525 (Linking).

Ushiyama, T., H. Ueyama, K. Inoue, J. Nishioka, I. Ohkubo and S. Hukuda, (1998). Estrogen receptor gene polymorphism and generalized osteoarthritis, *J Rheumatol*. Vol 25, No. 1, pp. 134-7. ISSN 0315-162X (Print) 0315-162X (Linking).

Vaes, R. B., F. Rivadeneira, J. M. Kerkhof, A. Hofman, H. A. Pols, A. G. Uitterlinden and J. B. van Meurs, (2009). Genetic variation in the GDF5 region is associated with osteoarthritis, height, hip axis length and fracture risk: the Rotterdam study, *Ann Rheum Dis*. Vol 68, No. 11, pp. 1754-60. ISSN 1468-2060 (Electronic) 0003-4967 (Linking).

Wagener, R., S. K. Gara, B. Kobbe, M. Paulsson and F. Zaucke, (2009). The knee osteoarthritis susceptibility locus DVWA on chromosome 3p24.3 is the 5' part of the split COL6A4 gene, *Matrix Biol*. Vol 28, No. 6, pp. 307-10. ISSN

Valdes, A. M., N. K. Arden, A. Tamm, K. Kisand, S. Doherty, E. Pola, C. Cooper, K. R. Muir, I. Kerna, D. Hart, F. O'Neil, W. Zhang, T. D. Spector, R. A. Maciewicz and M. Doherty, (2010a). A meta-analysis of interleukin-6 promoter polymorphisms on risk of hip and knee osteoarthritis, *Osteoarthritis Cartilage*. Vol 18, No. 5, pp. 699-704. ISSN 1522-9653 (Electronic) 1063-4584 (Linking).

Valdes, A. M., R. J. Lories, J. B. van Meurs, H. Kerkhof, S. Doherty, A. Hofman, D. J. Hart, F. Zhang, F. P. Luyten, A. G. Uitterlinden, M. Doherty and T. D. Spector, (2009a). Variation at the ANP32A gene is associated with risk of hip osteoarthritis in women, *Arthritis Rheum*. Vol 60, No. 7, pp. 2046-54. ISSN 0004-3591.

Valdes, A. M., J. Loughlin, M. V. Oene, K. Chapman, G. L. Surdulescu, M. Doherty and T. D. Spector, (2007). Sex and ethnic differences in the association of ASPN, CALM1, COL2A1, COMP, and FRZB with genetic susceptibility to osteoarthritis of the knee, *Arthritis Rheum*. Vol 56, No. 1, pp. 137-46. ISSN 0004-3591 (Print) 0004-3591 (Linking).

Valdes, A. M., J. Loughlin, K. M. Timms, J. J. van Meurs, L. Southam, S. G. Wilson, S. Doherty, R. J. Lories, F. P. Luyten, A. Gutin, V. Abkevich, D. Ge, A. Hofman, A. G. Uitterlinden, D. J. Hart, F. Zhang, G. Zhai, R. J. Egli, M. Doherty, J. Lanchbury, et al., (2008). Genome-wide association scan identifies a prostaglandin-endoperoxide synthase 2 variant involved in risk of knee osteoarthritis, *Am J Hum Genet*. Vol 82, No. 6, pp. 1231-40. ISSN 1537-6605 (Electronic).

Valdes, A. M., T. D. Spector, S. Doherty, M. Wheeler, D. J. Hart and M. Doherty, (2009b). Association of the DVWA and GDF5 polymorphisms with osteoarthritis in UK populations, *Ann Rheum Dis*. Vol 68, No. 12, pp. 1916-20. ISSN 1468-2060 (Electronic) 0003-4967 (Linking).

Valdes, A. M., T. D. Spector, A. Tamm, K. Kisand, S. A. Doherty, E. M. Dennison, M. Mangino, I. Kerna, D. J. Hart, M. Wheeler, C. Cooper, R. J. Lories, N. K. Arden and M. Doherty, (2010b). Genetic variation in the SMAD3 gene is associated with hip and knee osteoarthritis, *Arthritis Rheum*. Vol 62, No. 8, pp. 2347-52. ISSN 1529-0131 (Electronic) 0004-3591 (Linking).

WellcomeTrustCaseControlConsortium, (2007). Genome-wide association study of 14,000 cases of seven common diseases and 3,000 shared controls, *Nature*. Vol 447, No. 7145, pp. 661-78. ISSN 0028-0836.

Vikkula, M., A. Palotie, P. Ritvaniemi, J. Ott, L. Ala-Kokko, U. Sievers, K. Aho and L. Peltonen, (1993). Early-onset osteoarthritis linked to the type II procollagen gene. Detailed clinical phenotype and further analyses of the gene, *Arthritis Rheum*. Vol 36, No. 3, pp. 401-9. ISSN 0004-3591 (Print) 0004-3591 (Linking).

Wu, Q., K. O. Kim, E. R. Sampson, D. Chen, H. Awad, T. O'Brien, J. E. Puzas, H. Drissi, E. M. Schwarz, R. J. O'Keefe, M. J. Zuscik and R. N. Rosier, (2008). Induction of an osteoarthritis-like phenotype and degradation of phosphorylated Smad3 by Smurf2 in transgenic mice, *Arthritis Rheum*. Vol 58, No. 10, pp. 3132-44. ISSN 0004-3591 (Print) 0004-3591 (Linking).

Zhai, G., D. J. Hart, B. S. Kato, A. MacGregor and T. D. Spector, (2007). Genetic influence on the progression of radiographic knee osteoarthritis: a longitudinal twin study, *Osteoarthritis Cartilage*. Vol 15, No. 2, pp. 222-5. ISSN 1063-4584 (Print) 1063-4584 (Linking).

Zhai, G., F. Rivadeneira, J. J. Houwing-Duistermaat, I. Meulenbelt, C. Bijkerk, A. Hofman, J. B. van Meurs, A. G. Uitterlinden, H. A. Pols, P. E. Slagboom and C. M. van Duijn, (2004). Insulin-like growth factor I gene promoter polymorphism, collagen type II alpha1 (COL2A1) gene, and the prevalence of radiographic osteoarthritis: the Rotterdam Study, *Ann Rheum Dis*. Vol 63, No. 5, pp. 544-8. ISSN 0003-4967 (Print) 0003-4967 (Linking).

Zhai, G., J. B. van Meurs, G. Livshits, I. Meulenbelt, A. M. Valdes, N. Soranzo, D. Hart, F. Zhang, B. S. Kato, J. B. Richards, F. M. Williams, M. Inouye, M. Kloppenburg, P. Deloukas, E. Slagboom, A. Uitterlinden and T. D. Spector, (2009). A genome-wide association study suggests that a locus within the ataxin 2 binding protein 1 gene is associated with hand osteoarthritis: the Treat-OA consortium, *J Med Genet*. Vol 46, No. 9, pp. 614-6.

Zhai, G., R. Wang-Sattler, D. J. Hart, N. K. Arden, A. J. Hakim, T. Illig and T. D. Spector, (2010). Serum branched-chain amino acid to histidine ratio: a novel metabolomic biomarker of knee osteoarthritis, *Ann Rheum Dis*. Vol 69, No. 6, pp. 1227-31. ISSN 1468-2060 (Electronic) 0003-4967 (Linking).

Zhang, Y., X. Feng, R. We and R. Derynck, (1996). Receptor-associated Mad homologues synergize as effectors of the TGF-beta response, *Nature*. Vol 383, No. 6596, pp. 168-72. ISSN 0028-0836 (Print) 0028-0836 (Linking).

13

Genetic Mouse Models for Osteoarthritis Research

Jie Shen[1], Meina Wang[1], Hongting Jin[1,2], Erik Sampson[1] and Di Chen[1,3]
[1]*Center for Musculoskeletal Research, Department of Orthopaedics and Rehablitation, University of Rochester, New York*
[2]*Institute of Orthopaedics and Traumatology, Zhejiang Chinese Medical University, Hangzhou*
[3]*Department of Biochemistry, Rush University Medical Center*
[1,3]*USA*
[2]*China*

1. Introduction

Osteoarthritis (OA), a degenerative joint disease, increases in prevalence with age, and affects majority of individuals over the age of 65. OA frequently affects several joints including the hands, knees, hips and spine, and is a leading cause of impaired mobility in the elderly. The major clinical symptoms include chronic pain, joint instability, stiffness and radiographic joint space narrowing (Felson, 2006; Goldring & Goldring, 2007).
During OA development, articular chondrocytes undergo hypertrophy leading to extracellular matrix degradation, articular cartilage breakdown and osteophyte formation in the margins of the articular cartilage (Felson, 2006; Goldring & Goldrig, 2007). The precise signaling pathways which are involved in the degradation of cartilage matrix and development of OA are poorly understood and there are currently no effective interventions to decelerate the progression of OA or retard the irreversible degradation of cartilage except for total joint replacement surgery (Krasnokutsky et al., 2007). In this chapter, we will summarize important molecular mechanisms related to OA pathogenesis and provide new insights into potential molecular targets for the prevention and treatment of OA.

2. Characteristics of articular cartilage

The skeleton is an organ composed of two distinct tissues: bone and cartilage. Bones are rigid mineralized organs formed in a variety of shapes. Normal articular cartilage, emerging during the postnatal stage as a permanent tissue distinct from the growth plate cartilage, is an extremely smooth, hard and white tissue that lines the surface of all the diathrodial joints. Articular cartilage facilitates interactions between two bones in a joint with a low coefficient of friction. Water, type II collagen (Col2), and proteoglycans are the principle components of articular cartilage. Of the wet mass, 65%~80% of cartilage is water, 10%~20% is Col2, and 4%~7% is aggrecan. Other collagens and proteoglycans such as types V, VI, IX, X, XI, XII, XIV collagens (Eyre et al., 2002) and decorin, biglycan, fibromodulin, lumican, epiphycan, and perlecan (Knudson & Knudson, 2001) also contribute a small part (less than 5%) of the normal cartilage composition. The articular chondrocyte is the only cell type in articular cartilage and as such is the major player in cartilage development and maintenance.

During articular cartilage development, articular chondrocytes establish the cartilage matrix by synthesizing and depositing collagens and proteoglycans. The collagen/proteoglycan matrix consists of a highly dense meshwork of collagen fibrils including the major collagen type II (Col2) and minor collagen types IX, and XI embedded in gel-like negatively-charged proteoglycans (Kannu et al., 2009). This hydrated architecture of the matrix provides the articular cartilage with tensile and resilient strength which allows joints to maintain proper biomechanical function (Iozzo, 2000).

As articular cartilage matures, articular chondrocytes maintain the cartilage by synthesizing matrix components (Col2 and proteoglycans) and matrix degrading enzymes with minimal turnover of cells and matrix. The existing collagen network becomes cross-linked, and articular cartilage matures into a permanent tissue with the ability to absorb and respond to mechanical stress (Verzijl et al., 2000). Under normal conditions, articular chondrocytes become arrested at a pre-hypertrophic stage of differentiation, thereby persisting throughout postnatal life to maintain normal articular cartilage structure (Pacifici et al., 2005).

3. Progression of osteoarthritis

Articular cartilage can be damaged by normal wear and tear or pathological processes such as abnormal mechanical loading or injury. Because articular cartilage is an avascular tissue, and chondrocytes possess little regenerative capacity and are arrested before terminal hypertrophic differentiation, articular cartilage has very limited capacity to repair after damage.

During the early stages of OA, the cartilage surface is still intact. The molecular composition and organization of the extracellular matrix is altered first (Glodring & Glodring, 2010). The articular chondrocytes, which possess little regenerative capacity and have a low metabolic activity in normal joints, exhibit a transient proliferative response and increase matrix synthesis (Col2, aggrecan etc.) attempting to initiate repair caused by pathological stimulation. This response is characterized by chondrocyte cloning to form clusters and hypertrophic differentiation, including expression of hypertrophic markers such as *Runx2*, *ColX*, and *Mmp13*. Changes in the composition and structure of the articular cartilage further stimulate chondrocytes to produce more catabolic factors involved in cartilage degradation. As proteoglycans and then the collagen network break down (Mort & Billington, 2001), cartilage integrity is disrupted. The articular chondrocytes will then undergo apoptosis and the articular cartilage will eventually be completely lost. The reduced joint space resulting from total loss of cartilage will cause friction between bones, leading to pain and limited joint mobility. Other signs of OA, including subchondral sclerosis, bone eburnation, osteophyte formation, as well as loosening and weakness of muscles and tendons will also appear.

4. Genetic contribution to osteoarthritis

The etiology of OA is multi-factorial, including obesity, joint mal-alignment, and prior joint injury or surgery. These factors can be segregated into categories such as mechanical influences, the effects of aging and genetic factors. Meniscal injuries are among the most common causes of OA in younger populations. The meniscus is a C-shaped structure that functions as shock-absorbing, load bearing, stability enhancing, and lubricating cushion in the knee joint. Studies show that loss of intact meniscus function leads to OA in humans due to joint instability and abnormal mechanical loading (Ding et al., 2007; Hunter et al., 2006). Recently, the meniscal-ligamentous injury (MLI) induced-OA model is becoming a well-established mouse model which mimics clinical situation allowing us to study the development and progression of trauma-induced OA on defined genetic backgrounds (Clements et al., 2003; Sampson et al., 2011). In this model, the ligation of the medial collateral ligament coupled with disruption of the meniscus from its anterior-medial attachment can reproducibly induce OA over a 3 month time period.

There are rare cases of OA involving mutations of *types II, IX* and *XI collagen* (Li et al., 2007; Kannu et al., 2009). In addition, OA progression is also affected by pro-inflammatory factors such as prostaglandins, TNF-α, interleukin-1, interleukin-6 and nitric oxide. However, there is no evidence supporting a critical role for these factors in the development of severe OA (Kawaguchi, 2009). As articular chondrocytes inappropriately undergo endochondral ossification-like maturation in the context of OA, however, several genetic mouse models have been developed and demonstrated potential roles of affected genes in OA pathogenesis.

4.1 TGF-β signaling

Chondrocyte differentiation and maturation during endochondral ossification are tightly regulated by several key growth factors and transcription factors, including members of the transforming growth factor β (TGF-β) super family, fibroblast growth factors (FGFs), indian hedgehog (Ihh), parathyroid hormone-related protein (PTHrP), and Wnt signaling proteins (Blaney Davidson et al., 2007; Kolpakova & Olsen, 2005; Komori, 2003; Kronenberg, 2003; Ornitz, 2005). The inhibition of TGF-β signaling represents a potential mechanism in the development of OA because TGF-β inhibits chondrocyte hypertrophy and maturation (Blaney Davidson et al., 2007). There are three isoforms of TGF-β, TGF-β1, 2 and 3, which can bind to the type II receptor to activate the canonical TGF-β/Smad signaling cascade. In the canonical pathway, TGF-β binds to the type II receptor which then phosphorylates type I transmembrane serine/threonine kinase receptors. The type I receptor subsequently phosphorylates Smads 2 and 3 (R-Smad) at a conserved SSXS motif at the C-terminus of Smads 2 and 3. The activated R-Smads thus dissociate from the receptor complex and form a heteromeric complex with the common Smad, Smad4. This heteromeric Smad complex then enters the nucleus and associates with other DNA binding proteins to regulate target gene transcription (Miyazawa et al., 2002).

Deletion of any TGF-β isoform gene could result in embryonic lethality and loss of TGF-β2 or TGF-β3 results in defects in bone development affecting the forelimbs, hindlimbs and craniofacial bones, suggesting that TGF-β plays an important role in skeletogenesis (Nicole & kerstin, 2000). Recent genetic manipulation of TGF-β signaling members also demonstrated that TGF-β signaling plays a critical role during OA development. Transgenic mice that over-express the dominant-negative type II TGF-β receptor (dn*Tgfbr2*) in skeletal tissue exhibit articular chondrocyte hypertrophy with increased type X collagen expression, cartilage disorganization and progressive degradation (Serra et al., 1997). Consistent with these findings, Smad3 knockout mice show progressive articular cartilage degradation resembling human OA (Yang et al., 2001). In order to overcome embryonic lethality and redundancy, we generated chondrocyte-specific *Tgfbr2* conditional knockout mice (*Tgfbr2* cKO or *Tgfbr2*^{Col2CreER} mice) in which deletion of the *Tgfbr2* gene is mediated by Cre recombinase driven by the chondrocyte-specific Col2a1 promoter in a tamoxifen (TM)-inducible manner (Chen et al, 2007; Zhu et al, 2008, 2009). These mice exhibit typical clinical features of OA, including cell cloning, chondrocyte hypertrophy, cartilage surface fibrillation, vertical clefts and severe articular cartilage damage as well as the formation of chondrophytes and osteophytes (Shen et al., unpublished data). In addition, the relationship between TGF-β signaling and OA is strengthened by the discovery that a single nucleotide polymorphism (SNP) in the human Smad3 gene is linked to the incidence of hip and knee OA in a 527 patient cohort (Valdes et al., 2010).

4.2 Wnt/β-catenin signaling

The canonical Wnt/β-catenin signaling pathway, which controls multiple developmental processes in skeletal and joint patterning, may also be involved in the progression of OA. *In vitro* studies show that over-expression of constitutively active β-catenin leads to loss of the chondrocyte phenotype including reduced Sox9 and Col2 expression in chick chondrocytes (Yang, 2003). When Wnt binds its receptor Frizzled and the co-receptor protein LRP5/6, the signaling protein Dishevelled (Dsh) is activated, leading to inactivation of the serine/threonine kinase GSK-3β, thus inhibiting the ubiquitination and degradation of β-catenin. β-catenin then accumulates in the nucleus and binds LEF-1/TCF to regulate the expression of Wnt target genes. In the absence of the Wnt ligand, cytosolic β-catenin binds the APC-Axin-GSK-3β degradation complex, and GSK-3β in this complex phosphorylates β-catenin to induce its proteosomal degradation. The degradation of β-catenin represses the expression of Wnt responsive genes, allowing binding of the corepressor Groucho to the transcription factors LEF-1/TCF.

Genome-wide scans, candidate gene association analyses and single nucleotide polymorphism (SNP) studies have demonstrated the association of hip OA with the Arg324Gly substitution mutation in the sFRP3 protein that antagonizes the binding of Wnt ligands to the Frizzled receptors. The mutation of sFRP3 causes increased levels of active β-catenin, promoting aberrant articular chondrocyte hypertrophy and thereby leading to hip and knee OA in patients (Loughlin et al., 2004; Lane et al., 2006; Loughlin et al., 2000; Min et al., 2005). Consistent with this finding, *Frzb* knockout mice are more sensitive to chemical-induced OA (Lories et al., 2007).

Since human genetic association studies suggest that Wnt/β-catenin signaling may play a critical role in the pathogenesis of OA, we have generated chondrocyte-specific *β-catenin* conditional activation (cAct) mice. These mice show high expression of β-catenin in articular chondrocytes leading to abnormal articular chondrocyte maturation and progressive loss of the articular cartilage surface in 5- and 8-month old mice (Zhu et al., 2009). The role of Wnt/β-catenin signaling in cartilage degeneration is further demonstrated in other animal models. Chondrocyte-specific Col2a1-Smurf2 transgenic mice develop an OA-like phenotype due to up-regulation of β-catenin caused by Smurf2-induced ubiquitination and degradation of GSK-3β (Wu et al., 2009). Furthermore, over-expression of Wnt-induced signaling protein 1 (WISP-1) in the mouse knee joint also leads to cartilage destruction (Blom et al., 2009). Consistent with these findings, it has been reported that a panel of Wnt signaling-related genes, including WISP-1 and β-catenin, were significantly up-regulated in knee joints and disc samples from patients with OA and disc degenerative disease (DDD) (Blom et al., 2009; Tang et al., unpublished data).

4.3 Indian hedgehog (Ihh) signaling

The Indian hedgehog (Ihh)/parathyroid hormone-related protein (PTHrP) negative-feedback loop is critical for chondrocyte differentiation during endochondral bone formation. Articular chondrocytes undergo cellular changes reminiscent of terminal growth plate chondrocyte differentiation during OA (Kronenberg, 2003). These observations suggest a pivotal role for Ihh signaling in OA development. Ihh is a major Hh ligand in chondrocytes, which binds with the Patched-1 (PTCH1) receptor to release its inhibition on Smoothened (SMO). SMO can then activate the glioma-associated oncogene homolog (Gli) family of transcription factors to initiate transcription of specific downstream target genes, including Hh signaling pathway members *Gli1*, *Ptch1* and hedgehog-interacting protein (*HHIP*).

Immunohistochemical studies demonstrated that Ihh signaling activation positively correlates with the severity of OA in human OA knee joint tissues and high expression of GLI1, PTCH and HHIP was found in surgically induced murine OA articular cartilage. Activation of Ihh signaling in mice with chondrocyte-specific over-expression of the *Gli2* or *Smo* genes induced a spontaneous OA-like phenotype with high MMP-13, ADAMTS5 and ColX expression. In contrast, deletion of the *Smo* gene or treatment with a pharmacological inhibitor of Ihh attenuated the severity of OA induced by MLI injury (Lin et al., 2009).

4.4 HIF-2α

The HIF proteins, including HIF-1, 2 and 3, are the basic helix-loop-helix transcription factors which function differently under normoxic and hypoxic conditions (Semenza, 2000; Lando et al., 2002; Bracken et al., 2003; Schofield and Ratcliffe, 2004). HIF-1α, in the articular cartilage, acts as an anabolic signal by stimulating specific extracellular matrix synthesis (Pfander et al., 2003; Duval et al., 2009). In contrast, HIF-2α (encoded by *EPAS1*) is a potential catabolic regulator of articular cartilage and induces articular cartilage degeneration (Saito et al., 2010; Yang et al., 2010). Promoter assays suggest that NF-κB signaling could significantly induce HIF-2α expression and then HIF-2α specifically regulate transcription of several catabolic genes such as *Mmp13* (Saito et al., 2010). Genetic screen using the human osteoarhritic cartilage UniGene library suggests that HIF-2α is a potential catabolic regulator of articular cartilage (Yang et al., 2010). Based on the Japanese population ROAD study, a functional SNP in human *EPAS1* proximal promoter region was associated with knee osteoarthritis in a 397 patient cohort (Muraki et al., 2009; Saito et al., 2010). Consistent with this finding, , HIF-2α expression was markedly increased in OA patients with degenerative cartilage (Saito et al., 2010; Yang et al., 2010). Chondrocyte-specific *Epas1* transgenic mice could spontaneously develop osteoarthritis phenotype with increased MMP-13 and ColX expression in articular cartilage. In addition, *Epas1* heteozygous deficient mice showed resistance to cartilage degeneration induced by meniscus surgery (Saito et al., 2010; Yang et al., 2010). Therefore, HIF-2α may be a critical transcription factor that targets several genes for osteoarthritis development.

4.5 Insulin-like growth factor (IGF)

The progressive nature of OA is charactized by a growing imbalance between anabolism and catabolism in articular cartilage. The three above-mentioned signaling pathways are mainly involved in regulation of articular chondrocyte catabolism. In contrast, insulin-like growth factor (IGF) is the most likely candidate affecting cartilage matrix synthesis (Guenther et al., 1982; McQuillan et al., 1986). The most important ligand in IGF signaling is IGF-1 which interacts with specific IGF membrane receptors as well as with the insulin receptor to activate their cytoplasmic tyrosine kinase domains and initiate the MAPK cascade and promote cell proliferation and differentiation. The action of IGF signaling on cellular anabolism is governed at different levels, including IGF ligand, receptors and IGF binding proteins (IGFBP) which modify the interaction of IGF with its receptor (Martel-Pelletier et al., 1998). In cartilage, IGF-1 is believed to stimulate synthesis of extracellular matrix proteins in chondrocytes (Schoenle et al., 1982; Trippel et al., 1989). The local production of IGF-1 is significantly increased in human OA synovial fluid, due to attempting to repair the damaged cartilage. However, the diseased cells are hypo-responsive to IGF-1 stimulation since highly-expressed IGFBP3 on the cell membrane interferes with the binding of IGF-1 to its receptor (Doré et al., 1994; Tardif et al., 1996). Moreover, the highly expressed IGF-1 may contribute to the subchondral bone sclerosis and osteophyte formation (Martel-Pelletier et al., 1998).

5. Cartilage degradation during OA

Articular chondrocytes, the only cell type in cartilage, are sensitive to altered mechanical loading pattern induced by obesity, injury and aging (Goldring & Goldring, 2007). Chondrocytes have receptors responding to mechanical stimulation, including integrins which serve as receptors for extracelluar matrix components such as fibronectin (FN) and type II collagen fragments (Millward-Sadler & Salter, 2004). In addition to these receptors, several signaling pathways mentioned above are mechano-responsive in chondrocytes as well, including TGF-β, Wnt and Ihh signaling (Blaney Davidson et al., 2006; Komm & Bex, 2006; Ng et al., 2006; Robinson et al., 2009). Activation of these signaling pathways induces the expression of matrix-degrading proteinases. Studies of large scale gene expression profiling from tissue samples of OA patients revealed two principle enzyme families responsible for cartilage degeneration during OA development: the matrix metalloproteinase (MMP) family members which target collagens and a disintegrin and metalloproteinase with thrombospondin motifs (ADAMTS) family members which mediate aggrecan degeneration (Aigner et al., 2006).

5.1 Collagenase: Matrix metalloproteinase

MMP-13 is a substrate-specific enzyme that targets collagen for degradation. Compared to other MMPs, MMP-13 expression is more restricted to connective tissues (Borden & Heller, 1997; Mengshol et al., 2000; Vincenti et al., 1998; Vincenti, 2001). MMP-13 preferentially cleaves Col2, which is most abundant in articular cartilage and in the nucleus pulposus, inner anulus fibrosus and cartilage endplate of the intervertebral disc. It also targets the degradation of other proteins in cartilage, such as aggrecan, types IV and IX collagen, gelatin, osteonectin and perlecan (Shiomi et al., 2010). MMP-13 has a much higher catalytic velocity rate compared with other MMPs over Col2 and gelatin, making it the most potent peptidolytic enzyme among collagenases (Knäuper et al., 1996; Reboul et al., 1996).

Clinical investigations revealed that patients with articular cartilage destruction had high MMP-13 expression (Roach et al., 2005), suggesting increased MMP-13 may be the cause of cartilage degradation. *Mmp13* deficient mice show no gross phenotypic abnormalities, and the only alteration is in growth plate architecture during early cartilage development (Inada et al., 2004; Stickens et al., 2004). However, transgenic mice with cartilage-specific *Mmp13*-overexpression develop spontaneous articular cartilage destruction characterized by excessive cleavage of Col2 and loss of aggrecan (Neuhold et al., 2001). In the above-mentioned *Tgfbr2* cKO and *β-catenin* cAct mouse models, MMP-13 expression is significantly increased (Shen et al., unpublished data; Zhu et al., 2009). These findings suggest that MMP-13 deficiency does not affect articular cartilage function during the postnatal and adult stages but abnormal up-regulation of MMP-13 can lead to cartilage destruction. Moreover, deletion of the *Mmp13* gene prevents articular cartilage erosion induced by meniscal injury (Little et al., 2009). Deletion of the *Mmp13* gene at least partially rescues the OA-like phenotype observed in *Tgfbr2* cKO and *β-catenin* cAct mice (Shen et al., unpublished data; Wang et al., unpublished data), suggesting that TGF-β/Smad3 and Wnt/β-catenin signaling play a critical role in the development of OA through up-regulation of MMP-13 expression.

5.2 Aggrecanse: ADAMTS

The ADAMTS family consists of large family members and they share several distinct protein modules as well. Studies show that ADAMTS4 and 5 expression levels are significantly increased during OA development. Single knockout of the *Adamts5* gene or double knockout of the *Adamts4* and *Adamts5* genes prevents cartilage degradation in surgery-induced and chemical-induced murine knee OA models (Glasson et al., 2005; Majumdar et al., 2007; Stanton et al., 2005). Interestingly, in *Tgfbr2* cKO, *β-catenin* and *Ihh* activation mouse models, ADAMTS5 was significantly increased in articular cartilage tissue, suggesting that maintaining proper ADAMTS5 levels are essential for normal articular cartilage function. Taken together, these findings indicate that catabolic enzymes play a significant role in OA progression and targeting these enzymes may be a viable therapeutic strategy to decelerate articular cartilage degradation.

6. Potential therapeutic approches

MMP-13 and ADAMTS5 are two potentially attractive targets for OA therapy. The inhibition of these enzymes and their regulatory mechanisms have been extensively studied. Tissue inhibitors of metalloproteinases (TIMP) are specific inhibitors which directly bind MMPs and ADAMTS in chondrocytes to prevent the destruction of articular cartilage (Stetler-Stevenson & Seo, 2005). A specific small molecule MMP-13 inhibitor can attenuate the severity of OA in the MLI-induced injury model as well (Wang et al., unpublished data). In addition to proteinase inhibitors, the transcription factor Runt domain factor-2 (Runx2) appears to be another potential target to regulate MMP-13 and ADAMTS5 *in vivo*. DNA sequence analysis of *Mmp13* and *Adamts5* promoters identified putative Runx2 binding sites in the promoter regions of these genes. In addition, Runx2 has an overlapping expression pattern with MMP-13 and ADAMTS5, almost exclusively in the developing cartilage and bone, suggesting that Runx2 may be an important transcription factor regulating tissue-specific expression of *Mmp13* and *Adamts5* in articular chondrocytes (Ducy et al., 1997; Enomoto et al., 2000; Inada et al., 1999; Komori et al., 1997). *In vitro* studies confirmed that MMP-13 and ADAMTS5 expression dramatically increase after alterations in TGF-β/Smad3,

Wnt/β-catenin and Ihh signaling pathways and concomitant up-regulation of Runx2 expression (Lin et al., 2009; Shen et al., unpublished data; Wang et al., unpublished data). Thus, manipulation of Runx2 expression *in vivo* could be an effective therapeutic strategy. During bone development, the temporal and spatial expression patterns of *Runx2* are regulated by cytokines and growth factors including TGF-β, BMP, and FGF (Kim et al., 2003; Takamoto et al., 2003; Tou et al., 2001; Zhou et al., 2000). In addition to gene expression, Runx2 protein levels are also regulated through post-translational mechanisms involving phosphorylation, ubiquitination and acetylation (Zhao et al., 2003, 2004; Jeon et al., 2006; Jonason et al., 2009; Shen et al., 2006a, 2006b; Shui et al., 2003; Zhang et al., 2009). We have recently found that cyclin D1 induces Runx2 ubiquitination and degradation in a phosphorylation-dependent manner leading to the inhibition of Runx2 transcriptional activity (Shen et al., 2006b). MicroRNA regulation is another important regulatory mechanism for protein translation. MicroRNA-140 (miR-140) is the first microRNA demonstrated to be involved in the pathogenesis of OA at least partially through regulation of ADAMTS5 mRNA expression. MiR-140 knockout mice are susceptible to age-related OA progression and conversely, over-expression of miR-140 in chondrocytes protects mice from OA development (Akhtar et al., 2010; Miyaki et al., 2009; Yamasaki et al., 2009).

7. Summary

Articular chondrocyte is the sensor of articular cartilage homeostasis, and plays a critical role in maintaining the normal physiological structure and function of articular cartilage. Recent studies demonstrate that articular chondrocyte homeostasis can be disrupted by multiple factors, including abnormal mechanical loading, and aging. Additionally, genetic alterations in TGF-β/Smad, Wnt/β-catenin and Ihh signaling pathways can disrupt the balance between anabolic and catabolic activity in articular cartilage and result in irreversible degradation of the extracellular matrix. Thus far, most of the mouse models of osteoarthritis converge at the up-regulation of catabolic enzymes, such as MMP-13 and ADAMTS5, suggesting that these enzymes may serve as potential therapeutic targets in regulation of the progression of OA. In addition, manipulation of the above-mentioned signaling pathways in articular chondrocytes could also play a role in articular cartilage regeneration.

8. References

Aigner, T.; Fundel, K.; Saas, J.; Gebhard, P.M.; Haag, J.; Weiss, T.; Zien, A.; Obermayr, F.; Zimmer, R.; Bartnik, E. (2006). Large-scale gene expression profiling reveals major pathogenetic pathways of cartilage degeneration in osteoarthritis. *Arthritis Rheu*, 54: 3533-3544.

Akhtar, N.; Rasheed, Z.; Ramamurthy, S.; Anbazhagan, A.N.; Voss, F.R.; Haqqi, T.M. (2010). MicroRNA-27b regulates the expression of MMP-13 in human osteoarthritis chondrocytes. *Arthritis Rheum*, 62: 1361-1371.

Blaney Davidson, E.N.; van der Kraan, P.M. & van den Berg, W.B. (2007). TGF-beta and osteoarthritis. *Osteoarthritis Cartilage*, 15: 597-604.

Blaney Davidson, E.N.; Vitters, E.L.; van der Kraan, P.M.; van den Berg, W.B. (2006). Expression of transforming growth factor-b (TGFβ) and the TGFβ signalling molecule SMAD-2P in spontaneous and instability-induced osteoarthritis: role in cartilage degradation, chondrogenesis and osteophyte formation. *Ann Rheum Dis*, 65: 1414-1421.

Blom, A.B.; Brockbank, S.M.; van Lent, P.L.; van Beuningen, H.M.; Geurts, J.; Takahashi, N.; van der Kraan, P.M.; van de Loo, F.A.; Schreurs, B.W.; Clements, K.; Newham, P.; van den Berg, W.B. (2009). Involvement of the Wnt signaling pathway in experimental and human osteoarthritis: prominent role of Wnt-induced signaling protein 1. *Arthritis Rheum*, 60: 501-512.

Borden, P. & Heller, R.A. (1997). Transcriptional control of matrix metalloproteinases and the tissue inhibitors of matrix metalloproteinases. *Crit Rev Eukaryotic Gene Expr*, 7: 159-178.

Bracken, C.P.; Whitelaw, M.L.; Peet, D.J. (2003). The hypoxia-inducible factors: key transcriptional regulators of hypoxic responses. *Cell Mol Life Sci*, 60: 1376-1393.

Chen, M.; Lichtler, A.C.; Sheu, T.; Xie, C.; Zhang, X.; O'Keefe, R.J.; Chen, D. (2007). Generation of a transgenic mouse model with chondrocyte-specific and tamoxifen-inducible expression of Cre recombinase. *Genesis*, 45: 44-50.

Clements, K.M.; Price, J.S.; Chambers, M.G.; Visco, D.M.; Poole, A.R.; Mason, R.M. (2003). Gene deletion of either interleukin-1beta, interleukin-1beta-converting enzyme, inducible nitric oxide synthase, or stromelysin 1 accelerates the development of knee osteoarthritis in mice after surgical transaction of the medial collateral ligament and partial medial meniscectomy. *Arthritis Rheum*, 48: 3452-3463.

Ding, C.H.; Martel-Pelletier, J.; Pelletier, J.P.; Abram, F.; Raynauld, J.P.; Cicuttini, F.; Jones, G. (2007). Meniscal tear as an osteoarthritis risk factor in a largely non-osteoarthritic cohort: a cross-sectional study. *J Rheumatol*, 34: 776-784.

Doré, S.; Pelletier, J.P.; Di Battista, J.A.; Tardif, G.; Brazeau, P.; Martel-Pelletier, J. (1994). Human osteoarthritic chondrocytes possess an increased number of insulin-like growth factor 1 binding sites but are unresponsive to its stimulation. Possible role of IGF-1- binding proteins. *Arthritis Rheum*, 37: 253-263.

Ducy, P.; Zhang. R.; Geoffroy, V.; Ridall, A.L.; Karsenty. G. (1997). Osf2/Cbfa1: a transcriptional activator of osteoblast differentiation. *Cell*, 89: 747-754.

Duval, E.; Leclercq, S.; Elissalde, J.M.; Demoor, M.; Galéra, P.; Boumédiene, K. (2009). Hypoxia-inducible factor 1alpha inhibits the fibroblast-like markers type I and type III collagen during hypoxia-induced chondrocyte redifferentiation: hypoxia not only induces type II collagen and aggrecan, but it also inhibits type I and type III collagen in the hypoxia-inducible factor 1 alpha-dependent redifferentiation of chondrocytes. *Arthritis Rheum*, 60: 3038-3048.

Enomoto, H.; Enomoto-Iwamoto, M.; Iwamoto, M.; Nomura, S.; Himeno, M.; Kitamura, Y.; Kishimoto, T.; Komori, T. (2000). Cbfa1 is a positive regulatory factor in chondrocyte maturation. *J Biol Chem*, 275: 8695-8702.

Eyre, D.R.; Wu, J.J.; Fermandes, R.J.; Pietka, T.A.; Weis, M.A. (2002). Recent developments in cartilage research: matrix biology of the collagen II/IX/Xi heterofibril network. *Biochem Soc Trans*, 30: 893-899.

Felson, D.T. (2006). Osteoarthritis of the knee. *NEJM*, 354: 841-848.

Glasson, S.S.; Askew, R.; Sheppard, B.; Carito, B.; Blanchet, T.; Ma, H.L.; Flannery, C.R.; Peluso, D.; Kanki, K.; Yang, Z.; Majumdar, M.K.; Morris, E.A. (2005). Deletion of active ADAMTS5 prevents cartilage degradation in a murine model of osteoarthritis. *Nature*, 434: 644-648.

Goldring, M.B. & Goldring, S.R. (2007). Osteoarthritis. *J Cel Physiol*, 213: 626-634.

Goldring, M.B. & Goldring, S.R. (2010). Articular cartilage and subchondral bone in the pathogenesis of osteoarthritis. *Ann N Y Acad Sci*, 1192: 230-237.

Guenther, H.L.; Guenther, H.E.; Froesch, E.R.; Fleisch, H. (1982). Effect of insulin-like growth factor on collagen and glycosaminoglycan synthesis by rabbit articular chondroytes in culture. *Experientia*, 38: 979-981.

Hunter, D.J.; Zhang, Y.Q.; Niu, J.B.; Tu, X.; Amin, S.; Clancy, M.; Guermazi, A.; Grigorian, M.; Gale, D.; Felson, D.T. (2006). The Association of Meniscal Pathologic Changes With Cartilage Loss in Symptomatic Knee Osteoarthritis. *Arthritis Rheum*, 54: 795-801.

Inada, M.; Yasui, T.; Nomura, S.; Miyake, S.; Dequchi, K.; Himeno, M.; Sato, M.; Yamagiwa, H.; Kimura, T.; Yasui, N.; Ochi, T.; Endo, N.; Kitamura, Y.; Kishimoto, T.; Komori, T. (1999). Maturational disturbance of chondrocytes in Cbfa1-deficient mice. *Dev Dyn*, 214: 279-290.

Inada, M.; Wang, Y.M.; Byrne, M.H.; Rahman, M.U.; Miyaura, C.; López-Otin, C.; krane, S.M. (2004). Critical roles for collagenase-3 (Mmp13) in development of growth plate cartilage and in endochondral ossification. *Proc Natl Acad Sci USA*, 101: 17192-17197.

Iozzo, R.V. Proteoglycans: Structure, Biology and Molecular Interactions. 2000; 1st Edition. Jefferson Medical College, Thomas Jefferson University, Philadelphia, Pennsylvania.

Jeon, E.J.; Lee, K.Y.; Choi, N.S.; Lee, M.H.; Kim, H.N.; Jin, Y.H.; Ryoo, H.M.; Choi, J.Y.; Yoshida, M.; Nishino, N.; Oh, B.C.; Lee, K.S.; Lee, Y.H.; Bae, S.C. (2006). Bone morphogenetic protein-2 stimulates Runx2 acetylation. *J Biol Chem*, 281: 16502-16511.

Jonason, J.H.; Xiao, G.; Zhang, M.; Xing, L.; Chen, D. (2009). Post-transcriptional regulation of runx2 in bone and cartilage. *J Dent Res*, 88: 693-703.

Kannu, P.; Bateman, J.F.; Belluoccio, D.; Fosang, A.J.; Savarirayan, R. (2009). Employing molecular genetics of chondrodysplasias to inform the study of osteoarthritis. *Arthritis Rheum*, 60: 325-334.

Kawaguchi, H. (2009). Regulation of osteoarthritis development by Wnt-beta-catenin signaling through the endochondral ossification process. *J Bone Miner Res*, 24: 8-11

Kim, H.J.; Kim, J.H.; Bae, S.C.; Choi, J.Y.; Kim, H.J.; Ryoo, H.M. (2003). The protein kinase C pathway plays a central role in the fibroblast growth factorstimulated expression and transactivation activity of Runx2. *J Biol Chem*, 278: 319-326.

Knäuper, V.; Lopez-Otin, C.; Smith, B.; Knight, G.; Murphy, G. (1996). Biochemical characterization of human collagenase-3. *J Biol Chem*, 271: 1544-1550.

Knudson, C.B. & Knudson, W. (2001). Cartilage proteoglycans. *Semin Cell Dev Biol*, 12: 69-78.

Kolpakova, E. & Olsen, B.R. (2005). Wnt/beta-catenin-a canonical tale of cell-fate choice in the vertebrate skeleton. *Dev Cell*, 8: 626-627.

Komm, B.S. & Bex, F.J. (2006). Wnt/β-Catenin signaling is a normal physiological response to mechanical loading in bone. *The Journal of Biological Chemistry*, 281: 31720-31728.

Komori, T.; Yagi, H.; Nomura, S.; Yamaquchi, A.; Sasaki, K.; Dequchi, K.; Shimizu, Y.; Bronson, R.T.; Gao, Y.H.; Inada, M.; Sato, M.; Okamoto, R.; Kitamura, Y.; Yoshiki, S.; Kishimoto, T. (1997). Targeted disruption of Cbfa1 results in a complete lack of bone formation owing to maturational arrest of osteoblasts. *Cell*, 89: 755-764.

Komori, T. (2003). Requisite roles of Runx2 and Cbfb in skeletal development. *J Bone Miner Metab*, 21: 193-197.

Krasonkutsky, S.; Samuels, J. & Abramson, S.B. (2007). Osteoarthritis in 2007. *Bulletin of the NYU Hospital for Joint Disease*, 65: 222-228.

Kronenberg, H.M. (2003). Developmental regulation of the growth plate. *Nature*, 423: 332-336.

Lando, D.; Peet, D.J.; Whelan, D.A.; Gorman, J.J.; Whitelaw, M.L. (2002). Asparagine hydroxylation of the HIF transactivation domain a hypoxic switch. *Science*, 295: 858-861.

Lane, N.E.; Lian, K.; Nevitt, M.C.; Zmuda, J.M.; Lui, L.; Li, J.; Wang, J.; Fontecha, M.; Umblas, N.; Rosenbach, M.; de Leon, P.; Corr, M. (2006). Frizzledrelated protein variants are risk factors for hip osteoarthritis. *Arthritis Rheum*, 54: 1246-1254.

Li, Y.; Xu, L. & Olsen, B.R. (2007). Lessons from genetic forms of osteoarthritis for the pathogenesis of the disease. *Osteoarthritis Cartilage*, 15: 1101–1105.

Lin, A.C.; Seeto, B.L.; Bartoszko, J.M.; Khoury, M.A.; Whetstone, H.; Ho. L.; Hsu, C.; Ali, A.S.; Alman, B.A. (2009). Modulating hedgehog signaling can attenuate the severity of osteoarthritis. *Nature Medicine*, 15: 1421-1426.

Little, C.B.; Barai, A.; Burkhardt, D.; Smith, S.M.; Fosang, A.J.; Werb, Z.; Shah, M.; Thompson, E.W. (2009). Matrix metalloproteinase 13-deficient mice are resistant to osteoarthritic cartilage erosion but not chondrocyte hypertrophy or osteophyte development. *Arthritis Rheum*, 60: 3723-3733.

Lories, R.J.; Peeters, J.; Bakker, A.; Tylzanowski, P.; Derese, I.; Schrooten, J.; Thomas, J.T.; Luyten, F.P. (2007). Articular cartilage and biomechanical properties of the long bones in Frzb-knockout mice. *Arthritis Rheum*, 56: 4095-4103.

Loughlin, J.; Mustafa, Z.; Smith, A.; Irven, C.; Carr, A.J.; Clipsham, K.; Chitnavis, J.; Bloomfield, V.A.; McCartney, M.; Cox, O.; Sinsheimer, J.S.; Sykes, B.; Chapman, K.E. (2000). Linkage analysis of chromosome 2q in osteoarthritis. *Rheumatology*, 39: 377-381.

Loughlin, J.; Dowling, B.; Chapman, K.; Marcelline, L.; Mustafa, Z.; Southam, L.; Ferreira, A.; Ciesielski, C.; Carson, D.A.; Corr, M. (2004). Functional variants within the secreted frizzled-related protein 3 gene are associated with hip osteoarthritis in females. *Proc Natl Acad Sci USA*, 101: 9757-9762.

Majumdar, M.K.; Askew, R.; Schelling, S.; Stedman, N.; Blanchet, T.; Hopkins, B.; Morris, E.A.; Glasson, S.S. (2007). Double-knockout of ADAMTS-4 and ADAMTS-5 in mice results in physiologically normal animals and prevents the progression of osteoarthritis. *Arthritis Rheum*, 56: 3670-3674.

Martel-Pelletier, J.; Di Battista, J.A.; Lajeunesse, D.; Pelletier, J.P. (1998). IGF/IGFBP axis in cartilage and bone in osteoarthritis pathogenesis. *Inflamm Res*, 47: 90-100.

McQuillan, D.J.; Handley, C.J.; Campbell, M.A.; Bolis, S.; Milway, V.E.; Herington, A.C. (1986). Stimulation of proteoglycan biosynthesis by serum and insulin-like growth factor-1 in cultured bovine articular cartilage. *Biochem J*, 240: 423-430.

Mengshol, J.A. ; Vincenti, M.P. ; Coon, C.I. ; Barchowsky, A.; Brinckerhoff, C.E. (2000). Interleukin-1 induction of collagenase 3 (matrix metalloproteinase 13) gene expression in chondrocytes requires p38, c-Jun N-terminal kinase, and nuclear factor kappaB: differential regulation of collagenase 1 and collagenase 3. *Arthritis Rheum*, 43: 801-811.

Millward-Sadler, S.J. & Salter, D.M. (2004). Integrin-dependent signal cascades in chondrocyte mechanotransduction. *Ann Biomed Eng*, 32: 435-446.

Min, J.L.; Meulenbelt, I.; Riyazi, N.; Kloppenburg, M.; Houwing-Duistermaat, J.J.; Seymour, A.B.; Pols, H.A.; van Duijn, C.M.; Slagboom, P.E. (2005). Association of the Frizzled-related protein gene with symptomatic osteoarthritis at multiple sites. *Arthritis Rheum*, 52: 1077-1080.

Miyaki, S.; Nakasa, T.; Otsuki, S.; Grogan, S.P.; Higashiyama, R.; Inoue, A.; Kato, Y.; Sato, T.; Lotz, M.K.; Asahara, H. (2009). MicroRNA-140 is expressed in differentiated human articular chondrocytes and modulates interleukin-1 responses. *Arthritis Rheum*, 60: 2723-2730.

Miyazawa, K.; Shinozaka, M.; Hara, T.; Furuya, T.; Miyazono, K. (2002). Two major Smad pathways in TFG-β superfamily signaling. *Genes to Cells*, 7: 1191-1204.

Mort, J.S. & Billington, C.J. (2001). Articular cartilage and changes in arthritis matrix degradation. *Arthritis Res*, 3: 337-341.

Muraki, S.; Oka, H.; Akune, T.; Mabuchi, A.; En-yo, Y.; Yoshida, M.; Saika, A.; Suzuki, T.; Yoshida, H.; Ishibashi, H.; Yamamoto, S.; Nakamura, K.; Kawaguchi, H.; Yoshimura, N. (2009). Prevalence of radiographic knee osteoarthritis and its association with knee pain in the elderly of Japanese population-based cohorts: the ROAD study. *Osteoarthritis Cartilage*, 17: 1137-1143.

Neuhold, L.A.; Killar, L.; Zhao, W.; Sung, M.L.; Warner, L.; Kulik, J.; Turner, J.; Wu, W.; Billinghurst, C.; Meijers, T.; Poole, A.R.; Babij, P.; DeGennaro, L.J. (2001). Postnatal expression in hyaline cartilage of constitutively active human collagenase-3 (MMP-13) induces osteoarthritis in mice. *J Clin Invest*, 107: 35-44.

Ng, T.C.; Chiu, K.W.; Rabie, A.B.; Hagg, U. (2006). Repeated mechanical loading enhances the expression of Indian hedgehog in condylar cartilage. *Front Biosci*, 11: 943-948.

Nicole, D. & Kerstin, K. (2000). Targeted mutations of transforming growth factor-β genes reveal important roles in mouse development and adult homeostasis. *Eur J Bioche*, 267: 6982-6988.

Ornitz, D.M. (2005). FGF signaling in the developing endochondral skeleton. *Cytokine Growth Factor Rev*, 16: 205-213.

Pacifici, M.; Koyama, E. & Iwamoto, M. (2005). Mechanismsof synovial joint and articular cartilage formation: recent advances, butmany lingeringmysteries. *Birth Defects Res. C Embryo Today*, 75: 237-248.

Pfander, D.; Cramer, T.; Schipani, E.; Johnson, R.S. (2003). HIF-1alpha controls extracellular matrix synthesis by epiphyseal chondrocytes. *J Cell Sci*, 116: 1819-1826.

Reboul, P.; Pelletier, J.P.; Tardif, G.; Cloutier, J.M.; Martel-Pelletier, J. (1996). The new collagenase, collagenase-3, is expressed and synthesized by human chondrocytes but not by synoviocytes: A role in osteoarthritis. *J Clin Invest*, 97: 2011-2019.

Roach, H.I.; Yamada, N.; Cheung, K.S.; Tilley, S.; Clarke, N.M.; Oreffo, R.O.; Kokubun, S.; Bronner, F. (2005). Association between the abnormal expression of matrix-degrading enzymes by human osteoarthritic chondrocytes and demethylation of specific CpG sites in the promoter regions. *Arthritis Rheum*, 52: 3110-3124.

Robinson, J.A.; Chatterjee-Kishore, M.; Yaworsky, P.J.; Cullen, D.M.; Zhao, W.G.; Li, C.; Kharode, Y.; Sauter, L.; Babij, P.; Brown, E.L.; Hill, A.A.; Akhter, M.P.; Johnson, M.L.; Recker, R.R.; Kannu, P.; Bateman, J.F.; Belluoccio, D. (2009). Employing molecular genetics of chondrodysplasias to inform the study of osteoarthritis. *Arthritis Rheum*, 60: 325–334.

Saito, T.; Fukai, A.; Mabuchi, A.; Ikeda, T.; Yano, F.; Ohba, S.; Nishida, N.; Akune, T.; Yoshimura, N.; Nakagawa, T.; Nakamura, K.; Tokunaga, K.; Chung, U.I.; Kawaguchi, H. (2010). Transcriptional regulation of endochondral ossification by HIF-2alpha during skeletal growth and osteoarthritis development. *Nat Med*, 16: 678-686.

Sampson, E.R.; Beck, C.A.; Ketz, J.; Canary, K.L.; Hilton, M.J.; Awad, H.; Schwarz, E.M.; Chen, D.; O'Keefe, R.J.; Rosier, R.N.; Zuscik, M.J. (2011). Establishment of quantitative methods for the assessment of murine arthritis. *The Journal of Orthopaedic Research*, Accepted.

Schoenle, E.; Zapf, J.; Humbel, R.E.; Froesch, E.R. (1982). Insulin-like growth factor I stimulates growth in hypophysectomized rats. *Nature*, 296: 252-253.

Schofield, C.J. & Ratcliffe, P.J. (2004). Oxygen sensing by HIF hydroxylases. *Nat Rev Mol Cell Biol*, 5: 343-354.

Semenza, G.L. (2000). HIF-1 and human disease: one highly involved factor. *Genes Dev*, 15: 1983-1991.

Serra, R.; Johnson, M.; Filvaroff, E.H.; LaBorde, J.; Sheehan, D.M.; Derynck, R.; Moses, H.L. (1997). Expression of a truncated, kinase-defective TGF-b type II receptor in mouse skeletal tissue promotes terminal chondrocyte differentiation and osteoarthritis. *J Cell Biol*, 139: 541-552.

Shen, R.; Chen, M.; Wang, Y.J.; Kaneki, H.; Xing, L.; O;Keefe, R.J.; Chen, D. (2006). Smad6 interacts with Runx2 and mediates Smad ubiquitin regulatory factor 1-induced Runx2 degradation. *J Biol Chem*, 281: 3569-3576.

Shen, R.; Wang, X.; Drissi, H.; Liu, F.; O'Kefe, R.J.; Chen, D. (2006). Cyclin D1-cdk4 induce runx2 ubiquitination and degradation. *J Biol Chem*, 281: 16347-16353.

Shiomi, T.; Lemaître, V.; D'Armiento, J.; Okada, Y. (2010). Matrix metalloproteinases, a disintegrin and metalloproteinases, and a disintegrin and metalloproteinases with thrombospondin motifs in non-neoplastic diseases. *Pathology International*, 60: 477-496.

Shui, C.; Spelsberg, T.C.; Riggs, B.L.; Khosla, S. (2003). Changes in Runx2/Cbfa1 expression and activity during osteoblastic differentiation of human bone marrow stromal cells. *J Bone Miner Res*, 18: 213-221.

Stanton, H.; Rogerson, F.M.; East, C.J.; Golub, S.B.; Lawlor, K.E.; Meeker, C.T.; Little, C.B.; Last, K.; Farmer, P.J.; Campbell, I.K.; Fourie, A.M.; Fosang, A.J. (2005). ADAMTS5 is the major aggrecanase in mouse cartilage in vivo and in vitro. *Nature*, 434: 648-652.

Stetler-Stevenson, W.G. & Seo, D.W. (2005). TIMP-2: an endogenous inhibitor of angiogenesis. *Trends in molecular medicine*, 11: 97-103.

Stickens, D.; Behonick, D.J.; Ortega, N.; Heyer, B.; Hartenstein, B.; Yu, Y.; Fosang, A.J.; Schorpp-Kistner, M.; Angel, P.; Werb, Z. (2004). Altered endochondral bone development in matrix metalloproteinase 13-deficient mice. *Development*, 131: 5883-5895.

Takamoto, M.; Tsuji, K.; Yamashita, T.; Sasaki, H.; Yano, T.; Taketani, Y.; Komori, T.; Nifuji, A.; Noda, M. (2003). Hedgehog signaling enhances core binding factor a1 and receptor activator of nuclear factor-kappaB ligand (RANKL) gene expression in chondrocytes. *J Endocrinol*, 177: 413-421.

Tardif, G.; Reboul, P.; Pelletier, J.P.; Geng, C.; Cloutier, J.M.; Martel-Pelletier, J. (1996). Normal expression of type 1 insulin-like growth factor receptor by human osteoarthritic chondrocytes with increased expression and synthesis of insulin-like growth factor binding proteins. *Arthritis Rheum*, 39: 968-978.

Tou, L.; Quibria, N.; Alexander, J.M. (2001). Regulation of human cbfa1 gene transcription in osteoblasts by selective estrogen receptor modulators (SERMs). *Mol Cell Endocrinol*, 183: 71-79.

Trippel, S.B.; Corvol, M.T.; Dumontier, M.F.; Rappaport, R.; Hung, H.H.; Mankin, H.J. (1989). Effect of somatomedin-C/insulin-like growth factor I and growth hormone on cultured growth plate and articular chondrocytes. *Pediatr Res*, 25: 76-82.

Valdes, A.M.; Spector, T.D.; Tamm, A.; Kisand, K.; Doherty, S.A.; Dennison, E.M.; Mangino, M.; Tamm, A.; Kerna, I.; Hart, D.J.; Wheeler, M.; Cooper, C.; Lories, R.J.; Arden, N.K.; Doherty, M. (2010). Genetic variation in the smad3 gene is associated with hip and knee osteoarthritis. *Arthritis Rheum*, 62: 2347-2352.

Verzijl, N.; DeGroot, J.; Thorpe, S.R.; Bank, R.A.; Shaw, J.N.; Lyons, T.J.; Bijlsma, J.W.; Lafeber, F.P.; Baynes, J.W.; TeKoppele, J.M. (2000). Effect of collagen turnover on the accumulation of advanced glycation end products. *J Biol Chem*, 275: 39027-39031.

Vincenti, M.P.; Coon, C.I.; Mengshol, J.A.; Yocum, S.; Mitchell, P.; Brinckerhoff, C.E. (1998). Cloning of the gene for interstitial collagenase-3 (matrix metalloproteinase-13) from rabbit synovial fibroblasts: differential expression with collagenase-1 (matrix metalloproteinase-1). *Biochem J*, 331: 341-346.

Vincenti, M.P. (2001). The matrix metalloproteinase (MMP) and tissue inhibitor of metalloproteinase (TIMP) genes. Transcriptional and posttranscriptional regulation, signal transduction and cell-type-specific expression. *Methods Mol Biol*, 151: 121-148.

Wu, Q.; Huang, J.H.; Sampson, E.R.; Kim, K.O.; Zuscik, M.J.; O'Keefe, R.J.; Chen, D.; Rosier; R.N. (2009). Smurf2 Induces degradation of GSK-3β and upregulates β-catenin in chondrocytes: A potential mechanism for Smurf2-induced degeneration of articular cartilage. *Exp Cell Res*, 315: 2386-2398.

Yamasaki, K.; Nakasa, T.; Miyaki, S.; Ishikawa, M.; Deie, M.; Adachi, N.; Yasunaga, Y.; Asahara, H.; Ochi, M. (2009). Expression of microRNA-146a in osteoarthritis cartilage. *Arthritis Rheum*, 60: 1035-1041.

Yang, X.; Chen, L.; Xu, X.; Li, C.; Huang, C.; Deng, C.X. (2001). TGF-β/Smad3 signals repress chondrocyte hypertrophic differentiation and are required for maintaining articular cartilage. *J Cell Biol*, 153: 35-46.

Yang, Y.Z. (2003). Wnts and Wing: Wnt signaling in vertebrate limb development and musculoskeletal morphogenesis. *Birth Defects Res*, 69: 305-317.

Yang, S.; Kim, J.; Ryu, J.H.; Oh, H.; Chun, C.H.; Kim, B.J.; Min, B.H.; Chun, J.S. (2010). Hypoxia-inducible factor-2alpha is a catabolic regulator of osteoarthritic cartilage destruction. *Nat Med*, 16: 687-693.

Zhang, M.; Xie, R.; Hou, W.; Wang, B.; Shen, R.; Wang, X.; Wang, Q.; Zhu, T.; Jonason, J.H.; Chen, D. (2009). PTHrP prevents chondrocyte premature hypertrophy by inducing cyclin D1-dependent Runx2 and Runx3 phosphorylation, ubiquitination and proteasome degradation. *J Cell Sci*, 122: 1382-1389.

Zhao, M.; Qiao, M.; Oyajobi, B.O.; Mundy, G.R.; Chen, D. (2003). E3 ubiquitin ligase Smurf1 mediates core-binding factor alpha 1/Runx2 degradation and plays a specific role in osteoblast differentiation. *J Biol Chem*, 278: 27939-27944.

Zhao, M.; Qiao, M.; Harris, S.E.; Oyajobi, B.O.; Mundy, G.R.; Chen, D. (2004). Smurf1 inhibits osteoblast differentiation and bone formation in vitro and in vivo. *J Biol Chem*, 279: 12854-12859.

Zhou, Y.X.; Xu, X.; Chen, L.; Li, C.; Brodie, S.G.; Deng, C.X. (2000). A Pro250Arg substitution in mouse Fgfr1 causes increased expression of Cbfa1 and premature fusion of calvarial sutures. *Hum Mol Genet*, 9: 2001-2008.

Zhu, M.; Chen, M.; Lichlter, A.C.; O'Keefe, R.J.; Chen, D. (2008). Tamoxifen-inducible Cre-recombination in articular chondrocytes of adult Col2a1-CreER^{T2} transgenic mice. *Osteoarthritis Cartilage*, 16: 129-130.

Zhu, M.; Tang, D.; Wu, Q.; Hao, S.; Chen, M.; Xie, C.; Rosier, R.N.; O'Keefe, R.J.; Zuscik, M.; Chen, D. (2009). Activation of β-catenin signaling in articular chondrocytes leads to osteoarthritis-like phenotype in adult β-catenin conditional activation mice. *J Bone Miner Res*, 24: 12-21.

Part 5

Metabolic

14

Cartilage Extracellular Matrix Integrity and OA

Chathuraka T. Jayasuriya and Qian Chen
Alpert Medical School of Brown Universit, Rhode Island Hospital
United States of America

1. Introduction

Articular cartilage tissue is mostly composed of extracellular matrix (ECM) in which a sparse population of cells (chondrocytes) reside. These cells produce both anabolic and catabolic factors that perpetuate a homeostatic process of ECM breakdown and repair termed cartilage turnover. This balance between tissue anabolism and catabolism is characteristic of normal articular cartilage. However, during osteoarthritis (OA), this process is disrupted due to disregulation of chondrocyte function. Although articular cartilage is anatomically classified as a single tissue type, it is divided into four zones defined by their physiological position relative to the joint surface. Likewise, the populations of chondrocytes housed within these zones and their respective ECMs often differ from one another in both appearance and organization. The calcified zone lies directly on top of the subchondral bone, which the cartilage tissue shields from physical forces. This zone contains a very small population of chondrocytes that are slowly being replaced by bone forming cells (osteoblasts) continuously throughout life. When compared to other cartilage zones, the calcified zone ECM is highly mineralized and contains the sparsest chondrocyte population. Osteoblasts from the neighboring subchondral bone secrete bone morphogenic factor (BMPs), and other factors such as stromal cell derived factor 1 (SDF-1) which promote chondrocyte hypertrophy and mineralization. The deep zone cartilage layer lies directly above the calcified zone and contains small vertical aggregates of chondrocytes embedded within a uniquely organized ECM which histologically resemble columnar structures. The middle zone is by far the largest layer containing round bodied chondrocytes and a well hydrated and robust collagen ECM network. Chondrocyte content increases gradually from the subchondral bone towards the articular surface that is in direct contact with the joint synovium. The superficial zone (A.K.A. tangential zone) makes up the articular surface and therefore contains the largest number of chondrocytes of all four zones. OA can affect just one or all four of these cartilage zones depending on the severity and pathological stage of the disease. Given its anatomical position, the superficial zone is often the first cartilage tissue zone to be exposed to injury or wear-and-tear due to excessive joint loading. Therefore this zone often appears to be the initial point of OA pathogenesis. During early stage OA, a sustained injury to the articular surface initially induces a mild but chronic inflammatory response (Martel-Pelletier et al., 2008) that slowly manifests into the disruption of cartilage homeostasis due to disredulation of chondrocyte function (Goldring & Marcu, 2009). As the disease persists, continued homeostatic imbalances eventually cause the release of excessive amounts of catabolic enzymes that break down the ECM resulting in lesion formation within the articular cartilage tissue. Similarly, the disregulated release of anabolic factors such as BMPs and IHH by chondrocytes can result in chondrocyte hypertrophy and eventually calcification of the cartilage ECM. Such changes often lead to osteophyte (bone spur) formation on the otherwise smooth articular surface making normal movement painful and destructive to the connective tissue demonstrating the importance of ECM microenvironment to cartilage tissue health.

2. Structure and function of cartilage ECM molecules and their mutations in degenerative joint diseases

Articular cartilage is an avascular aneural connective tissue composed of chondrocytes that produce and maintain a robust ECM protein network. During early bone development, mesenchymal stem cells of the chondrogenic progeny undergo differentiation into chondrocytes which proliferate, mature, and eventually calcify and undergo cell death as they are replaced by bone. This process leaves behind a layer of articullar cartilage that covers the surfaces of bones providing a low friction surface that can act as a weight/shear stress-bearing coat allowing for smooth joint transition during movement. Articular cartilage tissue has high water content contributing to its near frictionless nature.

2.1 Collagens

Articular cartilage ECM is composed mainly of three kinds of macromolecules: (1) collagens, (2) proteoglycans and (3) non-collagenous matrix proteins. Several collagens are cartilage specific including type II, VI, IX, X, and XI. Table 1 lists the most common cartilage ECM proteins and human diseases that result from their mutation, including their association with chondrodysplasia and OA.

2.1.1 Collagen II

Type II collagen makes up approximately 80 to 90 percent of all collagen content found in normal healthy articular cartilage tissue. In OA, tissue degradation is predominantly caused by the breakdown of cartilage ECM due to the overabundance of reactive proteases, many of which cleave type II collagen containing fibrils resulting in tissue destabilization due to reduction in tensile strength. Type II collagen is initially synthesized as pro-alpha-chains that are assembled into a triple helical structure by the globular domains that exist at both its N and C terminal ends. Two forms of pro-collagen are found in cartilage: Type IIA (COL2A1) and Type IIB. These trimeric type II collagen molecules crosslink with other collagens (i.e. type IX and XI) to form large fibrils that compose a web-like network, which binds to various ECM molecules. The stability of the triple helical structure provides the strength required by cartilage to resist tensile stress and also prevents type II collagen from being easily degraded by most endogenous proteases found in the tissue. Due to its long half-life (over 100 years under physiological conditions) and relative stability, the type II collagen network is never completely broken down or remodeled during normal cartilage homeostatic processes. Type II collagen mutations can cause a plethora of mild to severe phenotypes depending on the nature and location of the mutation. While heterozygous deletion of this gene in mice show a minimal phenotype, complete homozygous deletion predictably causes severe cartilage tissue disorganization and death shortly after birth (Li et al., 1995). In addition to being linked to the development of degenerative joint diseases such

Protein	Gene(s)	Human diseases caused by mutations	Chondrodysplasia	OA causative
Type II collagen	COL2A1	Stickler syndrome	Yes (mild)	May
		Achondrogenesis (type II)	Yes	No evidence
		Hypochondrogenesis	Yes	No evidence
		Spondyloepiphyseal dysplasia	Yes	May
		Spondyloepimetaphyseal dysplasia	Yes	May
Type VI collagen	COL6A1, COL6A2, COL6A3	Ullrich congenital muscular dystrophy	No evidence	No evidence
		Bethlem myopathy	No evidence	No evidence
Type IX collagen	COL9A1, COL9A2, COL9A3	Multiple epiphyseal dysplasia	Yes	May
		Lumbar disk disease	No evidence	No evidence
		Premature OA	No evidence	Yes
Type X collagen	COL10A1	Schmid metaphyseal dysplasia	Yes	No evidence
		Spondylometaphyseal dysplasia	Yes	May
Type XI collagen	COL11A1, COL11A2	Stickler syndrome	Yes (mild)	May
		Spondylomegaepiphyseal dysplasia	Yes	May
		Premature OA	No evidence	Yes
Aggrecan	ACAN	Several chondrodysplasias	Yes	May
Matrilin-3	MATN3	Multiple epiphyseal dysplasia	Yes	May
		Spondyloepimetaphyseal dysplasia	Yes	May
		Premature OA	No evidence	Yes
Cartilage oligomeric matrix protein	COMP	Pseudoachondroplasia	Yes	May
		Multiple epiphyseal dysplasia	Yes	May
Lubricin	PRG4	Camptodactyly-arthropathy-coxa vara-pericarditis syndrome	No evidence	No evidence

Table 1. Cartilage matrix proteins and common human diseases associated with their mutation, including their association with chondrodysplasia and osteoarthritis (OA)

as familial OA, various mutations in this molecule can cause more severe phenotypes such as Stickler syndrome, and several major chondrogenic defects (Byers, 2001). A mutation in the alpha helical domain causing a substitution of a glycine codon with a larger amino acid has been shown to disrupt proper alpha helix formation of type II collagen leading to severe chondrodysplasias and a significant reduction in cartilage tissue stability (Kuivaniemi et al., 1997; Prockop et al., 1997). Similarly in the 1990s, particular families were discovered to have missense mutation (R519C) causing the production of abnormal type II collagen pro-alpha-chains. These alpha chains formed protein dimers leading to mild chondrodysplasia followed by a unique form of familial OA (Byers, 2001; Eyre et al., 1991; Pun et al., 1994; Bleasel et al., 1998).

2.1.2 Collagen XI

Type XI collagen is the second most abundant collagen (3% of all collagens) found in adult articular cartilage and it is a core component of collagen fibrils. It is a heterotrimeric molecule composed of three alpha-chains. Interestingly, the first two chains are coded by the COL11A1 and COL11A2 genes respectively while the third chain is coded by COL2A1 and uniquely post transcriptionally modified (Martel-Pelletier et al., 2008). Type XI collagen makes hydroxylysine-based aldehyde cross-links with type II collagen to form collagen fibrils that stabilize articular cartilage (Cremer et al., 1988) and it has been suggested that the ratio of type XI to type II determines collagen fibril diameter and tensile strength. Like COL2A1, mutations in the type XI collagen genes can cause Stickler syndrome. A study done in 1995 also discovered that a single base pair deletion in the type XI collagen gene creates a frame shift resulting in a premature stop codon which is functionally equivalent to knocking out the gene itself (Li et al., 1995). Mice that are homozygous for this nonsense mutation develop serious chondrodysplasia and die at birth. Missense mutations in the COL11A2 gene have also been associated with spondylo-megaepiphyseal dysplasia (OSMED) (Vikkula et al., 1995) and mutations in both COL11A1 and COL11A2 can cause premature development of OA (Rodriguez et al., 2004).

2.1.3 Collagen IX

Type IX collagen is normally co expressed with type II collagen in hyaline cartilage. In adults, this collagen makes up about 1% of the collagen content found in the articular cartilage. Similar to type VI collagen, type IX collagen molecules exist in heterotrimeric form composed of three alpha-chains. Each of these heterotrimers has seven sites with which to form cross-links with other collagen molecules. Type IX collagen is found to be covalently bonded through aldimine-derived crosslinks to the surface of large type II collagen fibrils (Wu et al., 1992) and it is believed to constrain the lateral expansion of these fibrils (Blaschke et al., 2000; Gregory et al., 2000). Missense mutations in the type IX collagen genes have been associated with lumbar disk disease (LDD) (Zhu et al., 2011) and multiple epiphyseal dysplasia (MED) (Jackson et al., 2010) which indirectly leads to the development of OA. Surprisingly, mice deficient in type IX collagen exhibit normal signs of skeletal and chondral development; however they are afflicted by early joint cartilage degradation that resemble the formation of OA-like lesions (Hu et al., 2006).

2.1.4 Collagen VI

Hyaline cartilage contains a relatively low content of type VI collagen (less than 2% of all articular cartilage tissue collagens) that is found in all cartilage zones within the pericellular regions around chondrocytes (Pullig et al., 1999). Type VI collagen molecules are of heterotrimeric organization as they are composed of three non-identical alpha chains. Each chain contains a triple helical domain allowing for the formation of dimers and tetramers with each other (Engel et al., 1985; Furthmayr et al., 1983). Type VI collagen interacts with non-collagenous matrix proteins forming a network in the pericellular regions. It has been previously demonstrated that type VI collagen content is increased in certain patients suffering from OA. However, it is suspected that disregulated tissue homeostasis causes excessive collagen anabolism and deposition (Pullig et al., 1999). Mutations in the genes that code for the three type VI collagen alpha chains have been associated with noncartilage-specific abnormalities such as muscular dystrophy (Pace et al., 2008) and Bethlem myopathy (Lamandé et al., 1998). And a study conducted in 2009 demonstrated that COL6A1 homozygous knockout mice display lower bone mineral density and develop OA more rapidly than wild-type mice of the same genetic background (Alexopoulos et al., 2009).

2.1.5 Collagen X

Chondrocytes only express type X collagen within the hypertrophic zone of the growth plate (Linsenmayer et al., 1988). It is a homotrimer composed of three pro-alpha-chains each containing a C terminal alpha helical domain which allows these chains to assemble into short triple helixes (Wagner et al., 2000). It has been demonstrated that type X collagen expression and distribution is altered during OA such that these molecules are found among the noncalcified regions of the articular cartilage implying the occurrence of premature chondrocyte hypertrophy in these zones (von der Mark et al., 1992). Abnormalities in type X collagen can cause spinal and metaphyseal dysplasias (i.e. Schmid MCD) due to improper enchondral ossification (Bignami et al., 1992). A heterozygous missence mutation (Gly595Glu) in the COL10A1 gene was also previously found to correlate with spondylometaphyseal dysplasia (SMD) within a certain family (Ikegawa et al., 1998). And transgenic mice with deletions in the triple-helical domain of type X collagen develop SMD (Jacenko et al., 1993).

2.2 Proteoglycans

The second major structural components of articullar cartilage tissue are proteoglycans of which aggrecan is the most common. These ECM proteins predominantly help cartilage tissue to retain water and withstand compressive force during joint transition and loading.

2.2.1 Aggrecan

Aggrecan is a large chondroitin sulfate proteoglycan that consists of a 220 kDa protein core containing three globular domains (G1, G2 and G3) which allow it to form covalent bonds with its glycosaminoglycan (GAG) side chain components (Doege et al., 1991). Each GAG side chain is composed of a single keratin sulfate and two chondroitin sulfate domain regions all of which are adjacent to the G2 and G3 globular domains. The G1 domain is attached to a link protein that enables multiple aggrecan subunits to bind to a long nonsulfated glycosaminoglycan backbone known as hyluronic acid (HA). Thus aggrecan becomes trapped within the collagen network where some suspect that it acts to physically shield type II collagen from proteolytic cleavage (Pratta et al., 2003). Due to its overall negative charge, aggrecan draws water into the cartilage ECM allowing the tissue to swell. This swelling gives the tissue a spring-like quality helping it to withstand compressive forces that are applied to the joint during movement. Proteolytic cleavage of this vital ECM protein is mediated by proteases known as aggrecanases. During OA, the disregulation of aggrecanase synthesis and release causes much damage to aggrecan molecules and the cartilage tissue loses the ability to retain water as it suffers from a reduction in overall stability. As is the case with type II collagen and other major cartilage ECM proteins, deletions/mutations in aggrecan lead to severe chondrodysplasia which can often cause premature OA.

2.2.2 Hyaluronic acid

HA is a nonsulfated GAG that is covalently linked to aggrecan monomers and allows these subunits to aggregate in the cartilage ECM. HA species can have varying molecular mass depending on the length of the GAG. Their masses can range from as small as fifty to larger than thousands of Kilodaltons. The molecular weight of HA decreases during normal aging due to proteolytic cleavage and the cartilage tissue of young individuals tends to have larger species of HA compared to that of the elderly. In addition to the cartilage ECM, HA is also largely found in synovial fluid and contributes to its viscoelasticity. HA recognizes and specifically binds several different cell surface receptors (i.e. CD44, ICAM-1 and RHAMM) where it remains as a major component of the pericellular network surrounding chondrocytes. Due to its large size, HA can shield cells from coming into contact with inflammatory mediators such as cytokines and chemokines. It has also been suggested that HA can regulate collagenase and aggrecanase expression from chondrocytes and synovial cells. Previous studies have demonstrated that higher molecular mass species of HA can inhibit IL-1 mediated stimulation of certain MMPs and ADAMTS-4 by interacting with CD44 (Julovi et al., 2004; Wang et al., 2006; Theuns et al., 2008) while the opposite effect has been found to occur in the presence of smaller mass species (20 kDa) of this proteoglycan. Additionally, these larger species can also inhibit proteoglycan release from cartilage tissue ECM. HA is currently used as an intra-articularly therapy via joint injection for knee OA as this long proteoglycan is believed to decrease OA associated joint pain by increasing both the viscoelastic properties of synovial fluid and the lubrication of the articular surface preventing tissue tearing due to the friction generated during joint transition. (Moreland, 2003; Wobig et al., 1998; Altman & Moskowitz, 1998). Its efficacy in relieving OA related pain has been reported to be depend on the molecular mass of the HA chains as species of larger molecular mass were found to have a greater effect in reducing joint pain. Although the exact biological mechanism with which HA relieves OA associated joint pain remains to be elucidated, it is believed that this large proteoglycan supplements the natural synovial fluid increasing its viscoelasticity and reducing the friction generated during joint movement.

2.2.3 Leucine-rich small proteoglycans

Articullar cartilage also consists of a group of small proteoglycans classified for having seven to eleven leucine-rich repeats (SLRPs). The major cartilage SLRPs are decorin, biglycan, fibromodulin, lumican and epiphycan in the order of decreasing abundance. These small proteoglycans have several roles in maintaining cartilage tissue ECM organization and homeostasis such as interacting with various collagen species to strengthen the ECM network and protecting collagen fibrils from proteolytic cleavage by collagenases. The SLRPs decorin and biglycan are similar in structure as both consist of a leucine-rich core protein linked to either one (in the case of decorin) or two (in the case of biglycan) chondroitin/dermatan sulfate containing GAG chain(s). Previous literature has suggested that decorin can alter the cell cycle by modulating growth factor (i.e. TGF-β and EGF) signaling and it is currently studied in cancer research. Although similar in structure to decorin, biglycan has a different physiological role in ECM. It has been suggested that this proteoglycan modulates BMP-4 signaling during osteoblast differentiation (Chen et al., 2004). Biglycan is essential during skeletal development to maintain normal bone mineral density. Fibromodulin and lumican are SLRPs that competitively bind the same region of collagen fibrils helping to regulate fibril diameter and ECM network assembly (Svensson et al. 2000). Epiphycan is a dermatan sulfate proteoglycan with seven leucine-rich repeats believed to maintain joint integrity, yet little is known about its function and the biological mechanism with which it protects tissue. Mutations and/or deletions in SLRP genes are associated primarily with connective tissue and eye disorders. One recent study demonstrated that biglycan and epiphycan double knockout mice are normal at birth but develop several skeletal abnormalities later in life along with premature OA (Nuka et al., 2010). But there have yet to be more studies that suggest abnormalities in these genes are linked to degenerative joint diseases. Given the importance of SLRPs in regulating tissue homeostasis and matrix organization, this is quite surprising.

2.3 Non-collagenous matrix proteins

Other important non-collagenous matrix proteins found in articular cartilage include the matrilins (matrilin-1 and -3), the cartilage oligomeric matrix protein (COMP), and the lubricating protein predominantly secreted by chondrocytes of the superficial zone: lubricin.

2.3.1 Matrilins

The matrilins are a family of noncollagenous oligomeric ECM proteins that are found in a broad range of tissues including articular cartilage and bone (Deak et al., 1999; Wagener et al., 1997; Piecha et al., 1999; Klatt et al., 2001). There are currently four known members within this family. MATN1 and MATN3 are cartilage specific while MATN2 and MATN4 are found in many connective tissue types (van der Weyden et al. 2006; Wu et al., 1998; Piecha et al., 2002). It has been demonstrated that matrilins form a filamentous network pericellularly in the cartilage ECM (Klatt et al., 2000). Structurally, MATN1 consists of two Von Willebrand Factor A (vWFA) domains, one epidermal growth factor-like (EGF) domain, so named because they share a forty amino-acid long residue commonly found in epidermal growth factor protein, and one alpha helical coil-coiled oligomerization domain. Each vWFA domain contains a metal ion-dependant adhesion site (MIDAS) and previous studies have demonstrated that its mutation can abolish filamentous network formation resulting in abnormal ECM assembly (Chen et al., 1999). Its coil-coiled oligomerization domain allows it to form homotrimers with other MATN1 molecules or hetero-oligomers with MATN3. MATN1 is expressed by post proliferative chondrocytes that constitute the zone of maturation within the growth plate. MATN1 interacts with both type II collagen and aggrecan playing a role in organizing fibril formation. MATN1 knockout mice exhibit abnormal fibrillogenesis as their collagen fibrils become aggregated in a uniform directional orientation as opposed to the normal matrix network-like organization observed in wild-type animals.

Although mutations of MATN1 have not been associated with the development of degenerative joint diseases, MATN3 is the smallest and most recently discovered member of the matrilin family of ECM proteins. MATN3 contains a single vWFA domain, four EGF-like domains, and one alpha-helical oligomerization domain which allows it to form homo-oligomers with other MATN3 peptides and hetero-oligomers with MATN1 (Klatt et al., 2000). MATN3 is naturally found in the articular cartilage in its tetrameric form composed of four single oligomers covalently bound together by their alpha-helical oligomerization domains. Several known MATN3 mutations can lead to developmental abnormalities in articular cartilage and bone. These mutations can eventually either lead to OA directly, in the case of hand OA (Aeschlimann et al., 1993; Cepko et al., 1992) or indirectly, in the case of MED, which manifests with joint pain and early onset OA (Chen et al., 1992; Chen et al., 1993). A threonine to methionine missense mutation (T298M) in the first EGF-like domain of MATN3 has been found to correlate with the development of hand OA (Stefánsson et al., 2003) while a cystine to serine (C299S) missense mutation in this same region is common to many patients suffering from spondylo-epi-metaphyseal dysplasia (SEMD), which is a condition often leading to vertebral, epiphyseal/metaphyseal anomalies during development (Borochowitz et al., 2004). Likewise, an arginine to tryptophan missense mutation (R116W) in the vWFA domain has been associated with MED. It was discovered that this particular mutation prevents normal secretion of MATN3 from chondrocytes due to a dominant negative interaction between mutant and normal MATN3 quickly leading to an increase in MATN3 retention within the endoplasmic reticulum of these cells (Otten et al., 2005). Consequently, this reduction in the secretion of functional MATN3 is believed to contribute to MED. Interestingly, during advanced stages of OA, joint synovial fluid contains higher levels of cleaved ECM proteins including MATN3 oligomers due to the proteolysis of articular cartilage. One study has even shown that MATN3 mRNA is upregulated in some OA patients suggesting that the body may produce an excess of the protein (Pullig et al., 2002). Matrilin proteins are relatively well conserved between mice and humans making them ideal proteins to investigate in the mouse model. Complete homozygous deletion of the MATN3 gene in mice surprisingly results in no gross skeletal deformities at birth, but it does however result in the development of OA much earlier in life. MATN3 knockout mice were maintained in a C57BL/6J background and developed several signs of enhanced OA including osteophyte formation and the presence of large lesions in the superficial zone of the articular cartilage, which is the layer that is in direct contact with the knee joint synovium. Additionally, these knockout mice appear to have a higher bone mineral density (BMD) and lower overall cartilage proteoglycan content when compared to wild-type mice of the same genetic background. Perhaps the increase in BMD leads to over-loading of diarthroidial joints, which eventually manifests in the form of enhanced cartilage damage. Tentatively, MATN3's ability to prevent OA-like lesion formation in articular cartilage may also be related to its regulatory functions. The complete biological mechanism with which this ECM protein acts chondroprotectively remains to be elucidated.

2.3.2 COMP

Cartilage oligomeric matrix protein (COMP) is another non-collagenous ECM protein found in articular cartilage with a function that is not yet completely understood. It is a pentameric molecule which consists of five glycoprotein subunits held to one another by disulfide bonds.

Each subunit contains an EGF-like domain and a thrombospondin-like domain. Previous studies have shown that COMP can stimulate type II collagen fibrillogenesis (Rosenberg et al., 1998). In cartilage, COMP is found bound to types I, II, and IX collagen molecules. While COMP knockout mice exhibit normal chondral and skeletal development, various missense mutation in the COMP gene have been shown to cause severe chondrodysplasias such as pseudoachondroplasia (PSACH) and MED, which is accompanied by premature OA development. COMP is also used as a marker of OA pathogenesis because its concentration is commonly elevated in OA patients (Williams & Spector et al., 2008)

2.3.3 Lubricin

Lubricin is a large soluble proteoglycan that is highly expressed by synoviocytes and chondrocytes of superficial zone articular cartilage. It is found in the synovial fluid and it covers articular surfaces of joints acting as a lubricant that prevents friction induced tissue wear and tear during joint transition. Lubricin consists of a central core protein containing heavily glycosylated oligosaccharide side chains. The core protein contains two somatomedin B-like (SMB) domains, a single a hemopexin-like domain (PEX), and two glycosylated mucin-like domains (Rhee et al., 2005). It is coded by the PGR4 gene, which when knocked out results in cartilage degradation and synovial cell hyperplasia in mice. Mutations in this gene can cause camptodactyly-arthropathy-coxa vara-pericarditis syndrome (CACP), which is an autosomal recessive disease that causes synovial hyperplasia and joint degredation similar to the phenotype of mice that are completely deficient in this protein (Rhee et al., 2005).

3. Extracellular matrix breakdown during osteoarthritis

During cartilage turnover, ECM molecules are slowly broken down via proteolysis and replaced by newly synthesized ECM proteins secreted from nearby chondrocytes. The catabolic and anabolic processes of this turnover are balanced in normal cartilage so that the rate of proteolysis and ECM loss matches the rate of ECM synthesis. However, in OA cartilage, this balance is often observed to be shifted towards catabolism. Proteases act to degrade the ECM network by cleaving excessive amounts collagen and proteoglycans. These cleaved fragments are released into the cartilage matrix and some can even trigger further tissue catabolism by both known and unknown biological mechanisms. The degeneration of the joint cartilage is further enhanced by the lackluster process of tissue repair due to disregulated anabolism. During OA, the disregulation of common anabolic growth factors native to the articular cartilage (i.e. TGF-β, FGF and IGF) prevents adequate protection against the catabolic effects induced by proteases ultimately leading to an imbalanced cartilage turnover process that favors degradation.

3.1 Activation of matrix proteases: MMPs, ADAMTS family

OA is clinically characterized by its degenerative effect on major articular cartilage ECM components such as collagen fibrils and proteoglycans by proteolysis (Takaishi et al., 2008). This enhancement of articular cartilage ECM catabolism is mediated mostly by the matrix metalloproteinase (MMP) family of collagenases and the ADAMTS family of aggrecanases, which are often expressed by chondrocytes in response to inflammatory cytokines such as IL-1β (Martel-Pelletier et al., 2008; Glasson et al. 2005; Stanton et al.,

2005). MMPs are neutral zinc-dependent endoproteinases that, when activated, cleave and degrade ECM components during normal tissue turnover. The MMP family is divided into several categories based on their enzymatic activity: collagenases, gelatinases, stromelysins, and membrane-type MMPs (MT-MMPs). MMPs commonly involved in cartilage homeostasis are collagenases and gelatinases. Most MMPs are initially secreted as inactive pro-MMP proteins (zymogens) which are then activated by proteolytic cleavage themselves. Because of their catabolic activity, this family of proteases has received much attention in arthritis research. Both mRNA expression and enzymatic activity of certain metalloproteinase are increased in cartilage tissue during OA pathogenesis including: MMP-1 (Drummond et al., 1999), MMP-2 (Imai et al., 1997; Mohtai et al., 1993), MMP-3 (Okada et al., 1992), MMP-7 (Ohta et al., 1998), MMP-8 (Drummond et al., 1999), MMP-9 (Mohtai et al., 1993), MMP-10 and MMP-13 (Mitchell et al., 1996). Table 2 lists OA associated catabolic proteases and the matrix protein targets that they cleave.

OA associated proteinase	Matrix Substrate
MMP-1	Types I, II, III, VII, VIII, X collagen Aggrecan
MMP-2	Types IV, V, VII, X collagen Aggrecan, decorin
MMP-3	Types II, III, IV, V, IX, X collagen Aggrecan, decorin
MMP-7	Types IV, X collagen Aggrecan, versican
MMP-8	Types I, II, III collagen Aggrecan
MMP-9	Types IV, V collagen Decorin
MMP-10	Types III, IV, V collagen Aggrecan
MMP-13	Types II, III, IV, IX, X collagen Aggrecan
ADAMTS-4	Aggrecan Matrilin-3
ADAMTS-5	Aggrecan Brevican, matrilin-3

Table 2. Osteoarthritis (OA) associated MMPs and their cartilage extracellular matrix substrates.

3.1.1 MMP-1

MMP-1 is classified as a collagenase that shows preference for cleaving type III and type X collagens (Martel-Pelletier et al., 2008; Nwomeh et al., 2002) which, while not a major component of ECM, is still present in articular cartilage tissue. MMP-1 is stoichiometrically inhibited by tissue inhibitor of metalloproteinase (TIMP) 1 and 2.

3.1.2 MMP-2

MMP-2 (gelatinase A) is one of two gelatinases found in human tissues. It further degrades a broad range of collagen and proteoglycan species after these substrates have been initially cleaved by other protyolitic enzymes (i.e. collagenases and aggrecanases). During OA, most of the cartilage tissue damage caused by this metalloproteinase comes from its breakdown of aggrecan, decorin, type IV and X collagen. Active MMP-2 is present in superficial and transition zones of OA cartilage (Imai et al., 1997).

3.1.3 MMP-3

Similarly, MMP-3 is upregulated in early OA but mRNA levels subside during later stages. Immunohistochemical studies have previously demonstrated that MMP-3 is expressed primarily in the superficial and transition zone in early stage OA cartilage and MMP-3 staining positively correlates with tissue Mankin scores. In addition to degrading type IX collagen and certain proteoglycans (Martel-Pelletier et al., 2008; Okada et al., 1989), MMP-3 initiates a cascade that ultimately cleaves and activates pro-MMP-1.

3.1.4 MMP-7

Like MMP-2 and MMP-3, MMP-7 is mainly found in the superficial and transition zones of OA cartilage (Ohta et al., 1998). This metalloproteinase cleaves type IV and X collagens as well as various proteoglycans including aggrecan and versican. Additionally MMP-7 is involved in cleavage and activation of MMP-1, MMP-2, MMP-8 and MMP-9 pro-protein precursors (Dozier et al., 2006).

3.1.5 MMP-8

Unlike other OA associated metalloproteinases, MMP-8 is a collagenase that is produced by neutrophils in response to inflammatory cytokines. Although chondrocytes themselves produce very little of this catabolic enzyme (Stremme et al., 2003), inflammation of the synovium can cause the migration of neutrophils that synthesize and secrete it into and around the superficial zone of cartilage contributing to tissue destruction. MMP-8 cleaves type I, II, and III collagen species as well as various proteoglycans including aggrecan.

3.1.6 MMP-9

The second gelatinase common to human tissue is MMP-9 (gelatinase B) which prefers denatured collagen, mostly type IV and V, as a substrate for its catabolic activity (Okada et al., 1992). Its mRNA expression is minimal in normal articular cartilage but it is greatly elevated in fibrillated areas of OA cartilage.

3.1.7 MMP-10

MMP-10 is a collagenase that degrades collagens types III, IV, V and aggrecan (Nicholson et al., 1989; Fosang et al., 1991; Rechardt et al., 2000). It can also cleave and activate pro-MMP-1, -7, -8 and -9 (Nakamura et al., 1998).

3.1.8 MMP-13

Although many members of the MMP family are involved in cartilage ECM catabolism, no other MMP is as damaging to cartilage tissue during OA as is the collagenase MMP-13. Type

II collagen is the primary structural component of the articular cartilage ECM for which MMP-13 shows digestive preference over any other collagen type (Okada et al., 1992; Ohta et al., 1998). For this reason, it is the collagenase that causes the most cartilage ECM destruction during OA. In addition to type II collagen, it also cleaves type III, IV, IX and X collagen species endogenous to cartilage tissue. MMP-13 is normally expressed in many different tissues including skin, bone, muscle, and cartilage. Its expression normally coincides with type X collagen expression in cartilage undergoing hypertrophic differentiation (Kamekura et al., 2005). In normal healthy cartilage, the primary role of MMP-13 is to enable hypertrophic zone expansion as it denatures pre-existing type II collagen fibrils of the ECM. However, it has been shown that overexpression of MMP-13 in articular chondrocytes also induces OA phenotypic changes (Mitchell et al., 1996). Previous studies have attempted to use MMP-13 inhibitors such as pyrimidinetrione analogs (Drummond et al., 1999) and benzofuran (Blagg et al., 2005) to remedy OA induced cartilage damage. However, their responsiveness was found to be dose dependant and often caused unwanted musculoskeletal side effects (Wu et al., 2005).

3.1.9 Aggrecanases

Aggrecanase-1 (ADAMTS-4) and aggrecanase-2 (ADAMTS-5) are known to be the two most active aggrecanases that lead to articular cartilage ECM catabolism during both OA and rheumatoid arthritis (RA) (Tortorella et al., 1999; Abbaszade et al., 1999). ADAMTS-4 and -5 act on a specific cleavage site (Glu 373/Ala 374) truncating these large proteoglycan chains (Kuno et al. 2000; Rodrı´quez-Manzaneque et al., 2002). In addition to their primary activity of aggrecan cleavage, they have also been shown to cleave MATN3 tetramers at the alpha-helical oligomerization domain releasing MATN3 monomers into the extracellular space (Ahmad et al., 2009; Tahiri et al., 2008). Interestingly, a meniscal transaction induced OA model in mice showed that ADAMTS-5 KO mice sustain less damage to their articular cartilage than wild-type mice (Glasson et al., 2005) linking the expression of this aggrecanase to diminishing cartilage integrity.

3.2 Release and function of cleaved matrix proteins

Proteolytic cleavage of cartilage matrix constituents releases small oligomeric protein fragments into the extracellular space where they can mediate further tissue degradation. The release of oligomeric fragments produced during cleavage of ECM components such as fibronectin, HA, and type II collagen has previously been implicated in the enhancement of cartilage catabolism. Increasing concentrations of such fragments in synovial fluid samples of patients have been found to positively correlate with increasing grade of OA.

3.2.1 Fibronectin cleavage fragments

Fibronectin is a large (450 kDa) adhesive glycoprotein found in many tissues throughout the body including articular cartilage. While native fibronectin normally plays a role in cell-to-cell adhesion and migration, its smaller cleavage fragments (Fn-fs) have different properties and function. Due to enhanced proteolytic cleavage that characteristically occurs during OA and RA, elevated levels of Fn-fs (30 – 200 kDa) are commonly found in articular cartilage tissue and synovial fluid samples. Interestingly, injecting Fn-fs (but not native full length fibronectin) into the knees of rabbits causes up to a 50% depletion of total proteoglycan content in articular cartilage (Homandberg et al., 1993). These Fn-fs enhance the release of the catabolic cytokines: IL-1α/β, TNF-α, and IL-6, which greatly enhance the release of pro-MMP-2 and pro-MMP-3, while simultaneously suppressing the expression of aggrecan (Bewsey et al., 1996). The exact biological mechanism by which Fn-fs stimulate these catabolic effects is currently unknown however, the Fn-fs found in synovial fluid appear to bind and penetrate the articular cartilage surface of the superficial zone where they may then bind the fibronectin receptors of chondrocytes activating a cascade of events that result in the release of the aforementioned inflammatory cytokines (Xie & Homandberg, 1993). This is further supported by the finding that competitive inhibition of Fn-fs binding to the fibronectin receptor prevents Fn-fs associated catabolic activity (Homandberg & Hui, 1994).

3.2.2 Hyaluronan cleavage fragments

As previously discussed, injection of large molecular mass species of HA into the joint space of OA patients have been deemed therapeutic due to their pain relieving capabilities. However, cleavage of large HA species into smaller HA fragments (HA-fs) by proteolysis or oxidation generates oligomers that potentially have different properties than the original macromolecule (Soltés et al., 2007). CD44 is the primary cell membrane receptor that binds native HA. Adhesion to cells through CD44 allows HA to remain pericellular to chondrocytes where HA bound aggrecan aggregates can gather to draw water into the cartilage ECM giving the tissue compressive resistance required to withstand forces generated during joint loading and movement. However, HA-fs can competitively inhibit the interaction between CD44 and native high molecular weight HA species causing depletion of this (and other) proteoglycans within the cartilage ECM. Low mass (< 5 kDa) HA-fs can also induce MMP-3 and MMP-13 via Nf-kB activation by an unknown biological mechanism in explant culture experiments causing damage to cartilage tissue similar to the effect of Fn-fs. Additionally, HA-fs, but not native high molecular mass HA, have been known to activate iNOS in articular chondrocytes leading to enhanced production of NO ultimately causing further joint degredation.

3.2.3 Collagen cleavage fragments

During the normal pathophysiology of degenerative joint disease, type II collagen is also cleaved and partially degraded to produce smaller protein fragments with novel regulatory functions contributing to further tissue catabolism, as is the case with fibronectin and HA. Both the C-terminal and N-terminal ends of type II collagen monomers can be cleaved through proteolysis producing fragments termed CT and NT peptides, respectively. Such fragments have been shown to penetrate cartilage tissue and greatly enhance the mRNA expression of MMP-2, 3, 9, and 13 (Fichter et al., 2006) through MAPK p38 and NFκB signaling causing ECM breakdown and proteoglycan depletion (Guo et al., 2009). Similar to the way that HA-fs competitively inhibit HA interaction with CD44, it is surmised that type II collagen fragments can also bind chondrocyte cell membrane integrins preventing these receptors from interacting with type II collagen fibrils, thereby disrupting collagen network integrity. Annexin V is another chondrocyte cell membrane receptor that commonly interacts with native type II collagen. This interaction is vital for matrix vesicle mediated cartilage calcification. Like native type II collagen, the NT peptide can also regulate calcification by binding and activating this receptor. In high concentration, the NT peptide may potentially be responsible for pathological mineralization of the cartilage tissue as commonly seen in OA.

4. Extracellular matrix repair during osteoarthritis

In addition to ECM degradation due to the presence of reactive proteases, as well as their catabolic by-products (such as cleaved matrix protein fragments), OA is also characterized by a disregulation of important structural proteins as well as several important growth factors and their respective antagonists. This altered anabolism is most likely a compensatory reaction by chondrocytes attempting to repair OA induced tissue damage. However, the enhanced expression of some anabolic factors can trigger significant changes to cartilage homeostasis exacerbating the situation.

4.1 Altered expression of structural proteins

While proteolytic processing of collagens is a common characteristic of OA, some of these structural proteins exhibit increased expression and synthesis during disease pathogenesis. Type II, and VI collagens are both highly expressed in OA cartilage. The increase in these native collagen species also provide substrates for proteolysis which generates collagen fragments that have catabolic properties that ultimately results in MMP and NO release followed by proteoglycan depletion, as discussed previously. It is understandable how such events can mediate further tissue degradation during OA. Additionally, the expression and spatial distribution of type X collagen also changes in the OA joint. While typically type X collagen expression is only localized to the calcified zone, which lies right above the subchondral bone, this marker is also expressed by middle zone cartilage during OA pathogenesis. The appearance of type X collagen is often indicative of calcification, which seems to corroborate the increased tissue mineralization characteristic of later stages of this disease.

Although aggrecan expression is initially increased during early stage OA, during later stages of OA, its expression is downregulated in cartilage. Thus aggrecan depletion from cartilage tissue is not simply a result by ECM breakdown but it is also due to altered gene regulation. While the biological mechanism responsible for such alterations in gene regulation is not completely understood, it is at least partly due to cytokines and growth factors that are produced by chondrocytes, synoviocytes, and tissue localized immune cells during OA pathogenesis.

4.2 Altered expression of growth factors

The disregulation of potent growth factors during OA can significantly change tissue morphology.

4.2.1 BMPs & TGF-β

While members of the bone morphogenic protein (BMP) family are present in low amounts in normal articular cartilage, their expression is altered during OA. Normally, BMP-2, 4, 6, 7, 9, and 13 are expressed in articular cartilage. These growth factors stimulate chondrocytes to synthesize ECM constituents such as aggrecan and type II collagen to undergo chondrogenic differentiation. They play a role in cartilage repair and help to maintain joint integrity. Some members of the family such as BMP-7 can even inhibit inflammatory cytokine induced MMP synthesis in chondrocytes and synoviocytes. This family of growth factors also has endogenous inhibitors known as BMP antagonists. BMP antagonists are a group of proteins that function by directly binding BMPs as to prohibit them from interacting with their cognate receptors. This effectively prevents BMP signaling. During

OA, only BMP-2 is reported to be upregulated. However, BMP antagonists are also highly expressed in this disease. These antagonists alter normal cartilage homeostasis by inhibiting ECM anabolism mediated by all BMPs and significantly hindering cartilage tissue repair.

The expression and protein synthesis of the transforming growth factor beta (TGF-β) family are also altered during OA pathogenesis. Normal cartilage contains small amounts of these growth factors as they promote chondrocyte proliferation and chondrogenic differentiation. Similar to BMPs, they stimulate synthesis of ECM constituent proteins type II collagen and aggrecan. Additionally, TGF-β inhibits the expression and synthesis of MMP-1 and MMP-9. However, the exact function of TGF-β in the joint is still somewhat controversial due to its strong stimulation of MMP-13 and ADAMTS-4 expression in chondrocytes. OA cartilage displays a greater abundance of TGF-β than seen in normal non-diseased cartilage. This is consistent with the increase of both MMP-13 and ADAMTS-4 observed during disease progression. Inhibition of TGF-β has also been shown effective in preventing osteophyte formation in OA cartilage explants suggesting that this growth factor may play a role in inhibiting chondrocyte hypertrophy and premature ossification characteristic of OA (Scharstuhl et al., 2002).

4.2.2 IGFs, FGFs & HGF

Insulin-like growth factors (IGFs) and fibroblast growth factors (FGFs) are also two important proteins that are disregulated during OA. There are two types IGFs: IGF-1 and IGF-2. Both IGFs are present at higher levels in OA cartilage than normal. IGFs regulate homeostatic processes in many tissue types. In articular cartilage it promotes cell division, growth, and proteoglycan synthesis. A family of insulin-like growth factors binding proteins (IGFBPs) can modulate IGF activity by direct interaction. Out of the seven currently known IGFBPs (IGFBP-1 to 7), IGFBP-3 is the most common protein to modulate IGF activity. It has been shown that IGFBP-3 can inhibit the activity of both IGF-1 and IGF-2 in a dose dependant manner (Devi et al., 2001). In articular cartilage, IGFBP-3 has been found to increase in abundance with age. During OA pathogenesis, IGFBP-3 levels are increased even further potentially hindering the process of tissue repair. Like IGFs, FGFs are also upregulated during OA. This family of proteins includes 22 currently identified members. In cartilage biology, the most studied members are FGF-2, FGF-9, and FGF-18 due to their strong stimulation of matrix synthesis and tissue repair. However, the role of these growth factors during OA progression remains to be elucidated. Hepatocyte growth factor (HGF) is another potent multifunctional mitogenic protein that is disregulated in OA cartilage. Deep zone cartilage tissue normally contains two different truncated HGF isoforms (NK1 and NK2) (Guévremont et al., 2003). Although full length HGF is not produced by chondrocytes, osteoblasts from the subchondral bone produce HGF which may be processed in the nearby tissue generating these truncated peptides which diffuse into the calcified and deep zones of cartilage. MMP-13 expression is enhanced by chondrocytes and synoviocytes that come into contact with HGF. Its increasing abundance in OA cartilage can potentially enhance collagen fibril catabolism. Interestingly, HGF is also known for its ability to induce angiogenesis. It is unclear whether this function directly exacerbates the inflammation commonly characteristic of degenerative joint diseases.

5. Effect of major OA associated cytokines and chemokines on cartilage ECM

Unlike RA, OA is not traditionally classified an inflammatory arthropathy. It is unclear if the inflammation is intrinsic to osteoarthritis or a manifestation of associated crystal (e.g., calcium pyrophosphate or hydroxyapatite) arthritis complicating the osteoarthritis. It is characterized by mild yet chronic inflammation that indirectly plays a significant role in disease progression and tissue destruction. Pro-inflammatory cytokine and chemokine production by mononuclear cells, cells of the synovial membrane, and articular chondrocytes can disrupt normal cartilage homeostasis favoring proteoglycan depletion and tissue destruction. The two main pro-inflammatory cytokines noted for their destructive effects during OA are IL-1β and TNF-α.

5.1 IL-1β

IL-1β is expressed and released mainly by synoviocytes and mononuclear cells during joint inflammation, but studies have shown that articular chondrocytes of OA cartilage too upregulate its expression and synthesis. IL-1β exerts several significant catabolic and anti-anabolic effects that make it the most disease causative cytokine in OA. It induces expression of the collagenases, especially MMP-1, MMP-3, MMP-9 and MMP-13, which are believed to contribute significantly to the enhancement of articular cartilage catabolism that occurs during OA (Martel-Pelletier et al., 2008). The IL-1β pathway ultimately activates nuclear factor-κB (NFκB), which is necessary for the transcription of many genes relevant to OA and joint inflammation including MMPs (Park et al., 2004). It has been shown in murine articular cartilage explants that suppressing MMP production via IκB kinase inhibitiors is sufficient to reduce the degredation of both type II collagen and aggrecan (Pattoli et al., 2005).

The ability of IL-1β to downregulate the expression of type II collagen and aggrecan, the two main structural components of the articular cartilage ECM, further illustrates how this pathway can potentially hinder ECM repair in OA pathogenesis. It has been previously demonstrated that IL-1β induces a greater than twofold downregulation of both type II collagen and aggrecan expression in human chondrocytes (Toegal et al., 2008; Goldring et al., 1988). The production of type II collagen and aggrecan are important to the process of chondrogenesis during which mesenchymal stem cells of the chondrocyte lineage secrete the ECM protein components necessary to constitute articular cartilage. Even though chondrogenesis occurs primarily during development in humans, it can also be induced as a result of damage sustained to existing cartilage (as in the case of OA) (van Beuningen et al., 2000). IL-1β can inhibit chondrogenesis (Murakami et at., 2000) by downregulating the transcription factor SOX9 (Wehrli et al., 2003), which is a master regulator of the chondrogenesis pathway. Similarly, IL-1β downregulates the expression of certain TIMPs that normally bind and inhibit active MMPs (Martel-Pelletier et al., 2008). It is also known that the IL-1 receptor (IL-1RI) expression is higher in OA cartilage than in normal cartilage (Jacques et al., 2006) indicating the possibility that the IL-1β pathway is more active in OA chondrocytes. IL-1RI KO mice are resistant to the early development of OA (Jacques et al., 2006). All evidence point to IL-1β stimulation as a potential cause of articular cartilage ECM breakdown during OA. This is why it may be possible to regulate IL-1β activity, perhaps through endogenous pathway inhibition, to slow down OA development/progression.

5.1.1 IL-1RI and IL-1RA

The IL-1β pathway has several endogenous inhibitors (Martel-Pelletier et al., 2008; Arend et al., 2000). Normal signal transduction of this pathway is initiated upon ligand binding to the IL-1 receptor (IL-1RI). The ligand binding event enables IL-1RI to associate with another cell membrane bound protein known as the interleukin-1 receptor accessory protein (IL-1RAcP), which is necessary for pathway activation (Wesche et al., 1997). The association of these two membrane bound proteins allows for cross phosphorylation to occur in their transmembrane signaling domains initiating the signaling cascade that eventually leads to transcription of the proteases and cytokines described previously. Interleukin-1 receptor II (IL-1RII) is a cell membrane bound protein which competes with IL-1RI for IL-1 ligand binding (Gabay et al., 2010). IL-1RII is an IL-1RI protein mimic that does not contain a transmembrane signaling domain therefore it will not initiate signal transduction of the pathway and it is classified as an IL-1β pathway inhibitor. Two other endogenous inhibitors of this pathway are known as soluble interleukin-1 receptor II (sIL-1RII) and soluble interleukin-1 receptor accessory protein (sIL-1RAcP) (Gabay et al., 2010). These proteins mimic IL-1RI and IL-1RAcP respectively. sIL-1RII competes with IL-1RI to bind IL-1β, similarly sIL-1RAcP competes with IL-1RAcP to bind the IL-1RI.

The fifth, and arguable the most effective, inhibitor of this pathway is the IL-1RA. This protein is an IL-1α/β protein mimic and binds IL-1RI with a much higher affinity than does either IL-1α or IL-1β. IL-1RA bound IL-1RI cannot associate with IL-1RAcP and therefore is unable to initiate signal transduction of the IL-1β pathway. The IL-1RA gene can be alternatively spliced to form different isoforms. Currently four isoforms are known to exist in humans and two in mice. In humans, there are three intracellular isoforms of IL-RA (icIL-RA1, icIL-RA2, icIL-RA3) and one cell secreted isoform (sIL-1RA). The intracellular isoforms tend to be cell associated and stays in contact with the cell membrane of the cell from which it was produced. The secreted form of IL-1RA, however, can move into the extracellular space and proceed to inhibit the IL-1β signal transduction of cells that are further away. Several of these isoforms can be easily distinguished form one another due to their varying size: icIL-RA1/ icIL-RA2 (18-kDa), icIL-RA3 (16-kDa), and sIL-1RA (17-kDa) (Gabay et al., 2010).

IL-1RA is produced by many cell types including articular chondrocytes. It has been established that chondrocyte produced/secreted IL-1RA protein helps sustain articular cartilage integrity during both RA and OA induced inflammation. The later was demonstrated when chondrocytes taken from OA cartilage, which was transduced with IL-1RA, protected against IL-1-induced cartilage degradation in organ culture experiments (Baragi et al., 1995). Further support for the idea that IL-1RA is chondroprotective comes from IL-1RA knockout mice of multiple genetic backgrounds, which have been shown to develop early arthritis compared to wild-type mice of the same background (Arend et al., 2000). IL-RA knockout mice bred in both BALB/cA and MFIx129 backgrounds developed severe inflammatory arthritis. Additionally, IL-1β protein levels where elevated as high as three fold in these IL-1RA knock-out mice of both backgrounds while detectable levels of B-cells and T-cells remained constant between IL-1RA knock-out and wild-type mice (Nicklin et al., 2000).

In 1999, *in vivo* IL-1RA gene transfer experiments done in rabbits also demonstrated its potential to reduce OA severity. In these experiments, OA was artificially induced in the animals via meniscectomy after which local IL-1RA gene therapy by intra-articular plasmid injection was performed at 24 hour intervals 4 weeks post surgery. The animals were sacrificed exactly 4 weeks after the first injection and the joint synoviums were dissected and stained for IL-1RA. The level of IL-1RA present in the synoviums of these rabbits positively correlated with a reduction in articular cartilage lesions that resulted from OA indicating that IL-1RA was chondroprotective (Fernandes et al., 1999). A more recent study in 2005 looked at the levels of several potential chondrodestructive (IL-1α, IL-1β, TNF-α, etc.) as well as chondroprotective cytokines, one of which was sIL-1RA, in 31 patients who are at a higher risk of developing OA in one of their knees due to chronic anterior cruciate ligament (ACL) deficiency. This study found concentrations of IL-1β and TNF-α to be significantly higher in the ACL deficient vs. normal knees while the concentration of sIL-1RA decreased with increasing grades of articular chondral damage (Marks et al., 2005). Finally, a 2008 randomized double-blinded cohort study done in 167 patients with knee OA looked at the symptomatic effect of chromium sulfate induced autologous IL-1RA production and found a significant reduction of OA induced pain in the treated patients based on Knee injury and Osteoarthritis Outcome Score (KOOS) and Knee Society Clinical Rating System .

It is important to note that the chondroprotective effects of IL-1RA during OA are only observable when the protein is consistently present in the joint synovium of the arthritic joint. This explains why short-lived drugs such as AnikinRA (Cohen, 2004), which only last 4 hours post-intraarticular injection into human patients (as determined by serum analysis) have limited efficacy in treating OA progression (Chevalier et al., 2009). This is also most likely the underlying reason behind the success of longer lasting treatment options such as gene therapy and other methods aimed at increasing autologous IL-1RA production within the synovium of the OA joint.

5.2 TNF-α

Second only to IL-1β, TNF-α is a potent pro-inflammatory cytokine responsible for initiating much joint destruction during OA and other such joint degenerative diseases. TNF-α is currently looked on as a potential target for late stage OA therapy as its appearance in the joint is a telltale sign of advanced severity of the disease. In late stage OA, both TNF-α and its p55 receptor undergoes increased expression by articular chondrocytes and synoviocytes enhancing TNF-α pathway signaling. This leads to increased production of NO, ECM degrading enzymes, especially the highly catabolic collagenases MMP-3 and MMP-13, and other inflammatory cytokines like IL-1 and IL-6, which overall off-balances tissue homeostasis favoring ECM destruction. TNF-α also enhances the synthesis and release of the prostaglandin PGE2, which inhibits chondrocyte differentiation and maturation while simultaneously promoting MMP production and IL-6 expression. Additionally, circulating mononuclear cells that are localized to areas of inflammation that have undergone OA induced tissue injury also release TNF-α worsening joint inflammation and ultimately further favoring catabolism. Although commercially available TNF-α inhibitors are most efficacious for relieving of RA associated joint inflammation, it has been demonstrated that certain inhibitors, such as infliximab and etanercept, can suppress NO production in human cartilage (Vuolteenaho et al., 2002) making them potentially effective for treating OA. Despite these findings, only a handful of clinical studies have delved into testing the efficacy of this approach to OA treatment.

5.3 SDF-1

Recently, SDF-1 has received attention in arthritis research. Patients suffering from OA and RA display an increase of this chemokine in their synovial fluid. Although no evidence suggests that chondrocytes produce SDF-1, superficial and deep zone chondrocytes do however express the SDF-1 receptor (CXCR4) (Kanbe et al., 2002). Both synovial fibroblasts and osteoblasts from the subchondral bone produce SDF-1 and so it is also found in the deep zone of cartilage tissue. During OA pathogenesis, macrophages and lymphoid cells that have been localized to the inflamed synovium and/or joint cartilage will produce this chemokine. Since SDF-1 is known for its strong chemotactic abilities attracting lymphocytes to the site of joint inflammation, it has been implicated in enhancing cartilage tissue catabolism. In addition to its chemotactic ability, SDF-1 also stimulates the production of MMP-3 and MMP-13 by interacting with the CXCR4 receptors of articular chondrocytes (Kanbe et al., 2002; Chiu et al., 2007) contributing to collagen and proteoglycan cleavage.

6. Conclusion and future prospects in ECM biology and OA treatment

There are no FDA approved drugs specific for the treatment of OA. Currently, the most effective interventions merely alleviate OA symptoms. The three main interventions available are: (1) Supplements that attempt to enhance the body's endogenous cartilage regenerative capabilities, (2) Drugs that attempt to reduce OA associated pain, and (3) Surgical interventions such as total joint replacement, which is currently the most effective form of relieving the pain and inflammation occuring during the more severe later stages of this degenerative joint disease. Today, total joint replacement is a commonly performed routine surgery. It offers significant and permanent pain relief that other alternative therapies cannot provide, but it remains to be the last resort for late stage OA sufferers.

The use of anti-cytokine therapy to prevent cartilage tissue destruction has recently received attention in OA research. As previously discussed, OA induced ECM destruction most closely associates with induction of the IL-1β and TNF-α pathways. These major inflammatory cytokines stimulate mononuclear cells, synovial fibroblasts, and articular chondrocytes to release IL-6, NO, and chemokines that enhance joint damage. They additionally disregulate the release of anabolic growth factors and tissue destructive proteolytic enzymes from chondrocytes causing major alteration in the process of cartilage homeostasis. Numerous *in vitro* and *in vivo* studies conducted in animal models show that using IL-1Ra protein to inhibit IL-1β pathway activation has promise for preventing OA induced ECM degradation and inflammation. However, in human studies, the efficacy of IL-1 pathway inhibition for the purpose of OA therapy has been somewhat less successful. A paper published in 2009 reported the short-term efficacy of treating OA patients with recombinant IL-1Ra protein (Anakinra), which is a anti-inflammatory drug initially approved by the FDA for the treatment of RA. In this randomized double-blinded study, 160 knee OA sufferers were given 50 to 150 mg of Anakinra via intra-articular injection and their status was monitored for 4 weeks. During this time, knee joint pain was graded using the WOMAC pain index. Although there was no observable difference in cartilage destruction between the 150 mg Anakinra and placebo injected groups, Anakinra did prove to reduce OA associated knee joint pain on the fourth day after treatment. However, given the short half-life of this recombinant protein (approximately 5 hours), it did not have a significant beneficial effect after the fourth day (Chevalier et al., 2009). Similarly, inhibition of IL-1β and IL-1 receptor expression using a synthetic anti-inflammatory analgesic molecule named Diacerein has proved to have similar pain relieving effects with the additional benefit of preventing ECM catabolism to some degree. This drug also seems to have longer lasting therapeutic effects than Anakinra due to its relative stability (Pelletier et al., 2000).

As previously discussed, the intra-articular (or joint) injection of disease modifying ECM proteins such as lubricin and HA have been somewhat effective in reducing inflammation and tissue destruction. Similar use of various growth factors to repair OA induced ECM damage may be another promising avenue that warrants further investigation. Recent studies using "Preparations rich in growth factors" (PRGF), commonly consisting of platelet rich plasma (PRP), have demonstrated the efficacy of combining anabolic and anti-catabolic proteins to deliver a dual beneficial effect that reduces proteolytic ECM breakdown and promotes tissue repair in OA joints. Several studies conducted in the past decade have demonstrated that PRDF treatment reduces joint pain up to 5 weeks post injection while also showing signs that it may enhance regenerative capabilities of cartilage tissue. However, some of anabolic proteins used in these growth factor cocktails (i.e. TGF-β, IGF) are known to already be increased during OA pathogenesis. More studies need to be conducted in order to understand the mode by which such therapies are chondroprotective. Currently the use of PRP for the treatment of knee OA is in Phase 2 of clinical trials.

Localized intra-articular gene therapy is a very exciting and novel approach for treating degenerative joint diseases such as OA and RA. It provides a controlled method to sustain production of potentially therapeutic gene products that cannot be matched by more transient methods such as simple intra-articular injection. Sites of localized gene transfer include the synovium (most common target in past studies) as well as articular cartilage tissue itself. Thus far, gene candidates used for this approach include those that can potentially enhance ECM synthesis and repair and/or prevent ECM breakdown. IL-1Ra is an example of a chondroprotective gene that has been successfully utilized for gene transfer experiments in several animal models. These studies clearly show positive outcomes correlating with its expression within the joint including reduced inflammation and decreased tissue destruction (Calich et al., 2010). IGF-1 is another gene candidate that has been introduced into the knee joints of rabbits via adenovirus mediated gene transfer. These animals experienced enhanced ECM synthesis by the articular cartilage in their knee joints under both normal and inflamed conditions (Mi et al., 2000). The use of gene therapy for the treatment of OA has presented much promise; however, due to issues involving the practicality of its use, we are still a long time away from utilizing its full potential.

7. References

Abbaszade, I., Liu, RQ., Yang, F., Rosenfeld, SA., Ross, OH., Link, JR., et al. (1999). Cloning and characterization of ADAMTS11, an aggrecanase from the ADAMTS family. *J. Biol. Chem.*, Vol. 274, No. 33, (August 1999), pp. 23443–23450. ISSN 0021-9258

Aeschlimann, D., Wetterwald, A., Fleisch, H. & Paulsson, M. (1993). Expression of tissue transglutaminase in skeletal tissues correlates with events of terminal differentiation of chondrocytes. *Journal of Cell Biology*. Vol. 120, No. 6, (March 1993), pp. 1461-70, ISSN 0021-9525

Ahmad, R., Sylvester, J., Ahmad, M. & Zafarullah, M. (2009) Adaptor proteins and Ras synergistically regulate IL-1-induced ADAMTS-4 expression in human chondrocytes. *J. Immunol.*, Vol. 182, No.8 (April 2009), pp. 5081-5087, ISSN 1550-6606

Alexopoulos, LG., Youn, I., Bonaldo, P. & Guilak F. (2009). Developmental and osteoarthritic changes in Col6a1-knockout mice: biomechanics of type VI collagen in the cartilage pericellular matrix. *Arthritis Rheum.*, Vol. 60, No. 3, (March 2009), pp. 771-9, ISSN 0004-3591

Altman, RD. & Moskowitz, R. (1998). Intraarticular sodium hyaluronate (Hyalgan) in the treatment of patients with osteoarthritis of the knee: a randomized clinical trial. Hyalgan Study Group. *J Rheumatol.* Vol. 25, No. 11, (November 1998), pp. 2203-2212. ISSN 0315-162X

Arend, WP. & Gabay, C. (2000) Physiologic role of interleukin-1 receptor antagonist. *Arthritis Res.*, Vol. 2, No. 4, (May 2000), pp. 245-248, ISSN 1465-9905

Baragi, VM., Renkiewicz, RR., Jordan, H., Bonadio, J., Hartman, JW. & Roessler, BJ. (1995).Transplantation of transduced chondrocytes protects articular cartilage from interleukin 1-induced extracellular matrix degradation. *J. Clin. Invest.*, Vol. 96, No. 5, (November 1995), pp. 2454-2460, ISSN 0021-9738

Bewsey, KE., Wen, C., Purple, C. & Homandberg, GA. (1996). Fibronectin fragments induce the expression of stromelysin-1 mRNA and protein in bovine chondrocytes in monolayer culture. *Biochim Biophys Acta.*, Vol. 1317, No. 1, (October 1996), pp. 55-64, ISSN 0006-3002

Bignami, A., Asher, R. & Perides, G. (1992). The extracellular matrix of rat spinal cord: a comparative study on the localization of hyaluronic acid, glial hyaluronate-binding protein, and chondroitin sulfate proteoglycan. *Exp Neurol.*, Vol. 117, No. 1, (July 1992), pp. 90-3, ISSN 0014-4886

Blagg, JA., Noe, MC., Wolf-Gouveia, LA., Reiter, LA., Laird, ER., Chang, SP., et al. (2005) Potent pyrimidinetrione- based inhibitors of MMP-13 with enhanced selectivity over MMP-14. Bioorg. *Med. Chem. Lett.*, Vol. 15, No. 7 (April 2005), pp. 1807-1810, ISSN 0960-894X

Blaschke, UK., Eikenberry, EF., Hulmes, DJ., Galla, HJ. & Bruckner, P. (2000). Collagen XI nucleates self-assembly and limits lateral growth of cartilage fibrils. *J Biol Chem.* Vol. 275, No. 14, (April 2000), pp. 10370-10378, ISSN 0021-9258

Bleasel ,JF., Holderbaum, D., Brancolini, V., Moskowitz, RW., Considine, EL., Prockop, DJ., et al. (1998). Five families with arginine 519-cysteine mutation in COL2A1: evidence for three distinct founders. *Hum Mutat.* Vol. 12, No. 3, (October 1998), pp. 172-176, ISSN 1059-7794

Borochowitz, ZU., Scheffer, D., Adir, V., Dagoneau, N., Munnich, A. & Cormier-Daire, V. (2004) Spondylo-epi-metaphyseal dysplasia (SEMD) matrilin 3 type: homozygote matrilin 3 mutation in a novel form of SEMD. *J. Med. Genet.*, Vol. 41, No. 5, (May 2004), pp. 366–372, ISSN 1468-6244

Byers, PH. (2001). Folding defects in fibrillar collagens. *Philos Trans R Soc Lond B Biol Sci.*, Vol. 356, No. 1406, (February 2001), pp. 151-158, ISSN 0962-8436

Calich, AL., Domiciano, DS. & Fuller, R. (2010). Osteoarthritis: can anti-cytokine therapy play a role in treatment? *Clin Rheumatol.* Vol. 29, No. 5, (January 2010), pp. 451-455, ISSN 1434-9949

Cepko, C. L. Transduction of genes using retrovirus vectors. In: Current Protocols in Molecular Biology, edited by A. F.M., R. Brent, R. Kingston, D. D. Moore, J. G. Seidman, J. A. Smith and K. Struhl. New York: Greene Publishing Associates, 1992, p. 9.10-9.14.

Chen, Q., Fitch, JM., Linsenmayer, C. & Linsenmayer, TF. (1992) Type X collagen: covalent crosslinking to hypertrophic cartilage-collagen fibrils. *Bone & Mineral.* Vol. 17, No. 2, (May 1992), pp. 223-7, ISSN 0169-6009

Chen, Q., Fitch, JM., Gibney, E. & Linsenmayer, TF. (1993). Type II collagen during cartilage and corneal development: immunohistochemical analysis with an anti- telopeptide antibody. *Developmental Dynamics.* Vol. 196, No. 1, (January 1993), pp. 47-53, ISSN 1058-8388

Chen, Q., Zhang, Y., Johnson, DM. & Goetinck, PF. (1999). Assembly of a novel cartilage matrix protein filamentous network: molecular basis of differential requirement of von Willebrand factor A domains. *Mol Biol Cell.* Vol. 10, No. 7, (July 1999) pp. 2149-2162. ISSN 1059-1524

Chen, XD., Fisher, LW., Robey, PG. & Young, MF. (2004). The small leucine-rich proteoglycan biglycan modulates BMP-4-induced osteoblast differentiation. *FASEB J.*, Vol. 18, No. 9, (June 2004), pp. 948-58, ISSN 1530-6860

Chevalier, X., Goupille, P., Beaulieu, AD., Burch, FX., Bensen, WG., Conrozier, T. et al. (2009). Intraarticular injection of anakinra in osteoarthritis of the knee: a multicenter, randomized, double-blind, placebo-controlled study. *Arthritis Rheum.* Vol. 61, No. 3, (March 2009), pp. 344-352, ISSN 0004-3591

Chiu, YC., Yang, RS., Hsieh, KH., Fong, YC., Way, TD. & Lee, TS., (2007). Stromal cell-derived factor-1 induces matrix metalloprotease-13 expression in human chondrocytes. *Mol Pharmacol.*, Vol. 72, No. 3, (September 2007), pp. 695-703, ISSN 0026-895X

Cohen, SB. (2004) The use of anakinra, an interleukin-1 receptor antagonist, in the treatment of rheumatoid arthritis. *Rheum. Dis. Clin. N. Am.*, Vol. 30, No. 2 (May 2004), pp. 365-380, ISSN 0889-857X

Cremer, MA., Rosloniec, EF. & Kang AH. (1988). The cartilage collagens: a review of their structure, organization, and role in the pathogenesis of experimental arthritis in animals and in human rheumatic disease. *J Mol Med.*, Vol. 76, No. 3-4, (March 1988), pp. 275-88, ISSN 0946-2716

Deak, F., Wagener, R., Kiss, I. & Paulsson, M. (1999). The matrilins: a novel family of oligomeric extracellular matrix proteins. *Matrix Biol.*, Vol. 18, No. 1, (February 1999), pp.55–64, ISSN 0945-053X

Devi, GR., Graham, DL., Oh, Y. & Rosenfeld, RG. (2001). Effect of IGFBP-3 on IGF- and IGF-analogue-induced insulin-like growth factor-I receptor (IGFIR) signaling. *Growth Horm IGF Res.*, Vol. 11, No. 4, (August 2001), pp. 231-9, ISSN 1096-6374

Doege, KJ., Sasaki, M., Kimura, T. & Yamada, Y. (1991). Complete coding sequence and deduced primary structure of the human cartilage large aggregating proteoglycan, aggrecan. Human-specific repeats, and additional alternatively spliced forms. *J Biol Chem.*, Vol. 266, No. 2, (January 1991), pp. 894-902, ISSN 0021-9258

Dozier S., Escobar GP. & Lindsey ML. (2006) Matrix metalloproteinase (MMP)-7 activates MMP-8 but not MMP-13. *Med Chem.* Vol. 2, No. 5, (September 2006), pp. 523-526, ISSN 1573-4064

Drummond, AH., Beckett, P., Brown, PD., Bone, EA., Davidson, AH., Galloway, WA., et al. (1999). Preclinical and clinical studies of MMP inhibitors in cancer. *Ann N Y Acad Sci.*, Vol. 878, (June 1999), pp. 228-235, ISSN 0077-8923

Engel, J., Furthmayr, H., Odermatt, E., von der Mark, H., Aumailley, M., Fleischmajer, R., et al. (1985). Structure and macromolecular organization of type VI collagen. *Ann N Y Acad Sci.*, Vol. 460, (December 1985), pp. 25-37, ISSN 0077-8923

Eyre, DR., Weis, MA., & Moskowitz, RW. (1991). Cartilage expression of a type II collagen mutation in an inherited form of osteoarthritis associated with a mild chondrodysplasia. *J Clin Invest.*, Vol. 87, No. 1, (January 1991), pp. 357-361, ISSN 0021-9738

Fernandes, J., Tardif, G., Martel-Pelletier, J., Lascau-Coman, V., Dupuis, M., Moldovan, F., et al. (1999) In vivo transfer of interleukin-1 receptor antagonist gene in osteoarthritic rabbit knee joints: prevention of osteoarthritis progression. *Am. J. Pathol.*, Vol. 154, No. 4, (April 1999), pp.1159-1169, ISSN 0002-9440

Fichter, M., Korner, U., Schomburg, J., Jennings, L., Cole, AA., & Mollenhauer, J. (2006). Collagen degradation products modulate matrix metalloproteinase expression in cultured articular chondrocytes. *J Orthop Res.* Vol. 24, No. 1, (January 2006), pp. 63-70, ISSN 0736-0266

Fosang, AJ., Neame, PJ., Hardingham, TE., Murphy, G. & Hamilton, JA. (1991). Cleavage of cartilage proteoglycan between G1 and G2 domains by stromelysins. *J Biol Chem.* Vol. 266, No. 24, (August 1991), pp. 15579-15582, ISSN 0021-9258

Furthmayr, H., Wiedemann, H., Timpl, R., Odermatt, E. & Engel, J. (1983). Electron-microscopical approach to a structural model of intima collagen. *Biochem J. Vol.* 211, No. 2, (May 1983), pp. 303-311, ISSN 0264-6021

Gabay, C., Lamacchia, C. & Palmer, G. (2010). IL-1 pathways in inflammation and human diseases. Nat. Rev. *Rheumatol.*, Vol. 6, No. 4, (April 2010), pp. 232-41, ISSN 1759-4804

Glasson, SS., Askew, R., Sheppard, B., Carito, B., Blanchet, T., Ma, HL., et al. (2005) Depletion of active ADAMTS5 prevents cartilage degradation in murine model of osteoarthritis. *Nature.* Vol. 434, No. 7033 (March 2005), pp. 644-648, ISSN 1476-4687

Goldring, MB., Birkhead, J., Sandell, LJ., Kimura, T. & Krane, SM. (1988) Interleukin 1 suppresses expression of cartilage-specific types II and IX collagens and increases types I and III collagens in human chondrocytes. *J. Clin. Invest.*,Vol. 82, No. 6, (December 1988), pp. 2026-2037, ISSN 0021-9738

Goldring, MB. & Marcu, KB. (2009). Cartilage homeostasis in health and rheumatic diseases. *Arthritis Res Ther.* Vol. 11, No. 3, (May 2009), pp. 224, ISSN 1478-6362

Gregory, KE., Oxford, JT., Chen, Y., Gambee, JE., Gygi, SP., Aebersold, R., et al. (2000). Structural organization of distinct domains within the non-collagenous N-terminal region of collagen type XI. *J Biol Chem.* Vol. 275, No. 15, (April 2000), pp. 11498-11506, ISSN 0021-9258

Guévremont, M., Martel-Pelletier, J., Massicotte, F., Tardif, G., Pelletier, JP., Ranger, P., et al. (2003). Human adult chondrocytes express hepatocyte growth factor (HGF) isoforms but not HgF: potential implication of osteoblasts on the presence of HGF in cartilage. *J Bone Miner Res.*, Vol. 18, No. 6, (June 2003), pp. 1073-81, ISSN 0884-0431

Guo, D., Ding, L. & Homandberg, GA. (2009). Telopeptides of type II collagen upregulate proteinases and damage cartilage but are less effective than highly active fibronectin fragments. *Inflamm Res.*, Vol. 58, No. 3, (March 2009), pp. 161-9, ISSN 1420-908X

Homandberg, GA., Meyers, R. & Williams, JM. (1993). Intraarticular injection of fibronectin fragments causes severe depletion of cartilage proteoglycans in vivo. *J Rheumatol.* Vol. 20, No. 8, (August 1993), pp. 1378-1382, ISSN 0315-162X

Homandberg, GA. & Hui, F. (1994). Arg-Gly-Asp-Ser peptide analogs suppress cartilage chondrolytic activities of integrin-binding and nonbinding fibronectin fragments. *Arch Biochem Biophys.* Vol. 310, No. 1, (April 1994), pp. 40-48, ISSN 0003-9861

Hu, K., Xu, L., Cao, L., Flahiff, CM., Brussiau, J., Ho, K., et al. (2006). Pathogenesis of osteoarthritis-like changes in the joints of mice deficient in type IX collagen. *Arthritis Rheum.* Vol. 54, No. 9, (September 2006), pp. 2891-2900, ISSN 0004-3591

Ikegawa, S., Nishimura, G., Nagai, T., Hasegawa, T., Ohashi, H., Nakamura, Y. et al. (1998). Mutation of the type X collagen gene (COL10A1) causes spondylometaphyseal dysplasia. *Am J Hum Genet.*, Vol. 63, No. 6, (December 1998), pp. 1659-62, ISSN 0002-9297

Imai, K., Ohta, S., Matsumoto, T., Fujimoto, N., Sato, H., Seiki, M., et al. (1997). Expression of membrane-type 1 matrix metalloproteinase and activation of progelatinase A in human osteoarthritic cartilage. *Am. J. Pathol.*, Vol. 15, No. 1, (July 1997), pp. 245-256, ISSN 0002-9440

Jacenko O, LuValle PA & Olsen BR. (1993). Spondylometaphyseal dysplasia in mice carrying a dominant negative mutation in a matrix protein specific for cartilage-to-bone transition. *Nature.* Vol. 365, No. 6441, (September 1993), pp. 56-61, ISSN 0028-0836

Jackson, GC., Marcus-Soekarman, D., Stolte-Dijkstra, I., Verrips, A., Taylor, JA. & Briggs, MD. (2010). Type IX collagen gene mutations can result in multiple epiphyseal dysplasia that is associated with osteochondritis dissecans and a mild myopathy. *Am J Med Genet A.*, Vol. 152A, No. 4, (April 2010), pp. 863-9, ISSN 1552-4833

Jacques, C., Gosset, M., Berenbaum, F. & Gabay, C. (2006). The role of IL-1 and IL-1Ra in joint inflammation and cartilage degradation. *Vitam. Horm.*, Vol. 74, (December 2006), pp. 371-403, ISSN 0083-6729

Julovi, SM., Yasuda, T., Shimizu, M., Hiramitsu, T., & Nakamura, T. (2004). Inhibition of interleukin-1beta-stimulated production of matrix metalloproteinases by hyaluronan via CD44 in human articular cartilage. *Arthritis Rheum.* Vol. 50, No. 2, (February 2004), pp. 516-525, ISSN 0004-3591

Kamekura, S., Hoshi, K., Shimoaka, T., Chung, U., Chikuda, H., Yamada, T., et al. (2005) Osteoarthritis development in novel experimental mouse models induced by knee joint instability. *Osteoarthritis Cartil.*, Vol. 13, No. 7 (July 2005), pp. 632-641, ISSN 1063-4584

Kanbe, K., Takagishi, K. & Chen, Q. (2002). Stimulation of matrix metalloprotease 3 release from human chondrocytes by the interaction of stromal cell-derived factor 1 and CXC chemokine receptor 4. *Arthritis Rheum.*, Vol. 46, No. 1, (January 2002), pp. 130-7, ISSN 0004-3591

Klatt, AR., Nitsche, DP., Kobbe, B., Mörgelin, M., Paulsson, M. & Wagener, R. (2000) Molecular structure and tissue distribution of matrilin-3, a filament-forming extracellular matrix protein expressed during skeletal development. *Journal of Biological Chemistry.* Vol. 275, No. 6, (February 2000), pp. 3999-4006, ISSN 0021-9258

Klatt, AR., Nitsche, DP., Kobbe, B., Macht, M., Paulsson, M. & Wagener, R. (2001). Molecular structure, processing, and tissue distribution of matrilin-4. *J. Biol. Chem.*, Vol. 276, No. 20, (May 2001), pp. 17267–17275, ISSN 0021-9258

Kuivaniemi, H., Tromp, G., & Prockop, DJ. (1997). Mutations in fibrillar collagens (types I, II, III, and XI), fibril-associated collagen (type IX), and network-forming collagen (type X) cause a spectrum of diseases of bone, cartilage, and blood vessels. *Hum Mutat.*, Vol. 9, No. 4, (June 1997), pp. 300-315, ISSN 1059-7794

Kuno, K., Okada, Y., Kawashima, H., Nakamura, H., Miyasaka, M., Ohno, H., et al. (2000) ADAMTS-1 cleaves a cartilage proteoglycan, aggrecan. *FEBS Lett.*, Vol. 478, No. 3 (August 2000), pp. 241–245, ISSN 0014-5793

Lamandé, SR., Bateman, JF., Hutchison, W., McKinlay Gardner, RJ., Bower, SP., Byrne E., et al. (1998). Reduced collagen VI causes Bethlem myopathy: a heterozygous COL6A1 nonsense mutation results in mRNA decay and functional haploinsufficiency. *Hum Mol Genet.*, Vol. 7, No. 6 (June 1998), pp. 981-9, ISSN 0964-6906

Li, SW., Prockop, DJ., Helminen, H., Fässler, R., Lapveteläinen, T., Kiraly, K., et al. (1995). Transgenic mice with targeted inactivation of the Col2 alpha 1 gene for collagen II develop a skeleton with membranous and periosteal bone but no endochondral bone. *Genes Dev.*, Vol. 9, No. 22, (November 1995), pp. 2821-2830, ISSN 0890-9369

Li, Y., Lacerda, DA., Warman, ML., Beier, DR., Yoshioka, H., Ninomiya, Y., et al. (1995). A fibrillar collagen gene, Col11a1, is essential for skeletal morphogenesis. *Cell, Vol.* 80, No. 3, (February 1995), pp. 423-30, ISSN 0092-8674

Linsenmayer, TF., Eavey, RD. & Schmid, TM. (1988). Type X collagen: a hypertrophic cartilage-specific molecule. *Pathol Immunopathol Res.*, Vol. 7, No. 1-2, (1988), pp. 14-9, ISSN 0257-2761

Marks, PH. & Donaldson, ML. (2005) Inflammatory cytokine profiles associated with chondral damage in the anterior cruciate ligament-deficient knee. *Arthroscopy*. Vol. 21, No. 11, (November 2005), pp.1342-1347, ISSN 1526-3231

Martel-Pelletier, J., Boileau, C., Pelletier, JP. & Roughley, PJ. (2008). Cartilage in normal and osteoarthritis conditions. *Best Pract Res Clin Rheumatol*. Vol. 22, No. 2, (April 2008), pp. 351-384, ISSN 1521-6942

Mi, Z., Ghivizzani, SC., Lechman, ER., Jaffurs, D., Glorioso, JC., Evans, CH. et al. (2000). Adenovirus-mediated gene transfer of insulin-like growth factor 1 stimulates proteoglycan synthesis in rabbit joints. *Arthritis Rheum.* Vol. 43, No. 11, (November 2000), pp. 2563-2570, ISSN 0004-3591

Mitchell, PG., Magna, HA., Reeves, LM., Lopresti-Morrow, LL., Yocum, SA., Rosner, PJ., et al. (1996) Cloning, expression, and type II collagenolytic activity of matrix metalloproteinase-13 from human osteoarthritic cartilage. *J. Clin. Invest.*, Vol. 97, No. 3 (February 1996), pp. 761-768, ISSN 0021-9738

Mohtai,M., Smith, RL., Schurman, DJ., Tsuji, Y., Torti, FM., Hutchinson, NI., et al. (1993). Expression of 92-kD type IV collagenase/gelatinase (gelatinase B) in osteoarthritic cartilage and its induction in normal human articular cartilage by interleukin 1. *J. Clin. Invest.*, Vol. 92, No. 1, (July 1993), pp. 179-185, ISSN 0021-9738

Moreland, LW . (2003). Intra-articular hyaluronan (hyaluronic acid) and hylans for the treatment of osteoarthritis: mechanisms of action. *Arthritis Res Ther.* Vol 5, No. 2, (January 2003), pp. 54-67. ISSN 1478-6362

Murakami ,S., Lefebvre, V. & de Crombrugghe, B. (2000). Potent Inhibition of the Master Chondrogenic FactorSox9 Gene by Interleukin-1 and Tumor Necrosis Factor-α. *J. Biol. Chem.*, Vol. 275, No. 5, (February 2000), pp. 3687-92 , ISSN 0021-9258

Nakamura, H., Fujii, Y., Ohuchi, E., Yamamoto, E. & Okada, Y. (1998). Activation of the precursor of human stromelysin 2 and its interactions with other matrix metalloproteinases. *Eur J Biochem.* Vol. 253, No. 1, (April 1998), pp. 67-75, ISSN 0014-2956

Nicholson, R., Murphy, G. & Breathnach R. (1989). Human and rat malignant-tumor-associated mRNAs encode stromelysin-like metalloproteinases. *Biochemistry*. Vol. 28, No. 12, (June 1989), pp. 5195-5203, ISSN 0006-2960

Nicklin, MJ., Hughes, DE., Barton, JL., Ure, JM. & Duff, GW. (2000) Arterial inflammation in mice lacking the interleukin 1 receptor antagonist gene. *J. Exp. Med.*, Vol. 191, No. 2 (January 2000), pp. 303-312, ISSN 0022- 1007

Nuka, S., Zhou, W., Henry, SP., Gendron, CM., Schultz, JB., Shinomura, T., et al. (2010). Phenotypic characterization of epiphycan-deficient and epiphycan/biglycan double-deficient mice. *Osteoarthritis Cartilage.* Vol. 18, No. 1, (January 2010), pp. 88-96, ISSN 1522-9653

Nwomeh, BC., Liang, HX., Diegelmann, RF., Cohen, IK. & Yager, DR. (2002) Dynamics of the matrix metalloproteinases MMP-1 and MMP-8 in acute open human dermal wounds. *Wound Repair and Regeneration.* Vol. 6, No. 2, (March-April 2002), pp. 127-134, ISSN 1067-1927

Ohta, S., Imai, K., Yamashita, K., Matsumoto, T., Azumano, I. & Okada, Y. (1998) Expression of matrix metalloproteinase 7 (matrilysin) in human osteoarthritic cartilage. *Lab. Invest.*, Vol. 78, No. 1, (January 1998), pp. 79-87, ISSN 0023-6837

Okada, Y., Konomi, H., Yada, T., Kimata, K., and Nagase, H. (1989). Degradation of type IX collagen by matrix metalloproteinase 3 (stromelysin) from human rheumatoid synovial cells. FEBS Lett., Vol. 244, No. 2, (February 1989), pp. 473-476, ISSN 0014-5793

Okada, Y., Shinmei, M., Tanaka, O., Naka, K., Kimura, A., Nakanishi, I., et al. (1992). Localization of matrix metalloproteinase 3 (stromelysin) in osteoarthritic cartilage and synovium. *Lab. Invest.*, Vol. 66, No. 6, (June 1992), pp. 680-690, ISSN 0023-6837

Otten, C., Wagener, R., Paulsson, M. & Zaucke, F. (2005) Matrilin-3 mutations that cause chondrodysplasias interfere with protein trafficking while a mutation associated with hand osteoarthritis does not. *J. Med. Genet.*, Vol. 42, No. 10, (October 2005), pp. 774-779, ISSN 1468-6244

Pace, RA., Peat, RA., Baker, NL., Zamurs, L., Mörgelin, M., Irving, M., et al. (2008). Collagen VI glycine mutations: perturbed assembly and a spectrum of clinical severity. *Ann Neurol.*, Vol. 64, No. 3, (September 2008), pp. 294-303, ISSN 1531-8249

Park, MY., Jang, HD., Lee, SY., Lee, KJ. & Kim, E. (2004). Fas-associated factor-1 inhibits nuclear factor-kappaB (NF-kappaB) activity by interfering with nuclear translocation of the RelA (p65) subunit of NF-kappaB. *J Biol Chem.* Vol. 279, No. 4, (January 2004), pp. 2544-2549, ISSN 0021-9258

Pattoli, MA., MacMaster, JF., Gregor, KR. & Burke, JR. (2005) Collagen and aggrecan degradation is blocked in interleukin-1-treated cartilage explants by an inhibitor of

IkappaB kinase through suppression of metalloproteinase expression. *J. Pharmacol. Exp. Ther.*, Vol. 315, No. 1, (October 2005), pp. 382-388, ISSN 0022-3565

Pelletier, JP., Yaron, M., Haraoui, B., Cohen, P., Nahir, MA., Choquette, D. et al. (2000). Efficacy and safety of diacerein in osteoarthritis of the knee: a double-blind, placebo-controlled trial. The Diacerein Study Group. *Arthritis Rheum.* Vol. 43, No. 10, (October 2000), pp. 2339-2348, ISSN 0004-3591

Piecha, D., Muratoglu, S., Mörgelin, M., Hauser, N., Studer, D., Kiss, I. et al. (1999) Matrilin-2, a large, oligomeric matrix protein, is expressed by a great variety of cells and forms fibrillar networks. *J. Biol. Chem.*, Vol. 274, No. 19, (May 1999), pp. 13353–13361, ISSN 0021-9258

Piecha, D., Hartmann, K., Kobbe, B., Haase, I., Mauch, C., Krieg, T., et al. (2002) Expression of Matrilin-2 in Human Skin. *Journal of Investigative Dermatology.* Vol. 119, No. 1 (July 2002), pp. 38-43. ISSN 0022-202X

Pratta, MA., Yao, W., Decicco, C., Tortorella, MD., Liu, RQ., Copeland, RA., et al. (2003). Aggrecan protects cartilage collagen from proteolytic cleavage. *J Biol Chem.*, Vol. 278, No. 46, (November 2003), pp. 45539-45, ISSN 0021-9258

Prockop, DJ., Ala-Kokko, L., McLain, DA., & Williams, C. (1997). Can mutated genes cause common osteoarthritis? *Br J Rheumatol.*, Vol. 36, No. 8, (August 1997), pp. 827-829, ISSN 0263-7103

Pullig, O., Weseloh, G. & Swoboda, B. (1999). Expression of type VI collagen in normal and osteoarthritic human cartilage. *Osteoarthritis Cartilage*, Vol. 7, No. 2, (March 1999), pp. 191-202, ISSN 1063-4584

Pullig, O., Weseloh, G., Klatt, AR., Wagener, R. & Swoboda, B. (2002) Matrilin-3 in human articular cartilage: increased expression in osteoarthritis. *Osteoarthritis Cartilage.*, Vol. 10 No. 4, (April 2002) pp. 253-263, ISSN 1063-4584

Pun, YL., Moskowitz, RW., Lie, S., Sundstrom, WR., Block, SR., McEwen, C., et al. (1994). Clinical correlations of osteoarthritis associated with a single-base mutation (arginine519 to cysteine) in type II procollagen gene. A newly defined pathogenesis. *Arthritis Rheum.* Vol. 37, No. 2, (February 1994), pp. 264-269, ISSN 0004-3591

Rechardt, O., Elomaa, O., Vaalamo, M., Pääkkönen, K., Jahkola, T., Höök-Nikanne, J., et al. (2000). Stromelysin-2 is upregulated during normal wound repair and is induced by cytokines. *J Invest Dermatol.* Vol. 115, No. 5, (November 2000), pp. 778-787, ISSN 0022-202X

Rhee, DK., Marcelino, J., Al-Mayouf, S., Schelling, DK., Bartels, CF., Cui, Y., et al. (2005). Consequences of disease- causing mutations on lubricin protein synthesis, secretion, and post-translational processing. *J Biol Chem.*, Vol. 280, No. 35, (September 2005), pp. 31325-32, ISSN 0021-9258

Rodriguez, RR., Seegmiller, RE., Stark, MR. & Bridgewater, LC. (2004). A type XI collagen mutation leads to increased degradation of type II collagen in articular cartilage. *Osteoarthritis Cartilage*, Vol. 12, No. 4, (April 2004), pp. 314-20, ISSN 1063-4584

Rodríguez-Manzaneque, JC., Westling, J., Thai, SN., Luque, A., Knauper, V., Murphy, G., et al. (2002) ADAMTS1 cleaves aggrecan at multiple sites and is differentially inhibited by metalloproteinase inhibitors. *Biochem. Biophys. Res. Commun.*, Vol. 293, No. 1, (April 2002), pp. 501–508, ISSN 0006-291X

Rosenberg ,K., Olsson, H., Mörgelin, M. & Heinegård, D. (1998). Cartilage oligomeric matrix protein shows high affinity zinc-dependent interaction with triple helical collagen. *J Biol Chem.*, Vol. 273, No. 32, (August 1998), pp. 20397-403, ISSN 0021-9258

Scharstuhl, A., Glansbeek, HL., van Beuningen, HM., Vitters, EL., van der Kraan, PM. & van den Berg, WB. (2002). Inhibition of endogenous TGF-beta during experimental osteoarthritis prevents osteophyte formation and impairs cartilage repair. *J Immunol.*, Vol. 169, No. 1, (July 2002), pp. 507-14, ISSN 0022-1767

Soltés, L., Kogan, G., Stankovska, M., Mendichi, R., Rychlý, J., Schiller, J., et al. (2007). Degradation of high-molar-mass hyaluronan and characterization of fragments. *Biomacromolecules.*, Vol. 8, No. 9, (September 2007), pp. 2697-705, ISSN 1525-7797

Stanton, H., Rogerson, FM., East, CJ., Golub, SB., Lawlor, KE., Meeker, CT., et al. (2005) ADAMTS5 is the major aggrecanase in mouse cartilage in vivo and in vitro. *Nature.* Vol. 434, No. 7033, (March 2005), pp. 648-652, ISSN 1476-4687

Stefánsson, SE., Jónsson, H., Ingvarsson, T., Manolescu, I., Jónsson, HH., Olafsdóttir, G., et al. (2003) Genomewide scan for hand osteoarthritis: a novel mutation in matrilin-3. *Am. J. Hum. Genet.*, Vol. 72, No. 6, (June 2003), pp.1448–1459, ISSN 0002-9297

Stremme, S., Duerr, S., Bau, B., Schmid, E. & Aigner, T. (2003). MMP-8 is only a minor gene product of human adult articular chondrocytes of the knee. *Clin Exp Rheumatol.*, Vol. 21, No. 2, (March-April 2003), pp. 205-9, ISSN 0392-856X

Svensson, L., Närlid, I. & Oldberg, A. (2000). Fibromodulin and lumican bind to the same region on collagen type I fibrils. *FEBS Lett.*, Vol. 470, No. 2, (March 2000), pp. 178-82, ISSN 0014-5793

Tahiri, K., Korwin-Zmijowska, C., Richette, P., Héraud, F., Chevalier, X., Savouret, JF., et al. (2008) Natural chondroitin sulphates increase aggregation of proteoglycan complexes and decrease ADAMTS-5 expression in interleukin 1 beta-treated chondrocytes. *Ann. Rheum.* Dis., Vol. 67, No. 5, (May 2008), pp. 696-702, ISSN 1468-2060

Takaishi, H., Kimura, T., Dalal, S., Okada, Y. & D'Armiento, J. (2008) Joint diseases and matrix metalloproteinases: a role for MMP-13. *Current Pharm. Biotech.*, Vol. 9, No. 1 (February 2008), pp. 47-54, ISSN 1873-4316

Theuns, DA., Rivero-Ayerza, M., Goedhart, DM., Miltenburg, M. & Jordaens, LJ. (2008). Morphology discrimination in implantable cardioverter-defibrillators: consistency of template match percentage during atrial tachyarrhythmias at different heart rates. *Europace.*, Vol. 10, No. 9, (September 2008), pp. 1060-6, ISSN 1532-2092

Toegel, S., Wu, SQ., Piana, C., Unger, FM., Wirth, M., Goldring, MB., et al. (2008) Comparison between chondroprotective effects of glucosamine, curcumin, and diacerein in IL-1β-stimulated C-28/I2 chondrocytes. *Osteoarthritis and Cartilage.* Vol. 16, No. 10, (October 2008), pp. 1205-1212, ISSN 1522-9653

Tortorella, MD., Burn, TC., Pratta, MA., Abbaszade, I., Hollis, JM., Liu ,R., et al. (1999) Purification and cloning of aggrecanase-1: amember of the ADAMTS family of proteins. *Science.*Vol. 284, No. 5420, (June 1999), pp.1664–1666, ISSN 0036-8075

van Beuningen, HM., Glansbeek, HL., van der Kraan, PM. & van den Berg, WB. (2000) Osteoarthritis-like changes in the murine knee joint resulting from intra-articular transforming growth factor-beta injections. *Osteoarthritis and Cartilage.* Vol. 8, No. 1, (January 2000), pp. 25-33, ISSN 1063-4584 van der Weyden, L., Wei, L., Luo, J., Yang, X., Birk, DE., Adams, DJ., et al. (2006) Functional knockout of the matrilin- 3 gene causes premature chondrocyte maturation to hypertrophy and increases bone mineral density and osteoarthritis. *American Journal of Pathology*. Vol. 169, No. 2, (August 2006), pp. 515-527, ISSN 0002-9440

Vikkula, M., Mariman, EC., Lui, VC., Zhidkova, NI., Tiller, GE., Goldring, MB., et al. (1995). Autosomal dominant and recessive osteochondrodysplasias associated with the COL11A2 locus. *Cell.* Vol. 80, No. 3, (February 1995), pp. 431-437, ISSN 0092-8674

von der Mark, K., Kirsch, T., Nerlich, A., Kuss, A., Weseloh, G., Glückert, K., et al. (1992). Type X collagen synthesis in human osteoarthritic cartilage. Indication of chondrocyte hypertrophy. *Arthritis Rheum.*, Vol. 35, No. 7, (July 1992) pp. 806- 11, ISSN 0004-3591

Vuolteenaho, K., Moilanen, T., Hämäläinen, M., & Moilanen, E. (2002). Effects of TNFalpha-antagonists on nitric oxide production in human cartilage. *Osteoarthritis Cartilage*, Vol. 10, No. 4, (April 2002), pp. 327-32, ISSN 1063-4584

Wagener, R., Kobbe, B., & Paulsson, M. (1997). Primary structure of matrilin-3, a new member of a family of extracellular matrix proteins related to cartilage matrix protein (matrilin-1) and von Willebrand factor. *FEBS Lett.*, Vol. 413, No. 1, (August 1997), pp. 129–134, ISSN 0014-5793

Wagner, K., Pöschl, E., Turnay, J., Baik, J., Pihlajaniemi, T., Frischholz, S., et al. (2000). Coexpression of alpha and beta subunits of prolyl 4-hydroxylase stabilizes the triple helix of recombinant human type X collagen. *Biochem J.*, Vol. 352, No. 3 (December 2000), pp. 907-11, ISSN 0264-6021

Wang, CT., Lin, YT., Chiang, BL., Lin, YH. & Hou, SM. (2006). High molecular weight hyaluronic acid down-regulates the gene expression of osteoarthritis- associated cytokines and enzymes in fibroblast-like synoviocytes from patients with early osteoarthritis. *Osteoarthritis Cartilage*. Vol. 14, No 14, (December 2006), pp. 1237-1247, ISSN 1063-4584

Wehrli, BM., Huang, W., De Crombrugghe, B., Ayala, AG. & Czerniak, B. (2003) Sox9, a master regulator of chondrogenesis, distinguishes mesenchymal chondrosarcoma from other small blue round cell tumors. *Hum. Pathol.*, Vol. 34, No. 3, (March 2003), pp. 263-269, ISSN 0046-8177

Wesche, H., Korherr, C., Kracht, M., Falk, W., Resch, K., & Martin, MU. (1997). The interleukin-1 receptor accessory protein (IL-1RAcP) is essential for IL-1-induced activation of interleukin-1 receptor-associated kinase (IRAK) and stress-activated protein kinases (SAP kinases). *J. Biol. Chem.*, Vol. 272, No. 12, (March 1997), pp. 7727-31, ISSN 0021-9258

Williams, FM. & Spector, TD. (2008). Biomarkers in osteoarthritis. *Arthritis Res Ther*. Vol. 10, No. 1, (January 2008), pp. 101, ISSN 1478-6362

Wobig, M., Dickhut, A., Maier, R. & Vetter, G. (1998) Viscosupplementation with hylan G-F 20: a 26-week controlled trial of efficacy and safety in the osteoarthritic knee. *Clin Ther.* Vol. 20, No. 3, (June 1998), pp. 410-423. ISSN 0149-2918

Wu, J., Rush, TS 3rd., Hotchandani, R., Du, X., Geck, M., Collins, E., et al. (2005) Identification of potent and selective MMP-13 inhibitors. *Bioorg. Med. Chem. Lett.*, Vol. 15, No. 18, (September 2005), pp. 4105-4109, 0960-894X

Wu, JJ., Woods, PE. & Eyre, DR. (1992). Identification of cross-linking sites in bovine cartilage type IX collagen reveals an antiparallel type II-type IX molecular relationship and type IX to type IX bonding. *J Biol Chem.*, Vol. 267, No. 32, (November 1992), pp. 23007-14, ISSN 0021-9258

Wu, JJ. & Eyre, DR. (1998) Matrilin-3 forms disulfide-linked oligomers with matrilin-1 in bovine epiphyseal cartilage. *J. of Biol. Chem.* Vol. 273, No. 28, (July 1998), pp. 17433-17438 ISSN 0021-9258

Xie, D. & Homandberg, GA. (1993). Fibronectin fragments bind to and penetrate cartilage tissue resulting in proteinase expression and cartilage damage. *Biochim Biophys Acta.* Vol. 1182, No. 2, (September 1993), pp. 189-196, ISSN 0006-3002

Zhu, Y., Wu, JJ., Weis, MA., Mirza, SK. & Eyre, DR. (2011). Type IX Collagen Neo-Deposition in Degenerative Discs of Surgical Patients Whether Genotyped Plus or Minus for COL9 Risk Alleles. *Spine* (Phila Pa 1976)., Epub ahead of print. (February 2011), ISSN 1528-1159

15

Biochemical Mediators Involved in Cartilage Degradation and the Induction of Pain in Osteoarthritis

Michael B. Ellman[1,2], Dongyao Yan[1], Di Chen[1] and Hee-Jeong Im[1,2,3]

[1]Department of Biochemistry,
[2]Department of Orthopedic Surgery,
[3]Department of Internal Medicine,
Section of Rheumatology, Rush University Medical Center, Chicago, IL, USA

1. Introduction

Osteoarthritis, a debilitating degenerative joint disease predominantly found in elderly individuals, has become the principal source of physical disability resulting in increased health care costs and impaired quality of life in the United States. The pathogenesis of osteoarthritis (OA) involves the progressive deterioration of cartilage tissue, but many of the underlying biochemical and pathophysiological mechanisms involved in cartilage degradation and the induction of pain in this process remain largely unknown. Recent literature has focused on understanding many of these processes, with the intention of developing novel therapies aimed at slowing and/or reversing cartilage degradation and inducing symptomatic relief. This chapter provides an overview of several biochemical mediators involved in OA, with an emphasis on reviewing pertinent factors mediating cartilage breakdown and the induction of pain in degenerative conditions.

2. Anatomy

Articular cartilage lines the surfaces of joints and serves several important functions, including the provision of a smooth, low-friction surface, joint lubrication, and stress distribution with load bearing (1, 2). The components of articular cartilage include an elaborate mixture of water (65-80% of wet weight), collagen (10-20% of wet weight), proteoglycans (PGs; 10-15% of wet weight), and chondrocytes (5% of wet weight) (1). The extracellular matrix (ECM) includes collagen and PGs, principally aggrecan, with other proteins and glycoproteins in lesser amounts. This matrix allows normal cartilage to form the resilient, low-friction surface capable of absorbing shock with high impact mechanical loading (3).

Within the ECM, collagen fibers provide form, shape, and tensile strength to cartilage. The principal collagen fibers present in articular cartilage are type II fibers, with smaller quantities of types V, VI, IX, X, and XI (1). Collagen interacts to form fibrils that interact with and trap large aggregates of PGs, principally aggrecan. PGs bind water and help distribute stresses throughout the porous-permeable ECM under compressive loads. Aggrecan, the most abundant PG found in articular cartilage, is composed of a protein backbone bound by negatively-charged chondroitin sulfate and keratin sulfate groups. It binds with hyaluronic acid (HA) to form complexes within the ECM. Due to negatively-charged sulfated groups, these complexes electrostatically interact with cations, ultimately forming ion-dipole interactions with water, allowing cartilage to function as a hydrated tissue that resists compression.

The cellular makeup of cartilage consists of articular chondrocytes. Chondrocytes maintain and produce the components of the ECM that regulate cartilage homeostasis. They are mesenchymal in origin, few in number within the matrix, have a low rate of cell turnover, and receive nutrients and oxygen from the surrounding synovial fluid by means of diffusion (1). Further, they respond to a variety of factors, including matrix proteins, mechanical load, and soluble mediators such as growth factors and cytokines.

3. Metabolic disruption of cartilage homeostasis in osteoarthritis

Under normal conditions, chondrocytes maintain a dynamic equilibrium between synthesis and degradation of ECM components. In osteoarthritic states, however, there is a disruption of matrix equilibrium leading to progressive loss of cartilage tissue, clonal expansion of cells in the depleted regions, induction of oxidative states in a stressful cellular environment, and eventually, apoptosis of chondrocytes (2, 4). With progression, there is usually an increase in both degradation and synthesis within the joint, with an overall shift toward catabolism over anabolism. Chondrocyte metabolism is unbalanced due to excessive production of inflammatory cytokines and matrix-degrading enzymes, in conjunction with a downregulation of anabolic factors, eventually leading to destruction of the ECM and subsequent cartilage degradation. Oxidative stress elicited by reactive oxygen species (ROS) further disturbs cartilage homeostasis and promotes catabolism via induction of cell death, breakdown of matrix components, upregulation of latent matrix-degrading enzyme production, inhibition of ECM synthesis, and oxidation of intracellular and extracellular molecules (2).

One approach to slow or reverse catabolism involves attempts to downregulate the expression of catabolic factors and/or matrix-degrading enzymes, including matrix metalloproteases (MMPs) and a disintegrin-like and metalloprotease with thrombospondin motifs (ADAMTS family, aka aggrecanases)(5). In particular, MMP-13 is the most potent collagen type II-degrading enzyme in human articular cartilage (6). The regulation of matrix-degrading enzyme expression is stimulated by pro-inflammatory cytokines, growth factors, and metabolites, including lipopolysaccharide (LPS) (7), interleukin-1 (IL-1) (8), tumor necrosis factor-alpha (TNF-α) (8), fibroblast growth factor-2 (FGF-2, otherwise known as basic FGF) (9), and ROS (10). Equally important are attempts to upregulate anabolic factors in matrix homeostasis, including ECM components (e.g., aggrecan, collagen type II), growth factors (e.g. transforming growth factor (TGF)-β, bone morphogenetic proteins (BMPs), and insulin-like growth factor-1 (IGF-1)), and/or anti-destructive enzymes [e.g., tissue inhibitor of metalloproteases (TIMPs)] to prevent cartilage degradation.

4. Catabolic mediators in OA

Healthy articular chondrocytes and synoviocytes constitutively synthesize and secret a wide array of mediators to maintain their delicate homeostasis. When inappropriately regulated, a subset of mediators will drive detrimental catabolic processes in both cell populations, resulting in cartilage degeneration and chronic synovial inflammation. This section will summarize our current understanding of these key catabolic factors in OA pathogenesis.

4.1 Inflammatory mediators

Typical inflammatory mediators in OA include pro-inflammatory members from the interleukin family (IL-1, IL-6, and IL-17), TNF-α, and prostaglandin E2 (PGE2). The roles of these mediators have been extensively studied in arthritic tissues secondary to their high concentrations in degenerative states. Each of these mediators not only stimulates the production of cartilage-degrading proteases, but also upregulates other destructive factors via paracrine or autocrine mechanisms, thus perpetuating disease progression.

4.1.1 IL-1β

IL-1β is thought to play a prominent role in OA development. It demonstrates potent bioactivities in inhibiting ECM synthesis and promoting cartilage breakdown. Independent studies have shown that IL-1β represses the expression of essential ECM components, aggrecan and collagen type II, in chondrocytes (11-13). IL-1β also strikingly induces a spectrum of proteolytic enzymes, including collagenases (MMP-1 and MMP-13) and ADAMTS-4, in both chondrocytes and synovial fibroblasts. Aside from these direct effects, IL-1β induces a panel of cytokines, including IL-6, IL-8, and leukemia inducing factor (LIF), which produce additive or synergistic effects in the catabolic cascade (14). Further, IL-1β has been implicated in OA pathogenesis in numerous observational studies. Although less pronounced than what has been observed in rheumatoid arthritis patients, OA synovial fluids contains significantly higher levels of IL-1β compared to normal synovial fluid (15). Immunohistochemical analyses also reveal increased expression of IL-1β in OA cartilage and synovium (16, 17). Moreover, osteoarthritic chondrocytes exhibit heightened sensitivity to IL-1β stimulation, in part due to augmented IL-1 receptor type I expression (18). This pathological change renders OA chondrocytes even more susceptible to deleterious IL-1β attack. The significance of IL-1β in OA was further corroborated by *in vivo* studies and pharmaceutical efforts using IL-1 receptor antagonist (IL-1ra) as a potential therapeutic factor to prevent cartilage degeneration. As an inhibitory molecule of IL-1β, IL-1ra not only showed efficacy in OA animal models, but also improved clinical outcomes (19).

4.1.2 IL-6

Another constitutively expressed cytokine in human articular chondrocytes is IL-6 (20), yet only a fraction of OA patients contains increased IL-6 levels in arthritic cartilage and synovial fluid, suggesting that IL-6 may not be the ultimate driving force in this disease (21, 22). Nevertheless, *in vitro* studies demonstrate catabolic effects of IL-6 as this cytokine inhibits PG synthesis in chondrocytes, and this effect is potentiated by addition of soluble IL-6 receptor (sIL-6R) (23, 24). Combination treatment with IL-6 and sIL-6R has been shown to enhance aggrecanase-mediated PG depletion in cartilage (25). IL-6 also suppresses collagen type II expression (26), and to a lesser extent than IL-1β, dysregulates enzymatic antioxidant defense mechanisms in chondrocytes *via* modulation of key enzymes (27). Therefore, it is surprising that male IL-6$^{-/-}$ mice displayed more severe OA phenotypes compared with wild-type mice (28). In this report, de Hooge *et al* suggest that IL-6 exerted joint protection in aging murine OA joints. However, their findings differ qualitatively from those provided by Ryu *et al,* who reported that IL-6 promotes joint destruction in an instability-induced OA model (29). Further *in vivo* experiments are warranted to clarify such contradictions. Interestingly, a recent study suggested a mechanistic link between obesity and OA, based on the observation that the infrapatellar fat pad actively synthesizes IL-6 and sIL-6R in knee OA patients (30).

4.1.3 IL-17

The pro-inflammatory role of IL-17 is well-established in rheumatoid arthritis, but less so in OA. IL-17 is reported to exert stimulatory effects on MMP-3, MMP-13 and ADAMTS-4 expression in chondrocytes (31, 32). It directly inhibits PG synthesis, augments nitric oxide production, and triggers angiogenic factor release (33-35). Further, the IL-17 response can be amplified dramatically when other destructive cytokines, such as IL-1β and TNF-α, are present. In chondrocytes, IL-17-mediated type II collagen breakdown and MMP expression is synergistically enhanced by IL-1, IL-6, or TNF-α co-treatment (36). Likewise, synergy in nitric oxide production was observed when chondrocytes were treated with IL-17 and TNF-α (37). IL-17 also synergizes with IL-1β or TNF-α in PGE2 production in OA menisci *ex vivo* (38). Cytokine induction serves as a secondary mechanism in IL-17-mediated effects. In chondrocytes and synovial fibroblasts, IL-17 induces certain pro-inflammatory cytokines and chemokines, such as IL-1β, IL-6, and IL-8 (39, 40). In macrophages, IL-17 effectively upregulates IL-1 and TNF-α expression, which may contribute to chronic synovial inflammation observed in some OA patients (41). By way of adenovirus-mediated IL-17 overexpression, Koenders *et al.* showed that IL-17 is capable of causing joint inflammation and bone erosion by itself, and also synergizes with TNF-α (42). Conversely, IL-17 deficiency markedly mitigates the arthritic phenotype in a collagen-induced arthritis model, but whether IL-17 ablation also provides similar protection in OA models awaits investigation (43).

4.1.4 TNF-α

The relevance of TNF-α to OA pathogenesis is supported by the observation that TNF-α receptor expression is significantly upregulated in OA cartilage (44, 45). TNF-α concentration in synovial fluid also increases in patients with anterior cruciate ligament injury, suggesting this cytokine may play a role in OA development (46). Similar to IL-1β, TNF-α also promotes PG depletion (47-49). The induction of proteolytic enzymes MMP-3, MMP-9, and MMP-13 by TNF-α in chondrocytes may account for such an action (50, 51). TNF-α potently induces IL-6 and PGE2, which possibly results in secondary inflammatory events in the joint (47, 48, 52, 53). Another important process mediated by TNF-α is cell death. It appears that excessive exposure to TNF-α can elicit chondrocyte apoptosis, which will lead to local secondary necrosis and eventually a catabolic cascade due to absence of phagocytes in cartilage (54, 55). Consistent with these findings, TNF-α transgenic mice exhibit spontaneous cartilage damage and conspicuous occurrence of arthritis (54).

4.1.5 PGE2

PGE2 is yet another significant player in chondrocyte metabolism. Upregulated in OA, PGE2 inhibits PG and type II collagen synthesis with the highest cellular sensitivity among all prostanoids produced by chondrocytes (56, 57). Mechanistically, PGE2 appears to signal through the EP2 receptor to exert such inhibitory effects (58). Furthermore, EP4 receptor activation increases MMP-13 and ADAMTS-5 expression, thus promoting ECM degradation (59). Interestingly, some evidence suggests that specific EP2 activation enhances cartilage regeneration in rabbit models, indicating species differences in PGE2 responses (60). PGE2 also mediates or sensitizes chondrocytes to apoptosis (61, 62). Both IL-1 and TNF-α induce PGE2 production, with the former being more potent (63-65), and the involvement of PGE2 in IL-1β-induced MMP-3 and MMP-13 expression is demonstrated in PGE synthase-1 knockout chondrocytes. In these modified cells, the catabolic effects of IL-1β are dramatically reduced (66). However, another group claims that PGE2 acts as a secretagogue of IGF-1, which in turn mediates anabolism in chondrocytes (67). Whether this induction brings any benefit to OA cartilage is questionable, because IGF-1 non-responsiveness has been reported in OA chondrocytes (68).

4.2 Oxidative stress mediators, growth factors and glycoproteins

4.2.1 Nitric oxide

Nitric oxide (NO), a member of ROS, mediates the destructive actions of IL-1β and TNF-α in cartilage, including suppression of PG and collagen synthesis, as well as stimulation of MMPs (69-73). Spontaneous overproduction of NO produces similar effects in chondrocytes (73, 74), and prolonged exposure to NO together with other ROS can lead to apoptosis of articular cell types (62, 75, 76). NO is also partially responsible for the insensitivity of OA chondrocytes to IGF-1 (77). As a mediator downstream of IL-1, NO also inhibits BMP-2-mediated PG synthesis (78).

Inducible nitric oxide synthase (iNOS) is the major enzyme responsible for NO generation in articular cartilage. OA chondrocytes in the superficial zone express higher levels of iNOS (79, 80). Several destructive cytokines, including IL-1 and TNF-α, induce iNOS expression in articular cell types (81, 82). Forced expression of iNOS inhibits matrix synthesis in chondrocytes (74). Futher, in OA cartilage, iNOS inhibition gives rise to IL-10 induction and MMP-10 repression in the presence of IL-1β (83). More recently, iNOS was found to function as a crucial mediator downstream of the advanced glycation end products pathway and the leptin pathway in chondrocytes (84, 85). Pelletier *et al* provided compelling evidence regarding the importance of iNOS in OA progression. In their canine OA model, selective inhibition of iNOS resulted in marked attenuation of joint destruction (86). Intra-articular delivery of an iNOS inhibitor counteracts the acute effects mediated by IL-1β, reaffirming the catabolic role of iNOS in OA progression (87).

4.2.2 FGF-2

A series of studies have demonstrated that FGF-2 (otherwise known as basic FGF) acts as a catabolic growth factor in addition to its well-established mitogenic role in articular cartilage. Despite its positive effect on proliferation, FGF-2 inhibits IGF-1/BMP-7-enhanced PG deposition in human articular chondrocytes, and negatively affects the physical properties of normal cartilage (88, 89). FGF-2 alters the ratio of type II to type I collagen in articular chondrocytes, thus possibly leading to the formation of fibrocartilage, a poor substitute for hyaline cartilage (90, 91). In porcine chondrocytes, FGF-2 antagonizes IGF-1/TGF-β-mediated decorin and type II collagen production (92). Moreover, FGF-2 promotes cartilage degeneration *ex vivo* (93). A mechanistic explanation of FGF-2-mediated effects lies in its ability to upregulate MMP-13 and ADAMTS-5 (94, 95). FGF-2 orchestrates the MAPK, NFκB, and substance P signaling pathway to induce MMP-13 (5, 93, 94). It has also been shown that activation of FGF receptor 1 (FGFR1) is required for FGF-2-mediated MMP-13 and ADAMTS-5 induction (95).

Results acquired from comparative analyses suggest the biological relevance of FGF-2 to OA. FGF-2 levels in OA synovial fluids are significantly elevated compared to those in normal specimens (94). FGFR3 expression is markedly diminished in OA chondrocytes, which results in altered FGFR1 to FGFR3 ratios and may account for the inhibition of anabolism in the disease state (95). It should be noted that other studies indicate a chondroprotective role of FGF-2 in cartilage biology (96, 97). The discrepancies may arise from differences in cell origin (i.e. species, age, severity of OA, etc), and render future clarifications necessary.

4.2.3 Fibronectin

Fibronectin (Fn) is an adhesive glycoprotein found in cartilage and synovial membrane tissue (98). Evidence shows that Fn level is increased in OA cartilage as well as OA synovial fluid (99, 100). Heightened proteolytic activities in OA joints lead to the generation of Fn fragments (Fn-fs) of different sizes. Specifically, ADAMTS-8 was characterized as a fibronectinase in OA chondrocytes (101). Indeed, Fn-fs are found with increased abundance in OA synovial fluids and cartilage (99, 102). A 40-kDa collagen-binding Fn-f induces sustained PG degradation in both normal and OA cartilage (103). Furthermore, Fn-f stimulates type II collagen cleavage in an MMP-13-dependent manner (104). Preceding collagen disintegration, Fn-f disrupts the ECM by promoting the release of cartilage oligomeric matrix protein (COMP) and chondroadherin (105). Fn-f also augments cytokine, ROS, MMP and aggrecanase production in cartilage *ex vivo* and *in vitro* (10, 106-109). Stimulation of IL-1 leads to enhanced production of Fn-f, which exerts prolonged destructive effects (99).

4.2.4 Osteopontin

Osteopontin, a phosphorylated glycoprotein with cell and matrix binding affinities, has been characterized as a facilitator of osteoclast adhesion and an initiator of osteoid mineralization (110). Osteopontin deposition in cartilage exhibits a spatial pattern, based on the fact that it is mainly detected in chondrocytes residing in the upper deep zone (111). Comparative analyses reveal that, in contrast with healthy chondrocytes, OA chondrocytes express notable levels of osteopontin (111). Moreover, an apparent correlation exists between osteopontin level and the severity of OA lesions (111-113).

Nevertheless, the role of osteopontin in cartilage remains controversial. Osteopontin promotes calcium pyrophosphate dehydrate (CPPD) crystal formation in articular cartilage, suggesting that elevated osteopontin production in OA may be detrimental (114). Yet this stimulatory effect seems to depend on osteopontin concentration, because other studies demonstrate the opposite using higher concentrations of this protein (115). Another independent study also showed that osteopontin inhibits IL-1β-induced NO and PGE2 production in OA cartilage, suggesting an anti-catabolic role in cartilage homeostasis (116). Osteopontin deficiency exacerbates aging-induced and instability-induced OA in mice (117). Based on these apparently contradictory activities, it raises the possibility that osteopontin elicits different biological effects depending on the stages of OA.

4.2.5 Osteonectin

Osteonectin is a non-collagenous glycoprotein linking collagen fibrils to mineral in bone. It is also present in mineralizing chondroid bone (118). Articular chondrocytes synthesize osteonectin, and this process is regulated by endogenous stimuli. IL-1, TNF-α, and FGF-2, but not IL-6, greatly inhibit osteonectin expression (119, 120). IL-1 also impairs the glycosylation of osteonectin (120). On the other hand, TGF-β, PDGF, and IGF-1 upregulate osteonectin synthesis, even in the presence of IL-1 (119, 120). Osteonectin is localized to the superficial and middle zones of OA cartilage, while normal cartilage does not display such a pattern (120, 121). Osteonectin synthesis is also enhanced in OA synovial fibroblasts (120). Osteonectin induces collagenase expression in this cell type, which may contribute to cartilage damage (122).

4.3 Protective mediators in OA

In contrast to the aforementioned catabolic mediators in OA, several growth factors take on important anabolic roles in the joint, thus serving as potential targets for future therapeutic growth factor therapy in practice. While the literature has only begun to explore the *in vitro, in vivo,* and clinical effects of many of these factors, there is potential for these mediators to be major players in the treatment of degenerative joint diseases in the future. Multiple cytokines exert protection in articular joints, including IL-1 receptor antagonist (IL-1ra), IL-4, IL-10, IL-11, and IL-13. Perhaps the most well-studied anabolic factors to date include TGF-β, BMP-2, BMP-7, and IGF-1 (Table 1). We will also discuss two factors elucidated in our laboratory to have potent anabolic and anti-catabolic effects in human articular cartilage: resveratrol (RSV) and bovine lactoferricin (LfcinB).

4.3.1 Interleukins

The antagonistic effect of IL-1ra on IL-1 has been well established. By directly competing against IL-1 for its cognate receptor, IL-1ra effectively inhibits IL-1-mediated responses in chondrocytes, including PG depletion, MMP induction, and cytokine induction (123-125). IL-1ra expression is repressed by NO, which may blunt its action in OA cartilage (126). Not surprisingly, forced expression of IL-1ra confers resistance to IL-1 challenge in chondrocytes (127, 128). Both gene delivery and IL-1ra intra-articular injection have been shown to impede OA progression, indicating anti-IL-1 therapy is a viable option in OA disease modification (19, 129).

Protective roles of anti-inflammatory cytokines have also been linked to OA. An array of cytokines, including IL-4, IL-10, IL-11, and IL-13, has been shown to block the actions of catabolic cytokines *via* different mechanisms. IL-4 suppresses MMP-13, cathepsin B, and iNOS when cyclic tensile stress is applied on chondrocytes (130, 131). IL-4 has potent inhibitory effects on cartilage degradation in the presence of IL-1 and TNF-α (132). In synoviocytes, IL-4 downregulates apoptosis (133). IL-4 gene therapy appears to dampen inflammation in chondrocytes (134). Moreover, intra-articular injection of IL-4 results in notable amelioration of cartilage degenerative status (131).

IL-10 is upregulated in OA chondrocytes, and this phenomenon may represent a reparative effort (135). IL-10 suppresses IL-1 and TNF-α production (136). Compared to IL-1ra, IL-10 gene delivery into synoviocytes elicits moderate yet still significant protection on cartilage (137).

IL-1β	-: ↓ PG synthesis; ↓ type II collagen synthesis; ↑ MMPs; ↑ ADAMTS-4; ↑ ROS; ↑ IL-6; ↑ IL-8; ↑ LIF; ↑ synovial inflammation
IL-6	-: ↓ PG synthesis; ↓ type II collagen synthesis; ↑ PG depletion; dysregulation of antioxidant defense
IL-17	-: ↓ PG synthesis; ↑ type II collagen breakdown; ↑ MMPs; ↑ ADAMTS-4; ↑ NO; ↑ IL-1β; ↑ IL-6; ↑ IL-8; ↑ PGE2 (in menisci); ↑ TNF-α (in macrophage)
TNF-α	-: ↑ PG depletion; ↑ MMPs; ↑ IL-6; ↑ PGE2; ↑ chondrocyte apoptosis
PGE2	-: ↓ PG synthesis; ↓ type II collagen synthesis; ↑ MMPs; ↑ ADAMTS-5; ↑ chondrocyte apoptosis
NO	-: ↓ PG synthesis; ↓ type II collagen synthesis; ↑ MMPs; ↓ IGF-1 sensitivity; ↑ apoptosis
FGF-2	-: ↓ PG deposition; ↓ ratio of type II to type I collagen; ↑ MMP-13; ↑ ADAMTS-5
Fn-f	-: ↑ PG degradation; ↑ type II collagen cleavage; ↑ COMP and chondroadherin release; ↑ MMPs; ↑ aggrecanases; ↑ destructive cytokines
Osteopontin	-: ↑ CPPD formation +: ↓ NO; ↓ PGE2 (concentration-dependent)
Osteonectin	-: ↑ collagenases (in synovial fibroblasts)

(-) = Catabolic effects; (+) = Anabolic or anti-catabolic effects

Table 1. Effects of Catabolic Mediators in Articular Cartilage

IL-1ra	+: ↓ IL-1-mediated responses
IL-4	+: ↓ MMP-13; ↓ cathepsin B; ↓ iNOS; ↓ synovial fibroblast apoptosis; ↓ IL-1/TNF-α-mediated cartilage degradation
IL-10	+: ↓ IL-1; ↓ TNF-α; ↑ cartilage protection
IL-11	+: ↑ TIMP-1; ↓ pro-inflammatory cytokines; ↓ NO; ↓ TNF-α responses (synovial fibroblast)
IL-13	+: ↓ MMPs; ↓ IL-1β; ↓ TNF-α; ↑ IL-1ra; ↓ PGE2 and COX-2 (synovial fibroblasts); ↓ synoviocyte apoptosis
TGF-β	+: ↑ chondrocyte activity, ↑ PG synthesis, ↑ ECM synthesis; ↓IL-1, ↓ROS - : Osteophyte formation and synovial inflammation with prolonged exposure
BMP-2	+: ↑ ECM synthesis, ↑ collagen II expression - : +/- aggrecan degradation?
BMP-7	+: ↑ chondrocyte activity, ↑ PG synthesis, ↑ ECM synthesis; ↓cell proliferation; age-independent, ↑activity of other anabolic factors (IGF-1, BMPs), ↓MMPs, ↓IL-1 and IL-6; ↑ cartilage repair in vivo (sheep, rabbits) - : Unknown
IGF-1	+: ↑ ECM synthesis, ↑ PG synthesis; ↓apoptosis; + synergism with BMP-7 - : ↓effect with ↑ age and on OA cartilage
RSV	+: ↑ ECM synthesis, ↑ PG (aggrecan) synthesis; ↑ collagen II expression; ↓IL-1 & FGF-2 effects, + synergism with BMP-7 - : preliminary data; no in vivo studies
LfcinB	+: ↑ ECM synthesis, ↑ PG (aggrecan) synthesis; ↑ collagen II expression; ↓IL-1 & FGF-2 effects , + synergism with BMP-7 - : preliminary data; no *in vivo* studies

Table 2. Effects of Protective Mediators in Articular Cartilage

IL-11, an IL-6 family member, is believed to exert anti-catabolic and anti-inflammatory effects in articular joints, but remains poorly defined. IL-11 produced by articular chondrocytes stimulates the production of tissue inhibitor of metalloproteinase (TIMP) (138). IL-11 also downregulates pro-inflammatory cytokines and NO production (139). In OA synovial fibroblasts, IL-11 alone had no impact on PGE2 release, but shows anti-inflammatory properties in conjunction with TNF-α (140). In RA synovium, IL-11 directly inhibits MMP-1 and MMP-3 production, upregulates TIMP-1, and inhibits TNF-α production in the presence of soluble IL-11 receptor (141). Importantly, systemic treatment with IL-11 leads to a significant reduction in clinical and histological severity of established collagen-induced arthritis (CIA), suggesting an active role of IL-11 in joint homeostasis (142). IL-11 level is greatly increased in OA synovial fluid (143). However, IL-11 action is likely to be blunted due to the observation that the IL-11 receptor is markedly downregulated in OA chondrocytes (Im et al., unpublished data).

IL-13 downregulates MMP-13 expression in OA chondrocytes (144). Combined with IL-4, IL-13 abolishes IL-17 expression in RA synovial tissue (145). A more detailed study revealed that IL-13 represses IL-1β, TNF-α, and MMP-3, and simultaneously induces IL-1ra (146). IL-13, as well as IL-4 and IL-10, reduces TNF-α-induced PGE2 release and cyclooxygenase 2 (COX-2) in OA synovial fibroblasts (147). Similar to IL-4, IL-13 also inhibits synoviocyte apoptotic events (133). Nonetheless, IL-13 levels were found to be low in OA tissues (148). Whether IL-13 holds significance to OA pathogenesis needs to be further determined, especially in animal models.

4.3.2 TGF-β/BMP Superfamily

The TGF-β superfamily is composed of over 35 structurally-related members, with the majority of these members playing fundamental roles in development and homeostasis. In articular cartilage, three members of the TGF-β superfamily have been shown to play a significant role in cartilage homeostasis: TGF-β, BMP-2, and BMP-7. BMPs are structurally related to the transforming growth factor-β (TGF-β) superfamily and have wide-ranging biological activities, including the regulation of cellular proliferation, apoptosis, differentiation and migration, embryonic development and the maintenance of tissue homeostasis during adult life (149-151). It is now clear that they are expressed in a variety of tissues including adult articular cartilage.

4.3.2.1 TGF-β

Several studies demonstrate an anabolic role of TGF-*β* in articular cartilage. TGF-*β* has been shown to upregulate chondrocyte synthetic activity and suppress the catabolic activity of IL-1 (152, 153). *In vitro*, TGF-*β* stimulates chondrogenesis of synovial lining and bone marrow-derived mesenchymal stem cells (154). Additionally, asporin inhibits TGF-β-mediated stimulation of cartilage matrix genes such as collagen type II and aggrecan, and inhibits accumulation of PGs (155). In both Japanese (155) and Han Chinese (156) populations, patients with an asporin polymorphism demonstrated increased prevelance of arthritic conditions, presumably via inhibition of TGF-*β* expression, suggesting a protective role of TGF-*β* in articular cartilage. These findings were corroborated in knockout mice, as mice deficient for TGF-*β* or Smad3 (downstream mediator of TGF-*β*) developed cartilage degeneration resembling human OA (157, 158). Other studies demonstrate a vital role of TGF-*β* in the suppression of NO and other ROS levels (159), as well as the upregulation of PG synthesis in calf-cartilage explants in a dose-dependent manner (152, 160).

However, the literature also suggests that TGF-β demonstrates nondesirable side effects in joint tissues. For example, upon sustained exposure to in the joint, TGF-β can actually induce the formation of OA-like tissue pathology via stimulation of osteophyte formation, stimulation of synovial inflammation and fibrosis, and attraction of inflammatory leukocytes to the synovial lining (152, 153, 161, 162). These contradictory findings warrant further investigation, and recent research efforts are focused on downstream receptor usage to help provide further clues (152). Nevertheless, given its deleterious effects not seen in other growth factor-based strategies, TGF-β therapy is not presently a viable option for use in articular cartilage repair or regeneration.

4.3.2.2 BMP-2

Several studies have analyzed the role of BMP-2 in cartilage and found promising results. The effect of BMP-2 on mesenchymal stem cells is similar to that of TGF-β, with increased production of ECM and decreased expression of collage type 1, theoretically suppressing the formation of fibrocartilage (149, 154). *In vitro* analysis reveals that BMP-2 stimulates matrix synthesis and reverses chondrocyte dedifferentiation as indicated by an increase in synthesis of cartilage-specific collagen type II in OA chondrocytes (163). In rabbit knees, BMP-2-impregnated collagen sponges implanted into full-thickness cartilage defects enhance cartilage repair compared with empty defects or defects filled with collagen sponge alone, with this effect remaining at one year after implantation (164). Interestingly, however, in an IL-1-induced cartilage degeneration model in mice, BMP-2 stimulated matrix production via increased collagen type II and aggrecan expression (anabolic activity), but also increased aggrecan degradation as well, revealing a possible catabolic or self-regulatory role (165). Further studies are indeed warranted to further elucidate the effects of BMP-2 on cartilage repair.

4.3.2.3 BMP-7

BMP-7 (also known as osteogenic protein-1), another member of the TGF-β superfamily, is perhaps the most well-studied anabolic growth factor in cartilage repair. It is expressed in cartilage and exerts potent anabolic effects by stimulating differentiation and metabolic functions of both osteocytes and chondrocytes (166). In bone, a variety of animal models have clearly demonstrated a therapeutic potential of BMP-7 in bone repair applications, paving the way for BMP-7 to be used as the first commercial BMP to be used for bone repair clinically (149). In articular cartilage, BMP-7 has potent anabolic effects by stimulating matrix biosynthesis in both human adult articular chondrocytes (167) and human IVD cells (168).

In vitro, BMP-7 has several anabolic and anti-catabolic effects on articular cartilage. It promotes cell survival and upregulates chondrocyte metabolism (169) and protein synthesis without creating uncontrolled cell proliferation and formation of osteophytes, unlike other chondrogenic growth factors (149, 151). In a comparison study examining BMP-2, -4, -6, and -7, as well as cartilage-derived morphogenetic protein (CDMP)-1 (also known as GDF-5, growth differentiation factor-5) and CDMP-2, PG synthesis was stimulated to a greater extent by BMP-2 and -4, and the most significant upregulation after stimulation with BMP-7 (150). Importantly, its actions in cartilage are age-independent as BMP-7 induced similar anabolic responses in normal and OA chondrocytes from both young and old donors without inducing chondrocyte hypertrophy or changes in phenotype (151, 170, 171). Chubinskaya and colleagues have revealed that the anabolic effect of BMP-7 extends beyond stimulation of cartilage ECM proteins and their receptors, but also modulates the expression of various anabolic growth factors as well (IGF-1, TGF-β/BMPs) (151). In addition to its anabolic capacity, BMP-7 effectively counteracts chondrocyte catabolism, revealing a potent anti-catabolic effect in human articular cartilage. BMP-7 inhibits the expression of pro-inflammatory cytokines (IL-1 and IL-6), inhibits endogenous expression of cytokines (ie. IL-6, IL-8, IL-11) and their downstream signaling molecules (receptors, transcription factors, and mitogen-activated kinases), and blocks both a baseline and cytokine-induced expression of MMP-1 and MMP-13 (151). BMP-7 has also been shown to enhance the gene expression of the anabolic molecule tissue inhibitor of metalloproteinase (TIMP) in normal and OA chondrocytes (151), and acts synergistically with the anabolic growth actors IGF-1 (169) and TGF-β (172).

Data from animal studies reveal that BMP-7 clearly has therapeutic potential for cartilage repair. In a large chondral defect study in sheep cartilage, BMP-7 was shown to induce significant cartilage repair in a model where no repair takes place in the controls (173). Studies evaluating models of OA, however, are less numerous, but BMP-7 has been shown to prevent development of damage and in some models reverse the damage (151). Finally, although BMP-7 is highly effective at stimulating bone repair, it does not appear to lead to osteophyte formation when administered into a joint, nor does it stimulate uncontrolled fibroblast proliferation (leading to fibrosis) (149). Studies have demonstrated that recombinant BMP-7 use has a relatively safe profile with few side effects in rabbits, dogs, goats and sheep. Overall, the data clearly indicate that BMP-7 has an important role in cartilage, both in normal homeostasis and in repair, but several unknowns continue to exist, such as concentration, dosing, the use of scaffolds, methods of administration, and possibly combinations with other factors.

4.3.3 IGF-1

IGF-1 is a single chain polypeptide that is structurally similar to insulin, a key growth factor that enhances PG synthesis in articular cartilage (174). Much like BMP-7, IGF-1 has a promising future in the field of cartilage repair and regeneration therapy. *In vitro*, IGF-1 induces anabolic and anti-catabolic effects in normal articular cartilage from a variety of species (53, 175). *In vivo* studies support *in vitro* findings, as IGF-1 deficiency in rats leads to the development of articular cartilage lesions (176). In animal models, IGF-1 enhances repair of extensive cartilage defects and protects synovial membrane tissue from chronic inflammation (177, 178). Other studies in spine cartilage demonstrate similar results. Osada *et al* showed that IGF-1 stimulates PG synthesis in bovine NP cells in serum-free conditions in a dose-dependent manner and proposed an autocrine/paracrine mechanism of action (179). Gruber and colleagues found that the addition of IGF-1 increased cell survival upon experimental induction of apoptosis in spine disc annulus fibrosus cells (180), consistent with the anti-catabolic capacity of IGF-1 in both intervertebral disc (IVD) and articular cartilage tissues.

Despite its potent anabolic and anti-catabolic effects on normal cartilage tissue, however, IGF-1 appears to have a diminished ability to stimulate ECM formation and decrease catabolism with both age (181, 182) and OA (68, 149, 181). There appears to be an uncoupling of IGF-1 responsiveness in OA, as IGF-1 is able to stimulate matrix synthesis but is unable to decrease matrix catabolism (183). Nevertheless, combination growth factor therapy with IGF-1 and BMP-7 results in greater repair potential than either factor alone

(169), and the effects of combination factor therapy on aged and old cartilage defects have yet to be determined.

4.3.4 Resveratrol

The phytoestrogen resveratrol (trans-3,4′,5-trihydroxystilbene; RSV) is a natural polyphenol compound found in peanuts, cranberries, and the skin of red grapes, and is thought to be one of the compounds responsible for the health benefits of moderate red wine consumption (184, 185). The anti-inflammatory, anti-oxidant, cardioprotective, and antitumor properties of RSV have been well-documented in a variety of tissues (186-194), and recent studies have begun to analyze the effects of RSV on cartilage homeostasis. Elmali *et al* reported a significant protective effect of RSV injections on articular cartilage degradation in rabbit models for OA and RA via histological analysis *in vivo* (195, 196). In human articular chondrocytes, Shakibaei (197) and Czaki (198) have elucidated both anti-apoptotic and anti-inflammatory regulatory mechanisms mediated by RSV. In our laboratory, we have demonstrated potent anabolic and anti-catabolic potential of RSV in bovine spine nucleus pulposus IVD tissue (199) and human adult articular chondrocytes (Im et al., unpublished data) via inhibition of matrix-degrading enzyme expression at the transcriptional and translational level. Further, combination therapy of RSV with BMP-7 induces synergistic effects on PG accumulation, and RSV reverses the catabolic effects of FGF-2 and IL-1 on matrix-degrading enzyme expression, PG accumulation, and the expression of factors (iNOS, IL-1, IL-6) associated with oxidative stress and inflammatory states (199). Future studies are needed to assess the appropriate dose, route of administration, and downstream effects of RSV, as well as elucidate its role in old or degenerative cartilage *in vivo*. Nevertheless, these findings reveal considerable promise for use of RSV as a unique biological therapy for treatment of cartilage degenerative diseases in the future.

4.3.5 Lactoferricin

Bovine lactoferricin (LfcinB) is a 25-amino acid cationic peptide with an amphipatic, anti-parallel β-sheet structure that is obtained by acid-pepsin hydrolysis of the N-terminal region of lactoferrin (Lf) found in cow's milk (200, 201). It exerts more potent biological effects than equimolar amounts of Lf, is cell membrane-permeable, and interacts electrostatically with negatively-charged matrix and cell surface glycosaminoglycans (GAGs), heparin and chondroitin sulfate (200, 201). The anti-inflammatory, anti-viral, anti-bacterial, anti-oxidant, anti-pain, and anti-cancer properties of LfcinB have been reported in a variety of tissues (202, 203). The natural anti-oxidative effect of LfcinB has also been reported, suggesting a possible chondroprotective biological role in articular cartilage (204), and several recent studies have attempted to elucidate the role of LfcinB in musculoskeletal disease. In a mouse collagen-induced and septic arthritis model, periarticular injection of human Lf substantially suppresses local inflammation (205). Further, in a rat adjuvant arthritis model, oral administration of bovine Lf suppresses the development of arthritis and hyperalgesia in the adjuvant-injected paw, suggesting Lf has preventative and therapeutic effects on the adjuvant-induced inflammation and pain (206). Human iron-free Lf delays the apoptosis of neutrophils isolated from synovial fluid of patients with established rheumatoid arthritis (207). Lf was also identified as a novel bone growth factor, as local injection of Lf above the hemicalvaria of adult mice in vivo results in substantial increases in the dynamic histomorphometric indices of bone formation and bone area (208).

Previously in our laboratory, LfcinB was found to exert potent anabolic and anti-catabolic effects in bovine nucleus pulposus matrix homeostasis in the IVD, similar to RSV (209). Similar to the IVD, we also found similar anabolic and anti-catabolic effects of LfcinB in human articular cartilage (Im et al, unpublished data). LfcinB reverses the catabolic effects of FGF-2 and IL-1 on matrix-degrading enzyme production, PG accumulation, and expression of factors associated with oxidative stress and inflammation, suggesting the promise of LfcinB as an anti-catabolic and anti-inflammatory molecule in human articular cartilage. Further, LfcinB abolishes the expression of iNOS, increases the expression of SOD-1, and antagonizes the catabolic effects mediated by bFGF and IL-1 on iNOS and SOD-1 expression, suggesting an anti-oxidative role of LfcinB in cartilage. Taken together, much like RSV, LfcinB may play an important role in prevention and treatment of diseases such as OA. Nevertheless, caution must be advised as further studies are warranted to determine, among other things, possible detrimental effects of its use *in vivo*.

5. Pain modulators in OA

Clinically, pain is the most prominent and disabling symptom of OA, and arthritic pain is associated with inferior functional outcomes and reduced quality of life compared with a range of other chronic conditions (210). Like other chronic pain conditions, OA pain is a complex integration of sensory, affective and cognitive processes that involves a variety of abnormal cellular mechanisms at both peripheral (joints) and central (spinal and supraspinal) levels of the nervous system. For the development of new therapies aimed at pain relief, a thorough understanding of the pathological mechanisms eliciting pain in OA is required. Unfortunately, many of these mechanisms remain elusive because the primary site of pathology (i.e., articular cartilage) does not have neuronal pain receptors that can directly detect tissue injury due to mechanical damage. The process by which painful mechanical stimuli from arthritic joints are converted into electrical signals that propagate along sensory nerves to the central nervous system remains to be fully explored.

Nociceptors are located throughout the joint in tissues peripheral to cartilage, including the joint capsule, ligaments, periosteum and subchondral bone. Joint cartilage and synovial injury influences peripheral afferent and dorsal root ganglion (DRG) neurons and sensitizes symptomatic pain perception through the dynamic interactions between neuropathic pathways and OA tissues. Nociceptive input from the joint is processed via different spinal cord pathways, and inflammation may potentially reduce the threshold for pain. The relative contribution of these processes into peripheral and central pathways appears to be strongly segmented (211), with intra-articular anesthetic studies in hip and knee OA suggesting a peripheral drive to pain in approximately 60% to 80% of patients, depending on the affected joint (212). In some individuals, however, central mechanisms such as dysfunction of descending inhibitory control or altered cortical processing of noxious information, may play a greater role (213). Therefore, research and pharmacotherapy for OA pain may be separated into two broad classes: central sensitization and peripheral sensitization, both leading to one final outcome: pain in a patient with OA.

A detailed overview of the multiple, complex pathways associated with OA pain, particularly relating to central sensitization mechanisms, is outside the scope of this chapter. For example, current targets of pharmacotherapy for OA pain are numerous and include opioids, kinins, cannabinoids, and their respective receptors, in addition to adrenergic receptors, glutamate receptors, specific ion channels, and neurotrophins. The literature is replete with data on the alteration of pain pathways via inhibition of both central and peripheral processes (211). Here, we will focus on select pro-inflammatory cytokines and mediators previously discussed in this chapter, and report their known roles in pain processing. Our laboratory and others have mechanistically linked OA to pathological changes in the metabolism of ECM proteins and inflammatory states that may be controlled by epigenetic, epigenomic, and systemic processes involved in pain processing (5, 9, 89, 93, 94, 199, 214, 215).

5.1 Cytokines

Inflammatory stimuli initiate a cascade of events, including the production of TNF-α, interleukins, chemokines, sympathetic amines, substance P, leukotrienes and prostaglandins, each demonstrating a complex interplay with other mediators to induce pain (211, 216). Cytokines stimulate hyperalgesia by a number of direct and indirect actions. Sensitization of primary afferent fibers for mechanical stimuli is thought to be induced by inflammatory mediators. IL-1β activates nociceptors directly via intracellular kinase activation, but it may also induce indirect nociceptor sensitization via the production of kinins and prostanoids (217).

IL-6, a well-known pro-inflammatory mediator, has been associated with hyperalgesia and hypersensitivity in articular cartilage (218). As previously discussed, IL-6 plays an important role in the pathogenesis of rheumatoid arthritis, and its concentration is elevated in the serum and synovial fluid of arthritic patients (219, 220). Interestingly, primary afferent neurons also respond to IL-6 (221), suggesting an important role of IL-6 in pain propagation in arthritic states.

TNF-α also activates sensory neurons directly via the receptors TNFR1 and TNFR2, and initiates a cascade of inflammatory reactions via the production of IL-1, IL-6 and IL-8 (217, 222). Direct TNF-α application in the periphery induces neuropathic pain, and this pain may be blocked by anti-inflammatory medications such as ibuprofen and celecoxib (223). Anti-TNF-α treatment with a TNF antibody produces a prolonged reduction of pain symptoms in OA (224), and neutralization of TNF-α in mice rescues both mechanical hyperalgesia (testing of withdrawal responses in behavioral experiments) and the inflammatory process (225). Taken together, TNF-α induces an algesic effect, at least in part, via both neuronal and inflammatory stimulation. Antagonists to TNF-α, such as etanercept or infliximab, may indeed serve as a potential therapeutic strategy to decrease OA pain clinically (211). Further controlled studies are needed to substantiate these promising preliminary data on TNF inhibitors in OA.

5.2 Prostanoids and PGE2

During pro-inflammatory states, numerous prostanoid cyclooxygenase (COX) enzyme products are produced and released, including PGE2, PGD2, PGF2a, thromboxane, and PGI2 (211). These factors serve as the premise for blocking the major synthetic enzymes COX-1 and COX-2 with selective or non-selective COX-inhibitor medications (ie. nonsteroidal anti-inflammatory drugs) (226). Of these mediators, PGE2 is considered to be the major contributor to inflammatory pain in arthritic conditions. PGE2 exerts its effects via a variety of E prostanoid (EP) receptors (EP1, EP2, EP3, EP4), which are present in both peripheral sensory neurons and the spinal cord (211). Activation of these receptors produces a variety of effects, ranging from calcium influx to cAMP activation or inhibition.

Peripherally, sensitization of nociceptors by PGE2 is caused by the cAMP-mediated enhancement of sodium currents after ion channel phosphorylation (227). However, in the spinal cord, PGE2 acts via different receptors than peripherally, suggesting further complexity in the prostanoid regulation of pain (228).

In our laboratory, we have assessed the role of PGE2 in human adult articular cartilage homeostasis and its relation to possible pain pathways (58). PGE2 utilizes the EP2 and EP4 receptors downstream to induce its downstream catabolic effects, and PGE2 may mediate pain pathways in articular cartilage via its stimulatory effect on the pain-associated factors IL-6 (218) and iNOS (229). Further, when combined with the catabolic cytokine IL-1, PGE2 synergistically upregulates both IL-6 and iNOS mRNA levels *in vitro* (58). Similar synergistic results were found with iNOS expression as well. Therefore, the EP2/4 receptor may be an important signaling initiator of the PGE2-signaling cascade and a potential target for therapeutic strategies aimed at preventing progression of arthritic disease and pain in the future.

As opposed to PGE2 EP receptor blockade, an alternative route of PGE2 inhibition is via the blockade of PGE synthase (PGES), a major route of conversion of prostaglandin H2 to PGE2 (211). Two isoforms of the enzyme have been identified, membrane or microsomal associated (mPGES-1) and cytosolic (cPGES/p23), which are linked with COX-2 and COX-1 dependent PGE2 production, respectively (230). Both isoforms are upregulated by inflammatory mediators, and gene deletion studies in mice indicate an important role for mPGES in acute and chronic inflammation and inflammatory pain, revealing a potential target for pain treatment in OA (211, 231).

6. Discussion

In summary, the literature reveals important roles of catabolic and anabolic growth factors and cytokines in articular cartilage homeostasis and the development of OA. Each factor discussed plays a critical role in cartilage, both in normal homeostasis and in repair. Currently, many of these specific roles remain unknown, but recent efforts have begun to increase our understanding. Catabolic factors include pro-inflammatory mediators (IL-1, IL-6, IL-17, TNF-α and PGE2), oxidative mediators (iNOS), glycoproteins (fibronectin, osteonectin, and osteopontin), and even growth factors (FGF-2). In contrast, anabolic mediators include select interleukins, TGF-β, IGF-1, BMPs (BMP-2 and BMP-7), RSV and LfcinB. Upregulation of catabolic processes and/or downregulation of anabolic processes leads to disruption of equilibrium with subsequent cartilage degradation and OA, and several of these pathways are known to induce pain in OA as well (ie. IL-1, IL-6, NO, TNF-α, PGE2). The goal of biologic therapy is to retard this process via inhibition of catabolic processes and upregulation of anabolic processes with the hope of clinically preserving joint cartilage, thereby slowing or preventing the process of OA.

Despite a tremendous research effort in recent years to elucidate these processes, however, biologic therapy for OA remains experimental in nature, and several unknowns exist. Given the wide array of interactions of growth factors that are necessary for proper cartilage development and homeostasis *in vivo*, it is unlikely that any single growth factor will lead to complete cartilage repair or affect the arthritic joint clinically, and rather a combination approach will be required (149). Further, appropriate dosing, scaffolds, and routes of administration must be determined before any of these factors plays a role clinically. Nevertheless, this chapter reviews several of the most well-studied biochemical mediators involved in OA and provides a framework for the understanding of potential biologic therapies in the treatment of degenerative joint disease in the future.

7. References

[1] Lewis PB, McCarty LP, 3rd, Kang RW, Cole BJ. Basic science and treatment options for articular cartilage injuries. J Orthop Sports Phys Ther. 2006;36(10):717-27.

[2] Sandell LJ, Aigner T. Articular cartilage and changes in arthritis. An introduction: cell biology of osteoarthritis. Arthritis Res. 2001;3(2):107-13.

[3] Valverde-Franco G, Binette JS, Li W, Wang H, Chai S, Laflamme F, et al. Defects in articular cartilage metabolism and early arthritis in fibroblast growth factor receptor 3 deficient mice. Hum Mol Genet. 2006;15(11):1783-92.

[4] Nakata K, Ono K, Miyazaki J, Olsen BR, Muragaki Y, Adachi E, et al. Osteoarthritis associated with mild chondrodysplasia in transgenic mice expressing alpha 1(IX) collagen chains with a central deletion. Proc Natl Acad Sci U S A. 1993;90(7):2870-4.

[5] Im HJ, Li X, Muddasani P, Kim GH, Davis F, Rangan J, et al. Basic fibroblast growth factor accelerates matrix degradation via a neuro-endocrine pathway in human adult articular chondrocytes. J Cell Physiol. 2008;215(2):452-63.

[6] Bau B, Gebhard PM, Haag J, Knorr T, Bartnik E, Aigner T. Relative messenger RNA expression profiling of collagenases and aggrecanases in human articular chondrocytes in vivo and in vitro. Arthritis Rheum. 2002;46(10):2648-57.

[7] Liu MH, Sun JS, Tsai SW, Sheu SY, Chen MH. Icariin protects murine chondrocytes from lipopolysaccharide-induced inflammatory responses and extracellular matrix degradation. Nutr Res.30(1):57-65.

[8] Iannone F, Lapadula G. The pathophysiology of osteoarthritis. Aging Clin Exp Res. 2003;15(5):364-72.

[9] Ellman MB, An HS, Muddasani P, Im HJ. Biological impact of the fibroblast growth factor family on articular cartilage and intervertebral disc homeostasis. Gene. 2008;420(1):82-9.

[10] Del Carlo M, Schwartz D, Erickson EA, Loeser RF. Endogenous production of reactive oxygen species is required for stimulation of human articular chondrocyte matrix metalloproteinase production by fibronectin fragments. Free Radic Biol Med. 2007;42(9):1350-8.

[11] Goldring MB, Birkhead J, Sandell LJ, Kimura T, Krane SM. Interleukin 1 suppresses expression of cartilage-specific types II and IX collagens and increases types I and III collagens in human chondrocytes. J Clin Invest. 1988;82(6):2026-37.

[12] Lefebvre V, Peeters-Joris C, Vaes G. Modulation by interleukin 1 and tumor necrosis factor alpha of production of collagenase, tissue inhibitor of metalloproteinases and collagen types in differentiated and dedifferentiated articular chondrocytes. Biochim Biophys Acta. 1990;1052(3):366-78.

[13] Richardson DW, Dodge GR. Effects of interleukin-1beta and tumor necrosis factor-alpha on expression of matrix-related genes by cultured equine articular chondrocytes. Am J Vet Res. 2000;61(6):624-30.

[14] Goldring MB. Osteoarthritis and cartilage: the role of cytokines. Curr Rheumatol Rep. 2000;2(6):459-65.

[15] Kapoor M, Martel-Pelletier J, Lajeunesse D, Pelletier JP, Fahmi H. Role of proinflammatory cytokines in the pathophysiology of osteoarthritis. Nat Rev Rheumatol.7(1):33-42.

[16] Benito MJ, Veale DJ, FitzGerald O, van den Berg WB, Bresnihan B. Synovial tissue inflammation in early and late osteoarthritis. Ann Rheum Dis. 2005;64(9):1263-7.

[17] Smith MD, Triantafillou S, Parker A, Youssef PP, Coleman M. Synovial membrane inflammation and cytokine production in patients with early osteoarthritis. J Rheumatol. 1997;24(2):365-71.

[18] Martel-Pelletier J, McCollum R, DiBattista J, Faure MP, Chin JA, Fournier S, et al. The interleukin-1 receptor in normal and osteoarthritic human articular chondrocytes. Identification as the type I receptor and analysis of binding kinetics and biologic function. Arthritis Rheum. 1992;35(5):530-40.

[19] Evans CH, Gouze JN, Gouze E, Robbins PD, Ghivizzani SC. Osteoarthritis gene therapy. Gene Ther. 2004;11(4):379-89.

[20] Guerne PA, Carson DA, Lotz M. IL-6 production by human articular chondrocytes. Modulation of its synthesis by cytokines, growth factors, and hormones in vitro. J Immunol. 1990;144(2):499-505.

[21] Doss F, Menard J, Hauschild M, Kreutzer HJ, Mittlmeier T, Muller-Steinhardt M, et al. Elevated IL-6 levels in the synovial fluid of osteoarthritis patients stem from plasma cells. Scand J Rheumatol. 2007;36(2):136-9.

[22] Moktar NM, Yusof HM, Yahaya NH, Muhamad R, Das S. The transcript level of interleukin-6 in the cartilage of idiopathic osteoarthritis of knee. Clin Ter.161(1):25-8.

[23] Guerne PA, Desgeorges A, Jaspar JM, Relic B, Peter R, Hoffmeyer P, et al. Effects of IL-6 and its soluble receptor on proteoglycan synthesis and NO release by human articular chondrocytes: comparison with IL-1. Modulation by dexamethasone. Matrix Biol. 1999;18(3):253-60.

[24] Jikko A, Wakisaka T, Iwamoto M, Hiranuma H, Kato Y, Maeda T, et al. Effects of interleukin-6 on proliferation and proteoglycan metabolism in articular chondrocyte cultures. Cell Biol Int. 1998;22(9-10):615-21.

[25] Flannery CR, Little CB, Hughes CE, Curtis CL, Caterson B, Jones SA. IL-6 and its soluble receptor augment aggrecanase-mediated proteoglycan catabolism in articular cartilage. Matrix Biol. 2000;19(6):549-53.

[26] Poree B, Kypriotou M, Chadjichristos C, Beauchef G, Renard E, Legendre F, et al. Interleukin-6 (IL-6) and/or soluble IL-6 receptor down-regulation of human type II collagen gene expression in articular chondrocytes requires a decrease of Sp1.Sp3 ratio and of the binding activity of both factors to the COL2A1 promoter. J Biol Chem. 2008;283(8):4850-65.

[27] Mathy-Hartert M, Hogge L, Sanchez C, Deby-Dupont G, Crielaard JM, Henrotin Y. Interleukin-1beta and interleukin-6 disturb the antioxidant enzyme system in bovine chondrocytes: a possible explanation for oxidative stress generation. Osteoarthritis Cartilage. 2008;16(7):756-63.

[28] de Hooge AS, van de Loo FA, Bennink MB, Arntz OJ, de Hooge P, van den Berg WB. Male IL-6 gene knock out mice developed more advanced osteoarthritis upon aging. Osteoarthritis Cartilage. 2005;13(1):66-73.

[29] Ryu JH, Yang S, Shin Y, Rhee J, Chun CH, Chun JS. Interleukin 6 plays an essential role in hypoxia-inducible factor-2alpha-induced experimental osteoarthritic cartilage destruction in mice. Arthritis Rheum.

[30] Distel E, Cadoudal T, Durant S, Poignard A, Chevalier X, Benelli C. The infrapatellar fat pad in knee osteoarthritis: an important source of interleukin-6 and its soluble receptor. Arthritis Rheum. 2009;60(11):3374-7.

[31] Sylvester J, Liacini A, Li WQ, Zafarullah M. Interleukin-17 signal transduction pathways implicated in inducing matrix metalloproteinase-3, -13 and aggrecanase-1 genes in articular chondrocytes. Cell Signal. 2004;16(4):469-76.

[32] Benderdour M, Tardif G, Pelletier JP, Di Battista JA, Reboul P, Ranger P, et al. Interleukin 17 (IL-17) induces collagenase-3 production in human osteoarthritic chondrocytes via AP-1 dependent activation: differential activation of AP-1 members by IL-17 and IL-1beta. J Rheumatol. 2002;29(6):1262-72.

[33] Pacquelet S, Presle N, Boileau C, Dumond H, Netter P, Martel-Pelletier J, et al. Interleukin 17, a nitric oxide-producing cytokine with a peroxynitrite-independent inhibitory effect on proteoglycan synthesis. J Rheumatol. 2002;29(12):2602-10.

[34] Honorati MC, Neri S, Cattini L, Facchini A. Interleukin-17, a regulator of angiogenic factor release by synovial fibroblasts. Osteoarthritis Cartilage. 2006;14(4):345-52.

[35] Attur MG, Patel RN, Abramson SB, Amin AR. Interleukin-17 up-regulation of nitric oxide production in human osteoarthritis cartilage. Arthritis Rheum. 1997;40(6):1050-3.

[36] Koshy PJ, Henderson N, Logan C, Life PF, Cawston TE, Rowan AD. Interleukin 17 induces cartilage collagen breakdown: novel synergistic effects in combination with proinflammatory cytokines. Ann Rheum Dis. 2002;61(8):704-13.

[37] Martel-Pelletier J, Mineau F, Jovanovic D, Di Battista JA, Pelletier JP. Mitogen-activated protein kinase and nuclear factor kappaB together regulate interleukin-17-induced nitric oxide production in human osteoarthritic chondrocytes: possible role of transactivating factor mitogen-activated protein kinase-activated proten kinase (MAPKAPK). Arthritis Rheum. 1999;42(11):2399-409.

[38] LeGrand A, Fermor B, Fink C, Pisetsky DS, Weinberg JB, Vail TP, et al. Interleukin-1, tumor necrosis factor alpha, and interleukin-17 synergistically up-regulate nitric oxide and prostaglandin E2 production in explants of human osteoarthritic knee menisci. Arthritis Rheum. 2001;44(9):2078-83.

[39] Shalom-Barak T, Quach J, Lotz M. Interleukin-17-induced gene expression in articular chondrocytes is associated with activation of mitogen-activated protein kinases and NF-kappaB. J Biol Chem. 1998;273(42):27467-73.

[40] Honorati MC, Bovara M, Cattini L, Piacentini A, Facchini A. Contribution of interleukin 17 to human cartilage degradation and synovial inflammation in osteoarthritis. Osteoarthritis Cartilage. 2002;10(10):799-807.

[41] Jovanovic DV, Di Battista JA, Martel-Pelletier J, Jolicoeur FC, He Y, Zhang M, et al. IL-17 stimulates the production and expression of proinflammatory cytokines, IL-beta and TNF-alpha, by human macrophages. J Immunol. 1998;160(7):3513-21.

[42] Koenders MI, Marijnissen RJ, Devesa I, Lubberts E, Joosten LA, Roth J, et al. TNF / IL-17 interplay induces S100A8, IL-1beta, and MMPs, and drives irreversible cartilage destruction In Vivo: Rationale for combination treatment during arthritis. Arthritis Rheum.

[43] Nakae S, Nambu A, Sudo K, Iwakura Y. Suppression of immune induction of collagen-induced arthritis in IL-17-deficient mice. J Immunol. 2003;171(11):6173-7.

[44] Westacott CI, Atkins RM, Dieppe PA, Elson CJ. Tumor necrosis factor-alpha receptor expression on chondrocytes isolated from human articular cartilage. J Rheumatol. 1994;21(9):1710-5.

[45] Webb GR, Westacott CI, Elson CJ. Osteoarthritic synovial fluid and synovium supernatants up-regulate tumor necrosis factor receptors on human articular chondrocytes. Osteoarthritis Cartilage. 1998;6(3):167-76.

[46] Marks PH, Donaldson ML. Inflammatory cytokine profiles associated with chondral damage in the anterior cruciate ligament-deficient knee. Arthroscopy. 2005;21(11):1342-7.

[47] Shinmei M, Masuda K, Kikuchi T, Shimomura Y, Okada Y. Production of cytokines by chondrocytes and its role in proteoglycan degradation. J Rheumatol Suppl. 1991;27:89-91.

[48] Malfait AM, Verbruggen G, Veys EM, Lambert J, De Ridder L, Cornelissen M. Comparative and combined effects of interleukin 6, interleukin 1 beta, and tumor necrosis factor alpha on proteoglycan metabolism of human articular chondrocytes cultured in agarose. J Rheumatol. 1994;21(2):314-20.

[49] Steenvoorden MM, Bank RA, Ronday HK, Toes RE, Huizinga TW, DeGroot J. Fibroblast-like synoviocyte-chondrocyte interaction in cartilage degradation. Clin Exp Rheumatol. 2007;25(2):239-45.

[50] Muller RD, John T, Kohl B, Oberholzer A, Gust T, Hostmann A, et al. IL-10 overexpression differentially affects cartilage matrix gene expression in response to TNF-alpha in human articular chondrocytes in vitro. Cytokine. 2008;44(3):377-85.

[51] Ray A, Bal BS, Ray BK. Transcriptional induction of matrix metalloproteinase-9 in the chondrocyte and synoviocyte cells is regulated via a novel mechanism: evidence for functional cooperation between serum amyloid A-activating factor-1 and AP-1. J Immunol. 2005;175(6):4039-48.

[52] Shinmei M, Masuda K, Kikuchi T, Shimomura Y. The role of cytokines in chondrocyte mediated cartilage degradation. J Rheumatol Suppl. 1989;18:32-4.

[53] Tyler JA. Insulin-like growth factor 1 can decrease degradation and promote synthesis of proteoglycan in cartilage exposed to cytokines. Biochem J. 1989;260(2):543-8.

[54] Polzer K, Schett G, Zwerina J. The lonely death: chondrocyte apoptosis in TNF-induced arthritis. Autoimmunity. 2007;40(4):333-6.

[55] Lee SW, Song YS, Lee SY, Yoon YG, Lee SH, Park BS, et al. Downregulation of Protein Kinase CK2 Activity Facilitates Tumor Necrosis Factor-alpha-Mediated Chondrocyte Death through Apoptosis and Autophagy. PLoS One.6(4):e19163.

[56] Mitrovic D, Lippiello L, Gruson F, Aprile F, Mankin HJ. Effects of various prostanoids on the in vitro metabolism of bovine articular chondrocytes. Prostaglandins. 1981;22(3):499-511.

[57] Amin AR, Dave M, Attur M, Abramson SB. COX-2, NO, and cartilage damage and repair. Curr Rheumatol Rep. 2000;2(6):447-53.

[58] Li X, Ellman M, Muddasani P, Wang JH, Cs-Szabo G, van Wijnen AJ, et al. Prostaglandin E2 and its cognate EP receptors control human adult articular cartilage homeostasis and are linked to the pathophysiology of osteoarthritis. Arthritis Rheum. 2009;60(2):513-23.

[59] Attur M, Al-Mussawir HE, Patel J, Kitay A, Dave M, Palmer G, et al. Prostaglandin E2 exerts catabolic effects in osteoarthritis cartilage: evidence for signaling via the EP4 receptor. J Immunol. 2008;181(7):5082-8.

[60] Otsuka S, Aoyama T, Furu M, Ito K, Jin Y, Nasu A, et al. PGE2 signal via EP2 receptors evoked by a selective agonist enhances regeneration of injured articular cartilage. Osteoarthritis Cartilage. 2009;17(4):529-38.

[61] Miwa M, Saura R, Hirata S, Hayashi Y, Mizuno K, Itoh H. Induction of apoptosis in bovine articular chondrocyte by prostaglandin E(2) through cAMP-dependent pathway. Osteoarthritis Cartilage. 2000;8(1):17-24.

[62] Notoya K, Jovanovic DV, Reboul P, Martel-Pelletier J, Mineau F, Pelletier JP. The induction of cell death in human osteoarthritis chondrocytes by nitric oxide is related to the production of prostaglandin E2 via the induction of cyclooxygenase-2. J Immunol. 2000;165(6):3402-10.

[63] Campbell IK, Piccoli DS, Hamilton JA. Stimulation of human chondrocyte prostaglandin E2 production by recombinant human interleukin-1 and tumour necrosis factor. Biochim Biophys Acta. 1990;1051(3):310-8.

[64] Tawara T, Shingu M, Nobunaga M, Naono T. Effects of recombinant human IL-1 beta on production of prostaglandin E2, leukotriene B4, NAG, and superoxide by human synovial cells and chondrocytes. Inflammation. 1991;15(2):145-57.

[65] Verbruggen G, Veys EM, Malfait AM, De Clercq L, Van den Bosch F, de Vlam K. Influence of human recombinant interleukin-1 beta on human articular cartilage. Mitotic activity and proteoglycan metabolism. Clin Exp Rheumatol. 1991;9(5):481-8.

[66] Gosset M, Pigenet A, Salvat C, Berenbaum F, Jacques C. Inhibition of matrix metalloproteinase-3 and -13 synthesis induced by IL-1beta in chondrocytes from mice lacking microsomal prostaglandin E synthase-1. J Immunol.185(10):6244-52.

[67] Di Battista JA, Dore S, Martel-Pelletier J, Pelletier JP. Prostaglandin E2 stimulates incorporation of proline into collagenase digestible proteins in human articular chondrocytes: identification of an effector autocrine loop involving insulin-like growth factor I. Mol Cell Endocrinol. 1996;123(1):27-35.

[68] Dore S, Pelletier JP, DiBattista JA, Tardif G, Brazeau P, Martel-Pelletier J. Human osteoarthritic chondrocytes possess an increased number of insulin-like growth factor 1 binding sites but are unresponsive to its stimulation. Possible role of IGF-1-binding proteins. Arthritis Rheum. 1994;37(2):253-63.

[69] Taskiran D, Stefanovic-Racic M, Georgescu H, Evans C. Nitric oxide mediates suppression of cartilage proteoglycan synthesis by interleukin-1. Biochem Biophys Res Commun. 1994;200(1):142-8.

[70] Hauselmann HJ, Oppliger L, Michel BA, Stefanovic-Racic M, Evans CH. Nitric oxide and proteoglycan biosynthesis by human articular chondrocytes in alginate culture. FEBS Lett. 1994;352(3):361-4.

[71] Vuolteenaho K, Moilanen T, Knowles RG, Moilanen E. The role of nitric oxide in osteoarthritis. Scand J Rheumatol. 2007;36(4):247-58.

[72] Tamura T, Nakanishi T, Kimura Y, Hattori T, Sasaki K, Norimatsu H, et al. Nitric oxide mediates interleukin-1-induced matrix degradation and basic fibroblast growth factor release in cultured rabbit articular chondrocytes: a possible mechanism of pathological neovascularization in arthritis. Endocrinology. 1996;137(9):3729-37.

[73] Abramson SB. Nitric oxide in inflammation and pain associated with osteoarthritis. Arthritis Res Ther. 2008;10 Suppl 2:S2.

[74] Studer R, Jaffurs D, Stefanovic-Racic M, Robbins PD, Evans CH. Nitric oxide in osteoarthritis. Osteoarthritis Cartilage. 1999;7(4):377-9.

[75] Borderie D, Hilliquin P, Hernvann A, Lemarechal H, Menkes CJ, Ekindjian OG. Apoptosis induced by nitric oxide is associated with nuclear p53 protein expression in cultured osteoarthritic synoviocytes. Osteoarthritis Cartilage. 1999;7(2):203-13.

[76] Del Carlo M, Jr., Loeser RF. Nitric oxide-mediated chondrocyte cell death requires the generation of additional reactive oxygen species. Arthritis Rheum. 2002;46(2):394-403.

[77] Studer RK, Levicoff E, Georgescu H, Miller L, Jaffurs D, Evans CH. Nitric oxide inhibits chondrocyte response to IGF-I: inhibition of IGF-IRbeta tyrosine phosphorylation. Am J Physiol Cell Physiol. 2000;279(4):C961-9.

[78] van der Kraan PM, Vitters EL, van Beuningen HM, van de Loo FA, van den Berg WB. Role of nitric oxide in the inhibition of BMP-2-mediated stimulation of proteoglycan synthesis in articular cartilage. Osteoarthritis Cartilage. 2000;8(2):82-6.

[79] Amin AR, Di Cesare PE, Vyas P, Attur M, Tzeng E, Billiar TR, et al. The expression and regulation of nitric oxide synthase in human osteoarthritis-affected chondrocytes: evidence for up-regulated neuronal nitric oxide synthase. J Exp Med. 1995;182(6):2097-102.

[80] Melchiorri C, Meliconi R, Frizziero L, Silvestri T, Pulsatelli L, Mazzetti I, et al. Enhanced and coordinated in vivo expression of inflammatory cytokines and nitric oxide synthase by chondrocytes from patients with osteoarthritis. Arthritis Rheum. 1998;41(12):2165-74.

[81] Amin AR, Attur M, Abramson SB. Nitric oxide synthase and cyclooxygenases: distribution, regulation, and intervention in arthritis. Curr Opin Rheumatol. 1999;11(3):202-9.

[82] Vuolteenaho K, Moilanen T, Hamalainen M, Moilanen E. Effects of TNFalpha-antagonists on nitric oxide production in human cartilage. Osteoarthritis Cartilage. 2002;10(4):327-32.

[83] Jarvinen K, Vuolteenaho K, Nieminen R, Moilanen T, Knowles RG, Moilanen E. Selective iNOS inhibitor 1400W enhances anti-catabolic IL-10 and reduces

destructive MMP-10 in OA cartilage. Survey of the effects of 1400W on inflammatory mediators produced by OA cartilage as detected by protein antibody array. Clin Exp Rheumatol. 2008;26(2):275-82.

[84] Huang CY, Hung LF, Liang CC, Ho LJ. COX-2 and iNOS are critical in advanced glycation end product-activated chondrocytes in vitro. Eur J Clin Invest. 2009;39(5):417-28.

[85] Vuolteenaho K, Koskinen A, Kukkonen M, Nieminen R, Paivarinta U, Moilanen T, et al. Leptin enhances synthesis of proinflammatory mediators in human osteoarthritic cartilage--mediator role of NO in leptin-induced PGE2, IL-6, and IL-8 production. Mediators Inflamm. 2009;2009:345838.

[86] Pelletier JP, Jovanovic D, Fernandes JC, Manning P, Connor JR, Currie MG, et al. Reduced progression of experimental osteoarthritis in vivo by selective inhibition of inducible nitric oxide synthase. Arthritis Rheum. 1998;41(7):1275-86.

[87] Presle N, Cipolletta C, Jouzeau JY, Abid A, Netter P, Terlain B. Cartilage protection by nitric oxide synthase inhibitors after intraarticular injection of interleukin-1beta in rats. Arthritis Rheum. 1999;42(10):2094-102.

[88] Sah RL, Trippel SB, Grodzinsky AJ. Differential effects of serum, insulin-like growth factor-I, and fibroblast growth factor-2 on the maintenance of cartilage physical properties during long-term culture. J Orthop Res. 1996;14(1):44-52.

[89] Loeser RF, Chubinskaya S, Pacione C, Im HJ. Basic fibroblast growth factor inhibits the anabolic activity of insulin-like growth factor 1 and osteogenic protein 1 in adult human articular chondrocytes. Arthritis Rheum. 2005;52(12):3910-7.

[90] Schmal H, Zwingmann J, Fehrenbach M, Finkenzeller G, Stark GB, Sudkamp NP, et al. bFGF influences human articular chondrocyte differentiation. Cytotherapy. 2007;9(2):184-93.

[91] Stewart K, Pabbruwe M, Dickinson S, Sims T, Hollander AP, Chaudhuri JB. The effect of growth factor treatment on meniscal chondrocyte proliferation and differentiation on polyglycolic acid scaffolds. Tissue Eng. 2007;13(2):271-80.

[92] Sonal D. Prevention of IGF-1 and TGFbeta stimulated type II collagen and decorin expression by bFGF and identification of IGF-1 mRNA transcripts in articular chondrocytes. Matrix Biol. 2001;20(4):233-42.

[93] Muddasani P, Norman JC, Ellman M, van Wijnen AJ, Im HJ. Basic fibroblast growth factor activates the MAPK and NFkappaB pathways that converge on Elk-1 to control production of matrix metalloproteinase-13 by human adult articular chondrocytes. J Biol Chem. 2007;282(43):31409-21.

[94] Im HJ, Muddasani P, Natarajan V, Schmid TM, Block JA, Davis F, et al. Basic fibroblast growth factor stimulates matrix metalloproteinase-13 via the molecular cross-talk between the mitogen-activated protein kinases and protein kinase Cdelta pathways in human adult articular chondrocytes. J Biol Chem. 2007;282(15):11110-21.

[95] Yan D, Muddasani P, Cool SM, van Wijnen AJ, Mikecz K, Murphy G, et al. Fibroblast Growth Factor Receptor 1 Is Principally Responsible For Fibroblast Growth Factor 2-Induced Catabolic Activities In Human Articular Chondrocytes. Arthritis Res Ther. 2011:In press.

[96] Sawaji Y, Hynes J, Vincent T, Saklatvala J. Fibroblast growth factor 2 inhibits induction of aggrecanase activity in human articular cartilage. Arthritis Rheum. 2008;58(11):3498-509.

[97] Chia SL, Sawaji Y, Burleigh A, McLean C, Inglis J, Saklatvala J, et al. Fibroblast growth factor 2 is an intrinsic chondroprotective agent that suppresses ADAMTS-5 and delays cartilage degradation in murine osteoarthritis. Arthritis Rheum. 2009;60(7):2019-27.

[98] Yasuda T. Cartilage destruction by matrix degradation products. Mod Rheumatol. 2006;16(4):197-205.

[99] Homandberg GA, Wen C, Hui F. Cartilage damaging activities of fibronectin fragments derived from cartilage and synovial fluid. Osteoarthritis Cartilage. 1998;6(4):231-44.

[100] Jones KL, Brown M, Ali SY, Brown RA. An immunohistochemical study of fibronectin in human osteoarthritic and disease free articular cartilage. Ann Rheum Dis. 1987;46(11):809-15.

[101] Zack MD, Malfait AM, Skepner AP, Yates MP, Griggs DW, Hall T, et al. ADAM-8 isolated from human osteoarthritic chondrocytes cleaves fibronectin at Ala(271). Arthritis Rheum. 2009;60(9):2704-13.

[102] Xie DL, Meyers R, Homandberg GA. Fibronectin fragments in osteoarthritic synovial fluid. J Rheumatol. 1992;19(9):1448-52.

[103] Chevalier X, Groult N, Emod I, Planchenault T. Proteoglycan-degrading activity associated with the 40 kDa collagen-binding fragment of fibronectin. Br J Rheumatol. 1996;35(6):506-14.

[104] Yasuda T, Poole AR. A fibronectin fragment induces type II collagen degradation by collagenase through an interleukin-1-mediated pathway. Arthritis Rheum. 2002;46(1):138-48.

[105] Johnson A, Smith R, Saxne T, Hickery M, Heinegard D. Fibronectin fragments cause release and degradation of collagen-binding molecules from equine explant cultures. Osteoarthritis Cartilage. 2004;12(2):149-59.

[106] Kang Y, Koepp H, Cole AA, Kuettner KE, Homandberg GA. Cultured human ankle and knee cartilage differ in susceptibility to damage mediated by fibronectin fragments. J Orthop Res. 1998;16(5):551-6.

[107] Long D, Blake S, Song XY, Lark M, Loeser RF. Human articular chondrocytes produce IL-7 and respond to IL-7 with increased production of matrix metalloproteinase-13. Arthritis Res Ther. 2008;10(1):R23.

[108] Saito S, Yamaji N, Yasunaga K, Saito T, Matsumoto S, Katoh M, et al. The fibronectin extra domain A activates matrix metalloproteinase gene expression by an interleukin-1-dependent mechanism. J Biol Chem. 1999;274(43):30756-63.

[109] Stanton H, Ung L, Fosang AJ. The 45 kDa collagen-binding fragment of fibronectin induces matrix metalloproteinase-13 synthesis by chondrocytes and aggrecan degradation by aggrecanases. Biochem J. 2002;364(Pt 1):181-90.

[110] Dodds RA, Connor JR, James IE, Rykaczewski EL, Appelbaum E, Dul E, et al. Human osteoclasts, not osteoblasts, deposit osteopontin onto resorption surfaces: an in vitro and ex vivo study of remodeling bone. J Bone Miner Res. 1995;10(11):1666-80.

[111] Pullig O, Weseloh G, Gauer S, Swoboda B. Osteopontin is expressed by adult human osteoarthritic chondrocytes: protein and mRNA analysis of normal and osteoarthritic cartilage. Matrix Biol. 2000;19(3):245-55.

[112] Honsawek S, Tanavalee A, Sakdinakiattikoon M, Chayanupatkul M, Yuktanandana P. Correlation of plasma and synovial fluid osteopontin with disease severity in knee osteoarthritis. Clin Biochem. 2009;42(9):808-12.

[113] Gao SG, Li KH, Zeng KB, Tu M, Xu M, Lei GH. Elevated osteopontin level of synovial fluid and articular cartilage is associated with disease severity in knee osteoarthritis patients. Osteoarthritis Cartilage.18(1):82-7.

[114] Rosenthal AK, Gohr CM, Uzuki M, Masuda I. Osteopontin promotes pathologic mineralization in articular cartilage. Matrix Biol. 2007;26(2):96-105.

[115] Gericke A, Qin C, Spevak L, Fujimoto Y, Butler WT, Sorensen ES, et al. Importance of phosphorylation for osteopontin regulation of biomineralization. Calcif Tissue Int. 2005;77(1):45-54.

[116] Attur MG, Dave MN, Stuchin S, Kowalski AJ, Steiner G, Abramson SB, et al. Osteopontin: an intrinsic inhibitor of inflammation in cartilage. Arthritis Rheum. 2001;44(3):578-84.

[117] Matsui Y, Iwasaki N, Kon S, Takahashi D, Morimoto J, Denhardt DT, et al. Accelerated development of aging-associated and instability-induced osteoarthritis in osteopontin-deficient mice. Arthritis Rheum. 2009;60(8):2362-71.

[118] Jundt G, Berghauser KH, Termine JD, Schulz A. Osteonectin--a differentiation marker of bone cells. Cell Tissue Res. 1987;248(2):409-15.

[119] Chandrasekhar S, Harvey AK, Johnson MG, Becker GW. Osteonectin/SPARC is a product of articular chondrocytes/cartilage and is regulated by cytokines and growth factors. Biochim Biophys Acta. 1994;1221(1):7-14.

[120] Nakamura S, Kamihagi K, Satakeda H, Katayama M, Pan H, Okamoto H, et al. Enhancement of SPARC (osteonectin) synthesis in arthritic cartilage. Increased levels in synovial fluids from patients with rheumatoid arthritis and regulation by growth factors and cytokines in chondrocyte cultures. Arthritis Rheum. 1996;39(4):539-51.

[121] Nanba Y, Nishida K, Yoshikawa T, Sato T, Inoue H, Kuboki Y. Expression of osteonectin in articular cartilage of osteoarthritic knees. Acta Med Okayama. 1997;51(5):239-43.

[122] Tremble PM, Lane TF, Sage EH, Werb Z. SPARC, a secreted protein associated with morphogenesis and tissue remodeling, induces expression of metalloproteinases in fibroblasts through a novel extracellular matrix-dependent pathway. J Cell Biol. 1993;121(6):1433-44.

[123] Arend WP, Welgus HG, Thompson RC, Eisenberg SP. Biological properties of recombinant human monocyte-derived interleukin 1 receptor antagonist. J Clin Invest. 1990;85(5):1694-7.

[124] Smith RJ, Chin JE, Sam LM, Justen JM. Biologic effects of an interleukin-1 receptor antagonist protein on interleukin-1-stimulated cartilage erosion and chondrocyte responsiveness. Arthritis Rheum. 1991;34(1):78-83.

[125] Woodell-May J, Matuska A, Oyster M, Welch Z, O'Shaughnessey K, Hoeppner J. Autologous protein solution inhibits MMP-13 production by IL-1beta and TNFalpha-stimulated human articular chondrocytes. J Orthop Res.

[126] Pelletier JP, Mineau F, Ranger P, Tardif G, Martel-Pelletier J. The increased synthesis of inducible nitric oxide inhibits IL-1ra synthesis by human articular chondrocytes: possible role in osteoarthritic cartilage degradation. Osteoarthritis Cartilage. 1996;4(1):77-84.

[127] Baragi VM, Renkiewicz RR, Jordan H, Bonadio J, Hartman JW, Roessler BJ. Transplantation of transduced chondrocytes protects articular cartilage from interleukin 1-induced extracellular matrix degradation. J Clin Invest. 1995;96(5):2454-60.

[128] Muller-Ladner U, Roberts CR, Franklin BN, Gay RE, Robbins PD, Evans CH, et al. Human IL-1Ra gene transfer into human synovial fibroblasts is chondroprotective. J Immunol. 1997;158(7):3492-8.

[129] Caron JP, Fernandes JC, Martel-Pelletier J, Tardif G, Mineau F, Geng C, et al. Chondroprotective effect of intraarticular injections of interleukin-1 receptor antagonist in experimental osteoarthritis. Suppression of collagenase-1 expression. Arthritis Rheum. 1996;39(9):1535-44.

[130] Doi H, Nishida K, Yorimitsu M, Komiyama T, Kadota Y, Tetsunaga T, et al. Interleukin-4 downregulates the cyclic tensile stress-induced matrix metalloproteinases-13 and cathepsin B expression by rat normal chondrocytes. Acta Med Okayama. 2008;62(2):119-26.

[131] Yorimitsu M, Nishida K, Shimizu A, Doi H, Miyazawa S, Komiyama T, et al. Intra-articular injection of interleukin-4 decreases nitric oxide production by chondrocytes and ameliorates subsequent destruction of cartilage in instability-induced osteoarthritis in rat knee joints. Osteoarthritis Cartilage. 2008;16(7):764-71.

[132] Yeh LA, Augustine AJ, Lee P, Riviere LR, Sheldon A. Interleukin-4, an inhibitor of cartilage breakdown in bovine articular cartilage explants. J Rheumatol. 1995;22(9):1740-6.

[133] Relic B, Guicheux J, Mezin F, Lubberts E, Togninalli D, Garcia I, et al. Il-4 and IL-13, but not IL-10, protect human synoviocytes from apoptosis. J Immunol. 2001;166(4):2775-82.

[134] Manning K, Rachakonda PS, Rai MF, Schmidt MF. Co-expression of insulin-like growth factor-1 and interleukin-4 in an in vitro inflammatory model. Cytokine.50(3):297-305.

[135] Iannone F, De Bari C, Dell'Accio F, Covelli M, Cantatore FP, Patella V, et al. Interleukin-10 and interleukin-10 receptor in human osteoarthritic and healthy chondrocytes. Clin Exp Rheumatol. 2001;19(2):139-45.

[136] Fernandes JC, Martel-Pelletier J, Pelletier JP. The role of cytokines in osteoarthritis pathophysiology. Biorheology. 2002;39(1-2):237-46.

[137] Zhang X, Mao Z, Yu C. Suppression of early experimental osteoarthritis by gene transfer of interleukin-1 receptor antagonist and interleukin-10. J Orthop Res. 2004;22(4):742-50.

[138] Maier R, Ganu V, Lotz M. Interleukin-11, an inducible cytokine in human articular chondrocytes and synoviocytes, stimulates the production of the tissue inhibitor of metalloproteinases. J Biol Chem. 1993;268(29):21527-32.

[139] Trepicchio WL, Dorner AJ. The therapeutic utility of Interleukin-11 in the treatment of inflammatory disease. Expert Opin Investig Drugs. 1998;7(9):1501-4.

[140] Alaaeddine N, Di Battista JA, Pelletier JP, Kiansa K, Cloutier JM, Martel-Pelletier J. Differential effects of IL-8, LIF (pro-inflammatory) and IL-11 (anti-inflammatory) on TNF-alpha-induced PGE(2)release and on signalling pathways in human OA synovial fibroblasts. Cytokine. 1999;11(12):1020-30.

[141] Hermann JA, Hall MA, Maini RN, Feldmann M, Brennan FM. Important immunoregulatory role of interleukin-11 in the inflammatory process in rheumatoid arthritis. Arthritis Rheum. 1998;41(8):1388-97.

[142] Walmsley M, Butler DM, Marinova-Mutafchieva L, Feldmann M. An anti-inflammatory role for interleukin-11 in established murine collagen-induced arthritis. Immunology. 1998;95(1):31-7.

[143] Trontzas P, Kamper EF, Potamianou A, Kyriazis NC, Kritikos H, Stavridis J. Comparative study of serum and synovial fluid interleukin-11 levels in patients with various arthritides. Clin Biochem. 1998;31(8):673-9.

[144] Tardif G, Pelletier JP, Dupuis M, Geng C, Cloutier JM, Martel-Pelletier J. Collagenase 3 production by human osteoarthritic chondrocytes in response to growth factors and cytokines is a function of the physiologic state of the cells. Arthritis Rheum. 1999;42(6):1147-58.

[145] Chabaud M, Durand JM, Buchs N, Fossiez F, Page G, Frappart L, et al. Human interleukin-17: A T cell-derived proinflammatory cytokine produced by the rheumatoid synovium. Arthritis Rheum. 1999;42(5):963-70.

[146] Jovanovic D, Pelletier JP, Alaaeddine N, Mineau F, Geng C, Ranger P, et al. Effect of IL-13 on cytokines, cytokine receptors and inhibitors on human osteoarthritis synovium and synovial fibroblasts. Osteoarthritis Cartilage. 1998;6(1):40-9.

[147] Alaaeddine N, Di Battista JA, Pelletier JP, Kiansa K, Cloutier JM, Martel-Pelletier J. Inhibition of tumor necrosis factor alpha-induced prostaglandin E2 production by the antiinflammatory cytokines interleukin-4, interleukin-10, and interleukin-13 in osteoarthritic synovial fibroblasts: distinct targeting in the signaling pathways. Arthritis Rheum. 1999;42(4):710-8.

[148] Woods JM, Haines GK, Shah MR, Rayan G, Koch AE. Low-level production of interleukin-13 in synovial fluid and tissue from patients with arthritis. Clin Immunol Immunopathol. 1997;85(2):210-20.

[149] Fortier LA, Barker JU, Strauss EJ, McCarrel TM, Cole BJ. The Role of Growth Factors in Cartilage Repair. Clin Orthop Relat Res.

[150] Chubinskaya S, Segalite D, Pikovsky D, Hakimiyan AA, Rueger DC. Effects induced by BMPS in cultures of human articular chondrocytes: comparative studies. Growth Factors. 2008;26(5):275-83.

[151] Chubinskaya S, Hurtig M, Rueger DC. OP-1/BMP-7 in cartilage repair. Int Orthop. 2007;31(6):773-81.

[152] van der Kraan PM, Blaney Davidson EN, van den Berg WB. A role for age-related changes in TGFbeta signaling in aberrant chondrocyte differentiation and osteoarthritis. Arthritis Res Ther.12(1):201.

[153] Blaney Davidson EN, van der Kraan PM, van den Berg WB. TGF-beta and osteoarthritis. Osteoarthritis Cartilage. 2007;15(6):597-604.

[154] Fan J, Gong Y, Ren L, Varshney RR, Cai D, Wang DA. In vitro engineered cartilage using synovium-derived mesenchymal stem cells with injectable gellan hydrogels. Acta Biomater.6(3):1178-85.

[155] Kizawa H, Kou I, Iida A, Sudo A, Miyamoto Y, Fukuda A, et al. An aspartic acid repeat polymorphism in asporin inhibits chondrogenesis and increases susceptibility to osteoarthritis. Nat Genet. 2005;37(2):138-44.

[156] Jiang Q, Shi D, Yi L, Ikegawa S, Wang Y, Nakamura T, et al. Replication of the association of the aspartic acid repeat polymorphism in the asporin gene with knee-osteoarthritis susceptibility in Han Chinese. J Hum Genet. 2006;51(12):1068-72.

[157] Yang X, Chen L, Xu X, Li C, Huang C, Deng CX. TGF-beta/Smad3 signals repress chondrocyte hypertrophic differentiation and are required for maintaining articular cartilage. J Cell Biol. 2001;153(1):35-46.

[158] Serra R, Johnson M, Filvaroff EH, LaBorde J, Sheehan DM, Derynck R, et al. Expression of a truncated, kinase-defective TGF-beta type II receptor in mouse skeletal tissue promotes terminal chondrocyte differentiation and osteoarthritis. J Cell Biol. 1997;139(2):541-52.

[159] Blaney Davidson EN, Scharstuhl A, Vitters EL, van der Kraan PM, van den Berg WB. Reduced transforming growth factor-beta signaling in cartilage of old mice: role in impaired repair capacity. Arthritis Res Ther. 2005;7(6):R1338-47.

[160] Morales TI. Transforming growth factor-beta 1 stimulates synthesis of proteoglycan aggregates in calf articular cartilage organ cultures. Arch Biochem Biophys. 1991;286(1):99-106.

[161] Bakker AC, van de Loo FA, van Beuningen HM, Sime P, van Lent PL, van der Kraan PM, et al. Overexpression of active TGF-beta-1 in the murine knee joint: evidence for synovial-layer-dependent chondro-osteophyte formation. Osteoarthritis Cartilage. 2001;9(2):128-36.

[162] Livne E, Laufer D, Blumenfeld I. Differential response of articular cartilage from young growing and mature old mice to IL-1 and TGF-beta. Arch Gerontol Geriatr. 1997;24(2):211-21.

[163] Gouttenoire J, Valcourt U, Ronziere MC, Aubert-Foucher E, Mallein-Gerin F, Herbage D. Modulation of collagen synthesis in normal and osteoarthritic cartilage. Biorheology. 2004;41(3-4):535-42.

[164] Arai Y, Kubo T, Kobayashi K, Takeshita K, Takahashi K, Ikeda T, et al. Adenovirus vector-mediated gene transduction to chondrocytes: in vitro evaluation of therapeutic efficacy of transforming growth factor-beta 1 and heat shock protein 70 gene transduction. J Rheumatol. 1997;24(9):1787-95.

[165] Blaney Davidson EN, Vitters EL, van Lent PL, van de Loo FA, van den Berg WB, van der Kraan PM. Elevated extracellular matrix production and degradation upon

bone morphogenetic protein-2 (BMP-2) stimulation point toward a role for BMP-2 in cartilage repair and remodeling. Arthritis Res Ther. 2007;9(5):R102.

[166] Im HJ, Pacione C, Chubinskaya S, Van Wijnen AJ, Sun Y, Loeser RF. Inhibitory effects of insulin-like growth factor-1 and osteogenic protein-1 on fibronectin fragment- and interleukin-1beta-stimulated matrix metalloproteinase-13 expression in human chondrocytes. J Biol Chem. 2003;278(28):25386-94.

[167] Flechtenmacher J, Huch K, Thonar EJ, Mollenhauer JA, Davies SR, Schmid TM, et al. Recombinant human osteogenic protein 1 is a potent stimulator of the synthesis of cartilage proteoglycans and collagens by human articular chondrocytes. Arthritis Rheum. 1996;39(11):1896-904.

[168] Imai Y, Okuma M, An HS, Nakagawa K, Yamada M, Muehleman C, et al. Restoration of disc height loss by recombinant human osteogenic protein-1 injection into intervertebral discs undergoing degeneration induced by an intradiscal injection of chondroitinase ABC. Spine (Phila Pa 1976). 2007;32(11):1197-205.

[169] Loeser RF, Pacione CA, Chubinskaya S. The combination of insulin-like growth factor 1 and osteogenic protein 1 promotes increased survival of and matrix synthesis by normal and osteoarthritic human articular chondrocytes. Arthritis Rheum. 2003;48(8):2188-96.

[170] Merrihew C, Kumar B, Heretis K, Rueger DC, Kuettner KE, Chubinskaya S. Alterations in endogenous osteogenic protein-1 with degeneration of human articular cartilage. J Orthop Res. 2003;21(5):899-907.

[171] Chubinskaya S, Kumar B, Merrihew C, Heretis K, Rueger DC, Kuettner KE. Age-related changes in cartilage endogenous osteogenic protein-1 (OP-1). Biochim Biophys Acta. 2002;1588(2):126-34.

[172] Miyamoto C, Matsumoto T, Sakimura K, Shindo H. Osteogenic protein-1 with transforming growth factor-beta1: potent inducer of chondrogenesis of synovial mesenchymal stem cells in vitro. J Orthop Sci. 2007;12(6):555-61.

[173] Jelic M, Pecina M, Haspl M, Kos J, Taylor K, Maticic D, et al. Regeneration of articular cartilage chondral defects by osteogenic protein-1 (bone morphogenetic protein-7) in sheep. Growth Factors. 2001;19(2):101-13.

[174] Luyten FP, Hascall VC, Nissley SP, Morales TI, Reddi AH. Insulin-like growth factors maintain steady-state metabolism of proteoglycans in bovine articular cartilage explants. Arch Biochem Biophys. 1988;267(2):416-25.

[175] Sah RL, Chen AC, Grodzinsky AJ, Trippel SB. Differential effects of bFGF and IGF-I on matrix metabolism in calf and adult bovine cartilage explants. Arch Biochem Biophys. 1994;308(1):137-47.

[176] Ekenstedt KJ, Sonntag WE, Loeser RF, Lindgren BR, Carlson CS. Effects of chronic growth hormone and insulin-like growth factor 1 deficiency on osteoarthritis severity in rat knee joints. Arthritis Rheum. 2006;54(12):3850-8.

[177] Goodrich LR, Hidaka C, Robbins PD, Evans CH, Nixon AJ. Genetic modification of chondrocytes with insulin-like growth factor-1 enhances cartilage healing in an equine model. J Bone Joint Surg Br. 2007;89(5):672-85.

[178] Fortier LA, Mohammed HO, Lust G, Nixon AJ. Insulin-like growth factor-I enhances cell-based repair of articular cartilage. J Bone Joint Surg Br. 2002;84(2):276-88.

[179] Osada R, Ohshima H, Ishihara H, Yudoh K, Sakai K, Matsui H, et al. Autocrine/paracrine mechanism of insulin-like growth factor-1 secretion, and the effect of insulin-like growth factor-1 on proteoglycan synthesis in bovine intervertebral discs. J Orthop Res. 1996;14(5):690-9.

[180] Gruber HE, Norton HJ, Hanley EN, Jr. Anti-apoptotic effects of IGF-1 and PDGF on human intervertebral disc cells in vitro. Spine (Phila Pa 1976). 2000;25(17):2153-7.

[181] Loeser RF, Shanker G, Carlson CS, Gardin JF, Shelton BJ, Sonntag WE. Reduction in the chondrocyte response to insulin-like growth factor 1 in aging and osteoarthritis: studies in a non-human primate model of naturally occurring disease. Arthritis Rheum. 2000;43(9):2110-20.

[182] Boehm AK, Seth M, Mayr KG, Fortier LA. Hsp90 mediates insulin-like growth factor 1 and interleukin-1beta signaling in an age-dependent manner in equine articular chondrocytes. Arthritis Rheum. 2007;56(7):2335-43.

[183] Morales TI. The quantitative and functional relation between insulin-like growth factor-I (IGF) and IGF-binding proteins during human osteoarthritis. J Orthop Res. 2008;26(4):465-74.

[184] Wang Z, Huang Y, Zou J, Cao K, Xu Y, Wu JM. Effects of red wine and wine polyphenol resveratrol on platelet aggregation in vivo and in vitro. Int J Mol Med. 2002;9(1):77-9.

[185] Orallo F, Alvarez E, Camina M, Leiro JM, Gomez E, Fernandez P. The possible implication of trans-Resveratrol in the cardioprotective effects of long-term moderate wine consumption. Mol Pharmacol. 2002;61(2):294-302.

[186] Haider UG, Sorescu D, Griendling KK, Vollmar AM, Dirsch VM. Resveratrol suppresses angiotensin II-induced Akt/protein kinase B and p70 S6 kinase phosphorylation and subsequent hypertrophy in rat aortic smooth muscle cells. Mol Pharmacol. 2002;62(4):772-7.

[187] Bhat KPL, Kosmeder JW, 2nd, Pezzuto JM. Biological effects of resveratrol. Antioxid Redox Signal. 2001;3(6):1041-64.

[188] Bertelli AA, Ferrara F, Diana G, Fulgenzi A, Corsi M, Ponti W, et al. Resveratrol, a natural stilbene in grapes and wine, enhances intraphagocytosis in human promonocytes: a co-factor in antiinflammatory and anticancer chemopreventive activity. Int J Tissue React. 1999;21(4):93-104.

[189] Fremont L. Biological effects of resveratrol. Life Sci. 2000;66(8):663-73.

[190] Huang KS, Lin M, Cheng GF. Anti-inflammatory tetramers of resveratrol from the roots of Vitis amurensis and the conformations of the seven-membered ring in some oligostilbenes. Phytochemistry. 2001;58(2):357-62.

[191] Jang M, Cai L, Udeani GO, Slowing KV, Thomas CF, Beecher CW, et al. Cancer chemopreventive activity of resveratrol, a natural product derived from grapes. Science. 1997;275(5297):218-20.

[192] Martinez J, Moreno JJ. Effect of resveratrol, a natural polyphenolic compound, on reactive oxygen species and prostaglandin production. Biochem Pharmacol. 2000;59(7):865-70.

[193] Ignatowicz E, Baer-Dubowska W. Resveratrol, a natural chemopreventive agent against degenerative diseases. Pol J Pharmacol. 2001;53(6):557-69.

[194] Leiro J, Alvarez E, Arranz JA, Laguna R, Uriarte E, Orallo F. Effects of cis-resveratrol on inflammatory murine macrophages: antioxidant activity and down-regulation of inflammatory genes. J Leukoc Biol. 2004;75(6):1156-65.

[195] Elmali N, Esenkaya I, Harma A, Ertem K, Turkoz Y, Mizrak B. Effect of resveratrol in experimental osteoarthritis in rabbits. Inflamm Res. 2005;54(4):158-62.

[196] Elmali N, Baysal O, Harma A, Esenkaya I, Mizrak B. Effects of resveratrol in inflammatory arthritis. Inflammation. 2007;30(1-2):1-6.

[197] Shakibaei M, John T, Seifarth C, Mobasheri A. Resveratrol inhibits IL-1 beta-induced stimulation of caspase-3 and cleavage of PARP in human articular chondrocytes in vitro. Ann N Y Acad Sci. 2007;1095:554-63.

[198] Csaki C, Keshishzadeh N, Fischer K, Shakibaei M. Regulation of inflammation signalling by resveratrol in human chondrocytes in vitro. Biochem Pharmacol. 2008;75(3):677-87.

[199] Li X, Phillips FM, An HS, Ellman M, Thonar EJ, Wu W, et al. The action of resveratrol, a phytoestrogen found in grapes, on the intervertebral disc. Spine (Phila Pa 1976). 2008;33(24):2586-95.

[200] Gitay-Goren H, Soker S, Vlodavsky I, Neufeld G. The binding of vascular endothelial growth factor to its receptors is dependent on cell surface-associated heparin-like molecules. J Biol Chem. 1992;267(9):6093-8.

[201] Baker EN, Baker HM. A structural framework for understanding the multifunctional character of lactoferrin. Biochimie. 2009;91(1):3-10.

[202] Mader JS, Richardson A, Salsman J, Top D, de Antueno R, Duncan R, et al. Bovine lactoferricin causes apoptosis in Jurkat T-leukemia cells by sequential permeabilization of the cell membrane and targeting of mitochondria. Exp Cell Res. 2007;313(12):2634-50.

[203] Gifford JL, Hunter HN, Vogel HJ. Lactoferricin: a lactoferrin-derived peptide with antimicrobial, antiviral, antitumor and immunological properties. Cell Mol Life Sci. 2005;62(22):2588-98.

[204] Henrotin YE, Bruckner P, Pujol JP. The role of reactive oxygen species in homeostasis and degradation of cartilage. Osteoarthritis Cartilage. 2003;11(10):747-55.

[205] Guillen C, McInnes IB, Vaughan D, Speekenbrink AB, Brock JH. The effects of local administration of lactoferrin on inflammation in murine autoimmune and infectious arthritis. Arthritis Rheum. 2000;43(9):2073-80.

[206] Hayashida K, Kaneko T, Takeuchi T, Shimizu H, Ando K, Harada E. Oral administration of lactoferrin inhibits inflammation and nociception in rat adjuvant-induced arthritis. J Vet Med Sci. 2004;66(2):149-54.

[207] Wong SH, Francis N, Chahal H, Raza K, Salmon M, Scheel-Toellner D, et al. Lactoferrin is a survival factor for neutrophils in rheumatoid synovial fluid. Rheumatology (Oxford). 2009;48(1):39-44.

[208] Cornish J, Callon KE, Naot D, Palmano KP, Banovic T, Bava U, et al. Lactoferrin is a potent regulator of bone cell activity and increases bone formation in vivo. Endocrinology. 2004;145(9):4366-74.

[209] Kim JS, Ellman MB, An HS, Yan D, van Wijnen AJ, Murphy G, et al. Lactoferricin mediates anabolic and anti-catabolic effects in the intervertebral disc. J Cell Physiol.

[210] Sprangers MA, de Regt EB, Andries F, van Agt HM, Bijl RV, de Boer JB, et al. Which chronic conditions are associated with better or poorer quality of life? J Clin Epidemiol. 2000;53(9):895-907.

[211] Dray A, Read SJ. Arthritis and pain. Future targets to control osteoarthritis pain. Arthritis Res Ther. 2007;9(3):212.

[212] Creamer P, Hunt M, Dieppe P. Pain mechanisms in osteoarthritis of the knee: effect of intraarticular anesthetic. J Rheumatol. 1996;23(6):1031-6.

[213] Kosek E, Ordeberg G. Lack of pressure pain modulation by heterotopic noxious conditioning stimulation in patients with painful osteoarthritis before, but not following, surgical pain relief. Pain. 2000;88(1):69-78.

[214] Loeser RF, Yammani RR, Carlson CS, Chen H, Cole A, Im HJ, et al. Articular chondrocytes express the receptor for advanced glycation end products: Potential role in osteoarthritis. Arthritis Rheum. 2005;52(8):2376-85.

[215] Li X, An HS, Ellman M, Phillips F, Thonar EJ, Park DK, et al. Action of fibroblast growth factor-2 on the intervertebral disc. Arthritis Res Ther. 2008;10(2):R48.

[216] Schaible HG, Richter F, Ebersberger A, Boettger MK, Vanegas H, Natura G, et al. Joint pain. Exp Brain Res. 2009;196(1):153-62.

[217] Sommer C, Kress M. Recent findings on how proinflammatory cytokines cause pain: peripheral mechanisms in inflammatory and neuropathic hyperalgesia. Neurosci Lett. 2004;361(1-3):184-7.

[218] Brenn D, Richter F, Schaible HG. Sensitization of unmyelinated sensory fibers of the joint nerve to mechanical stimuli by interleukin-6 in the rat: an inflammatory mechanism of joint pain. Arthritis Rheum. 2007;56(1):351-9.

[219] Arvidson NG, Gudbjornsson B, Elfman L, Ryden AC, Totterman TH, Hallgren R. Circadian rhythm of serum interleukin-6 in rheumatoid arthritis. Ann Rheum Dis. 1994;53(8):521-4.

[220] Desgeorges A, Gabay C, Silacci P, Novick D, Roux-Lombard P, Grau G, et al. Concentrations and origins of soluble interleukin 6 receptor-alpha in serum and synovial fluid. J Rheumatol. 1997;24(8):1510-6.

[221] Obreja O, Biasio W, Andratsch M, Lips KS, Rathee PK, Ludwig A, et al. Fast modulation of heat-activated ionic current by proinflammatory interleukin 6 in rat sensory neurons. Brain. 2005;128(Pt 7):1634-41.

[222] Ohtori S, Takahashi K, Moriya H, Myers RR. TNF-alpha and TNF-alpha receptor type 1 upregulation in glia and neurons after peripheral nerve injury: studies in murine DRG and spinal cord. Spine (Phila Pa 1976). 2004;29(10):1082-8.

[223] Schafers M, Marziniak M, Sorkin LS, Yaksh TL, Sommer C. Cyclooxygenase inhibition in nerve-injury- and TNF-induced hyperalgesia in the rat. Exp Neurol. 2004;185(1):160-8.

[224] Grunke M, Schulze-Koops H. Successful treatment of inflammatory knee osteoarthritis with tumour necrosis factor blockade. Ann Rheum Dis. 2006;65(4):555-6.

[225] Inglis JJ, Notley CA, Essex D, Wilson AW, Feldmann M, Anand P, et al. Collagen-induced arthritis as a model of hyperalgesia: functional and cellular analysis of the analgesic actions of tumor necrosis factor blockade. Arthritis Rheum. 2007;56(12):4015-23.

[226] Yaksh TL, Dirig DM, Conway CM, Svensson C, Luo ZD, Isakson PC. The acute antihyperalgesic action of nonsteroidal, anti-inflammatory drugs and release of spinal prostaglandin E2 is mediated by the inhibition of constitutive spinal cyclooxygenase-2 (COX-2) but not COX-1. J Neurosci. 2001;21(16):5847-53.

[227] England S, Bevan S, Docherty RJ. PGE2 modulates the tetrodotoxin-resistant sodium current in neonatal rat dorsal root ganglion neurones via the cyclic AMP-protein kinase A cascade. J Physiol. 1996;495 (Pt 2):429-40.

[228] Bar KJ, Natura G, Telleria-Diaz A, Teschner P, Vogel R, Vasquez E, et al. Changes in the effect of spinal prostaglandin E2 during inflammation: prostaglandin E (EP1-EP4) receptors in spinal nociceptive processing of input from the normal or inflamed knee joint. J Neurosci. 2004;24(3):642-51.

[229] Castro RR, Cunha FQ, Silva FS, Jr., Rocha FA. A quantitative approach to measure joint pain in experimental osteoarthritis--evidence of a role for nitric oxide. Osteoarthritis Cartilage. 2006;14(8):769-76.

[230] Claveau D, Sirinyan M, Guay J, Gordon R, Chan CC, Bureau Y, et al. Microsomal prostaglandin E synthase-1 is a major terminal synthase that is selectively up-regulated during cyclooxygenase-2-dependent prostaglandin E2 production in the rat adjuvant-induced arthritis model. J Immunol. 2003;170(9):4738-44.

[231] Trebino CE, Stock JL, Gibbons CP, Naiman BM, Wachtmann TS, Umland JP, et al. Impaired inflammatory and pain responses in mice lacking an inducible prostaglandin E synthase. Proc Natl Acad Sci U S A. 2003;100(15):9044-9.

16

Proteases and Cartilage Degradation in Osteoarthritis

Judith Farley, Valeria M. Dejica and John S. Mort
Genetics Unit, Shriners Hospital for Children and Department of Surgery, McGill University
Canada

1. Introduction

Osteoarthritis, the most common joint disease, affecting millions people world-wide, involves the degradation of the articular cartilage which provides frictionless contact between the bones in a joint during movement. To a first approximation, this tissue is composed of two components, a collagen framework and entrapped proteoglycans. The framework consists of type II collagen fibrils built on a type XI collagen core, and decorated with type IX collagen molecules and small proteoglycans. These composite fibrils give the tissue its integrity, tensile strength and ability to retain large proteoglycan aggregates. The extremely large size of the proteoglycan aggregates and their high negative charge endows them with an immense hydration capacity, giving cartilage the ability to absorb compressive loading by the slow displacement of bound water. Partial destruction or loss of the proteoglycans is the first step in the deterioration of cartilage as seen in arthritis. Subsequently, irreversible loss of collagen occurs leading to permanent cartilage degeneration. While glycosylhydrolases and free radicals could also participate, it is believed that proteolytic enzymes are the main agents responsible for the degradation of cartilage components in osteoarthritis. Currently two classes of proteases are thought to be the major mediators of collagen and proteoglycan cleavage. Collagen degradation was thought to be majorly due to the action of MMP (matrix metalloproteinase) collagenases while members of both MMP and ADAMTS (**a** **d**isintegrin **a**nd **m**etalloproteinase with **t**hrombo**s**pondin motifs) families are important mediators of the degradation of proteoglycans which due to their extended core protein conformation are susceptible to the action of many proteases (Mort and Billington, 2001). Recently however, there is increasing evidence for the role of the cysteine protease cathepsin K in collagen degradation in articular cartilage (Konttinen et al., 2002).

The cleavage of cartilage proteins often occurs at specific sites on these molecules depending on the particular protease mediating the event. This results in the generation of characteristic N- and C-terminal epitopes that can be used for the production of antibodies specific for these cleavage products (anti-neoepitope antibodies) (Mort et al., 2003). A series of such antibodies has been produced and their specificities validated. These allow evaluation of the roles of different proteases in the degradation of collagen and proteoglycans in mouse models of osteoarthritis and in human and equine osteoarthritic cartilage using immunohistochemical methods and immunoassays.

2. Matrix metalloproteinases

Matrix metalloproteinases (MMPs) are a family of functionally and structurally related zinc endopeptidases that cleave proteins of the extracellular matrix, including collagens, elastin, matrix glycoproteins and proteoglycans (Martel-Pelletier et al., 2001) and are considered to be responsible for much of the degeneration of articular cartilage.

Most MMPs are composed of three distinct domains: an amino-terminal propeptide involved in the maintenance of enzyme latency; a catalytic domain that binds zinc and calcium ions and a hemopexin-like domain that is located at the carboxy terminal zone of the protease and that plays a role in substrate binding (Nagase, 1997). All MMPs are synthesized as preproenzymes and most of them are either secreted from the cell or bound to the plasma membrane in an inactive or proenzyme state. Several proteolytic cleavages are required to activate them and are critical steps leading to extracellular matrix breakdown (Nagase, 1997). Most of the MMPs are optimally active at neutral pH (Martel-Pelletier et al., 2001).

The human genome codes for 24 MMPs which can be classified depending on which components of the cartilage matrix they degrade (Birkedal-Hansen et al., 1993; Lee and Murphy, 2004). The MMPs that are the most important in cartilage extracellular matrix degradation are the collagenases (MMP-1, -8 and -13), the stromelysins (MMP-3, -10 and -11) the gelatinases (MMP-2 and –9), matrilysin (MMP-7) and the membrane type MMPs, in particular MMP-14 which can also act as a collagenase (Nagase and Woessner, 1999).

2.1 Collagenases

Matrix metalloproteinases with collagenolytic abilities are termed collagenases. These proteases mediate the initial cleavage of the collagen triple helix, occurring at three quarters of the distance from the amino-terminal end of each chain, forming collagen fragments of three-quarter and one-quarter length (Harris and Krane, 1974) (Fig.1). This site is susceptible to cleavage due to a reduced proline and hydroxyproline content which results in lowering of the stability of the triple helix. The collagenases are able to unwind this region of the triple helix and cleave all three collagen strands (Chung et al., 2004). This initial cleavage allows other MMPs to further degrade these unwound collagen molecules (Burrage et al., 2006). There are 3 collagenases: collagenase-1 or interstitial collagenase (MMP-1); collagenase-2 or neutrophil collagenase (MMP-8); and collagenase-3 (MMP-13). In addition, MMP-2 and MMP-14 also have the ability to cleave triple helical collagen.

2.1.1 Collagenase-1 (MMP-1)

Collagenase-1, which is primarily produced by synoviocytes (Wassilew et al., 2010), has been found in increased concentration in synovial fluid of patients suffering from joint injuries and osteoarthritis (Tchetverikov et al., 2005). It can also degrade aggrecan and different types of collagen: type I, II, III, VII, X, IX and denatured type II (Martel-Pelletier et al., 2001; Poole et al., 2001). This collagenase preferentially degrades type III collagen and its expression is mainly found in the superficial zone of articular cartilage in well-established osteoarthritis (Freemont et al., 1997). Even though its affinity towards type II collagen is lower than for collagenase-3, it is found in higher concentration in osteoarthritic joints (Vincenti and Brinckerhoff, 2001). *In vitro* studies showed that human chondrocytes can produce significantly more collagenase-1 than collagenase-3 following stimulation with proinflammatory cytokines, namely TNF-α and IL-1 (Yoshida et al., 2005).

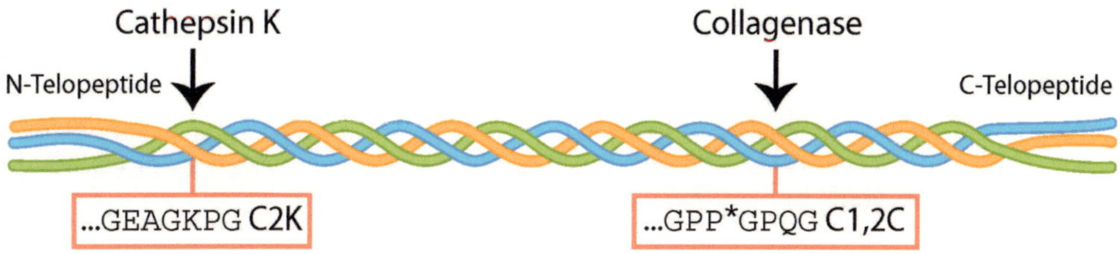

Fig. 1. Cleavage sites on type II collagen.
The type II collagen triple helix and non-helical telopeptides are indicated schematically. In reality there are many more turns in the triple helix. The ¾ / ¼ cleavage site for collagenases and the cleavage site for cathepsin K towards the N-terminus (Kafienah et al., 1998) are indicated along with the peptide sequences used to produce anti-neoepitope antibodies for the cleavage products. Asterisk indicates modification of proline to hydroxyproline.

2.1.2 Collagenase-2 (MMP-8)

Collagenase-2, which is mainly the product of neutrophils, degrades type I collagen with high specificity, but also cleaves collagen type II, III, VIII, X, aggrecan and link protein (Poole, 2001). It has been shown that collagenase-2 protein and mRNA are also produced by normal human chondrocytes (Cole et al., 1996), though recent data show that mRNA expression is very minor in normal and osteoarthritic chondrocytes (Stremme et al., 2003). Collagenase-2 is able to cleave the aggrecan molecule at the aggrecanase-site, between Glu^{373}-Ala^{374}, but cleaves preferentially between Asn^{341}-Phe^{342}, the MMP-site (Fosang et al., 1994) (Fig. 2).

2.1.3 Collagenase-3 (MMP-13)

Collagenase-3 was first cloned from human breast carcinoma in 1994 (Freije et al., 1994). It is predominantly a product of chondrocytes (Reboul et al., 1996) and has been shown to be expressed in human osteoarthritic cartilage (Mitchell et al., 1996), subchondral bone and hyperplasic synovial membrane in an osteoarthritis mouse model (Salminen et al., 2002). This collagenase is mostly expressed by chondrocytes surrounding osteoarthritic lesions (Shlopov et al., 1997) and can be found in superficial (Wu et al., 2002) and deep layers of osteoarthritic cartilage (Freemont et al., 1999; Moldovan et al., 1997). Matrix metalloproteinase-13 expression is strongly induced by interleukin-1 (IL-1), an important proinflammatory cytokine encountered in osteoarthritis (Gebauer et al., 2005; Vincenti and Brinckerhoff, 2001). Collagenase-3 degrades type II collagen preferentially, but also cleaves collagens type I, III, VII and X, aggrecan and gelatins (Poole et al., 2001). *In vitro* studies have shown that MMP-13 can cleave type II collagen about 5 times faster than type I collagen and about 6 times faster than type III collagen (Knäuper et al., 1996). Because type II collagen is its preferred substrate and because it can cleave type II collagen a least 5 to10 times faster than collagenase-1, collagenase-3 is considered to be one of the most important MMPs in osteoarthritis (Mitchell et al., 1996). It is also the collagenase with the most efficient gelatinolytic activity (Knäuper et al., 1996).
Many different *in vivo* studies have shown the importance of MMP-13 in osteoarthritis. Administration of specific MMP-13 inhibitors to animal models of osteoarthritis has shown a significant reduction in the severity of the pathology (Baragi et al., 2009; Johnson et al., 2007; Settle et al., 2010). Its importance in osteoarthritis was demonstrated, in a transgenic

mouse line expressing constitutively active human MMP-13 in hyaline cartilage where excessive MMP-13 expression resulted in articular cartilage degradation and joint pathology similar to osteoarthritis (Neuhold et al., 2001). Recently, MMP-13 knockout mice have been developed and surgical induction of osteoarthritis by destabilisation of the medial meniscus in these animals demonstrated that structural cartilage damage is dependent on MMP-13 activity (Little et al., 2009).

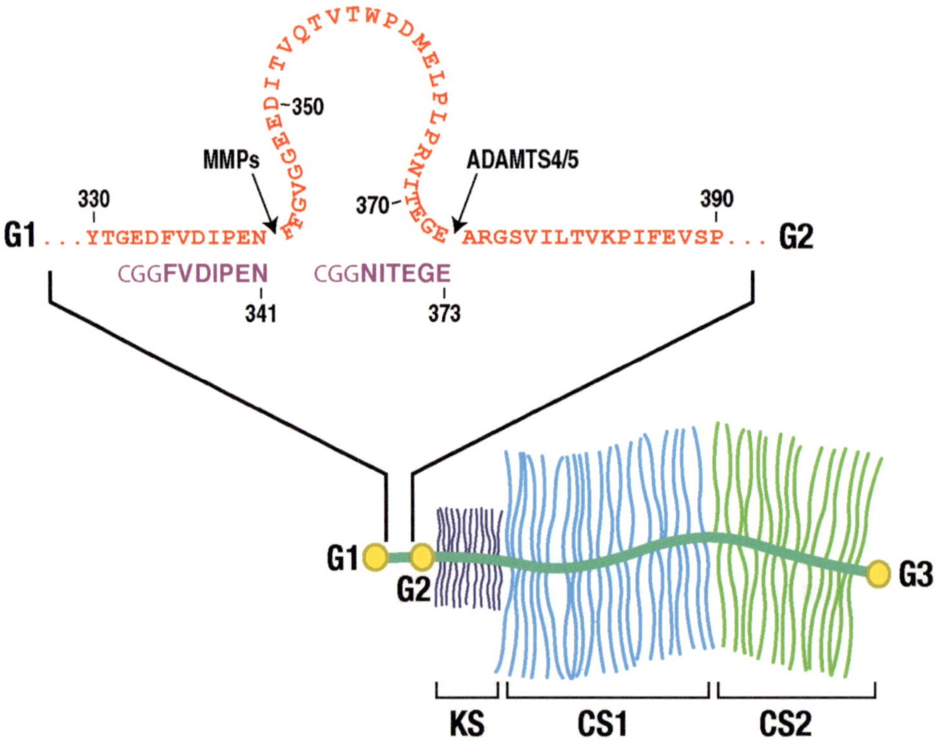

Fig. 2. Peptides used to generate anti-neoepitope antibodies to metalloproteinase cleavage products of aggrecan in the interglobular domain.
The domain structure of the aggrecan molecule is illustrated. The core protein (green) consists of two globular domains (G1 and G2) separated by an interglobular domain. A region rich in keratan sulfate (KS) follows along with two extended chondroitin sulfate rich regions (CS1 and CS2) which are substituted with glycosaminoglycan chains (blue). The CS1 region consists of a series of tandem repeats which can vary in number (Doege et al., 1997). The interglobular domain is susceptible to proteolytic attach. The sites of cleavage by MMPs and aggrecanases are indicated along with the sequences of peptides used to prepare anti-neoepitope antibodies which recognize the new C-termini of the G1-containing fragments that remain in the tissue following cleavage.

2.2 Gelatinases

Gelatinases are proteases that can further degrade denatured collagen, once the triple helix has been cleaved by collagenases. There are two gelatinases: gelatinase-A also termed 72 kDa or MMP-2 and gelatinase-B also termed 92 kDa or MMP-9.

2.2.1 Gelatinase-A (MMP-2)

Gelatinase-A degrades FACIT (fibril-associated collagens with interrupted triple helices) (Gordon and Hahn, 2010) collagens such as type IV collagen in the basement membrane and is a very efficient gelatinase degrading denatured fibrillar collagens and aggrecan (Poole, 2001). Gelatinase-A is mostly important in the completion of collagen degradation after specific cleavage of the triple helical region of fibrillar collagen molecules by collagenases (Nagase, 1997). This enzyme also cleaves the aggrecan molecule at the Asn^{341}-Phe^{342} site close to the G1 domain (Fosang et al., 1992) (Fig.2) and is mostly expressed in late stage osteoarthritis (Aigner et al., 2001).

It has been shown that in the horse, several joint cells, like chondrocytes and synovial fibroblasts, can produce gelatinase-A *in vitro* (Clegg et al., 1997a) and that the enzyme activity is increased in synovial fluid of joints of animals suffering from osteoarthritis (Clegg et al., 1997b). The activity of gelatinase-A was found to be increased in synovial fluid and synoviocytes of dogs with osteoarthritis, but was also detected in healthy joints (Volk et al., 2003). Recently, it has be shown that gelatinase-A deficiency in humans causes a disorder characterized by osteolysis and arthritis termed multicentric osteolysis with arthropathy, a disease that can be reproduced in gelatinase-A knockout mice (Mosig et al., 2007). Even if this enzyme seems to be implicated in the pathogenesis of osteoarthritis, it also plays a direct role in skeletal development.

2.2.2 Gelatinase-B (MMP-9)

Gelatinase-B has similar activities to MMP-2 but it can also act as an elastase. Though involved in collagen destruction, its collagenase action is at a very much lower level than that of gelatinase-A (Soder et al., 2006). Gelatinase-B can also cleave the aggrecan molecule at the same site as gelatinase-A, the Asn^{341}-Phe^{342} site (Fosang et al., 1992) (Fig. 2). This enzyme has been found in synovial fluid of humans (Koolwijk et al., 1995) and horses (Clegg et al., 1997b) with osteoarthritis, and its activity is increased in synovial fluid and synoviocytes of dogs (Volk et al., 2003) suffering from the same disease. Equine chondrocytes are also able of producing gelatinase-B *in vitro* (Clegg et al., 1997a).

2.3 Stromelysins

There are three stromelysins: stromelysin-1 or MMP-3, stromelysin-2 or MMP-10 and stromelysin-3 or MMP-11.

2.3.1 Stromelysin-1 (MMP-3)

Stromelysin-1 can degrade aggrecan, denatured collagens and interhelical collagen domains, as well as aggrecan and link protein. Importantly, stomelysin-1 can cleave the aggrecan molecule at the MMP site, at the Asn^{341}-Phe^{342} bond, to liberate the G1 domain from the remainder of the molecule (Flannery et al., 1992) (Fig.2). It has been shown that stromelysin-1 can activate the pro forms of collagenases and that this activation is a key step in cartilage degradation (Suzuki et al., 1990). In osteoarthritic cartilage, stromelysin-1 is localized in chondrocytes of the superficial and transition zone (Okada et al., 1992) and its strongest mRNA expression is found in early degenerative articular cartilage (Bau et al., 2002). In a rabbit model of surgically induced osteoarthritis, stromelysin-1 was found to be upregulated in the synovium initially, and in chondrocytes in the later phases of the disease (Mehraban et al., 1998), indicating that both cell types can produce stromelysin-1. It has been shown that in humans, the plasma level of stromelysin-1 was a significant predictor of joint space narrowing in knee osteoarthritis

(Lohmander et al., 2005). The concentration of this enzyme in human joint fluid can distinguish disease joints form healthy joints (Lohmander et al., 1993a). Another indication of the action of stromelysin-1 in the development of osteoarthritis is the significant decrease in severity of joint pathology in 2-year-old MMP-3 knockout mice (Blaney Davidson et al., 2007)

2.3.2 Stromelysins-2 and -3 (MMP-10 and MMP-11)

Stromelysin-2 has similar activities to MMP-3. This stromelysin can also activate procollagenases, and has been identified recently in synovial fluid and tissues from osteoarthritis patients, demonstrating the importance of this protease in articular cartilage degradation processes (Barksby et al., 2006).
Stromelysin-3 has been more implicated in general proteolysis, and shown to be up-regulated in osteoarthritic chondrocytes (Aigner et al., 2001). Unlike other MMPs, stromelysin-3 is activated intracellularly by the serine protease, furin, which processes many other proteins into their mature/active forms. MMP-11 is then secreted from cells in its active form (Pei and Weiss, 1995).

2.4 Other MMPs

Matrilysin (MMP-7), the smallest of the MMPs, lacking a hemopexin domain, is a protease that degrades aggrecan, gelatin, type IV collagen and link protein. Matrilysin cleaves the aggrecan molecule at the MMP-site (Fosang et al., 1992) and is mainly expressed in the superficial and transitional zones of osteoarthritic chondrocytes (Ohta et al., 1998). Matrilysin is the MMP with the highest specific activity against many extracellular matrix components (Murphy et al., 1991) and can also activate the zymogens of MMP-1 and MMP-9 (Imai et al., 1997).
There are six membrane-type matrix metalloproteinases (MT-MMPs) (Nagase and Woessner, 1999). Only MT1-MMP and MT3-MMP have been implicated in osteoarthritis (Burrage et al., 2006). The most important is MT1-MMP (MMP-14), expressed in human articular cartilage (Büttner et al., 1997) and synovial membrane. It degrades aggrecan, but also collagen type I, II, III and gelatin. It has been shown that MT1-MMP is highly expressed in osteoarthritic cartilage and could be responsible for the activation of progelatinase A in the extracellular matrix (Imai et al., 1995).

3. Aggrecanases

Aggrecanases are members of the '**A** **D**isintegrin **A**nd **M**etalloproteinase with **T**hrombospondin motifs' (ADAMTS) family of proteins. Synthesized as inactive pre-proenzymes, the ADAMTSs have a catalytic domain containing a zinc binding motif with 3 histidine residues, HEXXHXXGX-XH, and a critical methionine residue located in a 'Met-turn' downstream of the third zinc-binding histidine (Kuno et al., 1997). The propeptide is removed by the action of the proprotein convertase proteases furin (Koo et al., 2007) or PACE-4 (Malfait et al., 2008). Currently there are 19 ADAMTS genes known in humans, numbered ADAMTS-1 to ADAMTS-20, the same gene product being described as ADAMTS-5 and ADAMTS-11 (Porter et al., 2005).
The degradation of aggrecan leads to articular cartilage softening and loss of fixed charges (Maroudas, 1976). Two major cleavage sites of the aggrecan molecule are situated in the IGD region of the core protein, allowing aggrecan molecules lacking the G1 domain to freely exit the cartilage matrix and so to no longer contribute to cartilage function (Sandy et al., 1991). The first cleavage site at the Asn^{341}-Phe^{342} bond, creating the neoepitope VDIPEN, was found to be

generated by MMPs (Flannery et al., 1992; Fosang et al., 1991; Fosang et al., 1992). The second site at the Glu^{373}-Ala^{374} bond, creating the NITEGE neoepitope, was found to result from aggrecan cleavage by enzymes that were called aggrecanases (Sandy et al., 1991). There are 4 other aggrecanase cleavage sites situated in the GAG rich region (CS2) of aggrecan molecules between the globular domains G2 and G3 (Glu^{1545}-Gly^{1546}, Glu^{1714}-Gly^{1715}, Glu^{1819}-Ala^{1820}, and Glu^{1919}-Leu^{1920}, human sequences) (Tortorella et al., 2000) and a fifth cleavage site closer to the G3 domain that has been identified recently in bovine cartilage (Durigova et al., 2008). It was shown that aggrecan cleavage at the aggrecanase sites is responsible for cartilage degradation, *in vitro*, (Malfait et al., 2002; Tortorella et al., 2001) and, *in vivo*, ((Janusz et al., 2004), and that aggrecan neoepitopes generated by aggrecanases are found in synovial fluids of patients suffering from osteoarthritis (Lohmander et al., 1993b; Sandy et al., 1992). Moreover, it was also shown that contrary to MMP-inhibitors, aggrecanase inhibitors can block aggrecan degradation in human osteoarthritic cartilage (Malfait et al., 2002), demonstrating the importance of aggrecanases in cartilage matrix destruction.

The ongoing search for activities responsible for cartilage matrix degradation indicates that the ADAMTS family members are the most important aggrecanases. Of all of the ADAMTS enzymes, the phylogenetically closely related ADAMTS-1, -4, -5, -8, -9, -15 and -20 (Collins-Racie et al., 2004) are considered to be potential aggrecanases. All of the ADAMTS messenger RNAs except ADAMTS-7 were found to be present normal and/or osteoarthritic cartilage from hip or knee joints (Collins-Racie et al., 2004; Kevorkian et al., 2004; Naito et al., 2007). They have been shown to be able to cleave the aggrecan molecule at the Glu^{373}-Ala^{374} bond, except for ADAMTS-20 for which this cleavage site has not been tested to date (Collins-Racie et al., 2004; Rodríguez-Manzaneque et al., 2002; Somerville et al., 2003; Tortorella et al., 2000; Tortorella et al., 2002). The only 3 ADAMTSs that have been shown to be able to cleave aggrecan at the 4 aggrecanase sites located in the GAG rich region are ADAMTS-1, -4 and -5 (Rodríguez-Manzaneque et al., 2002; Tortorella et al., 2002), making them potent aggrecanases.

3.1 Aggrecanase-1 (ADAMTS-4)

Aggrecanase-1 has been well studied and evidence for its importance in aggrecan catabolism in cartilage is becoming stronger. ADAMTS-4 protein has been shown to be co-localized with aggrecan degradation products *in vitro* and *in vivo* (Naito et al., 2007). Selective inhibition of ADAMTS-4 and ADAMTS-5 has been shown to block the degradation of type II collagen by its protective effect on aggrecan molecules (Pratta et al., 2003). However, even if ADAMTS-4 has been shown to be able to cleave the aggrecan molecule *in vitro* (Tortorella et al., 2001), studies carried out with ADAMTS-4 knockout mice failed to show a protection against aggrecan loss after destabilizing knee surgery (Glasson et al., 2005). A similar study by Stanton et al. showed that, *in vitro*, ADAMTS-4 expression is not induced by IL-1α in mice suggesting that ADAMTS-4 may not be an important aggrecanase in osteoarthritis in mice (Stanton et al., 2005). However, in human osteoarthritis, ADAMTS-4 seems to play an important role in aggrecan degradation. In fact, this aggrecanase is induced in human cartilage, *in vitro*, by proinflammatory cytokines (Song et al., 2007), and is increased in osteoarthritic cartilage (Naito et al., 2007; Roach et al., 2005).

3.2 Aggrecanase-2 (ADAMTS-5)

ADAMTS-5 has also been well studied and its importance in aggrecan catabolism in cartilage has been shown. As mentioned for ADAMTS-4, selective inhibition of ADAMTS-

4 and ADAMTS-5 has been shown to have a protective effect on aggrecan molecules (Pratta et al., 2003). Studies carried out with ADAMTS-5 knockout and ADAMTS-4/-5 double knockout mice showed that these animals are more resistant to cartilage degradation after destabilizing knee surgery (Glasson et al., 2005; Majumdar et al., 2007; Stanton et al., 2005). In vitro, ADAMTS-5 expression is induced by IL-1α in mice, demonstrating its importance in osteoarthritis in that species (Stanton et al., 2005). ADAMTS-5 is also important in osteoarthritis in humans, its expression is high in human osteoarthritic cartilage and it is responsible for aggrecan degradation in normal and diseased cartilage (Bau et al., 2002; Plaas et al., 2007; Song et al., 2007). However, in the human, putative damaging polymorphisms in the ADAMTS-5 gene did not show any modification in susceptibility to osteoarthritis (Rodriguez-Lopez et al., 2008). The search for the most important aggrecanase in human osteoarthritis is still going strong (Fosang and Rogerson, 2010).

3.3 ADAMTS-1

ADAMTS-1 mRNA and protein are present in normal and OA cartilage (Kevorkian et al., 2004). This enzyme can cleave aggrecan at the Glu^{373}-Ala^{374} bond and at 4 additional aggrecanase sites between G2 and G3 (Rodríguez-Manzaneque et al., 2002). Concerning the expression of ADAMTS-1 in inflammatory conditions, ADAMTS-1 expression in articular chondrocytes is downregulated *in vitro* by human recombinant interleukin-1β (IL-1β) (Wachsmuth et al., 2004). An ADAMTS-1-KO mouse (Mittaz et al., 2004) showed that overall, ADAMTS-1 does not seem to be a key enzyme in normal and diseased cartilage, or in bone development and growth (Little et al., 2005).

4. Cathepsins

While the triple helical regions of the fibrillar collagens such as types I and II are resistant to the action of most proteases except the MMP collagenases (Nagase and Fushimi, 2008) which make an initial cleavage at the three quarter point, the cysteine protease, cathepsin K, is also able to degrade triple helical collagens (Garnero et al., 1998). Rather, this protease appears to erode the collagen fibrils from their termini, gradually reducing the chains to peptides with concomitant unwinding of the triple helix. Unlike the MMPs, cathepsins are single domain proteases which do not rely on additional modules to bind to their extracellular matrix substrates (Turk et al., 2001). However, the collagenolytic activity of cathepsin K is dependent on the presence of chondroitin 4-sulfate CS (Li et al., 2000) a major component of the aggrecan molecule which forms well-defined complexes with the enzyme (Cherney et al., 2011). While it was originally assumed that cathepsin K is unique to the osteoclast (and this cell does indeed contain huge amounts of the protease), many other cell types are now known to produce the enzyme (Anway et al., 2004; Sukhova et al., 1998). Its increasing abundance in chondrocytes close to the articular surface (Konttinen et al., 2002) suggests that its action may contribute to cartilage fibrillation seen with aging and joint disease.

5. Anti-neoepitope antibodies

The anti-cleavage site (anti-neoepitope) antibody approach has proven very productive as a means of detecting specific cleavage products in the extracellular matrix, thus demonstrating the action of one or a particular group of proteases (Mort et al., 2003; Mort and Buttle, 1999). In addition, since these cleavage products can accumulate in body fluids - synovial fluid, blood or urine - their quantitation can represent a measure of disease activity.

Our work has centered on aggrecan fragments generated by the action of MMPs and aggrecanases (ADAMTS family members, particularly ADAMTS-4 and -5) (Hughes et al., 1995; Sztrolovics et al., 2002) (Fig. 2) and on collagen cleavage epitopes generated by the action of collagenases (Billinghurst et al., 1997; Lee et al., 2009; Song et al., 1999) as well as the degradation of collagen in cartilage by cathepsin K (Dejica et al., 2008; Vinardell et al., 2009) (Fig. 1).

6. Immunohistochemical demonstration of protease action in cartilage

Anti-neoepitope antibodies can be used to demonstrate the effects of increased MMP activities in articular cartilage. This is illustrated in sections of joints of mice lacking the endogenous MMP inhibitor, tissue inhibitor of metalloproteinases-3 (TIMP-3). *Timp3*$^{-/-}$ mice are phenotypically normal, although old animals show some lung pathology (Leco et al., 2001) (Fig.3). However, detailed examination of the articular cartilage of adult animals demonstrates a decrease in glycosaminoglycan content (weaker Safranin O staining) and damage to the articular surface. Compared to wild type animals, there is a dramatic increase in the staining of the articular cartilage with an anti-VDIPEN antibody (Lee et al., 1998) which recognizes the G1 domain of aggrecan that remain located in the tissue following cleavage by MMPs. Although the aggrecanase cleavage site in mouse aggrecan generates the G1 terminating in the sequence ...NVTEGE rather than ...NITEGE, the antibody raised to the human epitope is fully functional with the mouse epitope and can be used to investigate the role of aggrecanases in cartilage degeneration in animal models of arthritis (van Lent et al., 2008).

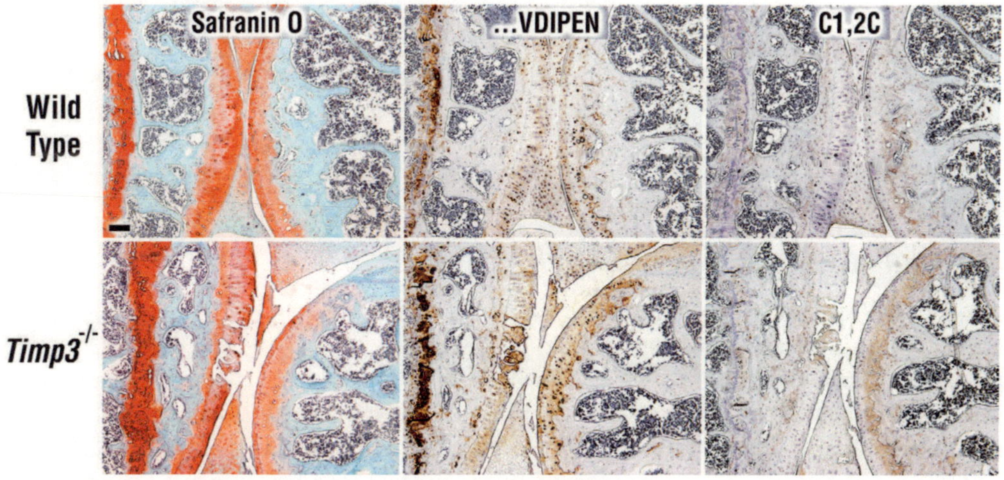

Fig. 3. Effect of increased MMP activity in mouse cartilage.

Hind joint sections of wild type and *Timp3*$^{-/-}$ 1-year-old FVB mice. Paraffin embedded samples were stained with Safranin O and Fast Green which identifies areas of fixed negative charge, or incubated with rabbit antibodies to either VDIPEN or the collagen epitope C1,2C, followed by a secondary horse radish peroxidase coupled system. Intense staining of the growth plate is visible on the left of the sections for glycosaminoglycans (Safranin O) and for the VDIPEN epitope indicating normal turnover of aggrecan. The magnification bar represents 100 µm.

Staining for the cleavage product for type II collagen by collagenases (the C1,2C epitope, Fig. 1) was also increased in the joints from *Timp3-/-* animals (Fig. 3) illustrating the broad inhibitory potential of TIMP-3.

Recently we have generated an antibody which is able to recognize and quantitate a cleavage product of type II collagen generated on the cleavage of the triple helical region by the action of cathepsin K (Dejica et al., 2008). Immunohistochemical studies demonstrated regions of cartilage reflecting cathepsin K activity (Fig. 4). Staining was dramatically increased in cartilage taken from osteoarthritis patients compared to that obtained from individuals with macroscopically normal tissue. The cleavage products are localized towards the articular surface in similar sites to those identified as due to the action of MMP collagenases as determined using the polyclonal antibody C1,2C which recognizes the C-terminal neoepitope of the 3/4 cleavage fragment (Wu et al., 2002). These areas of collagen degradation co-localize with the sites rich in cathepsin K (Konttinen et al., 2002; Vinardell et al., 2009).

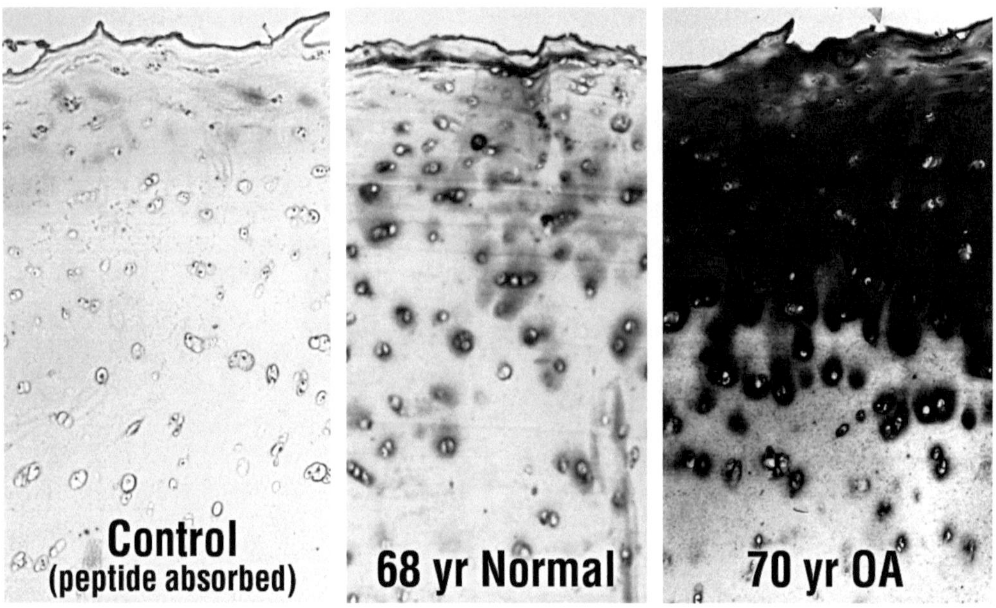

Fig. 4. Localization of cathepsin K generated type II cleavage products in cartilage from normal individuals and osteoarthritis (OA) patients.
Frozen sections were treated with chondroitinase ABC to remove glycosaminoglycans and stained using a rabbit antibody raised against the C2K epitope and a horse radish peroxidase labeled second step system. The reaction product was silver enhanced (Gallyas and Merchenthaler, 1988). A control section where the first step antibody was absorbed with the immunizing peptide is included.

The C2K epitope can be released from the tissue by digestion with chymotrypsin and quantitated using a competitive ELISA. Using this approach we demonstrated increased levels of cathepsin K-generated type II collagen fragments in cartilage from osteoarthritis patients relative to normal individuals. In addition, when cartilage was maintained in organ culture for two weeks in the presence of a specific cathepsin K inhibitor, a reduction in the levels of this epitope was observed, indicating that relatively short periods of cathepsin K activity produce detectable levels of this epitope (Dejica et al., 2008).

Together these results indicate that in addition to its critical role in bone resorption (Brömme and Lecaille, 2009; Tezuka et al., 1994), cathepsin K acts along with the MMPs and ADAMTS family members in the destruction of cartilage in osteoarthritis.

7. Acknowledgements

Work by the authors was supported by grants from the Canadian Arthritis Network of Centres of Excellence, the Canadian Institutes of Health Research and the Shriners of North America.

8. References

Aigner T.; Zien A.; Gehrsitz A.; Gebhard P.M. & McKenna L. (2001) Anabolic and catabolic gene expression pattern analysis in normal versus osteoarthritic cartilage using complementary DNA-array technology. *Arthritis Rheum.* Vol.44, pp. 2777-2789

Anway M.D.; Wright W.W.; Zirkin B.R.; Korah N.; Mort J.S. & Hermo L. (2004) Expression and location of cathepsin K in adult rat Sertoli cells. *Biol. Reprod.* Vol.70, pp. 562-569

Baragi V.M.; Becher G.; Bendele A.M.; Biesinger R.; Bluhm H.; Boer J.; Deng H.; Dodd R.; Essers M.; Feuerstein T.; Gallagher B.M., Jr.; Gege C.; Hochgurtel M.; Hofmann M.; Jaworski A.; Jin L.; Kiely A.; Korniski B.; Kroth H.; Nix D.; Nolte B.; Piecha D.; Powers T.S.; Richter F.; Schneider M.; Steeneck C.; Sucholeiki I.; Taveras A.; Timmermann A.; Van V.J.; Weik J.; Wu X. & Xia B. (2009) A new class of potent matrix metalloproteinase 13 inhibitors for potential treatment of osteoarthritis: Evidence of histologic and clinical efficacy without musculoskeletal toxicity in rat models. *Arthritis Rheum.* Vol.60, pp. 2008-2018

Barksby H.E., Milner J.M.; Patterson A.M.; Peake N.J.; Hui W.; Robson T.; Lakey R.; Middleton J.; Cawston T.E.; Richards C.D. & Rowan A.D. (2006) Matrix metalloproteinase 10 promotion of collagenolysis via procollagenase activation: implications for cartilage degradation in arthritis. *Arthritis Rheum.* Vol.54, pp. 3244-3253

Bau B.; Gebhard P.M.; Haag J.; Knorr T.; Bartnik E. & Aigner T. (2002) Relative messenger RNA expression profiling of collagenases and aggrecanases in human articular chondrocytes in vivo and in vitro. *Arthritis Rheum.* Vol.46, pp. 2648-2657

Billinghurst R.C.; Dahlberg L.; Ionescu M.; Reiner A.; Bourne R.; Rorabeck C.; Mitchell P.; Hambor J.; Diekmann O.; Tschesche H.; Chen J.; Van Wart H. & Poole A.R. (1997) Enhanced cleavage of type II collagen by collagenases in osteoarthritic articular cartilage. *J. Clin. Invest.* Vol.99, pp. 1534-1545

Birkedal-Hansen H.; Moore W.G.I.; Bodden M.K.; Windor L.J.; Birkedal-Hansen B.; DeCarlo A. & Engler J.A. (1993) Matrix metalloproteinases: a review. *Crit. Rev. Oral Biol. Med.* Vol.4, pp. 197-250

Blaney Davidson E.N.; Vitters E.L.; van Lent P.L.; van de Loo F.A.; van den Berg W.B. & van der Kraan P.M. (2007) Elevated extracellular matrix production and degradation upon bone morphogenetic protein-2 (BMP-2) stimulation point toward a role for BMP-2 in cartilage repair and remodeling. *Arthritis Res. Ther.* Vol.9, pp. R102

Brömme D. & Lecaille F. (2009) Cathepsin K inhibitors for osteoporosis and potential off-target effects. *Expert Opin. Investig. Drugs* Vol.18, pp. 585-600

Burrage P.S.; Mix K.S. & Brinckerhoff C.E. (2006) Matrix metalloproteinases: role in arthritis. *Front. Biosci.* Vol.11, pp. 529-543

Büttner F.H.; Chubinskaya S.; Margerie D.; Huch K.; Flechtenmacher J.; Cole A.A.; Kuettner K.E. & Bartnik E. (1997) Expression of membrane type 1 matrix metalloproteinase in human articular cartilage. *Arthritis Rheum.* Vol.40, pp. 704-709

Cherney M.M.; Lecaille F.; Kienitz M.; Nallaseth F.S.; Li Z.; James M.N.G. & Brömme D. (2011) Structure-activity analysis of cathepsin K/chondroitin 4-sulfate interactions. *J. Biol. Chem.* Vol.286, pp. 8988-8998

Chung L.; Dinakarpandian D.; Yoshida N.; Lauer-Fields J.L.; Fields G.B.; Visse R. & Nagase H. (2004) Collagenase unwinds triple-helical collagen prior to peptide bond hydrolysis. *EMBO J.* Vol.23, pp. 3020-3030

Clegg P.D.; Burke R.M.; Coughlan A.R.; Riggs C.M. & Carter S.D. (1997a) Characterisation of equine matrix metalloproteinase 2 and 9; and identification of the cellular sources of these enzymes in joints. *Equine Vet. J.* Vol.29, pp. 335-342

Clegg P.D.; Coughlan A.R.; Riggs C.M. & Carter S.D. (1997b) Matrix metalloproteinases 2 and 9 in equine synovial fluids. *Equine Vet. J.* Vol.29, pp. 343-348

Cole A.A.; Chubinskaya S.; Schumacher B.; Huch K.; Cs-Szabo G.; Yao J.; Mikecz K.; Hasty K.A. & Kuettner K.E. (1996) Chondrocyte matrix metalloproteinase-8. Human articular chondrocytes express neutrophil collagenase. *J. Biol. Chem.* Vol.271, pp. 11023-11026

Collins-Racie L.A.; Flannery C.R.; Zeng W.; Corcoran C.; Annis-Freeman B.; Agostino M.J.; Arai M.; DiBlasio-Smith E.; Dorner A.J.; Georgiadis K.E.; Jin M.; Tan X.Y.; Morris E.A. & LaVallie E.R. (2004) ADAMTS-8 exhibits aggrecanase activity and is expressed in human articular cartilage. *Matrix Biol.* Vol.23, pp. 219-230

Dejica V.M.; Mort J.S.; Laverty S.; Percival M.D.; Antoniou J.; Zukor D.J. & Poole A.R. (2008) Cleavage of type II collagen by cathepsin K in human osteoarthritic cartilage. *Am. J. Pathol.* Vol.173, pp. 161-169

Doege K.J.; Coulter S.N.; Meek L.M.; Maslen K. & Wood J.G. (1997) A human-specific polymorphism in the coding region of the aggrecan gene. Variable number of tandem repeats produce a range of core protein sizes in the general population. *J. Biol. Chem.* Vol.272, pp. 13974-13979

Durigova M.; Soucy P.; Fushimi K.; Nagase H.; Mort J.S. & Roughley P.J. (2008) Characterization of an ADAMTS-5-mediated cleavage site in aggrecan in OSM-stimulated bovine cartilage. *Osteoarthritis Cartilage* Vol.16, pp. 1245-1252

Flannery C.R.; Lark M.W. & Sandy J.D. (1992) Identification of a stromelysin cleavage site within the interglobular domain of human aggrecan. Evidence for proteolysis at this site *in vivo* in human articular cartilage. *J. Biol. Chem.* Vol.267, pp. 1008-1014

Fosang A.J.; Last K.; Neame P.J.; Murphy G.; Knäuper V.; Tschesche H.; Hughes C.E.; Caterson B. & Hardingham T.E. (1994) Neutrophil collagenase (MMP-8) cleaves at the aggrecanase site E^{373}-A^{374} in the interglobular domain of cartilage aggrecan. *Biochem. J.* Vol.304, pp. 347-351

Fosang A.J.; Neame P.J.; Hardingham T.E.; Murphy G. & Hamilton J.A. (1991) Cleavage of cartilage proteoglycan between G1 and G2 domains by stromelysins. *J. Biol. Chem.* Vol.266, pp. 15579-15582

Fosang A.J.; Neame P.J.; Last K.; Hardingham T.E.; Murphy G. & Hamilton J.A. (1992) The interglobular domain of cartilage aggrecan is cleaved by PUMP, gelatinases, and cathepsin B. *J. Biol. Chem.* Vol.267, pp. 19470-19474

Fosang A.J. & Rogerson F.M. (2010) Identifying the human aggrecanase. *Osteoarthritis Cartilage* Vol.18, pp. 1109-1116

Freemont A.J.; Byers R.J.; Taiwo Y.O. & Hoyland J.A. (1999) In situ zymographic localisation of type II collagen degrading activity in osteoarthritic human articular cartilage. *Ann. Rheum. Dis.* Vol.58, pp. 357-365

Freemont A.J.; Hampson V.; Tilman R.; Goupille P.; Taiwo Y. & Hoyland J.A. (1997) Gene expression of matrix metalloproteinases 1, 3, and 9 by chondrocytes in osteoarthritic human knee articular cartilage is zone and grade specific. *Ann. Rheum. Dis.* Vol.56, pp. 542-549

Freije J.M.P.; Díez-Itza I.; Balbín M.; Sánchez L.M.; Blasco R.; Tolivia J. & López-Otín C. (1994) Molecular cloning and expression of collagenase-3, a novel human matrix metalloproteinase produced by breast carcinomas. *J. Biol. Chem.* Vol.269, pp. 16766-16773

Gallyas F. & Merchenthaler I. (1988) Copper-H_2O_2 oxidation strikingly improves silver intensification of the nickel-diaminobenzidine (Ni-DAB) end-product of the peroxidase reaction. *J. Histochem. Cytochem.* Vol.36, pp. 807-810

Garnero P.; Borel O.; Byrjalsen I.; Ferreras M.; Drake F.H.; McQueney M.S.; Foged N.T.; Delmas P.D. & Delaissé J.M. (1998) The collagenolytic activity of cathepsin K is unique among mammalian proteinases. *J. Biol. Chem.* Vol.273, pp. 32347-32352

Gebauer M.; Saas J.; Sohler F.; Haag J.; Soder S.; Pieper M.; Bartnik E.; Beninga J.; Zimmer R. & Aigner T. (2005) Comparison of the chondrosarcoma cell line SW1353 with primary human adult articular chondrocytes with regard to their gene expression profile and reactivity to IL-1beta. *Osteoarthritis Cartilage* Vol.13, pp. 697-708

Glasson S.S.; Askew R.; Sheppard B.; Carito B.; Blanchet T.; Ma H.L.; Flannery C.R.; Peluso D.; Kanki K.; Yang Z.; Majumdar M.K. & Morris E.A. (2005) Deletion of active ADAMTS5 prevents cartilage degradation in a murine model of osteoarthritis. *Nature* Vol.434, pp. 644-648

Gordon M.K. & Hahn R.A. (2010) Collagens. *Cell Tissue Res.* Vol.339, pp. 247-257

Harris E.D. & Krane S.M. (1974) Collagenases. *N. Engl. J. Med.* Vol.291, pp. 605-609

Hughes C.E.; Caterson B.; Fosang A.J.; Roughley P.J. & Mort J.S. (1995) Monoclonal antibodies that specifically recognize neoepitope sequences generated by 'aggrecanase' and matrix metalloproteinase cleavage of aggrecan: application to catabolism *in situ* and *in vitro*. *Biochem. J.* Vol.305, pp. 799-804

Imai K.; Ohta S.; Matsumoto T.; Fujimoto N.; Sato H.; Seiki M. & Okada Y. (1997) Expression of membrane-type 1 matrix metalloproteinase and activation of progelatinase A in human osteoarthritic cartilage. *Am. J. Pathol.* Vol.151, pp. 245-256

Imai K.; Yokohama Y.; Nakanishi I.; Ohuchi E.; Fujii Y.; Nakai N. & Okada Y. (1995) Matrix metalloproteinase 7 (matrilysin) from human rectal carcinoma cells. Activation of the precursor, interaction with other matrix metalloproteinases and enzymic properties. *J. Biol. Chem.* Vol.270, pp. 6691-6697

Janusz M.J.; Little C.B.; King L.E.; Hookfin E.B.; Brown K.K.; Heitmeyer S.A.; Caterson B.; Poole A.R. & Taiwo Y.O. (2004) Detection of aggrecanase- and MMP-generated catabolic neoepitopes in the rat iodoacetate model of cartilage degeneration. *Osteoarthritis Cartilage* Vol.12, pp. 720-728

Johnson A.R.; Pavlovsky A.G.; Ortwine D.F.; Prior F.; Man C.F.; Bornemeier D.A.; Banotai C.A.; Mueller W.T.; McConnell P.; Yan C.; Baragi V.; Lesch C.; Roark W.H.; Wilson M.; Datta K.; Guzman R.; Han H.K. & Dyer R.D. (2007) Discovery and characterization of a novel inhibitor of matrix metalloprotease-13 that reduces cartilage damage in vivo without joint fibroplasia side effects. *J. Biol. Chem.* Vol.282, pp. 27781-27791

Kafienah W.; Brömme D.; Buttle D.J.; Croucher L.J. & Hollander A.P. (1998) Human cathepsin K cleaves native type I and II collagens at the N-terminal end of the triple helix. *Biochem. J.* Vol.331, pp. 727-732

Kevorkian L.; Young D.A.; Darrah C.; Donell S.T.; Shepstone L.; Porter S.; Brockbank S.M.; Edwards D.R.; Parker A.E. & Clark I.M. (2004) Expression profiling of metalloproteinases and their inhibitors in cartilage. *Arthritis Rheum.* Vol.50, pp. 131-141

Knäuper V.; López-Otín C.; Smith B.; Knight C.G. & Murphy G. (1996) Biochemical characterization of human collagenase-3. *J. Biol. Chem.* Vol.271, pp. 1544-1550

Konttinen Y.T.; Mandelin J.; Li T.F.; Salo J.; Lassus J.; Liljestrom M.; Hukkanen M.; Takagi M.; Virtanen I. & Santavirta S. (2002) Acidic cysteine endoproteinase cathepsin K in the degeneration of the superficial articular hyaline cartilage in osteoarthritis. *Arthritis Rheum.* Vol.46, pp. 953-960

Koo B.H.; Longpre J.M.; Somerville R.P.T.; Alexander J.P.; Leduc R. & Apte S.S. (2007) Regulation of ADAMTS9 secretion and enzymatic activity by its propeptide. *J. Biol. Chem.* Vol.282, pp. 16146-16154

Koolwijk P.; Miltenburg A.M.M.; van Erck M.G.M.; Oudshoorn M.; Niedbala M.J.; Breedveld F.C. & van Hinsbergh V.W.M. (1995) Activated gelatinase-B (MMP-9) and urokinase-type plasminogen activator in synovial fluids of patients with arthritis. Correlation with clinical and experimental variables of inflammation. *J. Rheumatol.* Vol.22, pp. 385-393

Kuno K.; Kanada N.; Nakashima E.; Fujiki F.; Ichimura F. & Matsushima K. (1997) Molecular cloning of a gene encoding a new type of metalloproteinase-disintegrin family protein with thrombospondin motifs as an inflammation associated gene. *J. Biol. Chem.* Vol.272, pp. 556-562

Leco K.J.; Waterhouse P.; Sanchez O.H.; Gowing K.L.M.; Poole A.R.; Wakeham T.W.; Mak T.W. & Khokha R. (2001) Spontaneous air space enlargement in the lungs of mice lacking tissue inhibitor of metalloproteinases-3 (TIMP-3). *J. Clin. Invest.* Vol.108, pp. 817-829

Lee E.R.; Lamplugh L.; Kluczyk B.; Leblond C.P. & Mort J.S. (2009) Neoepitopes reveal the features of type II collagen cleavage and the identity of a collagenase involved in the transformation of the epiphyses anlagen in development. *Dev. Dyn.* Vol.238, pp. 1547-1563

Lee E.R.; Lamplugh L.; Leblond C.P.; Mordier S.; Magny M.-C. & Mort J.S. (1998) Immunolocalization of the cleavage of the aggrecan core protein at the Asn^{341}-Phe^{342} bond, as an indicator of the location of the metalloproteinases active in the lysis of the rat growth plate. *Anat. Rec.* Vol.252, pp. 117-132

Lee M.H. & Murphy G. (2004) Matrix metalloproteinases at a glance. *J. Cell Sci.* Vol.117, pp. 4015-4016

Li Z.; Hou W.S. & Brömme D. (2000) Collagenolytic activity of cathepsin K is specifically modulated by cartilage-resident chondroitin sulfates. *Biochemistry* Vol.39, pp. 529-536

Little C.B.; Barai A.; Burkhardt D.; Smith S.M.; Fosang A.J.; Werb Z.; Shah M. & Thompson E.W. (2009) Matrix metalloproteinase 13-deficient mice are resistant to osteoarthritic cartilage erosion but not chondrocyte hypertrophy or osteophyte development. *Arthritis Rheum.* Vol.60, pp. 3723-3733

Little C.B.; Mittaz L.; Belluoccio D.; Rogerson F.M.; Campbell I.K.; Meeker C.T.; Bateman J.F.; Pritchard M.A. & Fosang A.J. (2005) ADAMTS-1-knockout mice do not exhibit abnormalities in aggrecan turnover *in vitro* or *in vivo*. *Arthritis Rheum.* Vol.52, pp. 1461-1472

Lohmander L.S.; Brandt K.D.; Mazzuca S.A.; Katz B.P.; Larsson S.; Struglics A. & Lane K.A. (2005) Use of the plasma stromelysin (matrix metalloproteinase 3) concentration to predict joint space narrowing in knee osteoarthritis. *Arthritis Rheum.* Vol.52, pp. 3160-3167

Lohmander L.S.; Hoerrner L.A. & Lark M.W. (1993a) Metalloproteinases, tissue inhibitor, and proteoglycan fragments in knee synovial fluid in human osteoarthritis. *Arthritis Rheum.* Vol.36, pp. 181-189

Lohmander L.S.; Neame P.J. & Sandy J.D. (1993b) The structure of aggrecan fragments in human synovial fluid: evidence that aggrecanase mediates cartilage degradation in inflammatory joint disease, joint injury and osteoarthritis. *Arthritis Rheum.* Vol.36, pp. 1214-1222

Majumdar M.K.; Askew R.; Schelling S.; Stedman N.; Blanchet T.; Hopkins B.; Morris E.A. & Glasson S.S. (2007) Double-knockout of ADAMTS-4 and ADAMTS-5 in mice results in physiologically normal animals and prevents the progression of osteoarthritis. *Arthritis Rheum.* Vol.56, pp. 3670-3674

Malfait A.M.; Arner E.C.; Song R.H.; Alston J.T.; Markosyan S.; Staten N.; Yang Z.; Griggs D.W. & Tortorella M.D. (2008) Proprotein convertase activation of aggrecanases in cartilage in situ. *Arch. Biochem. Biophys.* Vol.478, pp. 43-51

Malfait A.M.; Liu R.Q.; Ijiri K.; Komiya S. & Tortorella M.D. (2002) Inhibition of ADAM-TS4 and ADAM-TS5 prevents aggrecan degradation in osteoarthritic cartilage. *J. Biol. Chem.* Vol.277, pp. 22201-22208

Maroudas A.I. (1976) Balance between swelling pressure and collagen tension in normal and degenerate cartilage. *Nature* Vol.260, pp. 808-809

Martel-Pelletier J.; Welsch D.J. & Pelletier J.P. (2001) Metalloproteases and inhibitors in arthritic diseases. *Best Pract. Res. Clin. Rheumatol.* Vol.15, pp. 805-829

Mehraban F.; Lark M.W.; Ahmed F.N.; Xu F. & Moskowitz R.W. (1998) Increased secretion and activity of matrix metalloproteinase-3 in synovial tissues and chondrocytes from experimental osteoarthritis. *Osteoarthritis Cartilage* Vol.6, pp. 286-294

Mitchell P.G.; Magna H.A.; Reeves L.M.; Lopresti-Morrow L.L.; Yocum S.A.; Rosner P.J.; Geoghegan K.F. & Hambor J.E. (1996) Cloning, expression, and type II collagenolytic activity of matrix metalloproteinase-13 from human osteoarthritic cartilage. *J. Clin. Invest.* Vol.97, pp. 761-768

Mittaz L.; Russell D.L.; Wilson T.; Brasted M.; Tkalcevic J.; Salamonsen L.A.; Hertzog P.J. & Pritchard M.A. (2004) Adamts-1 is essential for the development and function of the urogenital system. *Biol. Reprod.* Vol.70, pp. 1096-1105

Moldovan F.; Pelletier J.P.; Hambor J.; Cloutier J.M. & Martel-Pelletier J. (1997) Collagenase-3 (matrix metalloprotease 13) is preferentially localized in the deep layer of human arthritic cartilage in situ: in vitro mimicking effect by transforming growth factor beta. *Arthritis Rheum.* Vol.40, pp. 1653-1661

Mort J.S. & Billington C.J. (2001) Articular cartilage and changes in arthritis: matrix degradation. *Arthritis Res.* Vol.3, pp. 337-341

Mort J.S. & Buttle D.J. (1999) The use of cleavage site specific antibodies to delineate protein processing and breakdown pathways. *J. Clin. Pathol. :Mol. Pathol.* Vol.52, pp. 11-18

Mort J.S.; Flannery C.R.; Makkerh J.; Krupa J.C. & Lee E.R. (2003) The use of anti-neoepitope antibodies for the analysis of degradative events in cartilage and the molecular basis for neoepitope specificity. *Biochem. Soc. Symp.* Vol.70, pp. 107-114

Mosig R.A.; Dowling O.; DiFeo A.; Ramirez M.C.; Parker I.C.; Abe E.; Diouri J.; Aqeel A.A.; Wylie J.D.; Oblander S.A.; Madri J.; Bianco P.; Apte S.S.; Zaidi M.; Doty S.B.; Majeska R.J.; Schaffler M.B. & Martignetti J.A. (2007) Loss of MMP-2 disrupts skeletal and craniofacial development and results in decreased bone mineralization, joint erosion and defects in osteoblast and osteoclast growth. *Hum. Mol. Genet.* Vol.16, pp. 1113-1123

Murphy G.; Cockett M.I.; Ward R.V. & Docherty A.J.P. (1991) Matrix metalloproteinase degradation of elastin, type IV collagen and proteoglycan. A quantitative comparison of the activities of 95 kDa and 72 kDa gelatinases, stromelysins-1 and -2 and punctuated metalloproteinase (PUMP). *Biochem. J.* Vol.277, pp. 277-279

Nagase H. (1997) Activation mechanisms of matrix metalloproteinases. *Biol. Chem.* Vol.378, pp. 151-160

Nagase H. & Fushimi K. (2008) Elucidating the function of non catalytic domains of collagenases and aggrecanases. *Connect. Tissue Res.* Vol.49, pp. 169-174

Nagase H. & Woessner J.F. (1999) Matrix metalloproteinases. *J. Biol. Chem.* Vol.274, pp. 21491-21494

Naito S.; Shiomi T.; Okada A.; Kimura T.; Chijiiwa M.; Fujita Y.; Yatabe T.; Komiya K.; Enomoto H.; Fujikawa K. & Okada Y. (2007) Expression of ADAMTS4 (aggrecanase-1) in human osteoarthritic cartilage. *Pathol. Int.* Vol.57, pp. 703-711

Neuhold L.A.; Killar L.; Zhao W.; Sung M.L.; Warner L.; Kulik J.; Turner J.; Wu W.; Billinghurst C.; Meijers T.; Poole A.R.; Babij P. & DeGennaro L.J. (2001) Postnatal expression in hyaline cartilage of constitutively active human collagenase-3 (MMP-13) induces osteoarthritis in mice. *J. Clin. Invest.* Vol.107, pp. 35-44

Ohta S.; Imai K.; Yamashita K.; Matsumoto T.; Azumano I. & Okada Y. (1998) Expression of matrix metalloproteinase 7 (matrilysin) in human osteoarthritic cartilage. *Lab. Invest.* Vol.78, pp. 79-87

Okada Y.; Shinmei M.; Tanaka O.; Naka K.; Kimura A.; Nakanishi I.; Bayliss M.T.; Iwata K. & Nagase H. (1992) Localization of matrix metalloproteinase 3 (stromelysin) in osteoarthritic cartilage and synovium. *Lab. Invest.* Vol.66, pp. 680-690

Pei D. & Weiss S.J. (1995) Furin-dependent intracellular activation of the human stromelysin-3 zymogen. *Nature* Vol.375, pp. 244-247

Plaas A.; Osborn B.; Yoshihara Y.; Bai Y.; Bloom T.; Nelson F.; Mikecz K. & Sandy J.D. (2007) Aggrecanolysis in human osteoarthritis: confocal localization and biochemical characterization of ADAMTS5-hyaluronan complexes in articular cartilages. *Osteoarthritis Cartilage* Vol.15, pp. 719-734

Poole, AR (2001) Cartilage in health and disease. In Arthritis and Allied Conditions (Koopman, W. J., ed.), 226-284, Lippincott, Williams and Wilkins, Baltimore

Poole A.R.; Kojima T.; Yasuda T.; Mwale F.; Kobayashi M. & Laverty S. (2001) Composition and structure of articular cartilage: a template for tissue repair. *Clin. Orthop.* pp. S26-S33

Porter S.; Clark I.M.; Kevorkian L. & Edwards D.R. (2005) The ADAMTS metalloproteinases. *Biochem. J.* Vol.386, pp. 15-27

Pratta M.A.; Yao W.; Decicco C.; Tortorella M.D.; Liu R.Q.; Copeland R.A.; Magolda R.; Newton R.C.; Trzaskos J.M. & Arner E.C. (2003) Aggrecan protects cartilage collagen from proteolytic cleavage. *J. Biol. Chem.* Vol.278, pp. 45539-45545

Reboul P.; Pelletier J.P.; Tardif G.; Cloutier J.M. & Martel-Pelletier J. (1996) The new collagenase, collagenase-3, is expressed and synthesized by human chondrocytes but not by synoviocytes. A role in osteoarthritis. *J. Clin. Invest.* Vol.97, pp. 2011-2019

Roach H.I.; Yamada N.; Cheung K.S.; Tilley S.; Clarke N.M.; Oreffo R.O.; Kokubun S. & Bronner F. (2005) Association between the abnormal expression of matrix-degrading enzymes by human osteoarthritic chondrocytes and demethylation of specific CpG sites in the promoter regions. *Arthritis Rheum.* Vol.52, pp. 3110-3124

Rodriguez-Lopez J.; Mustafa Z.; Pombo-Suarez M.; Malizos K.N.; Rego I.; Blanco F.J.; Tsezou A.; Loughlin J.; Gomez-Reino J.J. & Gonzalez A. (2008) Genetic variation including nonsynonymous polymorphisms of a major aggrecanase, ADAMTS-5, in susceptibility to osteoarthritis. *Arthritis Rheum.* Vol.58, pp. 435-441

Rodríguez-Manzaneque J.C.; Westling J.; Thai S.N.M.; Luque A.; Knäuper V.; Murphy G.; Sandy J.D. & Iruela-Arispe M.L. (2002) ADAMTS1 cleaves aggrecan at multiple sites and is differentially inhibited by metalloproteinase inhibitors. *Biochem. Biophys. Res. Commun.* Vol.293, pp. 501-508

Salminen H.J.; Säämänen A.-M.K.; Vankemmelbeke M.N.; Auho P.K.; Perälä M.P. & Vuorio E.I. (2002) Differential expression patterns of matrix metalloproteinases and their inhibitors during development of osteoarthritis in a transgenic mouse model. *Ann. Rheum. Dis.* Vol.61, pp. 591

Sandy J.D.; Flannery C.R.; Neame P.J. & Lohmander L.S. (1992) The structure of aggrecan fragments in human synovial fluid. Evidence for the involvement in osteoarthritis of a novel proteinase which cleaves the Glu 373-Ala 374 bond of the interglobular domain. *J. Clin. Invest.* Vol.89, pp. 1512-1516

Sandy J.D.; Neame P.J.; Boynton R.E. & Flannery C.R. (1991) Catabolism of aggrecan in cartilage explants. Identification of a major cleavage site within the interglobular domain. *J. Biol. Chem.* Vol.266, pp. 8683-8685

Settle S.; Vickery L.; Nemirovskiy O.; Vidmar T.; Bendele A.; Messing D.; Ruminski P.; Schnute M. & Sunyer T. (2010) Cartilage degradation biomarkers predict efficacy of a novel, highly selective matrix metalloproteinase 13 inhibitor in a dog model of osteoarthritis: Confirmation by multivariate analysis that modulation of type ii collagen and aggrecan degradation peptides parallels pathologic changes. *Arthritis Rheum.* Vol.62, pp. 3006-3015

Shlopov B.V.; Lie W.R.; Mainardi C.L.; Cole A.A.; Chubinskaya S. & Hasty K.A. (1997) Osteoarthritic lesions: involvement of three different collagenases. *Arthritis Rheum.* Vol.40, pp. 2065-2074

Soder S.; Roach H.I.; Oehler S.; Bau B.; Haag J. & Aigner T. (2006) MMP-9/gelatinase B is a gene product of human adult articular chondrocytes and increased in osteoarthritic cartilage. *Clin. Exp. Rheumatol.* Vol.24, pp. 302-304

Somerville R.P.T.; Longpre J.M.; Jungers K.A.; Engle J.M.; Ross M.; Evanko S.; Wight T.N.; Leduc R. & Apte S.S. (2003) Characterization of ADAMTS-9 and ADAMTS-20 as a distinct ADAMTS subfamily related to *Caenorhabditis elegans* GON-1. *J. Biol. Chem.* Vol.278, pp. 9503-9513

Song R.H.; Tortorella M.D.; Malfait A.M.; Alston J.T.; Yang Z.; Arner E.C. & Griggs D.W. (2007) Aggrecan degradation in human articular cartilage explants is mediated by both ADAMTS-4 and ADAMTS-5. *Arthritis Rheum.* Vol.56, pp. 575-585

Song X.Y.; Zeng L.; Jin W.; Thompson J.; Mizel D.E.; Lei K.; Billinghurst R.C.; Poole A.R. & Wahl S.M. (1999) Secretory leukocyte protease inhibitor suppresses the inflammation and joint damage of bacterial cell wall-induced arthritis. *J. Exp. Med.* Vol.190, pp. 535-542

Stanton H.; Rogerson F.M.; East C.J.; Golub S.B.; Lawlor K.E.; Meeker C.T.; Little C.B.; Last K.; Farmer P.J.; Campbell I.K.; Fourie A.M. & Fosang A.J. (2005) ADAMTS5 is the major aggrecanase in mouse cartilage in vivo and in vitro. *Nature* Vol.434, pp. 648-652

Stremme S.; Duerr S.; Bau B.; Schmid E. & Aigner T. (2003) MMP-8 is only a minor gene product of human adult articular chondrocytes of the knee. *Clin. Exp. Rheumatol.* Vol.21, pp. 205-209

Sukhova G.K.; Shi G.P.; Simon D.I.; Chapman H.A. & Libby P. (1998) Expression of the elastolytic cathepsins S and K in human atheroma and regulation of their production in smooth muscle cells. *J. Clin. Invest.* Vol.102, pp. 576-583

Suzuki K.; Enghild J.J.; Morodomi T.; Salvesen G. & Nagase H. (1990) Mechanisms of activation of tissue procollagenase by matrix metalloproteinase 3 (stromelysin). *Biochemistry* Vol.29, pp. 10261-10270

Sztrolovics R.; White R.J.; Roughley P.J. & Mort J.S. (2002) The mechanism of aggrecan release from cartilage differs with tissue origin and the agent used to stimulate catabolism. *Biochem. J.* Vol.362, pp. 465-472

Tchetverikov I.; Lohmander L.S.; Verzijl N.; Huizinga T.W.; TeKoppele J.M.; Hanemaaijer R. & Degroot J. (2005) MMP protein and activity levels in synovial fluid from patients with joint injury, inflammatory arthritis, and osteoarthritis. *Ann. Rheum. Dis.* Vol.64, pp. 694-698

Tezuka K.; Tezuka Y.; Maejima A.; Sato T.; Nemoto K.; Kamioka H.; Hakeda Y. & Kumegawa M. (1994) Molecular cloning of a possible cysteine proteinase predominantly expressed in osteoclasts. *J. Biol. Chem.* Vol.269, pp. 1106-1109

Tortorella M.D.; Liu R.Q.; Burn T.; Newton R.C. & Arner E. (2002) Characterization of human aggrecanase 2 (ADAM-TS5): substrate specificity studies and comparison with aggrecanase 1 (ADAM-TS4). *Matrix Biol.* Vol.21, pp. 499-511

Tortorella M.D.; Malfait A.M.; Deccico C. & Arner E. (2001) The role of ADAM-TS4 (aggrecanase-1) and ADAM-TS5 (aggrecanase-2) in a model of cartilage degradation. *Osteoarthritis Cartilage* Vol.9, pp. 539-552

Tortorella M.D.; Pratta M.; Liu R.Q.; Austin J.; Ross O.H.; Abbaszade I.; Burn T. & Arner E. (2000) Sites of aggrecan cleavage by recombinant human aggrecanase-1 (ADAMTS-4). *J. Biol. Chem.* Vol.275, pp. 18566-18573

Turk V.; Turk B. & Turk D. (2001) Lysosomal cysteine proteases: facts and opportunities. *EMBO J.* Vol.20, pp. 4629-4633

van Lent P.L.E.M.; Grevers L.; Blom A.B.; Sloetjes A.; Mort J.S.; Vogl T.; Nacken W.; van den Berg W.B. & Roth J. (2008) Myeloid-related proteins S100A8/S100A9 regulate joint inflammation and cartilage destruction during antigen-induced arthritis. *Ann. Rheum. Dis.* Vol.67, pp. 1750-1758

Vinardell T.; Dejica V.; Poole A.R.; Mort J.S.; Richard H. & Laverty S. (2009) Evidence to suggest that cathepsin K degrades articular cartilage in naturally occurring equine osteoarthritis. *Osteoarthritis Cartilage* Vol.17, pp. 375-383

Vincenti M.P. & Brinckerhoff C.E. (2001) Early response genes induced in chondrocytes stimulated with the inflammatory cytokine interleukin-1β. *Arthritis Res.* Vol.3, pp. 381-388

Volk S.W.; Kapatkin A.S.; Haskins M.E.; Walton R.M. & D'Angelo M. (2003) Gelatinase activity in synovial fluid and synovium obtained from healthy and osteoarthritic joints of dogs. *Am. J. Vet. Res.* Vol.64, pp. 1225-1233

Wachsmuth L.; Bau B.; Fan Z.; Pecht A.; Gerwin N. & Aigner T. (2004) ADAMTS-1, a gene product of articular chondrocytes in vivo and in vitro, is downregulated by interleukin 1beta. *J. Rheumatol.* Vol.31, pp. 315-320

Wassilew G.I.; Lehnigk U.; Duda G.N.; Taylor W.R.; Matziolis G. & Dynybil C. (2010) The expression of proinflammatory cytokines and matrix metalloproteinases in the synovial membranes of patients with osteoarthritis compared with traumatic knee disorders. *Arthroscopy* Vol.26, pp. 1096-1104

Wu W.; Billinghurst R.C.; Pidoux I.; Antoniou J.; Zukor D.; Tanzer M. & Poole A.R. (2002) Sites of collagenase cleavage and denaturation of type II collagen in aging and osteoarthritic articular cartilage and their relationship to the distribution of matrix metalloproteinase 1 and matrix metalloproteinase 13. *Arthritis Rheum.* Vol.46, pp. 2087-2094

Yoshida M.; Tsuji M.; Funasaki H.; Kan I. & Fujii K. (2005) Analysis for the major contributor of collagenase to the primary cleavage of type II collagens in cartilage degradation. *Mod. Rheumatol.* Vol.15, pp. 180-186

17

Simple Method Using Gelatin-Coated Film for Comprehensively Assaying Gelatinase Activity in Synovial Fluid

Akihisa Kamataki[1], Wataru Yoshida[1], Mutsuko Ishida[1], Kenya Murakami[1], Kensuke Ochi[2] and Takashi Sawai[1]
[1]*Iwate Medical University,*
[2]*Kawasaki Municipal Kawasaki Hospital*
Japan

1. Introduction

Rheumatoid arthritis (RA) is a chronic inflammatory disease that leads to the irreversible destruction of cartilage and bone. An important step in the destruction of tissue is the degradation of extracellular matrix (ECM), whose major components are type II collagen and aggrecan in cartilage, and type I collagen in bone. The synovial fluid of RA patients often contains high concentrations of proteinases, such as those of the matrix metalloproteinase (MMP) and a disintegrin-like and metalloproteinase with thrombospondin type 1 motif (ADAMTS) families, which induce ECM degradation either directly or indirectly and participate in joint destruction. MMP-1, MMP-8, and MMP-13, which function as collagenases, have proteolytic activity towards type I and type II collagen (Chakraborti et al., 2003; Murphy & Nagase, 2008). MMP-2 and MMP-9, termed gelatinases, degrade denatured collagen, while MMP-3 degrades several ECM proteins (Chakraborti et al., 2003). All of them have the gelatinase activity. ADAMTS-4 and ADAMTS-5 are major enzymes involved in the degradation of aggrecan (Arner, 2002) and have low levels of gelatinase activity (Gendron et al., 2007; Lauer-Fields et al., 2007).
The concentration and activity of MMP and ADAMTS enzymes in synovial fluid and serum are measurable using ELISA or enzyme-specific substrates. In particular, MMP-3 is often the target of laboratory tests as a biomarker for disease progression. However, for the elucidation of actual RA progression, it is important to measure the comprehensive activity of all enzymes.
In situ zymography is a method for assessing endogenous protease activity in tissue section (Yan & Blomme, 2003). Film *in situ* zymography (FIZ) using gelatin-coated film is a useful method for assessing the enzymes involved in arthritis (Yoshida et al., 2009). In this method, a frozen tissue section is adhered onto a gelatin-coated film and gelatin degradation loci on the film are then analyzed after a suitable incubation period. A locus of gelatin degradation represents an area where comprehensive enzymatic activity is high. This chapter describes a method for assaying the comprehensive gelatinase activity in synovial fluid using gelatin-coated films for FIZ.

2. Method for synovial fluid analysis using gelatin-coated film

2.1 Synovial fluid samples

Synovial fluid samples were obtained from RA patients, osteoarthritis (OA) patients. Patients provided written consent for collection of synovial fluid samples before the procedure. All RA patients fulfilled the American College of Rheumatology criteria for the classification of RA. OA was diagnosed according to clinical findings. All the OA samples we examined were grade III or IV according to the Kellgren/Lawrence radiographic grading system. This study were approved by the ethics committees at Iwate Medical University

2.2 Method

Gelatin-coated film (Zymo-film; Fuji Film Co., Tokyo, Japan) is adhered onto a slide glass and a silicon gasket with 12 wells (flexi PERM; Greiner Bio-One GmbH, Frickenhausen, Germany) is then attached onto the film using Vaseline (Fig. 1). Two-hundred microliters of a two-fold serial dilution of synovial fluid sample is added into each well. To prevent the sample from evaporating, a lid is placed on the gasket and a moist chamber is used for the incubation period. After overnight incubation at 37 °C, the gelatin-coated film is washed twice with PBS, stained with a 0.2% Ponceau S solution, and then dried at room temperature (Fig. 2).

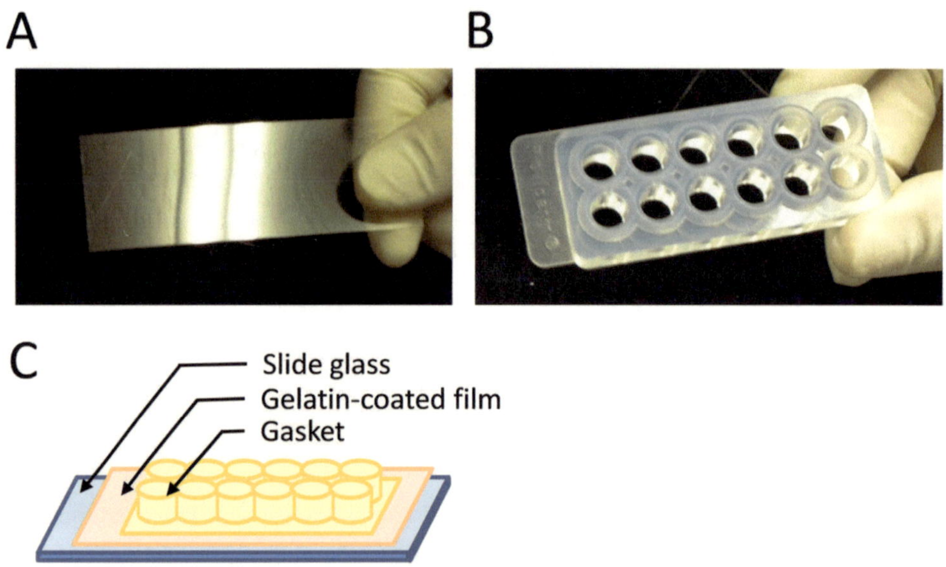

A: gelatin-coated film, B: gasket, C: illustration of the assembled detection system

Fig. 1. Gelatin-coated film and gasket

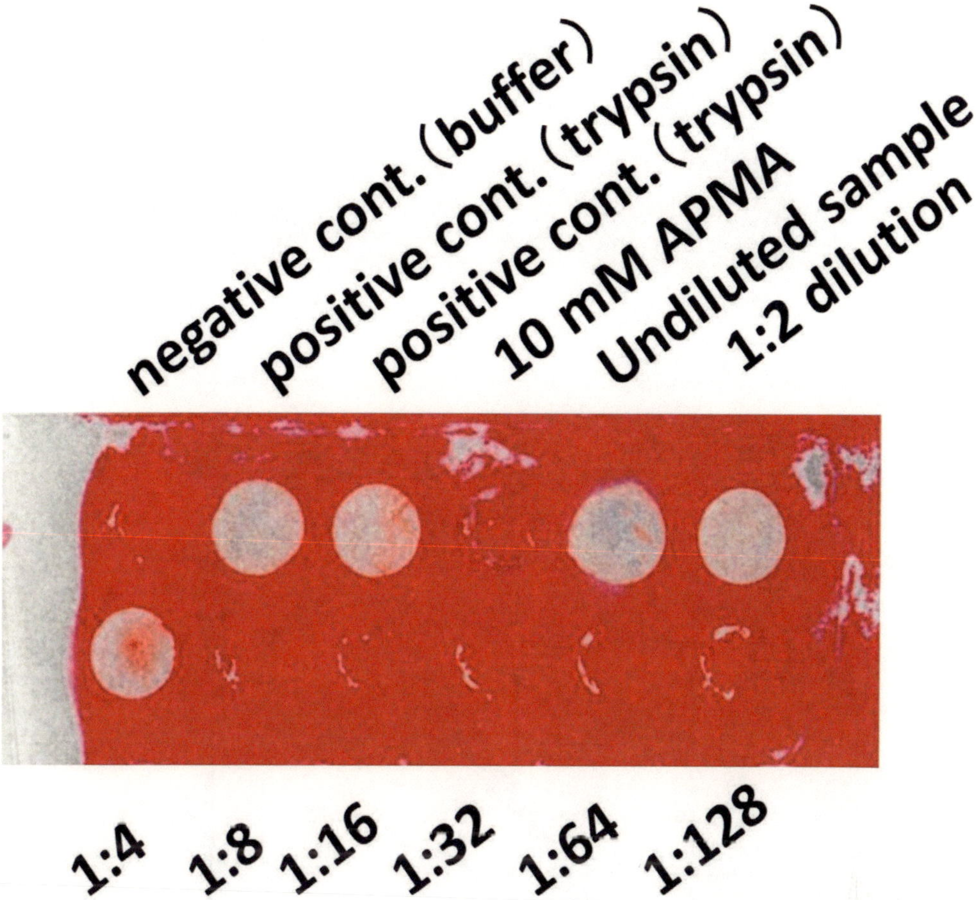

Gelatin-degraded spots are optically transparent. In this case, gelatinase activity was detected in the synovial fluid samples diluted up to 1:4.

Fig. 2. Ponceau S stained gelatin-coated film

PBS is used as a negative control, and a trypsin solution (1 and 10 μg/ml) is used as a positive control. To lower the viscosity of the synovial fluid, 15 units/μl hyaluronidase from *Streptomyces hyalyticus* (Sigma-Aldrich, St. Louis, MO, USA) is added to the synovial fluid samples. As p-aminophenylmercuric acetate (APMA) activates MMPs (Nagase et al., 1990, 1991), APMA is also added to the samples.

We demonstrated that six synovial fluid samples obtained from RA patients did not show gelatin degradation without APMA treatment (Fig. 3A, left, and Fig. 3B). However, treatment of the same samples with a final concentration of 1 mM APMA resulted in gelatin degradation (Fig. 3A, right, and Fig. 3B).

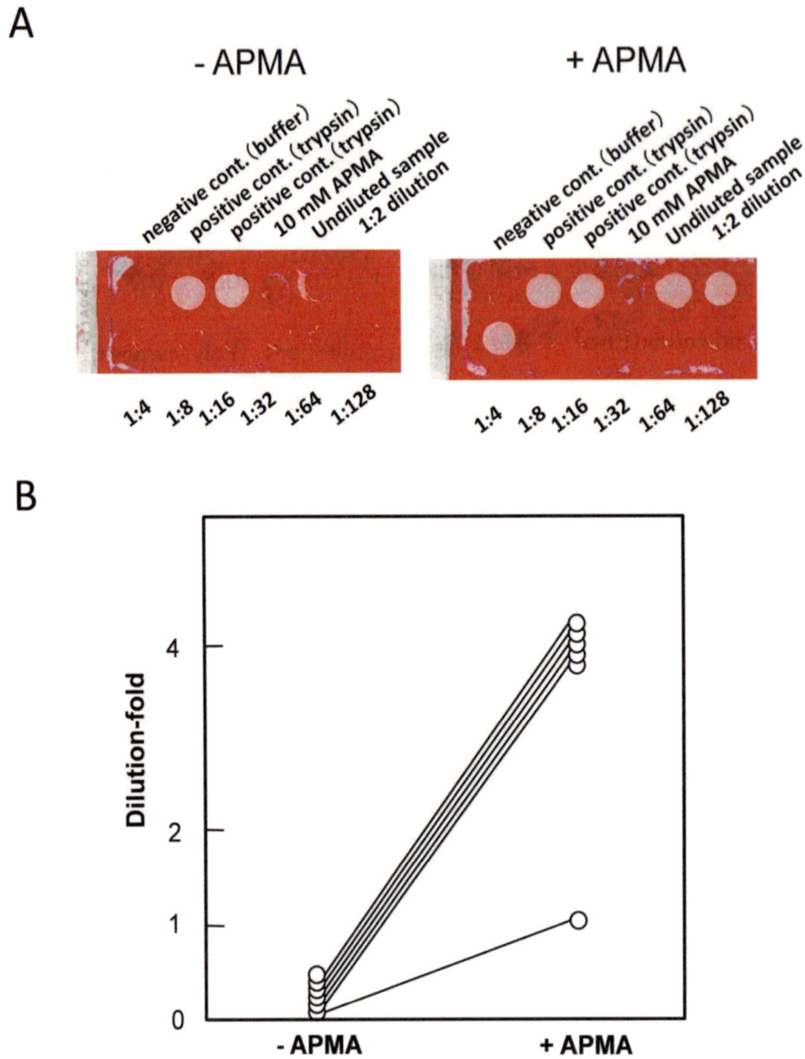

A. Gelatin-coated film incubated with synovial fluid treated with (right) and without (left) APMA. Without APMA treatment, even undiluted sample did not degrade the coated gelatin. With APMA treatment, samples diluted up to 1:4 showed gelatinase activity.
B. Change of gelatinase activity for six synovial fluid samples from RA patients following APMA treatment. The vertical axis shows the highest dilution-fold of samples that was positive for gelatinase activity. Zero indicates negative gelatinase activity.

Fig. 3. Gelatinase activity in synovial fluid samples with or without APMA treatment.

The optimal incubation time for the detection of gelatinase activity was determined by incubating synovial fluid samples for 3, 6, 12, 18, and 24 h on the gelatin-coated film. Only low levels of degradation levels were detected at 3 and 6 h (data not shown). The degradation levels at 18 and 24 h were constant for many samples (Fig. 4). In only one of seven samples, the degradation levels were elevated from 18 to 24 h. In the following experiments, the incubation time was fixed at 24 h.

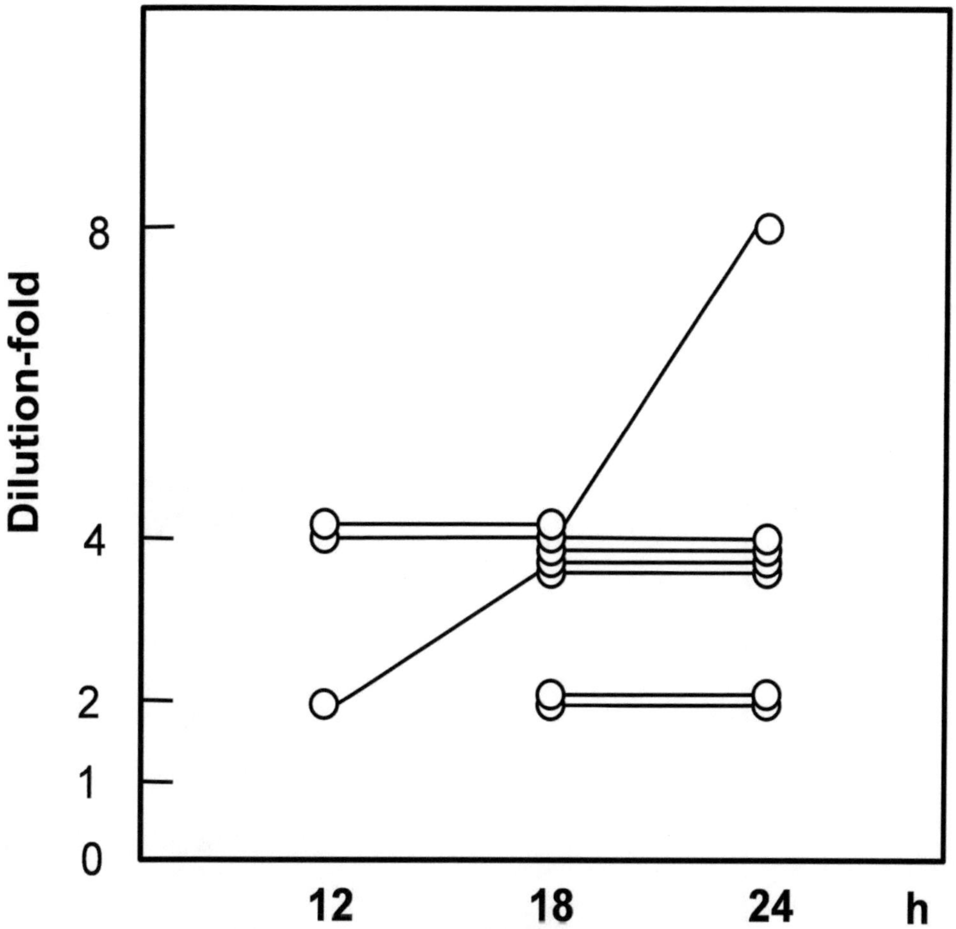

The vertical axis shows the highest dilution-fold of samples that was positive for gelatinase activity. Zero indicates negative gelatinase activity. Gelatin-coated films with synovial fluid samples were incubated for 12, 18, and 24 h.

Fig. 4. Gelatin degradation levels at various incubation times.

3. Comparison of gelatinase activity of RA and OA synovial fluid

Osteoarthritis (OA) is a disease of the joints and is caused by mechanical stress and an imbalance between catabolic and anabolic activities for cartilage (Sun, 2010). Although OA has a different etiology from RA, their mechanisms of pathogenesis are partly shared, with MMPs and ADAMTSs also playing a role in the development of OA (Huang & Wu, 2008; Murphy & Nagase, 2008; Sun, 2010). Therefore, the gelatinase activities of synovial fluid from RA and OA patients were analyzed and compared using the gelatin-coated film assay method. The synovial fluid from RA patients displayed higher proteinase activity than that from OA patients (Fig. 5), a result that is consistent with a previous study (Mahmoud et al., 2005).

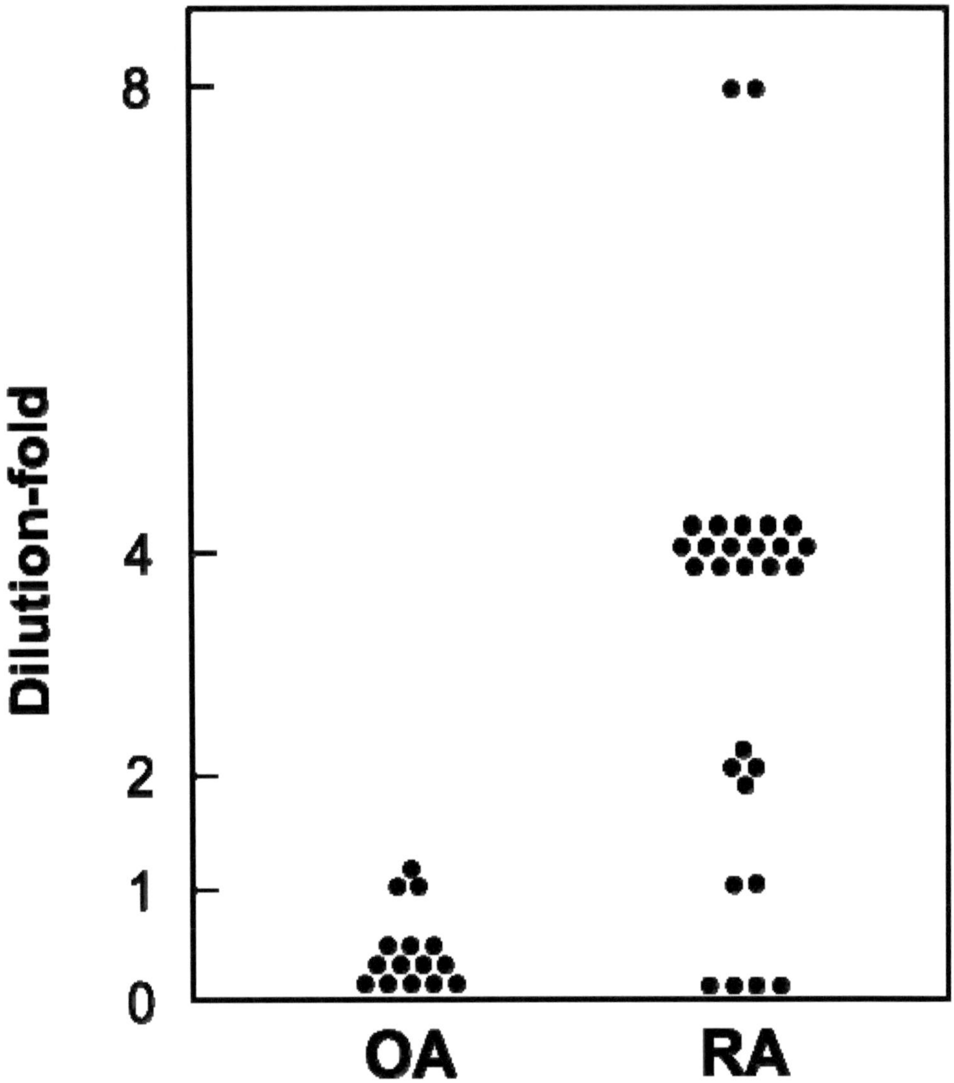

The vertical axis indicates the highest dilution-fold of sample that was positive for gelatinase activity. A value of zero indicates negative gelatinase activity. While only 3 of 15 (20%) samples from OA patients exhibited gelatinase activity, activity was detected in 24 of 28 (86%) samples from RA patients. Gelatinase activity was detected in two samples from RA patients diluted 1:8.

Fig. 5. Gelatinase activity of synovial fluid from OA and RA patients.

4. Correlation between gelatinase activity and biological marker

The concentration of proteases in serum and synovial fluid often correlates with that of biological markers. For example, MMP-3 levels significantly correlate with those of C-reactive protein (CRP) (Posthumus et al., 2003; Wassilew et al., 2010). On comparison of gelatinase activity with biological markers, it was demonstrated that samples with high gelatinase activity tended to have high CRP levels (Fig. 6).

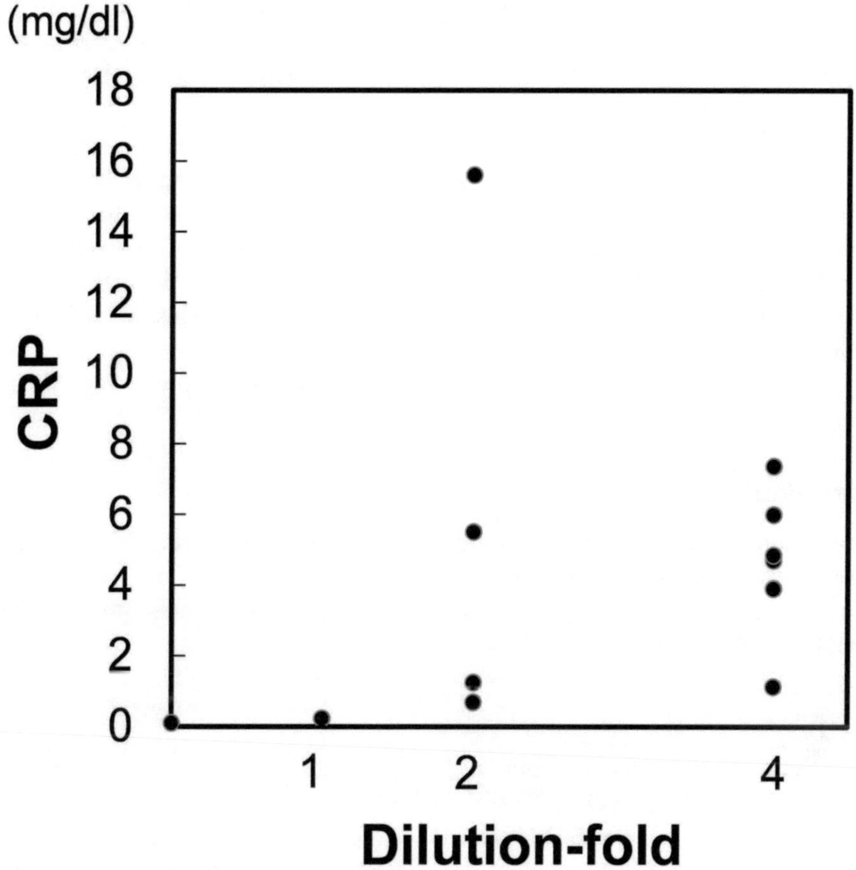

The horizontal axis represents the highest dilution-fold of synovial fluid sample that was positive for gelatinase activity from RA patients. The vertical axis indicates the CRP level.

Fig. 6. Correlation between gelatinase activity and CRP levels.

5. Conclusions

The protease MMP-3, which degrades several ECM proteins and activates a number of MMPs, is often a useful predictor of joint destruction (Mamehara et al., 2010; Yamanaka et al., 2000). However, other proteases present in synovial fluid are also involved in cartilage destruction and warrant measurement. Our method using gelatin coated-film allows the comprehensive assay of gelatinase activity, including MMP-3 and other proteases, and is thought to accurately reflect the pathological condition of RA and OA and serve as a useful tool for the prediction of joint destruction. Notably, the observed gelatinase activities of the synovial fluid from RA and OA patients assayed by this method were consistent with a previous report. Gelatinase activity measured by this method also correlated with CRP levels.

The benefits of this assay method include the capability to measure comprehensive enzyme activity and simplicity, as special instruments are not required. Despite these advantages, the detection sensitivity of the proposed method is not sufficient to detect the enzyme activities of many OA samples. Improvement of the detection sensitivity is the most important issue to address, and will provide detailed information about the gelatinase activity in synovial fluid and more closely reflect clinical conditions.

The developed assay method is expected to be a useful tool for predicting the effect of therapy for not only RA, but also OA.

6. Abbreviations

The abbreviations used are: RA, rheumatoid arthritis; OA, osteoarthritis; ECM, extracellular matrix; MMP, matrix metalloproteinase; ADAMTS, a disintegrin-like and metalloproteinase with thrombospondin type 1 motif; FIZ, film in situ zymography; APMA, p-Aminophenylmercuric acetate; CRP, C-reactive protein.

7. References

Arner EC. (2002). Aggrecanase-mediated cartilage degradation. Curr Opin Pharmacol. Vol. 2, No. 3, (Jun 2002) pp. 322-9. ISSN: 1471-4892

Chakraborti S, Mandal M, Das S, Mandal A, Chakraborti T. (2003). Regulation of matrix metalloproteinases: an overview. *Mol Cell Biochem*, Vol. 253, No. 1-2, (Nov 2003) pp. 269-85. ISSN: 0300-8177

Gendron C, Kashiwagi M, Lim NH, Enghild JJ, Thøgersen IB, Hughes C, Caterson B, Nagase H. (2007). Proteolytic activities of human ADAMTS-5: comparative studies with ADAMTS-4. *J Biol Chem*, Vol. 282, No. 25, (Jun 2007) pp. 18294-306. ISSN: 0021-9258

Huang K, Wu LD. (2008). Aggrecanase and aggrecan degradation in osteoarthritis: a review. J Int Med Res. Vol. 36, No. 6, (Nov-Dec 2008) pp. 1149-60. ISSN: 0300-0605

Lauer-Fields JL, Minond D, Sritharan T, Kashiwagi M, Nagase H, Fields GB. (2007). Substrate conformation modulates aggrecanase (ADAMTS-4) affinity and sequence specificity. Suggestion of a common topological specificity for functionally diverse proteases. *J Biol Chem*, Vol. 282, No. 1, (Jan 2007) pp. 142-50. ISSN: 0021-9258

Mahmoud RK, El-Ansary AK, El-Eishi HH, Kamal HM, El-Saeed NH. (2005). Matrix metalloproteinases MMP-3 and MMP-1 levels in sera and synovial fluids in patients with rheumatoid arthritis and osteoarthritis. *Ital J Biochem*, Vol. 54, No. 3-4, (Sep-Dec 2005) pp. 248-57, ISSN: 0021-2938

Mamehara A, Sugimoto T, Sugiyama D, Morinobu S, Tsuji G, Kawano S, Morinobu A, Kumagai S. (2010). Serum matrix metalloproteinase-3 as predictor of joint destruction in rheumatoid arthritis, treated with non-biological disease modifying anti-rheumatic drugs. *Kobe J Med Sci*, Vol. 56, No. 3, (Sep 2010) pp. E98-107. ISSN: 0023-2513

Murphy G, Nagase H. (2008). Reappraising metalloproteinases in rheumatoid arthritis and osteoarthritis: destruction or repair? Nat Clin Pract Rheumatol, Vol. 4, No. 3, (Mar 2008) pp. 128-35. ISSN: 1745-8382

Nagase H, Enghild JJ, Suzuki K, Salvesen G. (1990). Stepwise activation mechanisms of the precursor of matrix metalloproteinase 3 (stromelysin) by proteinases and (4-aminophenyl) mercuric acetate. *Biochemistry*, Vol. 29, No. 24 (Jun 1990) pp. 5783-9. ISSN: 0006-2960

Nagase H, Suzuki K, Enghild JJ, Salvesen G. (1991). Stepwise activation mechanisms of the precursors of matrix metalloproteinases 1 (tissue collagenase) and 3 (stromelysin). *Biomed Biochim Acta*, Vol. 50, No. 4-6, (1991) pp. 749-54. ISSN: 0232-766X

Posthumus MD, Limburg PC, Westra J, van Leeuwen MA, van Rijswijk MH. (2003). Serum matrix metalloproteinase 3 levels in comparison to C-reactive protein in periods with and without progression of radiological damage in patients with early rheumatoid arthritis. *Clin Exp Rheumatol*, Vol. 21, No. 4, (Jul-Aug 2003) pp. 465-72, ISSN: 0392-856X

Sun HB. (2010). Mechanical loading, cartilage degradation, and arthritis. *Ann N Y Acad Sci*, Vol. 1211, (Nov 2010) pp. 37-50. ISSN: 0077-8923

Wassilew GI, Lehnigk U, Duda GN, Taylor WR, Matziolis G, Dynybil C. (2010). The expression of proinflammatory cytokines and matrix metalloproteinases in the synovial membranes of patients with osteoarthritis compared with traumatic knee disorders. *Arthroscopy*, Vol. 26, No. 8, (Aug 2010) pp. 1096-104. ISSN: 0749-8063

Yamanaka H, Matsuda Y, Tanaka M, Sendo W, Nakajima H, Taniguchi A, Kamatani N. (2000). Serum matrix metalloproteinase 3 as a predictor of the degree of joint destruction during the six months after measurement, in patients with early rheumatoid arthritis. *Arthritis Rheum*, Vol. 43, No. 4, (Apr 2000) pp. 852-8, ISSN: 0004-3591

Yan SJ, Blomme EA. (2003). In situ zymography: a molecular pathology technique to localize endogenous protease activity in tissue sections. *Vet Pathol*, Vol. 40, No. 3 (May 2003) pp. 227-36. ISSN: 0300-9858

Yoshida W, Uzuki M, Nishida J, Shimamura T, Sawai T. (2009). Examination of in vivo gelatinolytic activity in rheumatoid arthritis synovial tissue using newly developed in situ zymography and image analyzer. *Clin Exp Rheumatol*, Vol. 27, No. 4, (Jul-Aug 2009) pp. 587-93. ISSN: 0392-856X

18

Toll-Like Receptors: At the Intersection of Osteoarthritis Pathology and Pain

Qi Wu and James L. Henry
Department of Psychiatry and Behavioural Neurosciences, McMaster University, Hamilton, Canada

1. Introduction

Osteoarthritis (OA) is a common chronic joint disease projected to affect an astounding 18% of the population in the western world by the year 2020 (Lawrence et al., 1998). In addition, it has a cost of $15.5 billion per year in the US alone, taking into account the accompanying disability and social consequences (Yelin and Callahan, 1995). Current hypotheses of OA pathology and OA pain tend to be exclusive to either. Here we present a hypothesis that is an attempt to identify a common aetiology for both.

2. OA pathology

The features of OA constitute a group of conditions that are diagnosed upon common pathological and radiological characteristics (Felson et al., 1997) and are believed to be caused by material failure of the cartilage network leading to tissue breakdown (Poole, 1999) or by injury of chondrocytes with increased degradative responses (Aigner and Kim, 2002).

3. OA pain

Pain has been defined as the primary symptom of OA (Creamer, 2000). Physicians typically rely on scores of pain and measures of joint function to make treatment decisions for OA (Swagerty, Jr. and Hellinger, 2001), as pain rather than joint pathology is more pronounced in this disorder.

4. Immunologic mechanisms in OA

OA has been considered to primarily affect cartilage and bone. However, there is increasing awareness that all tissues of the synovial joint, including synovium, ligaments and nerve terminals, are likely affected by this complex disease. Moreover, OA has been described as a non-inflammatory degenerative condition that is characterized by the imbalance of articular cartilage degradation and repair. Traumatic injury of the joint, either acute sport injuries or chronic aging accumulation is the leading cause of this imbalance. But genetic factors also play a role in some OA. Surprisingly, C-reactive protein (CRP), a systemic marker of inflammation, is increased in serum in OA patients at early phases (Saxne et al.,

2003b;Sowers et al., 2002) although it has been suggested that inflammation is actually related to complication by crystalline arthritis (Rothschild and Martin, 2006). This suggests the presence of low-grade inflammation at early stages of the disease process.

Recently, the research of the genetic linkages and the innate immune activation in OA further supports a possible pathogenic role of inflammation and a "chronic wound repair" type of immunologic mechanisms in OA (Kato et al., 2004;Scanzello et al., 2008). There have been reports about linkages between HLA haplotypes and OA, including the linkages of HLA-Cw1, 4, 10 (Wakitani et al., 2001), HLA B35-DQ1, B40-DQ1, DR2-DQ1 (Merlotti et al., 2003), HLA DR2, DR4 (Riyazi et al., 2003). These HLAs are polymorphologic molecules presenting antigens to T cells, which supports a role of immune activation at the onset of OA.

Synovial inflammation is milder than in rheumatoid arthritis (RA). Despite this, cellular infiltration of activated lymphocytes and neo-vascularisation are documented in many advanced OA, as well as patients at early stages (Walsh et al., 2007;Pearle et al., 2007;Saito et al., 2002;Saxne et al., 2003a). The severity of synovial inflammation defined by MRI is correlated with pain intensities in OA patients (Hill et al., 2007). Synovitis seen under arthroscopy is associated with cartilage degradation (Ayral et al., 2005).

Increased levels of immunoglobulins have been reported in OA. Jasin reported IgM and IgG levels in OA cartilage tissue are three times more than in normal cartilage tissue (Jasin, 1985). This suggests that antibodies are synthesized within the affected joint by infiltrating immune cells or that the cartilage is more permeable to immunoglobulins.

5. Toll-like receptors (TLRs)

TLRs are a group of pattern recognition receptors (Barton and Medzhitov, 2002), which gate the immune response. Up to now, a total of 13 TLRs have been identified -TLR1 to TLR10 in human; TLR1 to TLR13 (except TLR10) in murine (Beutler, 2005). A highly specific pattern governs the TLR recognition of various microbial ligands. Each of these TLRs responds only to a limited number of microbial ligands summarized in Table 1 of Akira and Takeda (2004).

TLRs adopt either the myeloid differentiation primary response gene 88 (MyD88)-dependent or MyD88-independent pathway following activation. TLR signalling pathways lead to the production of several critical transcription factors, including NF-κB, interferon regulatory factor (IRF) and activator protein-1 (AP-1). Three most common TLR-mediated signalling pathways are the MyD88-dependent and MyD88-independent release of NF-κB, and the MyD88-independent production of IRF. Each of TLRs seems to recruit different subsequent signalling pathways (Akira and Takeda, 2004). But detailed information remains unclear to us.

Mollen et al. (2006) proposed the theory of "TLRs and danger signalling": During tissue stress or injury, a variety of damage-associated molecules are actively secreted by stressed cells, passively released from necrotic cells, or originally from the degradation of the extracellular matrix. These damage-associated molecular patterns are recognized by TLRs in a similar manner as that of exogenous pathogen-associated molecular patterns.

A long list of damage-associated molecules have been proposed as putative endogenous TLR ligands (Beg, 2002), including hyaluronan, heparin sulphate, fibrinogen, high-mobility group protein (HMGB1), HSP 60, host mRNA, host chromatin and small ribonucleoprotein particles as well. Therefore, TLRs seem to be critical players in determining the nature of tissue injure, and initiating corresponding signalling pathways that result in distinct forms of pain.

Increasing evidence supports TLR4 as the main TLR sensing tissue damage in that it responds to a couple of endogenous ligands, such as HSP 60, fibrinogen, heparin sulphate and hyaluronan (Johnson et al., 2002;Ohashi et al., 2000;Smiley et al., 2001;Taylor et al., 2004a;Termeer et al., 2002). TLR4-dependent signalling pathway has been linked to sterile inflammation resulted from various neural and non-neural tissue injuries. Studies reveal that the production of inflammatory cytokines is compromised during tissue injuries in C3H/HeJ strain mice featured with TLR4 mutation - reduced TNF level in would incision (Bettinger et al., 1994); low circulating IL-6 in hemorrhagic shock (Prince et al., 2006); and decreased IL-1β expression at the nerve stump in sciatic nerve lesion (Boivin et al., 2007). As a consequence, the overall inflammatory response in TLR4-deficient animals is attenuated. Evidence includes reduced accumulation and activation of macrophages in injured nerve tissue (Boivin et al., 2007); less severe systemic inflammatory response (e.g. lower hepatic IL-6 level, less liver injury) after bilateral femur fracture with soft tissue crush injury (Levy et al., 2006).

TLR2 was implicated in the pathogenesis of arthritis (Cho et al., 2007). TLR2, IL-8, and vascular endothelial growth factor (VEGF) were upregulated in arthritic joints in human synovial tissue culture, which was block by anti-TLR2 antibodies. Interestingly, HMGB1 was up-regulated at the same time frame in arthritic joints in human (Kokkola et al., 2002;Taniguchi et al., 2003). HMGB1 has been proposed as the primary putative endogenous TLR2 ligand (Park et al., 2004;van Beijnum et al., 2008;Yu et al., 2006). Although there is no direct evidence for the involvement of HMGB1-TLR2-mediated pathway in arthritis, some results favour the notion. Park et al. (2006) showed the protein-protein interaction between HMGB1 and TLR2 was functional in term of initiating intracellular signal transductions. Yu et al. (2006) demonstrated that anti-TLR2 antibody blocked HMGB1-induced TLR2-dependent IL-8 release in HEK cells.

TLR3 and TLR9 are known to recognize microbial nucleic acids. However, host nucleic acids are also capable of initiating immune response via TLR activation - chromatin can induce the production of anti-DNA antibodies via a TLR9-dependent mechanism (Leadbetter et al., 2002). In Alzheimer's patients, TLR3 expression was identified in brains without previous viral infection (Jackson et al., 2006). The up-regulation of TLR3 expression might partly be explained by the finding that RNA is a constituent in senile plaques (Marcinkiewicz, 2002). The inflammatory nature of the disease may result from TLR3 activation by host RNA. Necrotic cells resulted from various processes including tissue injuries release host nucleic acids. Kariko et al. (2004) demonstrated that it was RNA released from necrotic cells that led to TLR3-dependent release of TNF-α. Necrotic cell lysates lost the capability to stimulate TNF-α release once they were pretreated with Benzonase, a potent and nonspecific nuclease that degrades all RNA into oligomers of 2–5 nucleotides in length.

6. TLR pathways in OA pathology

Age and joint trauma are two risk factors for the development and progression of OA. Endogenous damage-associated molecules, including hyaluronan, fibronectin, have been identified in OA in response to initial tissue injury. Hyaluronan is highly viscous polysaccharide found in the extracellular matrix, and is a major component of synovial fluid and cartilage, which plays an important role in the lubrication and shock absorption for the joint tissue. Its molecular weight/length is reduced in exercise and joint injury (Brown et al., 2007). In OA, both of the concentration and molecular weight of hyaluronan are reduced (Dahl et al., 1985). Hyaluronan fragments of specific sizes have been shown to promote angiogenesis and have immune regulatory effects mediated by the TLR-4 receptor (Taylor et al., 2004b). However, TLR-4 responses initiated by bacterial product lipopolysaccharide (LPS) and endogenous product hyaluronan are different, due to the recruitment of different accessory molecules, CD14 for the LPS-TLR-4 response and CD44 for the hyaluronan-TLR-4 response (Taylor et al., 2007). Fibronectin is another extracellular matrix component affected by both age and tissue injury, and the presence of fibronectin and a specific isoform containing the B sequence, Ed-B fibronectin, in osteoarthritic cartilage but not in normal cartilage has led to the suggestion that the isoform might play a role in extracellular matrix remodelling (Chevalier et al., 1996). In addition to the traditional integrin-mediated pathways, certain splice variants of fibronectin are also capable of activating a TLR-4 dependant pathway (Lasarte et al., 2007;Gondokaryono et al., 2007;Okamura et al., 2001).

Although TLRs are constitutively expressed on immune cells, the expression of TLR can be induced on other cell types as a result of IL-1 stimulation or TLR-4 activation (Matsumura et al., 2003;Kim et al., 2006;Ojaniemi et al., 2006). Radstake et al. (2004) reported the expression of TLR-2 and TLR-4 in osteoarthritic synovial membrane. Moreover, cultured synovial cells and chondrocytes from OA subjects show responsiveness to TLR-4 agonist LPS and TLR-2 agonist peptidoglycan (Kim et al., 2006;Kyburz et al., 2003;Ozawa et al., 2007). TLR-4 deficiency rescues cartilage and bone erosion in arthritis, while TLR-2 deficiency promotes the disease severity (Abdollahi-Roodsaz et al., 2008).

Activation of TLR-2 and TLR-4 recruits downstream adaptors such as MyD88 and Toll-interleukin 1 receptor domain containing adaptor protein (TIRAP), and ultimately leads to the activation of various transcription factors including IRFs, AP-1, and NF-κB. All TLR pathways are capable of activating NF-κB, and recent evidence suggests a role of NF-κB in OA. The activation of NF-κB requires the degradation of IκB bounding to it. Amos et al. (2006) showed that inhibiting NF-κB via over-expressing IκBα inhibited the production of many inflammatory and destructive mediators in OA, including TNF-α, IL-6, IL-8, oncostatin M, and metaloproteinase (MMP)-1, 3, 9, 13. The Bondeson group further showed that several MMPs and aggrecanases such as a disintegrin and metalloprotease with thrombospondin motifs 4 and 5 (ADAMTS 4, 5) are NF-κB dependent (Bondeson et al., 2007). MMP-1 and MMP-13 are capable of cleaving collagen type II, and MMP-3 cleaves other components of extracellular matrix, such as fibronectin and laminin (Yoshihara et al., 2000). ADAMTS4 and ADAMTS5 work together to cleave aggregating proteoglycan aggrecan in cartilage (Song et al., 2007;Lohmander et al., 1993). Chen et al. (2008) reported the suppression of early surgically induced OA, such as minimized synovitis and articular cartilage damage, by intra-articular delivery of NF-κBp65 specific siRNA NF-kB.

Several autoantibodies against degradative products of cartilage tissues have been identified in OA, in both humans and other animal species. These include antibodies against collagen 2 (Jasin, 1985;Niebauer et al., 1987;Osborne et al., 1995), cartilage link protein (Guerassimov et al., 1998), G1 domain proteoglycan aggrecan (Niebauer et al., 1987), cartilage intermediate layer protein (Tsuruha et al., 2001), human chondrocyte gp-39 homologous, YKL-39 (Tsuruha et al., 2002), and osteopontin (Sakata et al., 2001). Collagen II has been indentified as one of the major autoantigens in human and other animal models of RA, but much remains to be known about the autoantigen(s) driving the synovitis in OA. MyD88 dependent TLR signalling is critical for the induction of adaptive immune responses, including B-cell activation and antibody production (for review see Pasare and Medzhitov, 2005). Stimulating TLRs on B cells can result in polyclonal activation and production of low-affinity immunoglobulin M (IgM) antibodies, which may be one of mechanisms producing autoreactive antibodies (Iwasaki and Medzhitov, 2004).

7. TLR bridges traumatic injury and OA pain

Chronic pain can arise from a wide variety of causes - arthritis pain, low back pain, migraine, cancer pain, post-herpetic neuralgia, diabetic neuropathy, and others. Currently, chronic pain is explained more or less on the basis of structural abnormalities, such as osteoarthritis or herniated disk (Omoigui, 2007a). Chronic pain has not been able to be classified into well mechanism-based entities. To distinguish inflammatory pain from neuropathic pain is the best attempt so far. Hawker et al. (2008) revealed two distinct types of OA pain: an early predictable dull, aching, throbbing "background" pain and an unpredictable short episode of intense pain that develops later (Hawker et al., 2008). During the progression of OA, pain evolves from the "background" pain that is use-related in early OA (Kidd, 2006), to unpredictable short episodes of intense pain on top of the "background" pain in advanced OA (Hawker et al., 2008). However, the nature of the pain in OA still remains unclear (Hunter et al., 2008;Kidd, 2006;McDougall, 2006;Wu and Henry, 2010). Our poor understanding of chronic pain results in poor mechanism-based treatments, particularly for neuropathic pain (Gordon and Dahl, 2004;Colombo et al., 2006;Jackson, 2006;Rice and Hill, 2006;Dworkin et al., 2007).

One critical fact about chronic pain is that its nature is determined shortly after the initial insult. For example, nerve section induces neuropathic pain only, but never inflammatory pain, no matter how complicated the subsequent cytokine cascade is. Different types of tissue injury are associated with distinct forms of chronic pain. TLRs likely play an important role in the "judgment of pain" in various tissue injuries, as they are the most important interface initiating the release of cytokines following cellular response to distinct pathogen- or damage-associated molecular patterns, and they have limited yet highly specific subtypes associated with distinct intracellular signalling pathways.

The notion that inflammatory mechanisms are underlying all pain syndromes was recently proposed in two review papers (Moalem et al., 2005;Omoigui, 2007b). Alteration of the chemical environment surrounding sensory neurons changes nociception (Clatworthy et al., 1995) demonstrated that the development of the thermal hyperalgesia was tightly governed by peri-axonal inflammation. These findings lead to a re-examination of the significance of the accumulation of immune cells and inflammatory factors in nerve injuries. Cytokines likely play critical roles in the above processes. TNF-α, IL-1 and IL-6 have been shown to induced hyperalgesia if injected peripherally into the paw (Cunha et al., 1992;Ferreira et al., 1988), which can be blocked by the application of antibodies against each of these cytokines (Cunha et al., 1992;Schafers et al., 2001;Sommer et al., 1999). A second line of evidence is from inflammatory models of neuropathic pain. Those models are able to mimic neuropathic type of pain by means that are unlikely to injure sensory axons. Neuropathic pain can be induced by placing chromic gut thread next to sciatic nerve (Maves et al., 1993), by cutting ventral roots of spinal nerves which are motor efferents (Li et al., 2002;Sheth et al., 2002), by applying complete Freund's adjuvant (CFA) (Eliav et al., 1999) or zymosan (Chacur et al., 2001) around the intact sciatic nerve. Third line of evidence is from neurology clinics. Neurologists surprisingly found that pain is a common comorbidity in autoimmune diseases of nervous system: 65% of multiple sclerosis patients reported pain during the course of their disease (Kerns et al., 2002); 70-90% of Guillain-Barre syndrome patients complained pain (Pentland and Donald, 1994;Moulin et al., 1997).

A sundry of signalling pathways – such as PKA, PKC, PKG, ERK, P38 MAPK, NF-κB and JAK/STAT have been implicated to be involved in the development of chronic pain (Hanada and Yoshimura, 2002;Ji and Woolf, 2001;Obata and Noguchi, 2004). Among them, NF-κB, JAK/STAT and MAPK pathways are of particular importance in chronic pain: NF-κB pathway is the most important cellular pathway responsible for the production of inflammatory cytokines (Nguyen et al., 2002); JAK/STAT pathway is the primary pathway responsible for cytokine receptor signalling (Ihle, 1995); and MAPKs play a pivotal role in transducing extracellular stimuli into intracellular posttranslational and transcriptional responses, and are hot topics in recent pain mechanism studies, particularly ERK and P38 (Ji and Suter, 2007;Ma and Quirion, 2005;Obata and Noguchi, 2004). TLR signalling pathways have intensive crosstalk with the above mentioned pain-related pathways.

TLR and NF-κB pathway - Different adaptor molecules recruited by different TLRs result in differences in NF-κB activation. TLR signalling via the MyD88-dependent pathway leads to the early phase release of NF-κB. During TLR2 or TLR4 signalling, TIRAP/MAL is recruited to TIR domain, and then MyD88, whereas during TLR5, TLR7 or TLR9 signalling, MyD88 is recruited to TIR domain. Activation of MyD88-independent pathway downstream of TLR3 or TLR4 accounts for the late phase release of NF-κB, where TRIF is the key adaptor recruited.

TLR and IFN-JAK-STAT pathway – Type I IFNs previously were found mainly due to the activation of the MyD88-independent pathway which triggers the expression of IFN-β and chemokine genes (Sakaguchi et al., 2003). Recruitment of MyD88 by TLR7, TLR8 or TLR9 also results in the release of different set of type I IFNs, including both IFN-α and IFN-β species. (Honda et al., 2004;Takaoka and Yanai, 2006). The activation of IFN-receptors by Type I IFNs is an important mechanism linking TLR pathway and the JAK-STAT pathway (Akira and Takeda, 2004;Kawai and Akira, 2005), as the JAK-STAT pathway is one of the best characterized IFN-signalling pathways (Stark et al., 1998).

TLR and MAPK pathway - TGF-β–activated protein kinase 1 (TAK1) is a member of the MAP3K family, which is a key regulator of MAP kinase activity (Yamaguchi et al., 1995). TAK1 can be activated by TLR3 or TLR4 signalling via the MyD88-independent pathway. Moreover, another MAP3K, MEKK3 could be activated via the MyD88-dependent pathway. TLR4 but not TLR9 signalling via MEKK3 induced the activation of JNK/P38 but not ERK, suggesting differential activation of MAPKs during TLR signalling (Huang et al., 2004).

Accumulating evidence shows that TLRs are involved in chronic pain determination, likely at the level of primary sensory neurons. Dorsal root ganglion (DRG) neurons are located at the first stop of the sensory pathway. Different types of pain seem to affect different subgroups of DRG neurons. TLRs are constitutively expressed in immune cells. However, TLR expression is also found in CNS and PNS - in microglia, astrocytes (Bsibsi et al., 2002) and sensory ganglia neurons (Wadachi and Hargreaves, 2006). In polyarthritis models induced by CFA injection (Djouhri and Lawson, 1999;Xu et al., 2000), only A δ neurons and C neurons were significantly altered in electrophysiological properties, with C neurons the more severely altered. In complete sciatic nerve transection model (Abdulla and Smith, 2001), partial sciatic nerve transection model (Liu and Eisenach, 2005), or lumbar spinal nerve transection models (Kim et al., 1998;Liu et al., 2000;Ma et al., 2003;Sapunar et al., 2005;Stebbing et al., 1999), changes in A type neurons were common, even in the large size neurons. In some studies (Abdulla and Smith, 2001;Kim et al., 1998;Ma et al., 2003), changes in C neurons were also reported, but are less prominent than those in A neurons. Therefore, it seems that there are distinct changes in subgroups of DRG neurons in various chronic pain models resulted from different mechanisms, which can be regarded as pain manifestation at the neuronal level. Several TLRs have clearly established their correlation with hyperalgesia or allodynia. Compared with wild type mice, TLR2 knock-out mice showed reduced mechanical allodynia and thermal hyperalgesia after spinal nerve axotomy (Kim et al., 2007). Intrathecal administration of TLR3 antisense oligodeoxynucleotide (ODN) suppressed the spinal nerve ligation-induced tactile allodynia, whereas intrathecal injection of TLR3 agonist induced behavioural changes similar to the nerve-injury induced sensory hypersensitivity (Obata et al., 2008). TLR4 knock-out mice and the rats treated with TLR4 antisense ODN both showed significantly attenuated mechanical allodynia and thermal hyperalgesia in L5 spinal nerve transection (Tanga et al., 2005). TLR activation in microglia in spinal cord was proven to play a critical role in spinal nerve axotomy-induced sensory hypersensitivity (Kim et al., 2007;Tanga et al., 2005;Obata et al., 2008).

8. Conclusion

We propose a novel concept regarding the mechanism underlying the pain in OA induced by traumatic injuries. Following an initial trauma to the joint, two distinct yet interacting processes are initiated. One is neural injury of joint afferents and ensuing maladaptive changes of the nervous system, which results in pain in OA. The other is the cartilage degradation and bony changes in the joint, which generates characteristic pathology in OA. These two processes are likely initiated by damage-associated molecules produced during the initial joint injury, such as hyaluronan, fibronectin and proteoglycan aggrecan, mediated by pattern-recognition receptors like the TLRs. The TLR-dependent pathways lead to the activation of NF-κB and downstream transcription factors to produce various inflammatory and destructive mediators and autoantibodies. Thus, various downstream pathways, such as the MMP-mediated, ADAMTS-mediated, MAPK-mediated, are activated to generate a spectrum of osteoarthritic changes, both functional (pain) and structural (deficit in cartilage and bone deformity). TLRs, maybe other pattern-recognition receptors, are at the intersection of OA pathology and pain.

9. Acknowledgement

This work was supported by an operating grant from the Canadian Arthritis Network and the Canadian Institutes of Health Research as well as funds from McMaster University. QW was supported by the Canadian Pain Society, the Canadian Arthritis Network and the Canadian Institutes of Health Research.

10. List of abbreviations

AP-1, Activator Protein-1; **CFA,** Complete Freund's Adjuvant; **CRP,** C-Reactive Protein; **DRG,** Dorsal Root Ganglion; **HMGB,** High-Mobility Group Protein; **IRF,** Interferon Regulatory Factor; **LPS,** Lipopolysaccharide; **MyD88,** Myeloid Differentiation Primary Response Gene 88; **OA,** Osteoarthritis; **ODN,** Oligodeoxynucleotide; **RA,** Rheumatoid Arthritis; **TAK1,** Transforming Growth Factor (TGF)-β-Activated Protein Kinase 1; **TIRAP,**

Toll-**I**nterleukin 1 **R**eceptor (TIR) Domain Containing **A**daptor **P**rotein; **TLR**, **T**oll-like **R**eceptor ; **VEGF**, **V**ascular **E**ndothelial **G**rowth **F**actor

11. References

[1] Abdollahi-Roodsaz S, Joosten LA, Koenders MI, Devesa I, Roelofs MF, Radstake TR, Heuvelmans-Jacobs M, Akira S, Nicklin MJ, Ribeiro-Dias F, van den Berg WB (2008) Stimulation of TLR2 and TLR4 differentially skews the balance of T cells in a mouse model of arthritis. J Clin Invest 118:205-216.

[2] Abdulla FA, Smith PA (2001) Axotomy- and autotomy-induced changes in the excitability of rat dorsal root ganglion neurons. J Neurophysiol 85:630-643.

[3] Aigner T, Kim HA (2002) Apoptosis and cellular vitality: issues in osteoarthritic cartilage degeneration. Arthritis Rheum 46:1986-1996.

[4] Akira S, Takeda K (2004) Toll-like receptor signalling. Nat Rev Immunol 4:499-511.

[5] Amos N, Lauder S, Evans A, Feldmann M, Bondeson J (2006) Adenoviral gene transfer into osteoarthritis synovial cells using the endogenous inhibitor IkappaBalpha reveals that most, but not all, inflammatory and destructive mediators are NFkappaB dependent. Rheumatology (Oxford) 45:1201-1209.

[6] Ayral X, Pickering EH, Woodworth TG, Mackillop N, Dougados M (2005) Synovitis: a potential predictive factor of structural progression of medial tibiofemoral knee osteoarthritis -- results of a 1 year longitudinal arthroscopic study in 422 patients. Osteoarthritis Cartilage 13:361-367.

[7] Barton GM, Medzhitov R (2002) Toll-like receptors and their ligands. Curr Top Microbiol Immunol 270:81-92.

[8] Beg AA (2002) Endogenous ligands of Toll-like receptors: implications for regulating inflammatory and immune responses. Trends Immunol 23:509-512.

[9] Bettinger DA, Pellicane JV, Tarry WC, Yager DR, Diegelmann RF, Lee R, Cohen IK, DeMaria EJ (1994) The role of inflammatory cytokines in wound healing: accelerated healing in endotoxin-resistant mice. J Trauma 36:810-813.

[10] Beutler B (2005) The Toll-like receptors: analysis by forward genetic methods. Immunogenetics 57:385-392.

[11] Boivin A, Pineau I, Barrette B, Filali M, Vallieres N, Rivest S, Lacroix S (2007) Toll-like receptor signaling is critical for Wallerian degeneration and functional recovery after peripheral nerve injury. J Neurosci 27:12565-12576.

[12] Bondeson J, Lauder S, Wainwright S, Amos N, Evans A, Hughes C, Feldmann M, Caterson B (2007) Adenoviral gene transfer of the endogenous inhibitor IkappaBalpha into human osteoarthritis synovial fibroblasts demonstrates that several matrix metalloproteinases and aggrecanases are nuclear factor-kappaB-dependent. J Rheumatol 34:523-533.

[13] Brown MP, Trumble TN, Plaas AH, Sandy JD, Romano M, Hernandez J, Merritt KA (2007) Exercise and injury increase chondroitin sulfate chain length and decrease hyaluronan chain length in synovial fluid. Osteoarthritis Cartilage 15:1318-1325.

[14] Bsibsi M, Ravid R, Gveric D, van Noort JM (2002) Broad expression of Toll-like receptors in the human central nervous system. J Neuropathol Exp Neurol 61:1013-1021.

[15] Chacur M, Milligan ED, Gazda LS, Armstrong C, Wang H, Tracey KJ, Maier SF, Watkins LR (2001) A new model of sciatic inflammatory neuritis (SIN): induction of unilateral and bilateral mechanical allodynia following acute unilateral peri-sciatic immune activation in rats. Pain 94:231-244.
[16] Chen LX, Lin L, Wang HJ, Wei XL, Fu X, Zhang JY, Yu CL (2008) Suppression of early experimental osteoarthritis by in vivo delivery of the adenoviral vector-mediated NF-kappaBp65-specific siRNA. Osteoarthritis Cartilage 16:174-184.
[17] Chevalier X, Groult N, Hornebeck W (1996) Increased expression of the Ed-B-containing fibronectin (an embryonic isoform of fibronectin) in human osteoarthritic cartilage. Br J Rheumatol 35:407-415.
[18] Cho ML, Ju JH, Kim HR, Oh HJ, Kang CM, Jhun JY, Lee SY, Park MK, Min JK, Park SH, Lee SH, Kim HY (2007) Toll-like receptor 2 ligand mediates the upregulation of angiogenic factor, vascular endothelial growth factor and interleukin-8/CXCL8 in human rheumatoid synovial fibroblasts. Immunol Lett 108:121-128.
[19] Clatworthy AL, Illich PA, Castro GA, Walters ET (1995) Role of peri-axonal inflammation in the development of thermal hyperalgesia and guarding behavior in a rat model of neuropathic pain. Neurosci Lett 184:5-8.
[20] Colombo B, Annovazzi PO, Comi G (2006) Medications for neuropathic pain: current trends. Neurol Sci 27 Suppl 2:S183-S189.
[21] Creamer P (2000) Osteoarthritis pain and its treatment. Curr Opin Rheumatol 12:450-455.
[22] Cunha FQ, Poole S, Lorenzetti BB, Ferreira SH (1992) The pivotal role of tumour necrosis factor alpha in the development of inflammatory hyperalgesia. Br J Pharmacol 107:660-664.
[23] Dahl LB, Dahl IM, Engstrom-Laurent A, Granath K (1985) Concentration and molecular weight of sodium hyaluronate in synovial fluid from patients with rheumatoid arthritis and other arthropathies. Ann Rheum Dis 44:817-822.
[24] Djouhri L, Lawson SN (1999) Changes in somatic action potential shape in guinea-pig nociceptive primary afferent neurones during inflammation in vivo. J Physiol 520:565-576.
[25] Dworkin RH, O'connor AB, Backonja M, Farrar JT, Finnerup NB, Jensen TS, Kalso EA, Loeser JD, Miaskowski C, Nurmikko TJ, Portenoy RK, Rice AS, Stacey BR, Treede RD, Turk DC, Wallace MS (2007) Pharmacologic management of neuropathic pain: evidence-based recommendations. Pain 132:237-251.
[26] Eliav E, Herzberg U, Ruda MA, Bennett GJ (1999) Neuropathic pain from an experimental neuritis of the rat sciatic nerve. Pain 83:169-182.
[27] Felson DT, McAlindon TE, Anderson JJ, Naimark A, Weissman BW, Aliabadi P, Evans S, Levy D, LaValley MP (1997) Defining radiographic osteoarthritis for the whole knee. Osteoarthritis Cartilage 5:241-250.
[28] Ferreira SH, Lorenzetti BB, Bristow AF, Poole S (1988) Interleukin-1 beta as a potent hyperalgesic agent antagonized by a tripeptide analogue. Nature 334:698-700.
[29] Gondokaryono SP, Ushio H, Niyonsaba F, Hara M, Takenaka H, Jayawardana ST, Ikeda S, Okumura K, Ogawa H (2007) The extra domain A of fibronectin stimulates murine mast cells via toll-like receptor 4. J Leukoc Biol 82:657-665.
[30] Gordon DB, Dahl JL (2004) Quality improvement challenges in pain management. Pain 107:1-4.

[31] Guerassimov A, Zhang Y, Banerjee S, Cartman A, Webber C, Esdaile J, Fitzcharles MA, Poole AR (1998) Autoimmunity to cartilage link protein in patients with rheumatoid arthritis and ankylosing spondylitis. J Rheumatol 25:1480-1484.

[32] Hanada T, Yoshimura A (2002) Regulation of cytokine signaling and inflammation. Cytokine Growth Factor Rev 13:413-421.

[33] Hawker GA, Stewart L, French MR, Cibere J, Jordan JM, March L, Suarez-Almazor M, Gooberman-Hill R (2008) Understanding the pain experience in hip and knee osteoarthritis--an OARSI/OMERACT initiative. Osteoarthritis Cartilage 16:415-422.

[34] Hill CL, Hunter DJ, Niu J, Clancy M, Guermazi A, Genant H, Gale D, Grainger A, Conaghan P, Felson DT (2007) Synovitis detected on magnetic resonance imaging and its relation to pain and cartilage loss in knee osteoarthritis. Ann Rheum Dis 66:1599-1603.

[35] Honda K, Yanai H, Mizutani T, Negishi H, Shimada N, Suzuki N, Ohba Y, Takaoka A, Yeh WC, Taniguchi T (2004) Role of a transductional-transcriptional processor complex involving MyD88 and IRF-7 in Toll-like receptor signaling. Proc Natl Acad Sci U S A 101:15416-15421.

[36] Huang Q, Yang J, Lin Y, Walker C, Cheng J, Liu ZG, Su B (2004) Differential regulation of interleukin 1 receptor and Toll-like receptor signaling by MEKK3. Nat Immunol 5:98-103.

[37] Hunter DJ, McDougall JJ, Keefe FJ (2008) The symptoms of osteoarthritis and the genesis of pain. Rheum Dis Clin North Am 34:623-643.

[38] Ihle JN (1995) Cytokine receptor signalling. Nature 377:591-594.

[39] Iwasaki A, Medzhitov R (2004) Toll-like receptor control of the adaptive immune responses. Nat Immunol 5:987-995.

[40] Jackson AC, Rossiter JP, Lafon M (2006) Expression of Toll-like receptor 3 in the human cerebellar cortex in rabies, herpes simplex encephalitis, and other neurological diseases. J Neurovirol 12:229-234.

[41] Jackson KC (2006) Pharmacotherapy for neuropathic pain. Pain Pract 6:27-33.

[42] Jasin HE (1985) Autoantibody specificities of immune complexes sequestered in articular cartilage of patients with rheumatoid arthritis and osteoarthritis. Arthritis Rheum 28:241-248.

[43] Ji RR, Suter MR (2007) p38 MAPK, microglial signaling, and neuropathic pain. Mol Pain 3:33.

[44] Ji RR, Woolf CJ (2001) Neuronal plasticity and signal transduction in nociceptive neurons: implications for the initiation and maintenance of pathological pain. Neurobiol Dis 8:1-10.

[45] Johnson GB, Brunn GJ, Kodaira Y, Platt JL (2002) Receptor-mediated monitoring of tissue well-being via detection of soluble heparan sulfate by Toll-like receptor 4. J Immunol 168:5233-5239.

[46] Kariko K, Ni H, Capodici J, Lamphier M, Weissman D (2004) mRNA is an endogenous ligand for Toll-like receptor 3. J Biol Chem 279:12542-12550.

[47] Kato T, Xiang Y, Nakamura H, Nishioka K (2004) Neoantigens in osteoarthritic cartilage. Curr Opin Rheumatol 16:604-608.

[48] Kawai T, Akira S (2005) Toll-like receptor downstream signaling. Arthritis Res Ther 7:12-19.

[49] Kerns RD, Kassirer M, Otis J (2002) Pain in multiple sclerosis: a biopsychosocial perspective. J Rehabil Res Dev 39:225-232.
[50] Kidd BL (2006) Osteoarthritis and joint pain. Pain 123:6-9.
[51] Kim D, Kim MA, Cho IH, Kim MS, Lee S, Jo EK, Choi SY, Park K, Kim JS, Akira S, Na HS, Oh SB, Lee SJ (2007) A critical role of toll-like receptor 2 in nerve injury-induced spinal cord glial cell activation and pain hypersensitivity. J Biol Chem 282:14975-14983.
[52] Kim HA, Cho ML, Choi HY, Yoon CS, Jhun JY, Oh HJ, Kim HY (2006) The catabolic pathway mediated by Toll-like receptors in human osteoarthritic chondrocytes. Arthritis Rheum 54:2152-2163.
[53] Kim YI, Na HS, Kim SH, Han HC, Yoon YW, Sung B, Nam HJ, Shin SL, Hong SK (1998) Cell type-specific changes of the membrane properties of peripherally-axotomized dorsal root ganglion neurons in a rat model of neuropathic pain. Neuroscience 86:301-309.
[54] Kokkola R, Sundberg E, Ulfgren AK, Palmblad K, Li J, Wang H, Ulloa L, Yang H, Yan XJ, Furie R, Chiorazzi N, Tracey KJ, Andersson U, Harris HE (2002) High mobility group box chromosomal protein 1: a novel proinflammatory mediator in synovitis. Arthritis Rheum 46:2598-2603.
[55] Kyburz D, Rethage J, Seibl R, Lauener R, Gay RE, Carson DA, Gay S (2003) Bacterial peptidoglycans but not CpG oligodeoxynucleotides activate synovial fibroblasts by toll-like receptor signaling. Arthritis Rheum 48:642-650.
[56] Lasarte JJ, Casares N, Gorraiz M, Hervas-Stubbs S, Arribillaga L, Mansilla C, Durantez M, Llopiz D, Sarobe P, Borras-Cuesta F, Prieto J, Leclerc C (2007) The extra domain A from fibronectin targets antigens to TLR4-expressing cells and induces cytotoxic T cell responses in vivo. J Immunol 178:748-756.
[57] Lawrence RC, Helmick CG, Arnett FC, Deyo RA, Felson DT, Giannini EH, Heyse SP, Hirsch R, Hochberg MC, Hunder GG, Liang MH, Pillemer SR, Steen VD, Wolfe F (1998) Estimates of the prevalence of arthritis and selected musculoskeletal disorders in the United States. Arthritis Rheum 41:778-799.
[58] Leadbetter EA, Rifkin IR, Hohlbaum AM, Beaudette BC, Shlomchik MJ, Marshak Rothstein A (2002) Chromatin-IgG complexes activate B cells by dual engagement of IgM and Toll-like receptors. Nature 416:603-607.
[59] Levy RM, Prince JM, Yang R, Mollen KP, Liao H, Watson GA, Fink MP, Vodovotz Y, Billiar TR (2006) Systemic inflammation and remote organ damage following bilateral femur fracture requires Toll-like receptor 4. Am J Physiol Regul Integr Comp Physiol 291:R970-R976.
[60] Li L, Xian CJ, Zhong JH, Zhou XF (2002) Effect of lumbar 5 ventral root transection on pain behaviors: a novel rat model for neuropathic pain without axotomy of primary sensory neurons. Exp Neurol 175:23-34.
[61] Liu B, Eisenach JC (2005) Hyperexcitability of axotomized and neighboring unaxotomized sensory neurons is reduced days after perineural clonidine at the site of injury. J Neurophysiol 94:3159-3167.
[62] Liu CN, Wall PD, Ben-Dor E, Michaelis M, Amir R, Devor M (2000) Tactile allodynia in the absence of C-fiber activation: altered firing properties of DRG neurons following spinal nerve injury. Pain 85:503-521.

[63] Lohmander LS, Neame PJ, Sandy JD (1993) The structure of aggrecan fragments in human synovial fluid. Evidence that aggrecanase mediates cartilage degradation in inflammatory joint disease, joint injury, and osteoarthritis. Arthritis Rheum 36:1214-1222.

[64] Ma C, Shu Y, Zheng Z, Chen Y, Yao H, Greenquist KW, White FA, LaMotte RH (2003) Similar electrophysiological changes in axotomized and neighboring intact dorsal root ganglion neurons. J Neurophysiol 89:1588-1602.

[65] Ma W, Quirion R (2005) The ERK/MAPK pathway, as a target for the treatment of neuropathic pain. Expert Opin Ther Targets 9:699-713.

[66] Marcinkiewicz M (2002) BetaAPP and furin mRNA concentrates in immature senile plaques in the brain of Alzheimer patients. J Neuropathol Exp Neurol 61:815-829.

[67] Matsumura T, Degawa T, Takii T, Hayashi H, Okamoto T, Inoue J, Onozaki K (2003) TRAF6-NF-kappaB pathway is essential for interleukin-1-induced TLR2 expression and its functional response to TLR2 ligand in murine hepatocytes. Immunology 109:127-136.

[68] Maves TJ, Pechman PS, Gebhart GF, Meller ST (1993) Possible chemical contribution from chromic gut sutures produces disorders of pain sensation like those seen in man. Pain 54:57-69.

[69] McDougall JJ (2006) Pain and OA. J Musculoskelet Neuronal Interact 6:385-386.

[70] Merlotti D, Santacroce C, Gennari L, Geraci S, Acquafredda V, Conti T, Bargagli G, Canto ND, Biagi F, Gennari C, Giordano N (2003) HLA antigens and primary osteoarthritis of the hand. J Rheumatol 30:1298-1304.

[71] Moalem G, Grafe P, Tracey DJ (2005) Chemical mediators enhance the excitability of unmyelinated sensory axons in normal and injured peripheral nerve of the rat. Neuroscience 134:1399-1411.

[72] Mollen KP, Anand RJ, Tsung A, Prince JM, Levy RM, Billiar TR (2006) Emerging paradigm: toll-like receptor 4-sentinel for the detection of tissue damage. Shock 26:430-437.

[73] Moulin DE, Hagen N, Feasby TE, Amireh R, Hahn A (1997) Pain in Guillain-Barre syndrome. Neurology 48:328-331.

[74] Nguyen MD, Julien JP, Rivest S (2002) Innate immunity: the missing link in neuroprotection and neurodegeneration? Nat Rev Neurosci 3:216-227.

[75] Niebauer GW, Wolf B, Bashey RI, Newton CD (1987) Antibodies to canine collagen types I and II in dogs with spontaneous cruciate ligament rupture and osteoarthritis. Arthritis Rheum 30:319-327.

[76] Obata K, Katsura H, Miyoshi K, Kondo T, Yamanaka H, Kobayashi K, Dai Y, Fukuoka T, Akira S, Noguchi K (2008) Toll-like receptor 3 contributes to spinal glial activation and tactile allodynia after nerve injury. J Neurochem.

[77] Obata K, Noguchi K (2004) MAPK activation in nociceptive neurons and pain hypersensitivity. Life Sci 74:2643-2653.

[78] Ohashi K, Burkart V, Flohe S, Kolb H (2000) Cutting edge: heat shock protein 60 is a putative endogenous ligand of the toll-like receptor-4 complex. J Immunol 164:558-561.

[79] Ojaniemi M, Liljeroos M, Harju K, Sormunen R, Vuolteenaho R, Hallman M (2006) TLR-2 is upregulated and mobilized to the hepatocyte plasma membrane in the space of

Disse and to the Kupffer cells TLR-4 dependently during acute endotoxemia in mice. Immunol Lett 102:158-168.

[80] Okamura Y, Watari M, Jerud ES, Young DW, Ishizaka ST, Rose J, Chow JC, Strauss JF, III (2001) The extra domain A of fibronectin activates Toll-like receptor 4. J Biol Chem 276:10229-10233.

[81] Omoigui S (2007b) The biochemical origin of pain: the origin of all pain is inflammation and the inflammatory response. Part 2 of 3 - inflammatory profile of pain syndromes. Med Hypotheses 69:1169-1178.

[82] Omoigui S (2007a) The biochemical origin of pain--proposing a new law of pain: the origin of all pain is inflammation and the inflammatory response. Part 1 of 3--a unifying law of pain. Med Hypotheses 69:70-82.

[83] Osborne AC, Carter SD, May SA, Bennett D (1995) Anti-collagen antibodies and immune complexes in equine joint diseases. Vet Immunol Immunopathol 45:19-30.

[84] Ozawa T, Koyama K, Ando T, Ohnuma Y, Hatsushika K, Ohba T, Sugiyama H, Hamada Y, Ogawa H, Okumura K, Nakao A (2007) Thymic stromal lymphopoietin secretion of synovial fibroblasts is positively and negatively regulated by Toll-like receptors/nuclear factor-kappaB pathway and interferon-gamma/dexamethasone. Mod Rheumatol 17:459-463.

[86] Park JS, Svetkauskaite D, He Q, Kim JY, Strassheim D, Ishizaka A, Abraham E (2004) Involvement of toll-like receptors 2 and 4 in cellular activation by high mobility group box 1 protein. J Biol Chem 279:7370-7377.

[87] Pasare C, Medzhitov R (2005) Control of B-cell responses by Toll-like receptors. Nature 438:364-368.

[88] Pearle AD, Scanzello CR, George S, Mandl LA, DiCarlo EF, Peterson M, Sculco TP, Crow MK (2007) Elevated high-sensitivity C-reactive protein levels are associated with local inflammatory findings in patients with osteoarthritis. Osteoarthritis Cartilage 15:516-523.

[89] Pentland B, Donald SM (1994) Pain in the Guillain-Barre syndrome: a clinical review. Pain 59:159-164.

[90] Poole AR (1999) An introduction to the pathophysiology of osteoarthritis. Front Biosci 4:D662-D670.

[91] Prince JM, Levy RM, Yang R, Mollen KP, Fink MP, Vodovotz Y, Billiar TR (2006) Toll-like receptor-4 signaling mediates hepatic injury and systemic inflammation in hemorrhagic shock. J Am Coll Surg 202:407-417.

[92] Radstake TR, Roelofs MF, Jenniskens YM, Oppers-Walgreen B, van Riel PL, Barrera P, Joosten LA, van den Berg WB (2004) Expression of toll-like receptors 2 and 4 in rheumatoid synovial tissue and regulation by proinflammatory cytokines interleukin-12 and interleukin-18 via interferon-gamma. Arthritis Rheum 50:3856-3865.

[93] Rice AS, Hill RG (2006) New treatments for neuropathic pain. Annu Rev Med 57:535-551.

[94] Riyazi N, Spee J, Huizinga TW, Schreuder GM, de Vries RR, Dekker FW, Kloppenburg M (2003) HLA class II is associated with distal interphalangeal osteoarthritis. Ann Rheum Dis 62:227-230.

[95] Rothschild BM, Martin LD. Skeletal Impact of Disease. Albuquerque: New Mexico Museum of Natural History Press, 2006.

[96] Saito I, Koshino T, Nakashima K, Uesugi M, Saito T (2002) Increased cellular infiltrate in inflammatory synovia of osteoarthritic knees. Osteoarthritis Cartilage 10:156-162.
[97] Sakaguchi S, Negishi H, Asagiri M, Nakajima C, Mizutani T, Takaoka A, Honda K, Taniguchi T (2003) Essential role of IRF-3 in lipopolysaccharide-induced interferon-beta gene expression and endotoxin shock. Biochem Biophys Res Commun 306:860-866.
[98] Sakata M, Tsuruha JI, Masuko-Hongo K, Nakamura H, Matsui T, Sudo A, Nishioka K, Kato T (2001) Autoantibodies to osteopontin in patients with osteoarthritis and rheumatoid arthritis. J Rheumatol 28:1492-1495.
[99] Sapunar D, Ljubkovic M, Lirk P, McCallum JB, Hogan QH (2005) Distinct membrane effects of spinal nerve ligation on injured and adjacent dorsal root ganglion neurons in rats. Anesthesiology 103:360-376.
[100] Saxne T, Lindell M, Mansson B, Petersson IF, Heinegard D (2003a) Inflammation is a feature of the disease process in early knee joint osteoarthritis. Rheumatology (Oxford) 42:903-904.
[101] Saxne T, Lindell M, Mansson B, Petersson IF, Heinegard D (2003b) Inflammation is a feature of the disease process in early knee joint osteoarthritis. Rheumatology (Oxford) 42:903-904.
[102] Scanzello CR, Plaas A, Crow MK (2008) Innate immune system activation in osteoarthritis: is osteoarthritis a chronic wound? Curr Opin Rheumatol 20:565-572.
[103] Schafers M, Brinkhoff J, Neukirchen S, Marziniak M, Sommer C (2001) Combined epineurial therapy with neutralizing antibodies to tumor necrosis factor-alpha and interleukin-1 receptor has an additive effect in reducing neuropathic pain in mice. Neurosci Lett 310:113-116.
[104] Sheth RN, Dorsi MJ, Li Y, Murinson BB, Belzberg AJ, Griffin JW, Meyer RA (2002) Mechanical hyperalgesia after an L5 ventral rhizotomy or an L5 ganglionectomy in the rat. Pain 96:63-72.
[105] Smiley ST, King JA, Hancock WW (2001) Fibrinogen stimulates macrophage chemokine secretion through toll-like receptor 4. J Immunol 167:2887-2894.
[106] Sommer C, Petrausch S, Lindenlaub T, Toyka KV (1999) Neutralizing antibodies to interleukin 1-receptor reduce pain associated behavior in mice with experimental neuropathy. Neurosci Lett 270:25-28.
[107] Song RH, Tortorella MD, Malfait AM, Alston JT, Yang Z, Arner EC, Griggs DW (2007) Aggrecan degradation in human articular cartilage explants is mediated by both ADAMTS-4 and ADAMTS-5. Arthritis Rheum 56:575-585.
[108] Sowers M, Jannausch M, Stein E, Jamadar D, Hochberg M, Lachance L (2002) C-reactive protein as a biomarker of emergent osteoarthritis. Osteoarthritis Cartilage 10:595-601.
[109] Stark GR, Kerr IM, Williams BR, Silverman RH, Schreiber RD (1998) How cells respond to interferons. Annu Rev Biochem 67:227-264.
[110] Stebbing MJ, Eschenfelder S, Habler HJ, Acosta MC, Janig W, McLachlan EM (1999) Changes in the action potential in sensory neurones after peripheral axotomy in vivo. Neuroreport 10:201-206.

[111] Swagerty DL, Jr., Hellinger D (2001) Radiographic assessment of osteoarthritis. Am Fam Physician 64:279-286.

[112] Takaoka A, Yanai H (2006) Interferon signalling network in innate defence. Cell Microbiol 8:907-922.

[113] Tanga FY, Nutile-McMenemy N, DeLeo JA (2005) The CNS role of Toll-like receptor 4 in innate neuroimmunity and painful neuropathy. Proc Natl Acad Sci U S A 102:5856-5861.

[114] Taniguchi N, Kawahara K, Yone K, Hashiguchi T, Yamakuchi M, Goto M, Inoue K, Yamada S, Ijiri K, Matsunaga S, Nakajima T, Komiya S, Maruyama I (2003) High mobility group box chromosomal protein 1 plays a role in the pathogenesis of rheumatoid arthritis as a novel cytokine. Arthritis Rheum 48:971-981.

[115] Taylor KR, Trowbridge JM, Rudisill JA, Termeer CC, Simon JC, Gallo RL (2004a) Hyaluronan fragments stimulate endothelial recognition of injury through TLR4. J Biol Chem 279:17079-17084.

[116] Taylor KR, Trowbridge JM, Rudisill JA, Termeer CC, Simon JC, Gallo RL (2004b) Hyaluronan fragments stimulate endothelial recognition of injury through TLR4. J Biol Chem 279:17079-17084.

[117] Taylor KR, Yamasaki K, Radek KA, Di NA, Goodarzi H, Golenbock D, Beutler B, Gallo RL (2007) Recognition of hyaluronan released in sterile injury involves a unique receptor complex dependent on Toll-like receptor 4, CD44, and MD-2. J Biol Chem 282:18265-18275.

[118] Termeer C, Benedix F, Sleeman J, Fieber C, Voith U, Ahrens T, Miyake K, Freudenberg M, Galanos C, Simon JC (2002) Oligosaccharides of Hyaluronan activate dendritic cells via toll-like receptor 4. J Exp Med 195:99-111.

[119] Tsuruha J, Masuko-Hongo K, Kato T, Sakata M, Nakamura H, Nishioka K (2001) Implication of cartilage intermediate layer protein in cartilage destruction in subsets of patients with osteoarthritis and rheumatoid arthritis. Arthritis Rheum 44:838-845.

[120] Tsuruha J, Masuko-Hongo K, Kato T, Sakata M, Nakamura H, Sekine T, Takigawa M, Nishioka K (2002) Autoimmunity against YKL-39, a human cartilage derived protein, in patients with osteoarthritis. J Rheumatol 29:1459-1466.

[121] van Beijnum JR, Buurman WA, Griffioen AW (2008) Convergence and amplification of toll-like receptor (TLR) and receptor for advanced glycation end products (RAGE) signaling pathways via high mobility group B1 (HMGB1). Angiogenesis 11:91-99.

[122] Wadachi R, Hargreaves KM (2006) Trigeminal nociceptors express TLR-4 and CD14: a mechanism for pain due to infection. J Dent Res 85:49-53.

[123] Wakitani S, Imoto K, Mazuka T, Kim S, Murata N, Yoneda M (2001) Japanese generalised osteoarthritis was associated with HLA class I--a study of HLA-A, B, Cw, DQ, DR in 72 patients. Clin Rheumatol 20:417-419.

[124] Walsh DA, Bonnet CS, Turner EL, Wilson D, Situ M, McWilliams DF (2007) Angiogenesis in the synovium and at the osteochondral junction in osteoarthritis. Osteoarthritis Cartilage 15:743-751.

[125] Wu Q, Henry JL (2010) Changes in Aβ non-nociceptive primary sensory neurons in a rat model of osteoarthritis pain. Mol Pain 6:37.

[126] Xu GY, Huang LY, Zhao ZQ (2000) Activation of silent mechanoreceptive cat C and Adelta sensory neurons and their substance P expression following peripheral inflammation. J Physiol 528:339-348.

[127] Yamaguchi K, Shirakabe K, Shibuya H, Irie K, Oishi I, Ueno N, Taniguchi T, Nishida E, Matsumoto K (1995) Identification of a member of the MAPKKK family as a potential mediator of TGF-beta signal transduction. Science 270:2008-2011.

[128] Yelin E, Callahan LF (1995) The economic cost and social and psychological impact of musculoskeletal conditions. National Arthritis Data Work Groups. Arthritis Rheum 38:1351-1362.

[129] Yoshihara Y, Nakamura H, Obata K, Yamada H, Hayakawa T, Fujikawa K, Okada Y (2000) Matrix metalloproteinases and tissue inhibitors of metalloproteinases in synovial fluids from patients with rheumatoid arthritis or osteoarthritis. Ann Rheum Dis 59:455-461.

[130] Yu M, Wang H, Ding A, Golenbock DT, Latz E, Czura CJ, Fenton MJ, Tracey KJ, Yang H (2006) HMGB1 signals through toll-like receptor (TLR) 4 and TLR2. Shock 26:174-179.

19

Anion Channels in Osteoarthritic Chondrocytes

Elizabeth Perez-Hernandez[1], Nury Perez-Hernandez[2], Fidel de la C. Hernandez-Hernandez[3] and Juan B. Kouri-Flores[3]
[1]*Hospital de Ortopedia Dr. Victorio de la Fuente Narváez –IMSS,*
[2]*Departamento de Biomedicina Molecular, Escuela Nacional de Medicina y Homeopatía- IPN,*
[3]*Departamento de Infectómica y Patogénesis Molecular, CINVESTAV-IPN, México*

1. Introduction

Osteoarthritis (OA) is the most common form of arthritis and represents a global health problem. OA is estimated to affect 40% of the population over 70 years of age and is a major cause of pain and physical disability (Lawrence, 2008). This is a condition that predominantly involves hip, knee, spine, foot and hands. Several risk factors have been associated with the initiation and progression of OA, increasing age, sex, obesity, occupational loading, malalignment, articular trauma and crystal deposition.

OA is a chronic degenerative joint disorder characterized primarily by destruction of articular cartilage, formation of reparative fibrocartilage and subchondral bone remodelling. However, not only the cartilage and bone are affected, also the synovium and the joint-stabilizing structures such as ligaments and meniscus (Baker-LePain, 2010). Apparently, all the tissues of the joint respond to mechanical stress with the consequent loss of function and clinical deterioration.

The application of mechanical forces under physiological conditions is a preponderant factor in cartilage homeostasis. It is now well know, that environmental factors, such as compressive and tensile forces, load and shear stress have a significant influence on the chondrocyte metabolism. Also, conditions that alter the load distribution on the articular surface can induce the development of OA (Roos, 2005).

This degradative process of the cartilage in OA is a consequence of an imbalance between anabolism and catabolism of chondrocytes. Generally, chondrocytes respond with increased expression of inflammatory mediators and matrix-degrading proteinases (Kurz, 2005).

Other effect observed in chondrocytes under mechanical stimulation is the change in membrane and osmotic potential (Wright, 1992, Bush, 2001). In OA, chondrocytes undergo depolarization instead of hyperpolarization (Millward-Sadler, 2000), and the decrease of the osmotic potential has been associated with loss of volume control in early stages of OA (Stockwell, 1991, Bush, 2003). However, the sequence of mechanobiological events necessary for the maintenance of extracellular matrix (ECM) homeostasis and its involvement in the pathogenesis of OA is still poorly understood.

2. Articular cartilage structure

Articular cartilage is a specialized connective tissue that contains a single cell type, the chondrocytes, embedded in an ECM which is composed of water and macromolecules. Collagens, proteoglycans and noncollagenous proteins are the main components of matrix. The chondrocytes are highly differentiated cells and constitute 1% of the total cartilage volume (Stockwell, 1967). These cells are responsible of the production and organization of ECM. Cartilage is divided into four horizontal zones: superficial, transitional o middle, radial o deep, and calcified zones. Each of these layers has specific morphological and functional characteristics related to the metabolic activity.

In the superficial zone, chondrocytes are flattened and oriented parallel to the surface. This layer consists of a low proportion of proteoglycans, thin collagen fibers and higher water content (Weiss, 1968). Functionally, this zone is responsible of the highest resistance to compressive forces during joint movement.

The transitional or middle zone consist of rounded chondrocytes, a network of collagen fibers arranged radially and an increased proteoglycan content.

In the deep zone, the chondrocytes are grouped in perpendicular columns to the articular surface. This layer contains the highest proportion of aggrecan and long collagen fibers, approximately of 55 μm across (Minns, 1977).

The calcified zone links and anchors the articular cartilage to subchondral bone through collagen fibers arranged perpendicularly. The hypertrophic chondrocytes are scarce and located in uncalcified lacunae.

Also, the matrix is subdivided into the pericellular, territorial and interterritorial regions which are arranged around the chondrocytes. The pericellular matrix is composed for sulfated proteoglycans and glycoproteins. They provide protection to chondrocytes when exposed to chondrocyte load and maintain water homeostasis. Together, the chondrocyte and pericellular matrix constitute the chondron (Poole, 1997). Adjacent to this region, the territorial matrix contains a dense meshwork of collagen fibers that provide mechanical protection to the chondrocytes. The concentration of proteoglycans rich in chondroitin sulfate is higher in this region. In the interterritorial region predominates proteoglycans rich in keratan sulfate and the collagen fibers of largest diameter (Stockwell, 1990).

The biochemical properties of cartilage are dependent of the integrity of the matrix. In the ECM of mature mammalian articular cartilage, the collagen represents 50-60% dry weight. The network consists of collagen IX (1%), collagen XI (3%) and collagen II (≥90%) (Eyre, 1987). Type II collagen, a fibrillar protein, is composed of three identical α-1 chains in form triple helix and constitutes the basic structure of cartilage. Type XI collagen is probably copolymerized and type IX collagen is covalently linked to the type II collagen fibrils (Mendler, 1989). Among other types of collagen found in cartilage, type X collagen is described in the calcified zone (Gannon, 1991), type VI collagen promotes the chondrocyte-matrix attachment (Wu, 1987) and type III collagen is copolymerized and linked to collagen II (Wu, 1996). Generally, these collagen fibers provided to the cartilage the tensile stiffness and strength.

The second largest component of the ECM are the proteoglycans, which constitute 5 to 10% of the tissue wet weight. These are molecules consisting of glycosaminglycans (GAGs) chains bound to a protein core. Also, the aggrecan are composed of proteoglycan aggregates in association with hyaluronic acid (HA) and link protein (Hardingham, 1974). The keratan sulfate and chondroitin sulfate are the main types of GAGs. The anionic groups of aggrecan attract cations such as Na^+, this allows an osmotic imbalance and the accumulation of fluid in the ECM, which is critical for the biomechanical properties of cartilage. Collagen fibrils interact with aggrecan monomers in the keratan sulfate-rich regions (Hedlund, 1999). Other proteoglycans include decorin, biglycan, lumican and fibromodulin, consisting of small leucine-rich repeat. They bind to fibrillar collagen via its core protein regulating the fibril diameter and fibril-fibril interaction in the ECM.

In addition, there are nocollagenous proteins such as fibronectin and tenascin favoring chondrocyte-matrix interaction.

3. Chondrocytes mechanotransduction

The articular cartilage is continuously exposed to mechanical stress which significantly affects the response of chondrocytes to their environment (Grodzinsky, 2000). Under conditions of continuous compression, the chondrocytes undergo changes in potential membrane (Wright, 1992), matrix water content, ion concentrations and pH (Mobasheri, 1998; Mow, 1999). The process of converting physical forces into biochemical signals and the subsequent transduction into cellular responses is referred to as mechanotransduction (Huang, 2004).

Miscellaneous "mechanoreceptors" including ion channels and cell adhesion molecules, such as integrins have been described in chondrocytes. Thus far, α1β1 integrin, a receptor for collagen, α5β1 integrin, a receptor for fibronectin and αVβ5 integrin, a receptor for vitronectin have been implicated in the regulation of chondrocyte behaviour (Ostergaard, 1998; Loeser, 1995). Voltage-gated Na^+ and K^+ channels (Sugimoto, 1996), epithelial sodium channels (ENaC) (Mobasheri, 1999) and N-/L-type voltage-gated Ca^{2+} channels (Wang, 2000) have been considered as potential mechanosensitive ion channels.

3.1 Membrane potential

The negative resting membrane potential (RMP) in most cells, is the result from activity of K^+ (Wilson, 2004) and Cl^- channels (ClC) (Tsuga, 2002; Funabashi, 2010). In chondrocytes, the RMP ranging from -10.6 mV to -46 mV (Wright, 1992; Clark, 2010; Lewis 2011), and those values are determined by the influx and efflux of cations and anions in the cell membrane. Consequently, the stability of the ECM is linked to the ionic changes and the RMP in chondrocytes. Several studies related the use of ionic blockers such as lidocaine and verapamil, showed a decrease in the synthesis of GAGs (Wu, 2000; Mouw, 2007), inhibition of chondrocytes proliferation (Wohlrab, 2002) and induction of apoptosis (Wohlrab, 2005). The permeability of ion channels is regulated by chondrocyte channelome (Barret-Jolley, 2010).

The ion channels so far identified in chondrocytes are summarized in Table 1.

The membrane potential in articular chondrocytes is primarily related to the Cl^- conductance greater than K^+ conductance (Tsuga, 2002; Funabashi, 2010). More recently, it was showed the involvement of TRPV5 (gadolinium-sensitive cation channels) in the relatively positive RMP of the chondrocytes. Furthermore, has been suggested that the positive membrane potential is due to TRVP5 higher than that generated by potassium ions, which would allow efflux of potassium ions into the cell limiting the increase in cell volume in situations of reduced osmolarity (Lewis, 2011).

Ion channels	Reference
Voltage-gated K^+ channels	Walsh, 1992 Sugimoto, 1996 Wilson, 2004 Mobasheri, 2005 Ponce, 2006 Clark, 2010
Voltage-gated Na^+ channels	Sugimoto, 1996 Ramage, 2008
Voltage-gated Ca^{2+} channels	Shakibaei, 2003 Sanchez, 2004 Mancilla, 2007 Xu, 2009
Voltage-activated H^+ channels	Sanchez, 2006
Cl^- channels (ClC)	Sugimoto, 1996 Tsuga, 2002 Isoya, 2009 Okumura, 2009 Funabashi, 2010 Perez, 2010
ATP-dependent K^+ channels	Mobasheri, 2007
Ca^{2+}-dependent K^+ channels	Grandolfo, 1992 Long, 1994 Martina, 1997 Mozrzymas, 1997 Mobasheri, 2010
Transient receptor potential (TRP) channel	Sanchez, 2003 Phan, 2009 Lewis, 2010
Epithelial sodium channels (ENaC)	Trujillo, 1999 Shakibaei, 2003 Lewis, 2008

Table 1. Ion channels described in chondrocytes

Therefore, it has been proposed that the ClCs functions in chondrocytes could be involved in setting of the membrane potential or anionic osmolyte channels (Barret-Jolley, 2010).

3.2 Mechanotransduction in osteoarthritic chondrocytes

In vivo, the extracellular environment surrounding the chondrocytes is negatively charged and provides a high osmolarity, from 480 mOsm to 55 0mOsm under load (Urban, 1993; 1994; Xu, 2010). Under physiological conditions, chondrocytes are able to regulate their volume through osmotic pressure cycles (Bush, 2001). However, in OA, the chondrocytes have decreased osmotic potential and increased water content (Stockwell, 1991). Furthermore, in osteoarthritic chondrocytes described a high recovery of the increased volume, which promotes the progression of the disease (Jones, 1999; Bush, 2005).

In this matter, in the superficial and middle zones of normal cartilage and the zone of fibrillated osteoarthritic cartilage has been demonstrated the expression of ATP-dependent K^+ channels (Mobasheri, 2007). Under normal conditions, mechanical stimulation produces hyperpolarization of the membrane of chondrocytes, but in OA the depolarization is induced. According to studies preformed with sodium channel blockers, this response could be due to the involvement of Ca^{2+}-dependent K^+ channels (stretch-activated channels) in the process of chondrocyte mechanotransduction (Wright, 1996).

In osteoarthritic chondrocytes has been suggested that the response of membrane depolarization is due to the autocrine / paracrine activity of soluble factors. *In vitro*, mechanical stimulation of chondrocytes at 0.33 Hz induces membrane hyperpolarization due to IL-4 (Millward-Sadler, 1999) with the consequent increase in aggrecan mRNA levels. Interestingly, in osteoarthritic condrocytes, membrane depolarization is induced by proinflammatory cytokine IL-1 (Salter, 2002). Altered mechanotransduction in OA may contribute to the response of the chondrocyte favoring ECM degradation and disease progression.

Moreover, osmotic fluctuations, in addition to the volume change in chondrocytes (Bush, 2005; Kerrigan, 2006; Lewis, 2011) involve the filamentous actin restructuring (Chao, 2006; Erickson, 2003). Similarly, the osmotic stimulation of chondrocytes increases cytosolic calcium concentrations with the consequent regulation of metabolism, cell volume, and gene expression (Liu, 2006; Hardingham, 1999). In this case, a possible candidate in the chondrocyte mechanotransduction is the transient receptor potential vanilloid 4 channel (TRPV4), a Ca^{2+}-permeable, nonspecific cation channel (Liedtke, 2000; Phan, 2009).

4. Anion channels

The anion channels are a membranal class of porin ion channel that allow the passive diffusion of negatively charged ions along their electrochemical gradient. These channels allow the flow of monovalent anions such as I^-, NO_3^-, Br^-, and Cl, however, these are known as ClC (Fahlke, 2001). The ClC constitute a large family of Cl^- selective channels (Jentsch, 2002). In humans, have been described nine isoforms of ClCs. The first branch of this gene family encodes plasma membrane channels (ClC-1, -2, -Ka and -Kb) and others two branches (ClC-3, -4 and -5; ClC-6/-7) which encode for proteins found on intracellular vesicles (Jentsch, 2005).

In the plasma membrane, the main functions of ClCs are regulation cell volume and ionic homeostasis, transepithelial transport and excitability. Channels in intracellular organelles facilitate the exchange of anionic substrates between the biosynthetic compartments involved in acidification of vesicles in the endosomal pathway (Jentsch, 2002; 2007).

Different diseases have been associated with anionic channels. The loss of ClC-5 is related to Dent's disease (Lloyd, 1996), while the disruption of ClC-3, -6, or -7 in mice promotes the development of neurodegenerative disorders in the central nervous system (Kasper, 2005; Poët, 2006), and ClC-7 mutations have been related with osteopetrosis and lysosomal storage disease (Kasper, 2005; Poët, 2006).

4.1 ClC and chondrocytes proliferation

OA is a complex morphology reflect the severity of damage to articular structures. The histopathological parameters in OA include cartilage degradation with formation of fibrocartilage, fissures, denudation with exposure, repair and remodeling of subchondral bone. In addition, chondrocytes suffer proliferation and apoptosis (Pritzker, 2006) (Fig. 1).

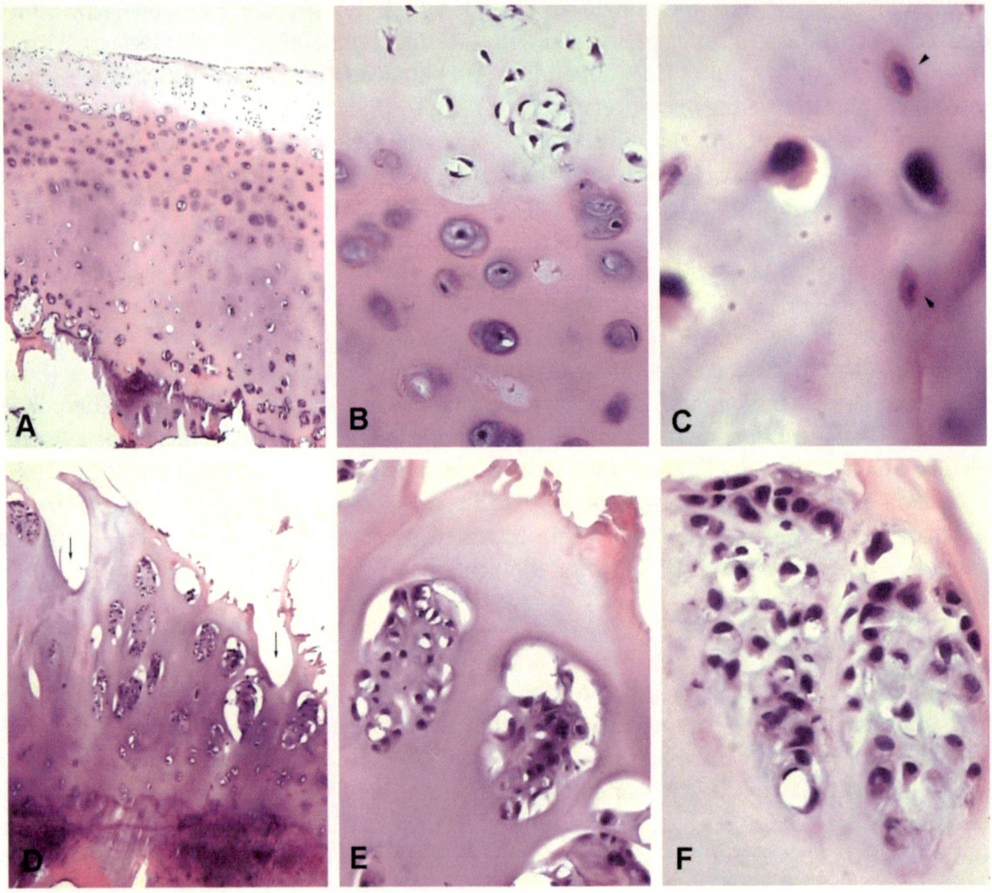

Fig. 1. OA cartilage morphology. A-B fibrillation zone, C apoptotic chondrocytes, D vertical fissures, E-F "clones" or chondrocytes aggregates. Hematoxylin and eosin staining. 10x, 20x and 40x.

This is a condition in which it was reported that the proliferative activity of chondrocytes is low compared with its absence in normal cartilage (Rothwell, 1973; Hulth, 1972). Apparently, the osteoarthritic chondrocytes have a greater access to proliferation factors due to alterations in the ECM (Lee, 1993). It is also possible that aggregates of chondrocytes or clones are a manifestation of the proliferative activity (Horton, 2005).

Moreover, apoptotic cell death is a mechanism widely described in association with OA (Blanco, 1998; Hashimoto, 1998a, 1998b; Kim, 2000; Kouri, 2000). The classic morphologic appearance of this process is characterized by fragmentation and nuclear condensation, and formation of apoptotic bodies (Aigner, 2002). In general, the response of osteoarthritic chondrocytes to the metabolic imbalance (Sandell, 2001), phenotypic modulation (Aigner, 1997) and cell death induces proliferation that compensate the cell loss and the demand of synthetic activity (Aigner, 2001; Rothwell, 1973; Hulth, 1972).

Processes such as proliferation and cell death have been linked to the involvement of ion channels. In this regard, it has been described the association between the activity of K^+ channels and the proliferation of Schwann cells and B lymphocytes (Deutsch, 1990), keratinocytes (Harmon, 1993), melanoma (Nilius, 1994), neuroblastoma and astrocytoma cells (Lee YS, 1993). It also has been associated intracellular free Ca^{2+} concentration and cell proliferation (Wohlrab, 1998).

In chondrocytes, there are changes in the membrane potential of human chondrocytes in response to modulators of ion channels such as tetraethylammonium (TEA), 4-aminopyridine (4-AP), 4′,4′diisothiocyanato-stilbene-2,2′-disulfonic acid (DIDS), 4-acetamido-4′-isothiocyano-2,2′-disulfonic acid (SITS), verapamil and lidocaine. About this, it was reported an increase in DNA synthesis with lidocaine and 4-AP after 12 days in chondrocytes culture (Wohlrab, 2002). Moreover, the exposure of chondrocytes to high concentrations of SITS induced necrosis while that the use of 4-AP caused cytotoxic effects and suppression of proliferation on the same system (Wohlrab, 2004).

4.2 CLIC proteins

The chloride intracellular channel (CLIC) proteins belong to the glutathione S-transferase (GST) superfamiliy and these are group of proteins with possible role of anion channels. However, they differ from classical GSTs because they contain an active site with cysteine residue, reactive for the protein itself and not through a thiol group (Littler, 2010). The CLICs are proteins highly conserved in vertebrates and these are referred to as CLIC1–CLIC6.

These proteins are present in soluble and membrane-inserted form. CLICs have been reported in membranous organelles, cytoplasmic and vesicular compartments and the nucleus (Valenzuela, 1997; Duncan, 1997; Chuang, 1999). The functions of CLICs include pH-dependent ion channel activity (Tulk, 2002; Littler, 2005) and enzymatic which likely to involve a glutathione (GSH) related cofactor (Littler, 2010). They could also be involved in maintaining the structure of intracellular organelles and their interaction with cytoskeleton proteins (Singh, 2007).

Functions of CLICs reported in the musculoskeletal system involve these proteins in the acidification processes in bone resorption (Edwards, 2006; Schlesinger, 1997). Despite their involvement in different systems with activities of ClC, has not been possible to attribute the channel protein function permanently.

CLICs proteins are implicated in cell cycle regulation, cell differentiation, and apoptosis. Specifically, CLIC4 has been linked to apoptosis and differentiation of fibroblasts into myofibroblasts (Fernandez-Salas, 2002; Ronnov-Jessen, 2002). In addition, it was reported that CLIC3 interacts with ERK7, a mitogen-activated protein kinase, allowing the regulation of the phosphatases or kinases (Qian, 1999).

4.3 CLIC6 protein

CLIC6 consist of 704 aminoacids with decapeptide repeats (Friedli, 2003) and and reportedly bind to the dopamine D(2)-like receptors (Griffon, 2003). It is also suggested that CLIC6 could be involved in the regulation of water and secretion of hormones (Nishizawa, 2000).

In chondrocytes, recently, we reported the identification of CLIC6 protein from proteomic analysis of rat normal articular cartilage (Perez, 2010). In human cartilage obtained from total knee arthroplasty, we found immunoreactivity for CLIC6 protein largely restricted to the aggregates of chondrocytes (clones or clusters) in the superficial zone (Fig. 2).

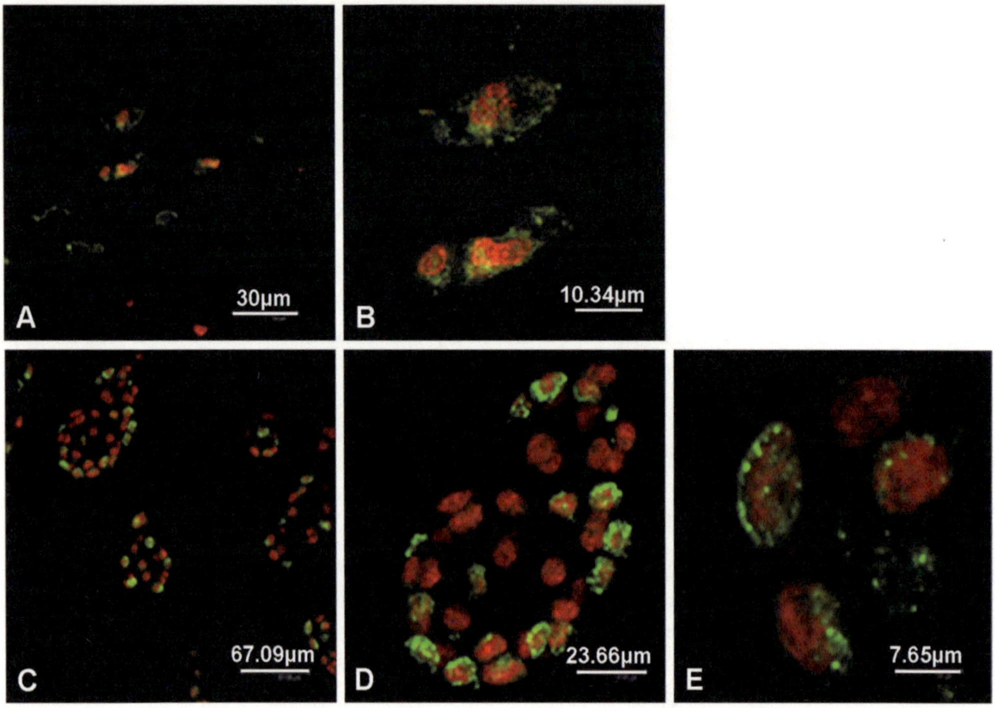

Fig. 2. CLIC6 immunostaining of NoAC and OAC. A-B Surface zone (NoAC), C-E Chondrocytes clusters (OAC). The anti-CLIC6 antibody was coupled to FITC (fluorescein-5-isothiocyanate) and the nucleus were counterstained with propidium iodide.

Immunolabelling was arranged in a coarse granular pattern located in the cytoplasm of most chondrocytes. Comparatively, chondrocytes of non osteoarthritic human articular cartilage (NoAC) showed scarse immunoreactivity predominantly in cells of superficial zones (unpublished data).

Although controversial, the formation of cell clusters in osteoarthritic cartilage (OAC) has been considered an event of repair and regeneration (Horton, 2005). However, electrophysiological and molecular investigations are required to define role of the CLIC6 protein on healthy and osteoarthritic chondrocytes.

5. Conclusion

The pathogenesis of OA includes homeostatic alterations that induce imbalance in the anabolic and catabolic processes. These have been associated with changes in the viability and chondrocytes proliferation. Previous studies have showed a low proliferative activity of OAC. However, the arrangement of the chondrocytes in groups (clones), a hallmark of OA, could possibly be considered a sign of proliferation.

CLIC6 protein expression in normal articular cartilage of rat, and immunolocalization in chondrocytes clusters removed from patients with OA, could suggest the involvement of this anion channel in the pathophysiologic processes of disease.

6. Acknowledgment

We wish to thank Jose C. Luna Muñoz, PhD, for image capture support at the Departamento de Fisiología y Unidad de Microscopia Confocal, CINVESTAV-IPN, México.

7. References

Aigner, T.; Dudhia, J. (1997). Phenotypic modulation of chondrocytes as a potential therapeutic target in osteoarthritis: a hypothesis. *Ann Rheum Dis.* Vol. 56, pp. 287-291.

Aigner, T.; Hemmel, M.; Neureiter, D.; Gebhard, P.M.; Zeiler, G.; Kirchner, T.; McKenna, L. (2001). Apoptotic cell death is not a widespread phenomenon in normal aging and osteoarthritis human articular knee cartilage: a study of proliferation, programmed cell death (apoptosis), and viability of chondrocytes in normal and osteoarthritic human knee cartilage. *Arthritis Rheum.* Vol. 44, pp. 1304-1312.

Aigner, T.; Kim, H.A. (2002). Apoptosis and cellular vitality: issues in osteoarthritic cartilage degeneration. *Arthritis Rheum.* Vol. 46, pp. 1986-1996.

Baker-LePain, J.C.; Lane, N.E. (2010). Relationship between joint shape and the development of osteoarthritis. *Curr Opin Rheumatol* Vol. 22, pp. 538–543.

Barrett-Jolley, R.; Lewis, R.; Fallman, R.; Mobasheri, A. (2010). The emerging chondrocyte channelome. *Front Physiol.* Vol. 1, pp. 135.

Blanco, F.J.; Guitian, R.; Vazquez-Martul, E.; de Toro, F.J.; Galdo, F. (1998). Osteoarthritis chondrocytes die by apoptosis. A possible pathway for osteoarthritis pathology. *Arthritis Rheum* Vol. 41, pp. 284–289.

Bush, P.G.; Hall, A.C. (2001). The osmotic sensitivity of isolated and in situ bovine articular chondrocytes. *J Orthop Res* Vol. 19, pp. 768-778.

Bush, P.G.; Hall, A.C. (2003). The volume and morphology of chondrocytes within non-degenerate and degenerate human articular cartilage. *Osteoarthritis Cartilage* Vol. 11, pp. 242-251.

Bush, P.G.; Hodkinson, P.D.; Hamilton, G.L.; Hall, A.C. (2005). Viability and volume of in situ bovine articular chondrocytes--changes following a single impact and effects of medium osmolarity. *Osteoarthritis Cartilage* Vol. 13, pp. 54-65.

Chao, P.H.; West, A.C.; Hung, C.T. (2006). Chondrocyte intracellular calcium, cytoskeletal organization, and gene expression responses to dynamic osmotic loading. *Am J Physiol Cell Physiol* Vol. 291, pp. C718–725.

Chuang, J.Z.; Milner, T.A.; Zhu, M.; Sung, C.H. (1999). A 29 kDa intracellular chloride channel p64H1 is associated with large dense-core vesicles in rat hippocampal neurons. *J Neurosci* Vol. 19, pp. 2919–2928.

Clark, R.B.; Hatano, N.; Kondo, C.; Belke, D.D.; Brown, B.S.; Kumar, S.; Votta, B.J.; Giles, W.R. (2010). Voltage-gated k+ currents in mouse articular chondrocytes regulate membrane potential. *Channels* Vol. 4, pp. 179-191.

Deutsch, C. (1990). K+ channels and mitogenesis, *Prog Clin Biol Res.* Vol. 334, pp. 251-271.

Duncan, R.R.; Westwood, P.K.; Boyd, A.; Ashley, R.H. (1997). Rat brain p64H1, expression of a new member of the p64 chloride channel protein family in endoplasmic reticulum. *J Biol Chem* Vol. 272, pp. 23880–23886.

Edwards, J.C.; Cohen, C.; Xu, W.; Schlesinger, P.H. (2006). c-Src control of chloride channel support for osteoclast HCl transport and bone resorption. *J Biol Chem* Vol. 281, pp. 28011–28022.

Erickson, G.R.; Northrup, D.L.; Guilak, F. (2003). Hypo-osmotic stress induces calcium-dependent actin reorganization in articular chondrocytes. *Osteoarthritis Cartilage* Vol. 11, pp. 187–197.

Eyre, D.R.; Wu, J.J. (1987). Type XI or 1α2α3α collagen. In *Structure and Function of Collagen Types*. R. Mayne, R.E. Burgeson (Ed), New York: Academic Press, pp. 261-281.

Fahlke, C. (2001) Ion permeation and selectivity in ClC-type chloride channels. *Am J Physiol Renal Physiol*. Vol. 280, pp. F748–F757.

Fernández-Salas, E.; Suh, K.S.; Speransky, V.V.; Bowers, W.L.; Levy, J.M.; Adams, T.; Pathak, K.R.; Edwards, L.E.; Hayes, D.D.; Cheng, C.; Steven, A.C.; Weinberg, W.C.; Yuspa, S.H. (2002). mtCLIC/CLIC4, an organellular chloride channel protein, is increased by DNA damage and participates in the apoptotic response to p53. *Mol Cell Biol* Vol. 22, pp. 3610–3620.

Friedli, M.; Guipponi, M.; Bertrand, S.; Bertrand, D.; Neerman-Arbez, M.; Scott, H.S.; Antonarakis, S.E.; Reymond, A. (2003). Identification of a novel member of the CLIC family, CLIC6, mapping to 21q22.12. *Gene*. Vol. 320, pp. 31–40.

Funabashi, K.; Fujii, M.; Yamamura, H.; Ohya, S.; Imaizumi, Y. (2010). Contribution of chloride channel conductance to the regulation of resting membrane potential in chondrocytes. *J Pharmacol Sci*. Vol. 113, pp. 94–99.

Gannon, J.M.; Walker, G.; Fischer, M.; Carpenter, R.; Thompson, R.C. Jr.; Oegema, T.R. Jr. (1991). Localization of type X collagen in canine growth plate and adult canine articular cartilage. *J Orthop Res* Vol. 9, pp. 485-494.

Grandolfo, M.; D'Andrea, P.; Martina, M.; Ruzzier, F.; Vittur, F. (1992). Calcium-activated potassium channels in chondrocytes. *Biochem Biophys Res Commun*. Vol. 182, pp. 1429–1434.

Griffon, N., Jeanneteau, F., Prieur, F., Diaz, J. and Sokoloff, P. (2003) CLIC6, a member of the intracellular chloride channel family, interacts with dopamine D(2)-like receptors. *Brain Res Mol Brain Res*. Vol. 117, pp. 47–57.

Grodzinsky AJ, Levenston ME, Jin M, Frank EH. (2000). Cartilage tissue remodeling in response to mechanical forces. *Annu Rev Biomed Eng*. Vol. 2, pp. 691–713.

Hardingham, T.E.; Muir, H. (1974). Hyaluronic acid in cartilage and proteoglycan aggregation. *Biochem J*. Vol. 139, pp. 565–581.

Hardingham, G.E.; Bading, H. (1999). Calcium as a versatile second messenger in the control of gene expression. *Microsc Res Tech* Vol. 46, pp. 348–355.

Harmon SC, Lutz D, Ducote J. (1993). Potassium channel openers stimulate DNA synthesis in mouse epidermal keratinocyte and whole hair follicle cultures. *Skin Pharmacol*. Vol. 6, pp. 170–178.

Hashimoto, S.; Ochs, R.L.; Komiya, S.; Lotz, M. (1998a). Linkage of chondrocyte apoptosis and cartilage degradation in human osteoarthritis. *Arthritis Rheum* Vol. 41, pp. 1632–1638.

Hashimoto, S.; Takahashi, K.; Amiel, D.; Coutts, R.D.; Lotz, M. (1998b). Chondrocyte apoptosis and nitric oxide production during experimentally induced osteoarthritis. *Arthritis Rheum* Vol. 41, pp. 1266–1274.

Hedlund, H.; Hedbom, E.; Heineg rd, D.; Mengarelli-Widholm, S.; Reinholt, F.P.; Svensson, O. (1999). Association of the aggrecan keratan sulfate-rich region with collagen in bovine articular cartilage. *J Biol Chem* Vol. 274, pp. 5777–5781.

Horton, W.E. Jr.; Yagi, R.; Laverty, D.; Weiner, S. (2005). Overview of studies comparing human normal cartilage with minimal and advanced osteoarthritic cartilage. *Clin Exp Rheumatol* Vol. 23, pp. 103–112.

Huang, H.; Kamm, R.D.; Lee, R.T. (2004). Cell mechanics and mechanotransduction: pathways, probes, and physiology. *Am J Physiol Cell Physiol.* Vol. 287, pp. C1-11.

Hulth, A.; Lindberg, L.; Telhag, H. (1972). Mitosis in human osteoarthritic cartilage. *Clin Orthop Rel Res* Vol. 84, pp. 197–199.

Isoya, E.; Toyoda, F.; Imai, S.; Okumura, N.; Kumagai, K.; Omatsu-Kanbe, M.; Kubo, M.; Matsuura, H.; Matsusue, Y. (2009). Swelling-activated Cl(-) current in isolated rabbit articular chondrocytes: inhibition by arachidonic acid. *J Pharmacol Sci.* Vol. 109, pp. 293–304.

Jentsch, T.J.; Stein, V.; Weinreich, F.; Zdebik, A.A. (2002). Molecular structure and physiological function of chloride channels. *Physiol Rev.* Vol. 82, pp. 503-568.

Jentsch, T.J.; Poët, M.; Fuhrmann, J.C.; Zdebik, A.A. (2005). Physiological functions of CLC Cl-–channels gleaned from human genetic disease and mouse models. *Annu Rev Physiol.* Vol. 67, pp. 779–807.

Jentsch, T.J. (2007) Chloride and the endosomal-lysosomal pathway: emerging roles of CLC chloride transporters. *J Physiol.* Vol. 578, pp. 633-40.

Jones, W.R.; Ting-Beall, H.P.; Lee, G.M.; Kelley, S.S.; Hochmuth, R.M.; Guilak, F. (1999). Alterations in the young's modulus and volumetric properties of chondrocytes isolated from normal and osteoarthritic human cartilage. *J Biomech* Vol. 32, pp. 119-127.

Kasper, D.; Planells-Cases, R.; Fuhrmann, J.C.; Scheel, O.; Zeitz, O.; Ruether, K.; Schmitt, A.; Poët, M.; Steinfeld, R.; Schweizer, M.; Kornak, U.; Jentsch, T.J. (2005). Loss of the chloride channel ClC-7 leads to lysosomal storage disease and neurodegeneration. *EMBO J.* Vol. 24, pp. 1079–1091.

Kerrigan, M.J.; Hook, C.S.; Qusous, A.; Hall, A.C. (2006). Regulatory volume increase (RVI) by in situ and isolated bovine articular chondrocytes. *J Cell Physiol* Vol. 209, pp. 481–492.

Kim, H.A.; Lee, Y.J.; Seong, S.C.; Choe, K.W.; Song, Y.W. (2000). Apoptotic chondrocyte death in human osteoarthritis. *J Rheum* Vol. 27, pp. 455–462.

Kouri, J.B.; Aguilera, J.M.; Reyes, J.; Lozoya, K.A.; Gonzalez S. (2000). Apoptotic chondrocytes from osteoarthrotic human articular cartilage and abnormal calcification of subchondral bone. *J Rheum* Vol. 27, pp. 1005–1019.

Kurz, B.; Lemke, A.K.; Fay, J.; Pufe, T.; Grodzinsky, A.J.; Schünke, M. (2005). Pathomechanisms of cartilage destruction by mechanical injury. *Ann Anat* Vol. 187, pp. 473–485.

Lawrence, R.C.; Felson, D.T.; Helmick, C.G.; Arnold, L.M.; Choi, H.; Deyo, R.A.; Gabriel, S.; Hirsch, R.; Hochberg, M.C.; Hunder, G.G.; Jordan, J.M.; Katz, J.N.; Kremers, H.M.; Wolfe, F. (2008). Estimates of the prevalence of arthritis and other rheumatic conditions in the United States. Part II. *Arthritis Rheum.* Vol. 58, pp. 26-35.

Lee, D.A.; Bentley, G.; Archer, C.W. (1993). The control of cell division in articular chondrocytes. *Osteoarthritis Cartilage* Vol. 1, pp. 137–146.

Lee, Y.S.; Sayeed, M.M.; Wurster, R.D. (1993). Inhibition of cell growth by K1 channel modulators is due to interference with agonist induced Ca2+ release. *Cell Signal* Vol. 5, pp. 803–809.

Lewis, R., Mobasheri, A., and Barrett-Jolley, R. (2008). Electrophysiological identification of epithelial sodium channels in canine articular chondrocytes. *Proc Physiol Soc.* Vol. 11, pp. C47.

Lewis, R.; Purves, G.; Crossley, J.; Barrett-Jolley, R. (2010). Modelling the membrane potential dependence on non-specific cation channels in canine articular chondrocytes. *Biophys J.* Vol. 98. (Suppl. 1), pp. 340A.

Lewis, R.; Asplin, K.E.; Bruce. G.; Dart, C.; Mobasheri, A.; Barrett-Jolley R. (2011). The role of the membrane potential in chondrocyte volume regulation. *J Cell Physiol.* Feb 15.

Liedtke W, Choe Y, Martí-Renom MA, Bell AM, Denis CS, Sali A, Hudspeth AJ, Friedman JM, Heller S. (2000). Vanilloid receptor-related osmotically activated channel (VR-OAC), a candidate vertebrate osmoreceptor. *Cell* Vol. 103, pp. 525–535.

Littler, D.R.; Assaad, N.N.; Harrop, S.J.; Brown, L.J.; Pankhurst, G.J.; Luciani, P.; Aguilar, M.I.; Mazzanti, M.; Berryman, M.A.; Breit, S.N.; Curmi, P.M. (2005). Crystal structure of the soluble form of the redox-regulated chloride ion channel protein CLIC4. *FEBS J.* Vol. 272, pp. 4996–5007.

Littler, D.R.; Harrop, S.J.; Goodchild, S.C.; Phang, J.M.; Mynott, A.V.; Jiang, L.; Valenzuela, S.M.; Mazzanti, M.; Brown, L.J.; Breit, S.N.; Curmi, P.M. (2010). The enigma of the CLIC proteins: Ion channels, redox proteins, enzymes, scaffolding proteins? *FEBS Lett.* Vol. 584, pp. 2093–2101

Liu, X.; Bandyopadhyay, B.C.; Nakamoto, T.; Singh, B.; Liedtke, W.; Melvin, J.E.; Ambudkar I. (2006). A role for AQP5 in activation of TRPV4 by hypotonicity: concerted involvement of AQP5 and TRPV4 in regulation of cell volume recovery. *J Biol Chem* Vol. 281, pp. 15485–15495.

Lloyd, S.E.; Pearce, S.H.; Fisher, S.E.; Steinmeyer, K.; Schwappach, B.; Scheinman, S.J.; Harding, B.; Bolino, A.; Devoto, M.; Goodyer, P.; Rigden, S.P.; Wrong, O.; Jentsch, T.J.; Craig, I.W.; Thakker, R.V. (1996). A common molecular basis for three inherited kidney stone diseases. *Nature* Vol. 379, pp. 445–449.

Loeser, R.F.; Carlson, C.S.; McGee, M.P. (1995). Expression of beta 1 integrins by cultured articular chondrocytes and in osteoarthritic cartilage. *Exp Cell Res* Vol. 217, pp. 248-257.

Long, K.J.; Walsh, K.B. (1994). Calcium-activated potassium channel in growth-plate chondrocytes: regulation by protein-kinase A. *Biochem Biophys Res Commun.* Vol. 201, pp. 776–781.

Mancilla, E.E.; Galindo, M.; Fertilio, B.; Herrera, M.; Salas, K.; Gatica, H.; Goecke, A. (2007). L-type calcium channels in growth plate chondrocytes participate in endochondral ossification. *J Cell Biochem.* Vol. 101, pp. 389–398.

Martina, M.; Mozrzymas, J.W.; Vittur, F. (1997). Membrane stretch activates a potassium channel in pig articular chondrocytes. *Biochim Biophys Acta.* Vol. 1329, pp. 205–210.

Mendler, M.; Eich-Bender, S.V.; Vaughan, L.; Winterhalter, K.M.; Bruckner P. (1989). Cartilage contains mixed fibrils of collagen types II, IX, and XI. *J Cell Biol* Vol. 108, pp. 191-197.

Millward-Sadler, S.J.; Wright, M.O.; Lee, H.S.; Nishida, K.; Caldwell, H.; Nuki, G.; Salter, D.M. (1999). Integrin-regulated secretion of interleukin 4: a novel pathway of mechanotransduction in human articular chondrocytes. *J Cell Biol* Vol. 145, pp. 183-189.

Millward-Sadler, S.J.; Wright, M.O.; Lee, H.S.; Caldwell, H.; Nuki, G.; Salter, D.M. (2000). Altered electrophysiological responses to mechanical stimulation and abnormal signaling through alpha5beta1 integrin in chondrocytes from osteoarthritic cartilage. *Osteoarthritis Cartilage* Vol. 8, pp. 272-278.

Minns, R.J.; Steven, F.S. (1977). The collagen fibril organization in human articular cartilage. *J Anat* Vol. 123, pp. 437- 457.

Mobasheri, A.; Mobasheri, R.; Francis, M.J.; Trujillo, E.; Alvarez de la Rosa, D.; Martín-Vasallo, P. (1998). Ion transport in chondrocytes: membrane transporters involved in intracellular ion homeostasis and the regulation of cell volume, free [Ca^{2+}] and pH. *Histol Histopathol.* Vol. 13, pp. 893–910.

Mobasheri, A.; Martín-Vasallo, P. (1999). Epithelial sodium channels in skeletal cells; a role in mechanotransduction? *Cell Biol Int.* Vol. 23, pp. 237–240.

Mobasheri, A.; Gent, T.C.; Womack, M.D.; Carter, S.D.; Clegg, P.D.; Barrett-Jolley, R. (2005). Quantitative analysis of voltage-gated potassium currents from primary equine (Equus caballus) and elephant (Loxodonta africana) articular chondrocytes. *Am J Physiol Regul Integr Comp Physiol.* Vol. 289, pp. R172–R180.

Mobasheri, A.; Gent, T.C.; Nash, A.I.; Womack, M.D.; Moskaluk, C.A.; Barrett-Jolley, R. (2007). Evidence for functional ATP-sensitive (K(ATP)) potassium channels in human and equine articular chondrocytes. *Osteoarthritis Cartilage.* Vol. 15, pp. 1–8.

Mobasheri, A.; Lewis, R.; Maxwell, J.E.; Hill, C.; Womack, M.; Barrett-Jolley, R. (2010). Characterization of a stretch-activated potassium channel in chondrocytes. *J Cell Physiol.* Vol. 223, pp. 511–518.

Mouw, J.K.; Imler, S.M.; Levenston, M.E. (2007). Ion-channel regulation of chondrocyte matrix synthesis in 3D culture under static and dynamic compression. *Biomech Model Mechanobiol* Vol. 6, pp. 33–41.

Mow, V.C.; Wang, C.C.; Hung, C.T. (1999). The extracellular matrix, interstitial fluid and ions as a mechanical signal transducer in articular cartilage. *Osteoarthritis Cartilage.* Vol. 7, pp. 41–58.

Mozrzymas, J.W.; Martina, M.; Ruzzier, F. (1997). A large-conductance voltage-dependent potassium channel in cultured pig articular chondrocytes. *Pflugers Arch.* Vol. 433, pp. 413–427.

Nilius, B.; Droogmans, G. (1994). A role for potassium channels in cell proliferation?. *News Physiol Sci.* Vol. 16:1–12.

Nishizawa, T., Nagao, T., Iwatsubo, T., Forte, J.G. and Urushidani, T. (2000) Molecular cloning and characterization of a novel chloride intracellular channel-related protein, parchorin, expressed in water-secreting cells. *J Biol Chem.* Vol. 275, pp. 11164–11173.

Okumura, N.; Imai, S.; Toyoda, F.; Isoya, E.; Kumagai, K.; Matsuura, H.; Matsusue, Y. (2009). Regulatory role of tyrosine phosphorylation in the swelling-activated chloride current in isolated rabbit articular chondrocytes. *J Physiol* Vol. 587, pp. 3761-3776.

Ostergaard, K.; Salter, D.M.; Petersen, J.; Bendtzen, K.; Hvolris, J.; Andersen, C.B. (1998). Expression of alpha and beta subunits of the integrin superfamily in articular cartilage from macroscopically normal and osteoarthritic human femoral heads. *Ann Rheum Dis* Vol. 57, pp. 303-308.

Pérez, E.; Gallegos, J.L.; Cortés, L.; Calderón, K.G.; Luna, J.C.; Cázares, F.E.; Velasquillo, M.C,; Kouri, J.B.; Hernández, F.C. (2010). Identification of latexin by a proteomic analysis in rat normal articular cartilage. *Proteome Sci.* Vol. 5, pp. 27.

Phan, M.N.; Leddy, H.A.; Votta, B.J.; Kumar, S.; Levy, D.S.; Lipshutz, D.B.; Lee, S.H.; Liedtke, W.; Guilak, F. (2009). Functional characterization of TRPV4 as an osmotically sensitive ion channel in porcine articular chondrocytes. *Arthritis Rheum.* Vol. 60, pp. 3028–3037.

Poët, M.; Kornak, U.; Schweizer, M.; Zdebik, A.A.; Scheel, O.; Hoelter, S.;Wurst, W.; Schmitt, A.; Fuhrmann, J.C.; Planells-Cases, R.; Mole, S.E.; Hübner, C.A.; Jentsch, T.J. (2006). Lysosomal storage disease upon disruption of the neuronal chloride transport protein ClC-6. *Proc Natl Acad Sci USA* Vol. 103, pp. 13854–13859.

Ponce, A. (2006). Expression of voltage dependent potassium currents in freshly dissociated rat articular chondrocytes. *Cell Physiol Biochem.* Vol. 18, pp. 35–46.

Poole, C.A. (1997). Articular cartilage chondrons: form, function and failure. *J Anat* Vol. 191, pp. 1–13.

Pritzker, K.P.; Gay, S.; Jimenez, S.A.; Ostergaard, K.; Pelletier, J.P.; Revell, P.A.; Salter, D.; van den Berg WB. (2006). Osteoarthritis cartilage histopathology: grading and staging. *Osteoarthritis Cartilage.* Vol. 14, pp. 13-29.

Qian, Z.; Okuhara, D.; Abe, M.K.; Rosner, M.R. (1999). Molecular cloning and characterization of a mitogen activated protein kinase-associated intracellular chloride channel. *J Biol Chem.* Vol. 274, pp. 1621–1627.

Ramage, L.; Martel, M.A.; Hardingham, G.E.; Salter, D.M. (2008). NMDA receptor expression and activity in osteoarthritic human articular chondrocytes. *Osteoarthritis Cartilage.* Vol. 16, pp. 1576–1584.

Ronnov-Jessen, L.; Villadsen, R.; Edwards, J.C.; Petersen, O.W. (2002). Differential expression of a chloride intracellular channel gene, CLIC4, in transforming growth factor-beta1-mediated conversion of fibroblasts to myofibroblasts. *Am J Pathol* Vol. 161, pp. 471–480.

Roos, E.M. (2005). Joint injury causes knee osteoarthritis in young adults. *Curr Opin Rheumatol* Vol. 17, pp. 195–200.

Rothwell, A.G.; Bentley, G. Chondrocyte multiplication in osteoarthritic articular cartilage. (1973). *J Bone Joint Surg Br.* Vol. 55, pp. 588–594.

Salter, D.M.; Millward-Sadler, S.J.; Nuki, G.; Wright, M.O. (2002). Differential responses of chondrocytes from normal and osteoarthritic human articular cartilage to mechanical stimulation. *Biorheology* Vol. 39, pp. 97-108.

Sanchez, J.C.; Danks, T.A.; Wilkins, R.J. (2003). Mechanisms involved in the increase in intracellular calcium following hypotonic shock in bovine articular chondrocytes. *Gen Physiol Biophys.* Vol. 22, pp. 487–500.

Sanchez, J. C., and Wilkins, R. J. (2004). Changes in intracellular calcium concentration in response to hypertonicity in bovine articular chondrocytes. *Comp Biochem Physiol A Mol Integr Physiol.* Vol. 137, pp. 173–182.

Sanchez, J.C.; Powell, T.; Staines, H.M.; Wilkins, R.J. (2006). Electrophysiological demonstration of voltage-activated H+ channels in bovine articular chondrocytes. *Cell Physiol Biochem.* Vol. 18, pp. 85-90.

Sandell, L.J.; Aigner, T. (2001). Articular cartilage and changes in arthritis. An introduction: cell biology of osteoarthritis. *Arthritis Res.* Vol. 3, pp. 107-113.

Schlesinger, P.H.; Blair, H.C.; Teitelbaum, S.L.; Edwards, J.C. (1997). Characterization of the osteoclast ruffled border chloride channel and its role in bone resorption. *J Biol Chem* Vol. 272, pp. 18636–18643.

Shakibaei, M.; Mobasheri, A. (2003). Beta1-integrins co-localize with Na, K-ATPase, epithelial sodium channels (ENaC) and voltage activated calcium channels (VACC) in mechanoreceptor complexes of mouse limb-bud chondrocytes. *Histol Histopathol.* Vol. 18, pp. 343–351.

Singh, H.; Cousin, M.A.; Ashley, R.H. (2007). Functional reconstitution of mammalian 'chloride intracellular channels' CLIC1, CLIC4 and CLIC5 reveals differential regulation by cytoskeletal actin. *FEBS J* Vo.l 274, pp. 6306–6316.

Stockwell, R.A. (1967). The cell density of human articular and costal cartilage. *J Anat* Vol. 101, pp. 753–763.

Stockwell, R.A. (1990). Morphology of cartilage. In *Maroudas A & Keuttner K* (eds.). Methods in cartilage research. San Diego: Academic Press, pp. 61–63.

Stockwell, R.A. (1991). Cartilage failure in osteoarthritis: Relevance of normal structure and function. *Clinical Anatomy* Vol. 4, pp. 161-191.

Sugimoto, T.; Yoshino, M.; Nagao, M.; Ishii, S.; Yabu, H. (1996). Voltage-gated ionic channels in cultured rabbit articular chondrocytes. *Comp Biochem Physiol C Pharmacol Toxicol Endocrinol.* Vol. 115, pp. 223–232.

Trujillo, E., Alvarez de la Rosa, D., Mobasheri, A., Gonzalez, T., Canessa, C. M., and Martin-Vasallo, P. (1999). Sodium transport systems in human chondrocytes. II. Expression of ENaC, Na+/K+/2Cl- cotransporter and Na+/H+ exchangers in healthy and arthritic chondrocytes. *Histol Histopathol.* Vol. 14, pp. 1023–1031.

Tsuga, K.; Tohse, N.; Yoshino, M.; Sugimoto, T.; Yamashita, T.; Ishii, S; Yabu, H. (2002). Chloride conductance determining membrane potential of rabbit articular chondrocytes. *J Membr Biol.* Vol. 185, pp. 75–81.

Tulk, B.M.; Kapadia, S.; Edwards, J.C. (2002). CLIC1 inserts from the aqueous phase into phospholipid membranes, where it functions as an anion channel. *Am J Physiol Cell Physiol.* Vol. 282, pp. C1103-1112.

Urban, J.P.; Hall, A.C.; Gehl, K.A. (1993). Regulation of matrix synthesis rates by the ionic and osmotic environment of articular chondrocytes. *J Cell Physiol.* Vol. 154, pp. 262–270.

Urban, J.P. (1994). The chondrocyte: a cell under pressure. *Br J Rheumatol.* Vol. 33, pp. 901–908.

Valenzuela SM, Martin DK, Por SB, Robbins JM, Warton K, Bootcov MR, Schofield PR, Campbell TJ, Breit SN. (1997). Molecular cloning and expression of a chloride ion channel of cell nuclei. *J Biol Chem* Vol. 272, pp. 12575–12582.

Walsh, K.B.; Cannon, S.D.; Wuthier, R.E. (1992). Characterization of a delayed rectifier potassium current in chicken growth plate chondrocytes. *Am J Physiol.* Vol. 262, pp. C1335–C1340.

Wang, X.T,; Nagaba, S.; Nagaba, Y.; Leung, S.W.; Wang, J.; Qiu, W.; Zhao, P.L.; Guggino, S.E. (2000). Cardiac L-type calcium channel alpha 1-subunit is increased by cyclic adenosine monophosphate: messenger RNA and protein expression in intact bone. *J Bone Miner Res.* Vol. 15, pp. 1275–1285.

Weiss, C.; Rosenberg, L.; Helfet, A.J. (1968). An ultrastructural study of normal young adult human articular cartilage. *J Bone Joint Surg Am* Vol. 50, pp. 663– 674.

Wilson, J.R.; Duncan, N.A.; Giles, W.R.; Clark, R.B. (2004). A voltage dependent K+ current contributes to membrane potential of acutely isolated canine articular chondrocytes. *J Physiol.* Vol. 557, pp. 93–104.

Wohlrab, D. (1998). Der Einfluß elektrophysiologischer Membraneigenschaften auf die Proliferation humaner Keratinozyten. Tectum, Marburg, pp. 1-89

Wohlrab, D.; Lebek, S.; Krüger, T.; Reichel, H. (2002). Influence of ion channels on the proliferation of human chondrocytes. *Biorheology* Vol. 39, pp. 55-61.

Wohlrab, D.; Vocke, M.; Klapperstuck, T.; Hein, W. (2004). Effects of potassium and anion channel blockers on the cellular response of human osteoarthritic chondrocytes. *J Orthop Sci.* Vol. 9, pp. 364–371.

Wohlrab, D.; Vocke, M.; Klapperstück, T.; Hein, W. (2005). The influence of lidocaine and verapamil on the proliferation, CD44 expression and apoptosis behavior of human chondrocytes. *Int J Mol Med.* Vol. 16, pp. 149-57.

Wright, M.O.; Stockwell, R.A.; Nuki, G. (1992). Response of the plasma membrane to applied hydrostatic pressure in chondrocytes and fibroblasts. *Connect Tissue Res* Vol. 28, pp. 49-70.

Wright, M.O.; Jobanputra, P.; Bavington, C.; Salter, D.M.; Nuki, G. (1996). The effects of intermittent pressurisation on the electrophysiology of cultured human articular chondrocytes: evidence for the presence of stretch activated membrane ion channels. *Clin Sci (Lond).* Vol. 90, pp. 61-71.

Wu, J.J.; Eyre, D.R.; Slayter, H.S. (1987). Type VI collagen of the intervertebral disc. Biochemical and electron microscopic characterization of the native protein. *Biochem J* Vol. 248, pp. 373-381.

Wu, J.J.; Murray, J.; Eyre, D.R. (1996). Evidence for copolymeric crosslinking between types II and III collagens in human articular cartilage. *Trans Orthop Res Soc* Vol. 21, pp. 42.

Wu, Q. Q., and Chen, Q. (2000). Mechanoregulation of chondrocyte proliferation, maturation, and hypertrophy: ion-channel dependent transduction of matrix deformation signals. *Exp Cell Res* Vol. 256, pp. 383–391.

Xu, J.; Wang, W.; Clark, C.C.; Brighton, C.T. (2009). Signal transduction in electrically stimulated articular chondrocytes involves translocation of extracellular calcium through voltage-gated channels. *Osteoarthritis Cartilage.* Vol. 17, pp. 397–405.

Xu, X.; Urban, J.P.; Tirlapur, U.K.; Cui, Z. (2010). Osmolarity effects on bovine articular chondrocytes during three-dimensional culture in alginate beads. *Osteoarthritis Cartilage* Vol. 18, pp. 433-439.

20

The Cholinergic System Can Be of Unexpected Importance in Osteoarthritis

Sture Forsgren
Department of Integrative Medical Biology, Anatomy Section, Umeå University, Umeå, Sweden

1. Introduction

The main belief is that joints such as the knee and ankle joints are not innervated by nerves with a cholinergic function. That includes the assumption that these joints are not innervated by the vagus nerve (van Maanen et al., 2009a, see also Grimsholm et al., 2008). Accordingly, there is actually no morphologic proof of a cholinergic innervation of the knee joint, nor of the ankle joint. Despite this fact, it is shown that electrical and pharmacological stimulation of the vagus nerve has a diminishing effect on carragenan-induced paw inflammation in rats (Borovikova et al., 2000a) and that interference with the effects of the vagus nerve leads to effects on the knee joint arthritis as seen experimentally (van Maanen et al., 2009b). There are also other findings which show the potential effects that interference with vagal effects has on joint inflammation. These will be discussed below.

It is actually strange that interference with cholinergic effects, as via manpulations of the vagus nerve, has effects in knee joint inflamed synovium without presence of a vagal nerve innervation. One possibility is that the effects are indirect, via an occurrence of vagal effects on other sites such as the spleen (Huston et al., 2006, see also van Maanen et al., 2009a). However, another possibility is that there is a non-neuronal production of acetylcholine (ACh) within the synovial tissue itself. This has actually been shown to be the case (Grimsholm et al., 2008) (see further in paragraph 3).

2. Non-neuronal ACh production – General aspects

It is nowadays known that there is a production of ACh in non-neuronal cells. The information has especially emerged via studies on expressions of the ACh-producing enzyme choline acetyltransferase (ChAT), but new knowledge on this topic has also become evident via studies of expressions of vesicular acetylcholine transporter (VAChT), carnitine acetyltransferase (CarAT), and the high-affinity choline transporter (CHT1). It is likely that the ACh produced in non-neuronal cells is released directly after synthesis, in contrast to the nerve-related ACh which is released via exocytosis.

Cell types for which ACh production has been shown are cells in the airways (Wessler et al., 2003, 2007), the keratinocytes of the skin (Grando et al., 1993, 2006), cells of the intestinal epithelium (Klapproth et al., 1997; Ratcliffe et al., 1998; Jönsson et al., 2007), cells of the urinary bladder wall (Lips et al., 2007; Yoshida et al., 2008), cells in blood vessel walls (Kirkpatrick et al., 2003; Lips et al., 2003) and certain cancer cells (Song et al., 2003, 2008;

Paleari et al., 2008). A further celltype for which there is evidence of ACh production is the tenocyte of human patellar (Danielson et al., 2006, 2007) and Achilles (Bjur et al., 2008) tenocytes. It was hereby found that the evidence was much stronger for chronic painful (tendinosis) tendons than normal pain-free tendons (Danielson et al., 2006, 2007; Bjur et al., 2008). Existence of a non-neuronal cholinergic system has also recently been shown for osteoblast-like cells (En-Nosse et al., 2009) and hepatocytes (Delbro et al., 2011).
Of special interest with respect to what will be discussed below, is the fact that inflammatory cells (Kawashima & Fuji, 2004) and fibroblasts (Fisher et al., 1993; Lips et al., 2003) show production of ACh. It should here be remembered that the tenocytes of human tendons in principle have fibroblast-like appearances.

3. Non-neuronal ACh production in synovium

It has previously been unclear as to whether there is a non-neuronal cholinergic system in synovial tissues. However, studies performed during recent years have provided evidence of ACh production in the synovial tissue of the human knee joint (Grimsholm et al., 2008). That was shown both via immunohistochemistry and in situ hybridization and was related to findings of ChAT expression in mononuclear-like as well as fibroblast-like cells (Grimsholm et al., 2008). The findings were shown both for synovial tissue of patients with rheumatoid arthritis (RA) as well as patients with osteoarthritis (OA). The occurrence of ChAT expression in mononuclear-like cells in OA synovium is shown below (Fig 1).

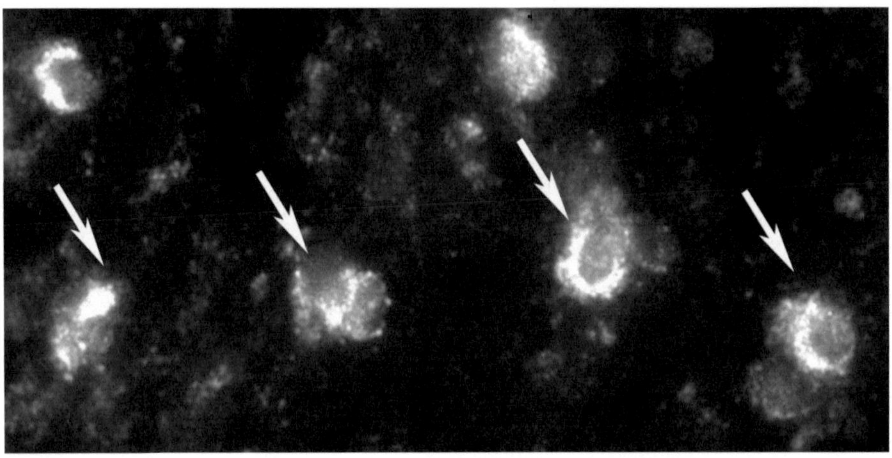

Fig. 1. Figure showing the expression of ChAT in mononuclear-like cells in the OA synovial tissue. Some of the immunoreactive cells are indicated with arrows.

4. Functions of non-neuronally produced ACh

The effects of the non-neuronal cholinergic system include functions on growth/differentiation and secretion and barrier functions (c.f. Wessler & Kirkpatrick, 2001, 2008). ACh has e.g. well-known effects on angiogenesis (Jacobi et al., 2002; Cooke et al., 2007). It is also known that an increased cell proliferation occurs in response to cholinergic stimulation (Mayerhofer & Fritz, 2002; Metzen et al., 2003; Oben et al., 2003). That includes proliferative effects on human fibroblasts (Matthiesen et al., 2006). Interestingly, it is also frequently emphasized that ACh not only is produced in immune cells but that it also has effects on these cells, ACh hereby modulating the activity of the immune cells via auto- and paracrine loops (Kawashima & Fuji, 2003, 2008). The findings that ACh hereby has anti-inflammatory effects, findings wich will be considered below, are especially interesting, but it is also possible that acute ACh stimulation can lead to proinflammatory effects (cf. Kawashima & Fuji, 2003).

5. Cholinergic anti-inflammatory pathway

A newly recognized concept is the "cholinergic anti-inflammatory pathway" (Borovikova et al., 2000b; Pavlov & Tracey, 2005; Tracey 2007). It is related to the occurrence of immunomodulatory effects of ACh released from cholinergic nerves. For example, as is commented on above, there occurs a suppression of the inflammation in the carrageenan paw edema in the rat in response to activation of this anti-inflammatory pathway via pharmalogic or electrical stimulation of the vagus nerve (Borovikova et al., 2000a). There is furthermore an attenuation in macrophage activation in response to electrical stimulation of the vagus nerve (de Jonge et al., 2005) and stimulation of the vagus nerve does on the whole improve survival in animal models of inflammation (e.g. Bernik et al., 2002). Neural inputs to immune cells can control cytokine production (Tracey, 2007). Concerning joints, there is evidence of a role of the cholinergic anti-inflammatory pathway in the murine CIA model of RA (van Maanen et al., 2010). Studies on the synovium in RA do nevertheless suggest that the cholinergic anti-inflammatory pathway might be suppressed in this condition (Goldstein et al., 2007).

It can be asked as to whether ACh originating from non-neuronal cells can be involved in the anti-inflammatory pathway. This can actually be the case. It is thus possible that neuronally released ACh triggers the release of ACh from these non-neuronal cells (Wessler & Kirkpatrick., 2008) and that effects via the non-neuronal cholinergic system even can occur independently of actions via cholinergic nerves (Kawashima & Fuji, 2003). Further evidence is the finding that ACh-induced modulation of immune functions in peripheral leukocytes occurs independently of neuronal innervation (Neumann et al., 2007). The non-neuronal ACh production in synovial tissue might therefore be of importance in the regulation of the processe that occur in this tissue in various forms of arthritis, including OA.

6. Involvement of the α7nAChR in anti-inflammatory effects

The nicotinic acetylcholine receptor AChRα7 (α7nAChR) is considered to be important in the cholinergic anti-inflammatory pathway (Wang et al., 2003; Kawashima & Fuji, 2008). The α7nAChR is thus shown to contribute to anti-inflammatory effects of ACh in several models (Tracey, 2002; Ulloa, 2005; de Jonge & Ulloa, 2007). α7nAChR agonists are furthermore shown to suppress the production of TNF alpha, IL-1, IL-6 and IL-8 and various other cytokines in macrophages after challenge with lipopolysaccharide (Borovikova et al., 2000a; Wang et al., 2003). An α7nAChR agonist is also shown to decrease the production of IL-6 by IL-1 stimulated fibroblast-like synoviocytes (Waldburger et al., 2008). The results of still other studies show that specific α7nAChR agonists can reduce TNFalpha-induced IL-6 as well as IL-8 production by fibroblast-like synoviocytes (van Maanen et al., 2009c).

7. Current study: Expression of α7nAChR in osteoarthritis

7.1 Introduction

Except for effects in the autonomic nervous system, ACh is reported to have proliferative and growth-promoting effects, effects in cancer progression and anti-inflammatory effects. As ACh has anti-inflammatory effects and effects in relation to growth/proliferation, it is of interest to consider its importance in arthritic processes. The findings that mononuclear- as well as fibroblast-like cells in the synovium of the knee joints of patients with RA as well as OA show ChAT, favouring ACh production, is therefore of interest (Grimsholm et al., 2008). The receptor through which the inflammatory-mediating effects of ACh is reported to be mainly mediated is the α7nAChR (Kawashima & Fuji., 2008). It is therefore of interest to note that expression of α7nAChR has been shown for the synovial tissue of patients with RA and psoriatic arthritis (van Maanen et al., 2009a; Westman et al., 2009) . The receptor was also to some extent noted for the synovium of healthy individuals (Westman et al., 2009). In studies on synovial tissue from 3 patients with OA, as well 3 patients with RA, it was shown that the α7nAChR was expressed in the synovial intimal lining (Waldburger et al., 2008). The details of receptor expression at the tissue level concerning OA has not been further studied. More information is therefore welcome concerning the situation in OA.

Therefore, the expression pattern of the α7nAChR in the knee synovial joint of patients with OA was examined in the present study.

7.2 Materials & methods

7.2.1 Patient material

Synovial biopsies were collected from the knee joint of six patients with OA. Four of these were females (range 58-81 years; mean age 68 years) and two were males (50 and 62 years of age). The biopsies were obtained during prosthesis operations. They thus corresponded to samples of cases with advanced and long-lasting OA. The OA patients fullfilled the criteria of Altman and co-writers (Altman et al., 1986). All study protocols were approved by the Regional Ethical Review Board in Umeå (EPN) (project nr. 05-016M). The experiments were conducted according to the principles expressed in the Declaration of Helsinki. Informed consent was obtained from all individuals.

7.2.2 Fixation and sectioning

Directly after the surgical procedures, the tissue samples were transported to the laboratory. They were fixed in 4% formaldehyde in 0.1 M phosphate buffer (pH 7.0) at 4°C for 24 h and were then washed in Tyrode's solution (pH 7.2) containing 10% (w/v) sucrose for 24 h, mounted on thin cardboard with OCT embedding medium (Miles Laboratories, Naperville, IL, USA) and frozen in propane chilled by liquid N_2. A series of 7 μm thick sections were cut on a cryostat and mounted on slides coated with chrome-alum gelatine for immunohistochemistry. Some of the sections were stained with haematoxylin-eosin (htx-eosin) for delineating tissue morphology.

7.2.3 Immunofluorescence staining

The sections were mounted in Vectashield hard set microscopy mounting medium (Dakopatts, Denmark). The immunohistochemical procedures were in principle as previously described (Bjur et al., 2008). In order to enhance specific immunoreactions, treatment with $KMnO_4$ was applied in accordance with developed procedues in the laboratory (Hansson & Forsgren., 1995).

The sections were incubated for 20 min in a 1% solution of Triton X-100 (Kebo lab, Stockholm) in 0.01 M phosphate buffer saline (PBS), pH 7.2, containing 0,1% sodium azide as preservative, and thereafter rinsed in PBS three times, 5 min each time. The sections were then incubated with 5% normal donkey serum in PBS. The sections were thereafter incubated with the primary antibody, diluted in PBS, in a humid environment. Incubation was performed for 60 min at 37°C. After incubation with specific antiserum, and three 5 min washes in PBS, another incubation in normal donkey serum followed, after which the sections were incubated with secondary antibody. As secondary antibody, a FITC-conjugated donkey anti-goat IgG (Jackson Immunoresearch, West Grove, PA), diluted 1:100, was used. Incubation with secondary antibody was performed for 30 min at 37°C. The sections were thereafter washed in PBS and then mounted in Vectashield Mounting Medium (H-1000) (Vector Laboratories, Burlingame, CA, USA). Examination was carried out in a Zeiss Axioscope 2 plus microscope equipped with an Olympus DP70 digital camera.

The primary antibody was an antibody against the nicotinic acetylcholine receptor AChRα7 (α7nAChR). This antibody is an affinity purified goat polyclonal antibody raised against a peptide mapping at the C-terminus of α7nAChR of human origin (Santa Cruz Biotechnology; sc-1447, dilution used 1:100). The outcome of immunostaining using the used protocol, including the currently used secondary antiserum, with primary antibody being substituted by PBS or normal serum, has been previously evaluated for human tissue (Danielson et al 2006a; Bjur et al., 2008) (control stainings). Sections of fixed rabbit muscle/inflammatory tissue were furthermore processed in parallel for control purposes, the same procedures as used here for demonstration of α7nAChR immunoreactions in the synovial tissue being used. It was hereby found that the inflammatory cells in the muscle inflammation (myositis) showed distinct α7nAChR immunoreactions, whilst the muscle tissue did not (not shown). Occurrence of α7nAChR immunoreactions for inflammatory cells in muscle inflammation (myositis) is a well-known fact (Leite et al., 2010).

7.3 Results

Mononuclear-like and fibroblast-like cells occurred to varying extents in the synovial samples. They mainly lay scattered in the tissue. The degree of the inflammatory response varied greatly.

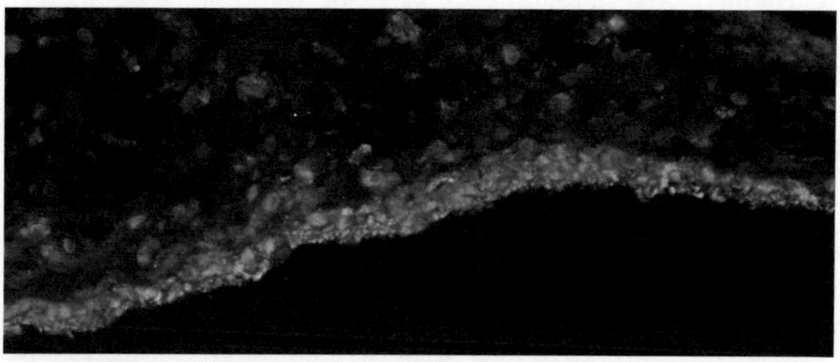

Fig. 2. Figure showing existence of marked α7nAChR immunoreactions in the synovial lining layer.

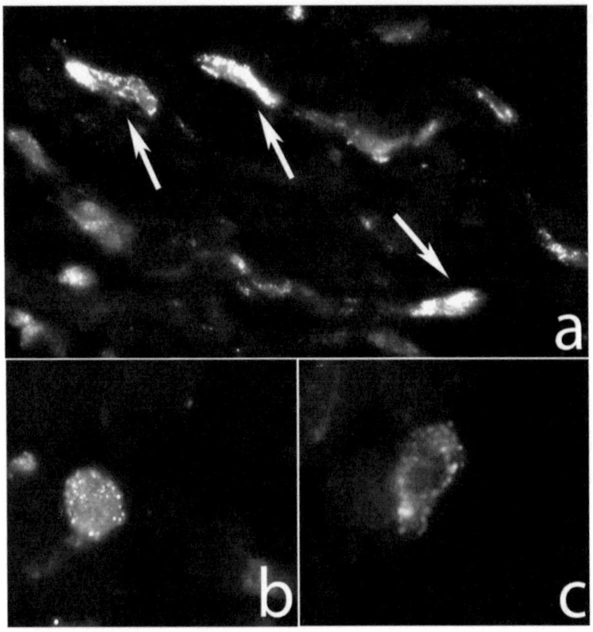

Fig. 3. Figure showing presence of α7nAChR immunoreactions in fibroblast-like (a) and mononuclear-like (b,c) cells in the synovial tissue. Arrows at fibroblast-like cells in (a).

Marked α7nAChR immunoreactions (IR) were seen in the synovial lining layer (Fig 2). α7nAChR IR were also seen for mononuclear-like and fibroblast-like cells (Fig 3).

7.4 Discussion

The observations show that there indeed is immunolabelling for the α7nAChR in the synovial tissue of patients with advanced OA. The findings are in line with recent findings of α7nAChR immunoreactions in the synovial lining layer for RA patients (van Maanen et al., 2009a) and similar findings made in another recent study on patients with RA and psoriatic arthritis (Westman et al., 2009). The observations are also in line with the findings of scattered cells showing fibroblast-like and mononuclear-like appearances exhibiting α7nAChR immunoreactions in RA and psoriatric arthritis (Westman et al., 2009). Furthermore, cultured RA fibroblast-like synoviocytes have been found to express α7nAChR (van Maanen et al., 2009a).

OA synovial intimal lining as well as cultured fibroblast-like synoviocytes obtained from synovial tissue from 3 OA patients express the α7nAChR (Waldburger et al., 2008). The present study thus extends the current knowledge in showing the expression patterns for mononuclear-like and fibroblast-like cells within the OA synovial tissue and is complementary concerning the delineation of the expression pattern for the synovial lining layer.

The existence of not only ACh production (Grimsholm et al., 2008) but also α7nAChR in fibroblast-like cells in the OA synovial tissue can be of functional importance. Stimulation of ACh receptors on pulmonary fibroblasts leads to an increase in collagen accumulation (Sekhon et al., 2002). It can also not be excluded that the α7nAChR may be related to attempts for repair. In studies on skin wound healing, it was thus shown that the α7nAChR is time-dependently expressed in distinct skin cell types, which may be closely involved in the repair processes of the skin wound (Fan et al., 2011). The α7nAChR is also described to contribute to the wound repair of respiratory epithelium (Tournier et al., 2006). Furthermore, an up-regulation of the cholinergic system is reported to be involved in the stimulation of collagen deposition during wound healing (Jacobi et al., 2002). The occurrence of anti-inflammatory effects via cholinergic effects on inflammatory cells is frequently doumented (e.g. Kawashima and Fuji., 2008). The in vitro studies performed by Waldburger and collaborators showed that both synovial fibroblast-like cells and peripheral macrophages respond to cholinergic stimulation leading to inhibition of pro-inflammatory cytokines (Waldburger et al., 2008).

8. Conclusion

The present study adds new information on the expression patterns of the α7nAChR for synovial tissue, namely for this tissue in OA. The results presented here, coupled to the finding that there is evidence favouring the occurrence of synthesis of ACh in OA synovial tissue (Grimsholm et al., 2008), imply that the non-neuronal cholinergic system should be further considered for the OA affected joint. It is likely that non-neuronal ACh can have its effects on the α7nAChR in the OA synovial tissue. Similarly, it is considered that the locally produced ACh in the airways targets ACh receptors located in the airway region where the ACh is produced (Racké et al., 2006).

One possibility is that the production of ACh in non-neuronal cells is related to the occurrence of a great demand on the tissue. That is discussed as one possibility to explain the much more marked ChAT expression in tenocytes of patients with chronic painful tendons than in tendons of normal subjects (Forsgren et al., 2009). Tissue organization and function is hereby influenced. Concerning OA, it would therefore be of interest to know if there is a cholinergic component concerning the cartilage destruction that occurs. It can hereby be noted that less cartilage destruction, as well as on the whole a milder arthritis, was observed for mice lacking the α7nAChR in studies on collagen-induced arthritis (Westman et al., 2010). It might be that the increased production of ACh in the tissue initially is an attempt to "rescue" the tissue, but that long-standing cholinergic upregulation can contribute to deterioration of the tissue. That was suggested to be the case for the chronic painful tendons (Forsgren et al., 2009). Effects of ACh on fibroblasts and myofibroblasts in chronic obstructive pulmonary disease are considered to be involved in remodelling of the tissue (Haag et al., 2008; Racké et al., 2008).

Interference with the effects of ACh, mainly via influences on the α7nAChR, may be a new strategy of value in the treatment of arthritis (van Maanen et al 2009b,c; Westman et al., 2009; Bruchfeld et al., 2010; Pan et al., 2010; Zhang et al., 2010). There are several lines of evidence which suggest that α7nAChR agonists can inhibit the proinflammatory cascade that occurs in arthritis. Selective α7nAChR agonist decreases the production of IL-6 by IL-6 stimulated fibroblast-like synoviocytes and the reduction of production from these cells of several cytokines/chemokines via ACh was blocked by a α7nAChR antagonist (Waldburger et al., 2008). It, however, remains to be clarified as to wheter α7nAChR agonist treatment is valuable in the chronic long-lasting stages of arthritis.

The overwhelming part of the studies favouring a functional importance of the cholinergic system and the possible usefulness of interfering with the α7nAChR are performed on RA. It should here be recalled that some RA specimens from chronic stages of severe RA contained an abundance of ChAT immunoreactive cells (fibroblast-like and monuclear-like cells) in our previous study (Grimsholm et al., 2008). The present study reinforces that a non-neuronal cholinergic system, including presence of the α7nAChR in the synovium, should be further considered also for OA.

9. Acknowledgements

The technical support of Ms. Ulla Hedlund is greatly acknowledged. Dr. Tore Dalén is gratefully acknowledged for supply of the samples. Professor Solbritt Rantapää-Dahlqvist and PhD Ola Grimsholm are acknowledged for the colloborative research in the initial studies on the non-neuronal cholinergic system of human synovium. Financial support has been given by the Faculty of Medicine, Umeå University.

10. References

Altman, R.; Asch, E.; Bloch, D.; Bole, G.; Borenstein, D.; Brandt, K.; Christy, W.; Cooke, TD.; Greenwald, R.; Hochberg, M.; et al. (1986). Development of criteria for the classification and reporting of osteoarthritis. Classification of osteoarthritis of the knee. Diagnostic and Therapeutic Criteria Committee of the American Rheumatism Association. *Arthritis and Rheumatism*, Vol.29, pp.1039-1049.

Bernik, TR.; Friedman, SG.; Ochani, M.; DiRaimo, R.; Ulloa, L.; Yang, H.; Sudan, S.; Czura, CJ.; Ivanova, SM. & Tracey KJ. (2002). Pharmalogical stimulation of the cholinergic anti-inflammatory patyhway. *Journal of Experimental Medicine*, Vol.195, pp. 781-788

Bjur, D.; Danielson, P.; Alfredson, H. & Forsgren, S. (2008). Presence of a non-neuronal cholinergic system and occurrence of up- and down-regulation of M2 muscarinic acetylcholine receptors: new aspects of importance regarding Achilles tendon tendinosis (tendinopathy). *Cell and Tissue Research*, Vol.331, pp. 385-400

Borovikova, LV.; Ivanova, S.; Zhang, M.; Yang, H.; Botchina, GI.; Watkins, LR.;Wang, H.; Abumrad, N.; Eaton, JW. & Tracey, KJ. (2000a). Vagus nerve stimulation attenuates the systemic inflammatory response to endotoxin. *Nature*, Vol.405, pp. 458-462

Borovikova, LV.; Ivanova, S.; Nardi, D.; Zhang, M.; Yang, H.; Ombrellino, M. & Tracey KJ. (2000b). Role of vagus nerve signaling in CNI-1493-mediated suppression of acute inflammation. *Autonomic Neuroscience* 2000, 85, 141-147

Bruchfeld, A.; Goldstein, RS.; Chavan, S.; Patel NB.;Rosas-Ballina, M.; Kohn, N.; Qureshi AR. & Tracey, KJ. (2010). Whole blood cytokine attenuation by cholinergic agionists ex vivo and relationship to vaghus nerve activity in rheumatoid arthritis. *Journal of Internal Medicine*, Vol.268, pp. 94-101

Cooke, JP. (2007). Angiogenesis and the role of the endothelial acetylcholine receptor. *Life Sciences*, Vol.80, pp. 2347-2351

Danielson, P.; Alfredson, H. & Forsgren, S. (2006). Immunohistochemical and histochemical findings favoring the occurrence of autocrine/paracrine as well as nerve-related cholinergic effects in chronic patellar tendon tendinosis. *Microscoscopy Research and Technique*, Vol.69, pp. 808-819

Danielson, P.; Alfredson, H. & Forsgren, S. (2007). In situ hybridization studies confirming recent findings of the existence of a local non-neuronal catecholamine production in human patellar tendinosis. *Microscopy Research and Technique*, Vol.70, pp. 908-911.

de Jonge, W.; van der Zanden, E.; The, FO.; Bijlsma, MF.; van Westerloo, DJ.; Bennink, RJ.; Barthoud, HR.; Uematsau, S.; Akira, S.; van den Wijngaard, RM. & Boeckxstaens, GE. (2005). Stimulation of the vagus nerve attenuates macrophage activation by activating the Jak2-STAT3 signaling pathway. *Nature Immunology*, Vol.6, pp. 844-851

de Jonge, WJ. & Ulloa, L. (2007). The α7 nicotinic acetylcholine receptor as a pharmalogical target for inflammation. *British Journal of Pharmacology*, Vol.151, pp. 915-929

Delbro, DS.; Hallsberg, L.; Wallin, M.; Gustafsson, BI. & Friman, S. (2011). Expression of the non-neuronal cholinergic system in rat liver. *APMIS*, Vol.119, pp. 227-228

En-Nosse, M.; Hartmann, S.; Trinkaus, K.; Alt, V.; Stigler, B.; Heiss, C.; Kilian, O.; Schnettler, R. & Lips, KS. (2009). Expression of non-neuronal cholinergic system in osteoblast-like cells and its involvement in osteogenesis. *Cell and Tissue Research*, Vol.338, pp. 203-215

Fan, YY.; Yu, TS.; Wang, T.; Liu, WW.; Zhao, R.; Zhang, ST.; Ma, WX.; Zheng, JL. & Guan, DW. (2011). Nicotinic acetylcholine receptor alpha7 subunit is time-dependently expressed in distinct cell types during skin wound healing in mice. *Histochemistry and Cell Biology*, publ online

Fisher, LJ.; Schinstine, M.; Salvaterra, P.; Dekker, AJ.; Thal, L. & Gage, FH. (1993). In vivo production and release of acetylcholine from primary fibroblasts genetically modified to express choline acetyltransferase. *Journal of Neurochemistry*, Vol.61, pp. 1323-1332.

Forsgren, S.; Grimsholm, O.; Jönsson, M.; Alfredson, H. & Danielson, P. (2009) New insight into the non-neuronal cholinergic system via studies on chronically painful tendons and inflammatory situations. Life Sciences, Vol.84, pp. 865-870

Grando, SA.; Kist, DA.; Qi, M. & Dahl, MV. (1993). Human keratinocytes synthesize, secrete, and degrade acetylcholine. *Journal of Investigative Dermatology*, Vol.101, pp. 32-36.

Grando, SA.; Pittelko, MR. & Schallreuter, KU. (2006). Adrenergic and cholinergic control in the biology of epidermis: physiological and clinical significance. *Journal of Investigative Dermatology*, Vol.126, pp. 1948-1965.

Goldstein, RS.; Bruchfeld, A.; Yang, L.; Qureshi, AR.; Gallowitsch-Puerta, M.; Patel NB.; Huston, BJ.; Chavan, S.; Rosas-Ballina, M.; Gregersen, PK.; Czura, CJ.; Sloan, RP.; Sama, AE. & Tracey, KJ. (2007) Cholinergic anti-inflammatory pathway activity and High Mobility Group Box-1 (HMGB1) serum levels in patients with rheumatoid arthritis. *Molecular Medicine*, Vol.13, pp. 210-215

Grimsholm, O.; Rantapää-Dahlqvist, S.; Dalén, T. & Forsgren, S. (2008). Unexpected findings of a marked non-neuronal cholinergic system in human knee joint synovial tissue. *Neuroscience Letters*, Vol.442, pp. 128-133

Haag, S.; Matthiesen, S.; Juergens, UR. & Racké, K. (2008). Muscarinic receptors mediate stimulation of collagen synthesis in human lung fibroblasts. *European Respiration Journal*, publ. online, 10.1183/09031936.00129307

Hansson, M. & Forsgren, S. (1995). Immunoreactive atrial and brain natriuretic peptides are co-localized in Purkinje fibres but not in the innervation of the bovine heart conduction system,. *Histochemical Journal*, Vol.27, pp. 222-230

Huston, JM.; Ochani, M.; Rosas-Ballina, M.; Liao, H.; Ochani, K.; Pavlov, VA.; Gallawitsch-Puerta, M.; Ashok, M.; Czura, CJ.; Foxwell, B.; Tracey. & Ulloa, L. (2006).

Splenectomy inactivates the cholinergic antiinflammatory pathway during lethal endotoxemia and polymicrobial sepsis. *Journal of Experimental Medicine*, vol.203, pp. 1623-1628

Jacobi, J.; Jang, JJ.; Sundram, U.; Dayoub, H.; Fajardo, LF. & Cooke, JP. (2002). Nicotine accelerates angiogenesis and wound healing in genetically diabetic mice. *American Journal of Pathology*, Vol.161, pp. 97-104

Jönsson, M.; Norrgård, Ö. & Forsgren, S. (2007). Presence of a marked non-neuronal cholinergic system in the human colon - Studies on the normal colon and the colon in ulcerative colitis. *Inflammatory Bowel Diseases*, Vol.13, pp. 1347-1356

Kawashima, K. & Fuji, T. (2003). The lymphocytic cholinergic system and its contribution to the regulation of immune activity. *Life Sciences*, Vol.74, pp. 675-696

Kawashima, K. & Fuji, T. (2004). Expression of non-neuronal acetylcholine in lymphocytes and its contribution to the regulation of immune function. *Frontieres in Biosciences*, Vol.9, pp. 2063-2085.

Kawashima, K. & Fuji, T. (2008). Basic and clinical aspects of non-neurional acetylcholine: Overview of non-neuronal cholinergic systems and their biological significance. Forum Minireview. *Journal of Pharmacological Sciences*, Vol.106, pp. 167-173

Kirkpatrick, CJ.; Bittinger, F.; Nozadze, K. & Wessler, I. (2003). Expression and function of the non-neuronal cholinergic ystem in endothelial cells. *Life Sciences*, Vol.72, pp. 2111-2116

Klapproth, H.; Reinheimer, T.; Metzen, J.; Münch, M.; Bittinger, F.; Kirkpatrick, CJ.; Höhle, KD.; Schermann, M.; Racke, K. & Wessler, I. (1997). Non-neuronal acetylcholine, a signaling molecule synthezised by surface cells of rat and man. *Naunyn-Schmiedeberg´s Archieves in Pharmacology*, Vol.355, pp. 515-523

Leite, PE.; Lagrota-Candido, J.; Moraes, L.; D´Elia, L.; Pinheiro, DF.; da Silva, RF.; Yamasaki, EN & Quirico-Santos, T. (2010). Nicotinic acetylcholine receptor activation reduces skeletal muscle inflammation of mdx mice. *Journal of Neuroimmunology*, Vol. 227, pp. 44-51

Lips, KS.; Pfeil, U.; Reiners, K.; Rimasch, C.; Kuchelmeister, K.; Braun-Dullaeus, RC.; Haberberger, RV.; Schmidt, R. & Kummer, W. (2003). Expression of the high-affinity choline transporter CHT1 in rat and human arteries. *Journal of Histochemistry and Cytochemistry*, Vol. 51, pp. 1645-1654

Lips, KS.; Wunsch, J.; Zargooni, S.; Bschleipfer, T.; Schukowski, K.; Weidner, M.; Wessler, I.; Schwantes, U.; Koepsell, H. & Kummer, W. (2007). Acetylcholine and Molecular Components of its Synthesis and Release Machinery in the Urothelium. *European Journal of Urology*, Vol.51, pp. 1042-1053

Matthiesen, S.; Bahulayan, A.; Kempkens, S.; Haag, S.; Fuhrmann, M.; Stichnote, C.; Juergens, UR. & Racke, K. (2006). Muscarinic receptors mediate stimulation of human lung fibroblast proliferation. *American Journal of Respiration and Cell Molecular Biology*, Vol. 35, pp. 621-627

Mayerhofer, A. & Fritz, S. (2002). Ovarian acetylcholine and muscarinic receptors: hints of a novel intrinsic ovarian regulatory system. *Microscoscopy Research and Technique*, Vol.59, pp. 503-508

Metzen, J.; Bittinger, F.; Kirkpatrick, J.; Kilbinger, H. & Wessler, I. (2003). Proliferative effect of acetylcholine on rat trachea epithelial cells is mediated by nicotinic receptors and muscarinic receptors of the M1-subtype. *Life Sciences*, Vol.72, pp. 2075-2080

Neumann, S.; Razen, M.; Habermehl, P.; Meyer, CU.; Zepp, F.; Kirkpatrick, CJ. & Wessler, I. (2007). The non-neuronal cholinergic system in peripheral blood cells: effects of nicotinic and muscarinic antagonists on phagocytosis, respiratory burst and migration. *Life Sciences*, Vol.80, pp. 2361-2364

Oben, JA.; Yang, S.; Lin, H.; Ono, M. & Diehl, AM. (2003). Acetylcholine promotes the proliferation and collagen gene expression of hepatic myofibroblastic stellate cells. *Biochemical and Biophysical Research Communications,* Vol.300, pp. 172-177

Pan, XH.; Zhang, J.; Yu, X.; Qin, L.; Kang, L. & Zhang, P. (2010). New therapeutic approaches for the treatment of rheumatoid arthritis may rise from the cholinergic anti-inflammatory pathway and antinociceptive pathway. *ScientificWorldJournal,* Vol.10, pp. 2248-2253

Paleari, L.; Grozio, A.; Cesario, A. & Russo, P. (2008). The cholinergic system and cancer. *Semininars in Cancer Biology*, Vol.18, pp. 211-217

Pavlov, VA. & Tracey, KJ. (2005). The cholinergic anti-inflammatory pathway. *Brain Behaviour Immunology*, Vol.19, pp. 493-499

Racké, K.; Juergens, UR. & Matthiesen, S. (2006). Control by cholinergic mechanisms. *European Journal of Pharmacology*, Vol.533, pp. 57-68

Racké, K.; Haag, S.; Bahulayan, A. & Warnken, M. (2008). Pulmonary fibroblasts, an emerging target for anti-obstructive drugs. *Naunyn Schmiedebergs Archives in Pharmacology*, Vol.378, pp. 193-201.

Ratcliffe, EM.; de Sa, DJ.; Dixon, MF. & Stead, RH. (1998). Choline acetyltransferase (ChAT) immunoreactivity in paraffin sections of normal and diseased intestines. *Journal of Histochemistry and Cytochemistry*, Vol.46, pp. 1223-1231

Sekhon, HS.; Keller, JA.; Proskocil, BJ.; Martin, EL. & Spindel, ER. (2002). Maternal nicotine exposure upregulates collagen gene expression in fetal monkey lung. Association with alpha7 nicotinic acetylcholine receptors. *American Journal of Respiration and Cell Molecular Biology*, Vol.26, pp. 31-41.

Song, P.; Sekhon, HS.; Keller, JA.; Blusztajn, JK.; Mark, GP. & Spindel, ER. (2003). Acetylcholine is synthesized by and acts as an autocrine growth factor for small cell lung carcinoma. *Cancer Research,* Vol. 63, 214-221.

Song, P. & Spindel, ER. (2008). Basic and clinical aspects of non-neuronal acetylcholine: expression of non-neuronal acetylcholine in lung cancer provides a new target for cancer therapy. *Journal of Pharmacological Sciences*, Vol.106, pp. 180-185.

Tournier, JM.; Maoche, K.; Coraux, C.; Zahm, JM.; Cloez-Tayarani, I.; Nawrocki-Raby, B.; Bonnomet, A.; Burlet, H.; Lebargy, F.; Polette, M. & Birembaut, P. (2006). Alpha3alpha5beta2-nicotinic acetylcholine receptor contributes to the wound repair of the respiratory epithelium by modulating intracellular calcium in migrating cells. *American Journal of Pathology*, Vol.168, pp. 55-68.

Tracey, KJ. (2002). The inflammatory reflex. *Nature*, Vol.420, pp. 853-859

Tracey, KJ. (2007). Physiology and immunology of the cholinergic antiinflammatory pathway. *Journal of Clinical Investigation*, Vol.117, pp. 289-296.

Ulloa, L. (2005). The vagus nerve and the nicotinic anti-inflammatory pathway. *Nature Review of Drug Discovery*, Vol.4, pp. 673-784

Van Maanen, MA.; Stoof, S.; Esmerij, P.; van der Zanden EP.; de Jonge, WJ.; Janssen, RA.; Fischer, DF.; Vandeghinste, N.; Brys, R.; Vervoordeldonk, MJ. & Tak, PP. (2009a). The alpha7 nicotinic acetylcholine receptor on fibroblast-like synoviocytes and in synovial tissue from rheumatoid arthritis patients: a possible role for a key neurotransmitter in synovial inflammation. *Arthritis and Rheumatism*, Vol.60, pp. 1272-1281

Van Maanen, MA.; Lebre, MC.; van der Poll, T.; LaRosa, GJ.; Elbaum, D.; Vervoordeldonk, MJ. & Tak, PP. (2009b). Stimulation of nicotinic acetylcholine receptors attenuates collagen-induced arthritis in mice. *Arthritis and Rheumatism*, Vol.60, pp. 114-122

Van Maanen, MA.; Vervoordeldonk, MJ. & Tak, PP. (2009c) The cholinergic anti-inflammatory pathway: towards innovative treatment of rheumatoid arthrits. *Nature Review in Rheumatology*, Vol.5, pp. 229-232

Van Maanen, MA.; Stoof, S.; LaRosa, G.; Vervoordeldonk, M. & Tak, PP. (2010). Role of the cholinergic system in rheumatoid arthritis: aggravation of arthritis in nicotinic acetylcholine receptor $\alpha 7$ subunit gene knockout mice. *Annals of Rheumatic Diseases*, Vol.69, pp. 1717-1723

Waldburger, JM.; Boyle, DL.; Pavlov, VA.; Tracey, KJ. & Firestein, GS. (2008). Acetylcholine regulation of synoviocyte expression by the alpha7 nicotinic receptor. *Arthritis and Rheumatism*, Vol.58, pp. 3439-3449

Wang, H.; Yu, M.; Ochani, M.; Amella, CA.; Tanovic, M.; Susarla, S.; Li, JH.; Wang, H.; Yang H.; Ulloa, L.; Al-Abed, Y.; Czura, CJ. & Tracey, KJ. (2003). Nicotinic acetylcholine receptor alpha7 subunit is an essential regulator of inflammation. *Nature*, vol.421, pp. 384-388

Westman, M.; Engström, M.; Catrina, AI. & Lampa, J. (2009). Cell specific synovial expression of nicotinic alpha 7 acetylcholine receptor in rheumatoid arthritis and psoriatic arthritis. *Scandinavian Journal of Immunology*, Vol.70, pp. 136-140

Westman, M.; Saha, S.; Morshed, M. & Lampa, J. (2010). Lack of acetylcholine nicotine alpha 7 receptor suppresses development of collagen-induced arthritis and adaptive immunity. *Clinical and Experimental Immunology*, Vol. 162, pp. 62-67

Wessler, I. & Kirkpatrick, CJ. (2001). The Non-neuronal cholinergic system: an emerging drug target in the airways. *Pulmonary Pharmacology and Therapy*, Vol.14, pp. 423-434

Wessler, I.; Kilbinger, H.; Bittinger, F.; Unger, R. & Kirkpatrick, J. (2003). The non-neuronal cholinergic system in humans: Expression, function and pathophysiology. *Life Sciences*, Vol.72, pp. 2055-2061

Wessler, I.; Bittinger, F.; Kamin, W.; Zepp, F.; Meyer, E.; Schad, A. & Kirkpatrick, CJ. (2007). Dysfunction of the non-neuronal cholinergic system in the airways and blood cells of patients with cystic fibrosis. *Life Sciences*, Vol.80, pp. 2253-2258

Wessler, I. & Kirkpatrick, CJ. (2008). Acetylcholine beyond neurons: the non-neuronal cholinergic system in humans. Review. *British Journal of Pharmacology*, Vol.154, pp. 1558-1571

Yoshida, M.; Masunaga, K.; Satoji, Y.; Maeda, Y.; Nagata, T. & Inadome, A. (2008). Basic and clinical aspects of non-neuronal acetylcholine: expression of non-neuronal acetylcholine in urothelium and its clinical significance. *Journal of Pharmacological Sciences*, Vol.106, pp. 193-198.

Zhang, P.; Qin, L. & Zhang, G. (2010). The potential application of nicotinic acetylcholine receptor agonists for the treatment of rheumatoid arthritis. *Inflammation Research*, publ online 2010

21

Transcriptional Regulation of Articular Chondrocyte Function and Its Implication in Osteoarthritis

Jinxi Wang[1,2], William C. Kramer[1] and John P. Schroeppel[1]
[1]*Department of Orthopaedic Surgery,*
[2]*Department of Biochemistry and Molecular Biology,*
University of Kansas Medical Center, Kansas City,
USA

1. Introduction

Osteoarthritis (OA) is characterized by joint pain and stiffness with radiographic evidence of joint space narrowing, osteophytes, and subchondral bone sclerosis. Current treatments primarily target symptomatic control of OA, including pharmacologic therapy, local joint injection, and surgical interventions. Pharmaceuticals such as nonsteroidal anti-inflammatory drugs (NSAIDs) and Acetaminophen are aimed to control inflammation and pain by blocking potent inflammatory cytokine pathways. Joint injections including glucocorticoids and hyaluranan-based formulations attempt to control inflammatory mediators locally and improve the glucosaminoglycan concentration within the joint space. Surgical procedures such as debridement, microfracture, osteochondral autografting, and autologous chondrocyte transplantation are currently employed to stimulate articular cartilage repair and delay the need for joint replacement. However, all these therapies are aimed at symptomatic control and have limited impact on impeding or reversing the progression to advanced OA. Therefore, interest has been high in development of structure or disease-modifying OA drugs (DMOADs) aimed at slowing, halting, or reversing the progression of structural damage of articular cartilage. A large number of candidate DMOADs have been tested but none have been approved by American or European regulatory agencies (Hellio Le Graverand-Gastineau, 2009; Lotz & Kraus, 2010).

A critical barrier in drug development for OA is that molecular and cellular mechanisms for the development of OA, especially the mechanisms that control the activity of adult articular chondrocytes, remain unclear. Overexpression of proinflammatory cytokines such as Interleukin-1β (IL-1β) and tumor necrosis factor-α (TNF-α) (Goldring, 2001; Fernandes et al., 2002), matrix-degrading proteinases such as matrix metalloproteinases (MMPs) (Burrage et al., 2006) and a disintegrin and metalloproteinase with thrombospondin motifs (ADAMTS) (Glasson et al., 2005; Karsenty, 2005; Stanton et al., 2005), and nitric oxide (Pelletier et al., 2000; Haudenschild et al., 2008; Lotz, 1999) may cause cartilage degradation. However, no single cytokine or proteinase can stimulate all the metabolic reactions observed in OA. Due to the involvement of multiple proteinases and proinflammatory cytokines in the pathogenesis of OA, a candidate DMOAD that inhibits a single proteinase or inflammatory cytokine is unlikely to produce long-term benefit if other catabolic factors are not blocked. Therefore, it is critical to identify which upstream factors regulate the expression of these catabolic molecules in articular cartilage and other joint tissues (e.g., synovium).

This chapter summarizes the recent advances in identification of potential upstream regulators such as transcription factors and specific growth factors that may control the expression of anabolic and/or catabolic molecules in articular cartilage and their functional implications in the pathogenesis and treatment of OA.

2. Dysfunction of adult articular chondrocytes and its significance in OA

It has been recognized that OA may develop as a result of: 1) abnormal loading on normal joint tissues (articular cartilage and subchondral bone); 2) normal/physiologic loading on abnormal/defective joint tissues; or 3) a combination of the two (Piscoya et al., 2005; Brandt et al., 2008; Segal et al., 2009; Buckwalter et al., 2004; Block & Shakoor, 2009; Drewniak et al., 2009; June & Fyhrie, 2008; Borrelli et al., 2009; van der Meulen & Huiskes, 2002; Rothschild & Panza, 2007). Dysfunction of articular chondrocytes may be the initial change in OA with normal loading on abnormal articular cartilage. For OA associated with abnormal loading on normal joint tissues, dysfunction of articular chondrocytes is not the initial cause. However, mechanical disruption of the extracellular matrix and abnormal mechanotransduction in articular chondrocytes during and after joint injury or malalignment may activate specific signaling pathways, leading to changes in gene expression and cartilage metabolism as a result of dysfunction of articular chondrocytes. In order to develop effective strategies for prevention and treatment of OA, it is critical to understand the regulatory mechanisms of articular chondrocyte function.

Mature cartilage exists in three main types: hyaline cartilage, fibrocartilage, and elastic cartilage. Hyaline cartilage is characterized by matrix containing type-II collagen (collagen-2) fibers, glycosaminoglycans, proteoglycans, and multiadhesive glycoproteins. Fibrocartilage is characterized by abundant type-I collagen (collagen-1) fibers in addition to the matrix material of hyaline cartilage. Elastic cartilage is characterized by elastic fibers and elastic lamellae in addition to the matrix material of hyaline cartilage. Elastic cartilage is found in the external ear, the wall of the external acoustic meatus, the eustacchium, and the epiglottis of the larynx (Ross & Pawlina, 2006). Hyaline cartilage is of particular focus here because it is the innate component of diarthrodial joint surface involved in OA. Normal articular cartilage is composed of hyaline cartilage, which is divided into four zones: 1) the superficial tangential zone, composed of thin tangential collagen fibrils and low aggrecan content, 2) the middle or transitional zone, composed of thick radial collagen bundles, 3) the deep zone, composed of even thicker radial bundles of collagen fibrils, and 4) the calcified cartilage zone located between the tidemark and the subchondral bone (Goldring & Marcu, 2009). The calcified zone persists after growth plate closure and serves as an important mechanical buffer between the uncalcified articular cartilage and the subchondral bone. Generally, cell density decreases and cell volume and relative proteoglycan content increase as the cartilage transitions from superficial to deep. Unlike those chondrocytes involved in endochondral ossification, the chondrocytes within normal articular cartilage do not undergo terminal differentiation, but persist and function to produce extracellular matrix and maintain cartilage homeostasis.

The extracellular matrix is produced and maintained by the chondrocyte. Articular cartilage is characterized by the absence of blood vessels or nerves. Due to the avascularity of articular cartilage, some nutrients are provided by diffusion of the synovial fluid. Articular chondrocytes have adapted to the very low oxygen tension (in the range of 1-7%) and low glucose levels with facilitated glucose transport via upregulation of hypoxia inducible factor-1 (HIF-1), expression of glucose transporter-1 and -3 (GLUT1 and GLUT3), and enhanced anaerobic glycolysis (Wilkins et al., 2000; Mobasheri et al., 2005; Clouet et al., 2009). Much like bone, the physiologic properties of articular cartilage are primarily related to the extracellular matrix, but homeostasis in adult articular cartilage relies on the function of articular chondrocytes. In healthy articular cartilage, chondrocytes maintain a very low turnover rate of its constituents with a good balance of anabolism vs. catabolism.

Articular cartilage undergoes changes in its material properties related to aging which are different from the disease process of OA, but may eventually predispose cartilage to OA or contribute to its progression. One such factor is the development of advanced glycation end products (AGEs), which enhance collagen cross-linking and make the tissue more brittle (Verzijl et al., 2002). Additionally, the ability of chondrocytes to respond to growth factor stimulation appears to decline with age, leading to decreased anabolism (Loeser & Shakoor, 2003). Chondrocytes also demonstrate increasing senescence with age due to erosion of telomere length related to oxidative stress.

OA is a disease process characterized radiographically by narrowing of joint space due to loss of articular cartilage, subchondral bone sclerosis, osteophyte formation, and subchondral cyst formation. In addition to bony changes evident on radiographs, OA also affects the synovium and surrounding connective tissue, indicating it is not simply a disease of articular cartilage (Brandt et al., 2006; Brandt et al., 2008). At the cellular and molecular level, OA is a disruption of normal cartilage homeostasis, generally leading to excessive catabolism relative to anabolism. Risk factors that contribute to development of OA include advanced age, joint trauma, irregular joint mechanics and malalignment, obesity, muscle weakness, and genetic predisposition. Although OA is not commonly referred to as an inflammatory arthropathy due to the lack of neutrophils in the synovial fluid and the absence of a systemic inflammatory response, inflammatory mediators clearly play a role in the progression of OA.

In early OA, global gene expression within the chondrocyte is activated following mechanical injury or biological abnormalities causing increased expression of inflammatory mediators, cartilage-degrading proteinases, and stress-response factors (Fitzgerald et al., 2004; Kurz et al., 2005). Loss of proteoglycans and cleavage of collagen-2 occurs initially at the surface of articular cartilage, causing an increase in water content and reduced tensile strength of the matrix (Goldring & Goldring, 2007). Chondrocyte clustering is one of the typical features of OA cartilage (Clouet et al., 2009). Chondrocytes initially attempt to synthesize and replace degraded extracellular matrix (ECM) components such as collagen-2, -9, and -11, aggrecan, and pericellular collagen-4 (Buckwalter et al., 2007). This compensatory synthesis of ECM components is most evident among the deeper regions of articular cartilage (Fukui et al., 2008). Among the factors stimulating anabolism are insulin-like growth factor-1 (IGF-1), members of the transforming growth factor-β (TGF-β) superfamily, and fibroblast growth factors (FGFs) (Fukui et al., 2003; Hermansson et al., 2004). These attempt to offset the degradation caused by inflammatory mediators such as IL-1β, TNF-a, MMPs (e.g., MMP-1, MMP-3, MMP-8, MMP-13, and MMP-14), aggrecanases (e.g., ADAMTS-4 and ADAMTS-5), and other catabolic cytokines and chemokines.

As OA progresses, the synthetic balance shifts to favor catabolism, which leads to cartilage degradation. Significant heterogeneity in the synthetic capacity of articular chondrocytes occurs in OA cartilage. Overall gene activation is increased in the deep zone, but is decreased in the superficial zone and areas in the mid zone with degradation (Fukui et al., 2008). Evidence of phenotypic modulation of endochondral ossification, such as collagen-1, -3, -10, is found in osteoarthritic cartilage, which is not characteristic of normal adult articular cartilage (Sandell & Aigner, 2001). OA changes also occur in the subchondral bone that accompanies articular cartilage loss. Subchondral plate thickness increases, the tidemark advances, and angiogenesis invades an otherwise avascular structure (Lane et al., 1977). Apoptosis of the chondrocyte is seen in OA cartilage, which is mediated in part, by the caspases and inflammatory mediators such as IL-1 and Nitric Oxide (NO) (Kim & Blanco, 2007).

Another indication of aberrant behavior of osteoarthritic chondrocytes is the presence of collagen-10 (a marker of hypertrophic chondrocytes) and other differentiation markers, including annexin VI , alkaline phosphatase (Alp), osteopontin (Opn), and osteocalcin (Pfander et al., 2001; Pullig et al., 2000a; Pullig et al., 2000b; von der Mark et al., 1992), indicating that OA cartilage cannot maintain the characteristics of the permanent cartilage but adds those of the embryonic or growth plate cartilage. These observations suggest that chondrocyte maturation is likely to be deeply involved in the pathogenesis of OA. Recent findings on the regulatory effects of transcription/growth factors on the function of adult articular chondrocytes and their significance in the pathogenesis of OA are discussed below.

3. Regulation of articular chondrocyte function and its implication in pathogenesis of OA

Many governing factors that are critical for skeletal development have also been found to have a significant involvement in adult chondrocyte homeostasis and pathophysiology of OA. For instance, during skeletal development, chondrocytes in the growth plate undergo hypertrophic and apoptotic changes and cartilage is degraded and replaced by bone. One of the current hypotheses is that OA reflects the inappropriate recurrence of the hypertrophic pathway in articular chondrocytes. To better understand the regulatory mechanisms of various transcription and non-transcription factors in articular chondrocyte function, it is necessary to include their regulatory roles in chondrocyte differentiation, endochondral ossification, and joint formation during skeletal development here in this chapter.

3.1 Chondrocyte differentiation and joint formation during skeletal development

3.1.1 Chondrocyte differentiation and endochondral ossification

Both the chondrocyte (cartilage-forming cell) and osteoblast (bone-forming cell) are derived from a common mesenchymal stem cell referred to as the osteochondroprogenitor cell. Limb development first begins with the formation of mesenchymal condensations and the subsequent formation of a surrounding cartilaginous envelope called the perichondrium. The progenitor cells proceed to form the anlagen, or cartilaginous template of each bone. Cartilage cells undergo proliferation, differentiation to functional chondrocytes, hypertrophic differentiation, apoptosis, calcification of cartilage, invasion of cartilage tissue by capillaries and chondroclasts (osteoclasts), and eventual resorption and replacement by newly formed bone. This process of bone formation is called endochondral ossification. The primary ossification center in the diaphysis of long bones is formed through endochondral ossification. A similar sequence of events occurs in the growth plate leading to rapid growth of the skeleton.

3.1.2 Joint formation

At the end of each long bone an interzone and secondary ossification center develop. The interzone is the first sign of joint development at each future joint location, which consists of closely associated mesenchymal cells. Articular chondrocytes may derive from a subset of interzone cells, especially from the intermediate layer. Physiological separation of the adjacent skeletal elements occurs with further development, which involves a process of cavitations within the interzone that leads to formation of a liquid-filled synovial space. Morphological and cytodifferentiation processes extending over developmental time eventually lead to maturation of the joint in which the proximal and distal ends acquire their reciprocal and interlocking shapes. The formation of hyaline articular cartilage and other joint-specific tissues makes the joint fully capable of providing its physiologic roles through life (Pacifici et al., 2005; Mitrovic, 1978).

3.1.3 Bone morphogenetic proteins (BMPs) and their antagonists in joint formation

BMPs are members of the TGF-β superfamily. BMP was originally identified as a secreted signaling molecule that could induce chondrocyte differentiation and endochondral bone formation. Subsequent molecular cloning studies have revealed that the BMP family consists of various molecules, including members of the growth and differentiation factor (GDF/Gdf) subfamily. BMP members have diverse biological activities during the development of various organs and tissues, as well as embryonic axis determination (Hogan, 1996; Sampath et al., 1990; Wozney et al., 1988). BMP2, BMP4, BMP7, and BMP14 (GDF5/Gdf5) are expressed in the perichondrium and are proposed to regulate cartilage formation and joint development (Francis-West et al., 1999; Macias et al., 1997; Zou et al., 1997; Tsumaki et al., 2002). Gdf5, also known as cartilage-derived morphogenetic protein 1 (CDMP-1), plays a role in chondrogenesis and chondrocyte metabolism, tendon and ligament tissue formation, and postnatal bone repair (Bos et al., 2008). Mutations of this gene are present in a number of developmental bone and cartilage diseases (Masuya et al., 2007; Bos et al., 2008). Gdf5 has at least two roles in skeletogenesis. At early stages, Gdf5 may stimulate recruitment and differentiation of chondrogenic cells when it is expressed throughout the condensations. At later stages, Gdf5 may promote interzone cell function and joint development when its expression becomes restricted to the interzone (Storm & Kingsley, 1999; Koyama et al., 2008).

Extracellular BMP antagonists such as Noggin and Chordin can block BMP signaling by binding to BMP and preventing BMP binding to specific cell surface receptors. *Noggin* is expressed in condensing limb mesenchyme in mouse embryos, and expression persists in differentiated chondrocytes. When the *Noggin* gene was ablated, the mesenchymal condensations became much larger and limb joints failed to form, indicating that *Noggin* is critical for normal development of both long bones and joints (Brunet et al., 1998). Subsequent work in chick embryos showed that expression of *Noggin, Chordin,* and BMP-2 characterizes the interzone once it is established, and that *Chordin* expression persists in older developing joints, while *Noggin* expression shifts to epiphyseal chondrocytes (Francis-West et al., 1999). These and other data are widely acknowledged to signify that the action of BMP antagonists is required to regulate the pace and extent of chondrogenesis in early developing long bones, and that sustained and more restricted expression and action of these factors in developing joints would maintain the mesenchymal character of interzone cells and permit normal progression of interzone function and joint formation (Hall & Miyake, 2000). Absence of joints in *Noggin*-null mice would thus be due to exuberant and nonphysiologic action by endogenous BMPs and, consequently, rapid and abnormal conversion of the entire mesenchymal condensations into chondrocytes. Though these conclusions are plausible and quite likely, what remains unclear is how the absence of *Noggin* leads to joint ablation; specifically, whether the interzone fails to form completely or whether it starts forming but cannot be sustained, whether other BMP inhibitors fail to be activated, or whether joint formation sites fail to respond to upstream patterning cues (Pacifici et al., 2005).

3.1.4 ERG regulates the differentiation of immature chondrocytes into permanent articular chondrocytes

The ERG (Ets-related gene) transcriptional activator belongs to the *Ets* gene family of transcription factors. ERG is not only expressed at the onset of joint formation, but persists once the articular layer has developed further. A variant of ERG named C-1-1 is expressed in most epiphyseal pre-articular/articular chondrocytes in developing long bones. When C-1-1 is mis-expressed in developing chick limbs, it is able to impose a stable and immature articular-like phenotype onto the entire limb chondrocyte population, effectively blocking maturation and endochondral ossification (Iwamoto et al., 2000). More recent studies found that limb long bone anlagen of transgenic mice expressing the ERG variant C-1-1 were entirely composed of chondrocytes actively expressing collagen-9 and aggrecan as well as articular markers such as Tenascin-C. Typical growth plates were absent and there was very low expression of maturation and hypertrophy markers, including Ihh, collagen-10, and Mmp13. There was a close spatio-temporal relationship in the expression of both ERG and GDF5 that is an effective inducer of ERG expression in developing mouse embryo joints. These results suggest that ERG is part of the molecular mechanisms driving the differentiation of immature chondrocytes into permanent articular chondrocytes, and may do so by acting downstream of GDF5 (Iwamoto et al., 2007).

These studies suggest that mesenchymal progenitor cells differentiate into two fundamentally distinct types of cartilage cells during skeletal development. The cartilage cells in the primary and secondary ossification centers and the growth plate undergo proliferation, differentiation to functional chondrocytes, hypertrophic differentiation, apoptosis, and eventual resorption and replacement by newly formed bone through the endochondral sequence of ossification. This type of cartilage is called temporal or replacement cartilage. In contrast, cartilage cells close to the surface of growing long bones divide and differentiate to form hyaline articular cartilage, which is termed permanent or persistent cartilage because articular chondrocytes normally do not undergo terminal differentiation or endochondral ossification and are not replaced by bone (Eames et al., 2004; Pacifici et al., 2005).

3.2 Transcriptional regulation of articular chondrocyte function

Factors that have been reported to regulate chondrocyte differentiation during development and articular chondrocyte function in the adult stage are discussed below.

3.2.1 Sox9

The transcription factor Sox9 is a member of the high mobility group (HMG) and appears to be an essential transcription factor driving chondrogenesis during development and growth (Bi et al., 1999). Sox9 is expressed predominantly by mesenchymal progenitor cells and proliferating chondrocytes, but is not found in hypertrophic chondrocytes or osteoblasts (Zou et al., 2006). Sox9 is critical for the differentiation of mesenchymal progenitor cells into chondrocytes during cartilage morphogenesis. Prechondrocytic mesenchymal cells lacking Sox9 are unable to differentiate into chondrocytes (Bi et al., 1999). Joint formation is defective in Sox9-deficient mouse embryos (Akiyama et al., 2002). Two other members of the Sox family, Sox5 and Sox6 may also be essential for cartilage formation (Smits et al., 2001). Sox9 up-regulates the expression of chondrocyte-specific marker genes encoding collagen-2, collagen-9, collagen-11, and aggrecan by binding to their enhancer sequences (Evangelou et al., 2009). Sox9 also acts cooperatively with Sox5 and Sox6, which are present after cell condensation during chondrocyte differentiation, to activate collagen-2 and aggrecan genes (Zou et al., 2006; Lefebvre et al., 1998; Leung et al., 1998). It has been reported that the Sox trio (Sox 5, Sox6, Sox9) inhibit terminal stages of chondrocyte differentiation (Ikeda et al., 2004; Saito et al., 2007); however, the precise underlying regulatory mechanism remains unclear. Recently, Amano *et al.* demonstrated that the Sox trio inhibited chondrocyte maturation and calcification by up-regulating parathyroid hormone related protein (PTHrP) (Amano et al., 2009). The anabolic effects of insulin-like growth factor-1 (IGF-1), bone morphogenetic protein-2 (BMP-2), and fibroblast growth factor-2 (FGF-2) on developing chondrocytes also appear to be mediated, in part, by Sox9 (Leung et al., 1998; Lefebvre et al., 1998; Goldring et al., 2008; Kolettas et al., 2001; Zehentner et al., 1999).

Despite the fact that Sox9 is critical for chondrocyte differentiation and cartilage morphogenesis during skeletal development (Bi et al., 1999), the expression and function of Sox9 in adult articular cartilage are controversial in literature. A gene expression study reported that Sox9 expression was lower in human OA cartilage (Brew et al., 2010). However, another study showed no significant difference in subcellular expression of Sox9 protein between osteoarthritic and normal control human cartilage. Sox9 overexpression did not correlate with collagen-2 expression in adult articular cartilage, suggesting that Sox9 is not a key regulator of collagen-2 expression in human adult articular chondrocytes (Aigner et al., 2003). Furthermore, *in vitro* studies showed that overexpression of Sox9 was unable to restore the chondrocyte phenotype of dedifferentiated osteoarthritic articular chondrocytes (Kypriotou et al., 2003). These studies suggest that although Sox9 plays a crucial role in chondrocyte differentiation during skeletal development, its regulatory effect on the function of adult articular chondrocytes and development of OA remains to be elucidated.

3.2.2 Runx2

The transcription factor Runx2 (also called Cbfa1, Osf2, or AML3) is a member of the Runt family of transcription factors. Runx2 has been identified as a master regulator of osteoblast differentiation. Runx2$^{-/-}$ mice died shortly after birth and exhibited a cartilaginous skeleton completely void of intramembranous and endochondral ossification due to the maturational arrest of osteoblasts. (Komori et al., 1999; Coffman, 2003; Takeda et al., 2001; Ducy et al., 1997; Komori et al., 1997; Otto et al., 1997). Histologic analyses of Runx2$^{-/-}$ mice have revealed delayed maturation of chondrocytes, indicating that Runx2 is involved in both osteogenesis and chondrogenesis (Inada et al., 1999). Eames et al. demonstrated the ability of Runx2 overexpression to change permanent cartilage (e.g., articular cartilage) to temporal cartilage (e.g., growth plate cartilage) (Eames et al., 2004). Among the chondrogenic phenotypes during endochondral ossification, Runx2 is expressed mainly in the prehypertrophic and, to a lesser extent, in the late hypertrophic chondrocytes (Takeda et al., 2001). Its expression coincides with Indian hedgehog (Ihh), collagen-10, and BMP-6. Matrix metalloproteinase-13 (MMP-13), which is expressed by terminal hypertrophic chondrocytes, is a downstream target of Runx2 (Hess et al., 2001). Growth arrest and DNA damage induceable-45β (GADD45β) has been described as a probable intermediate molecule in the interaction between Runx2 and MMP-13 (Goldring et al., 2006; Ijiri et al., 2008; Ijiri et al., 2005).

In adult mice, Runx2 is expressed in the articular cartilage of wild-type mice at the early stage of post-traumatic knee OA, induced by surgical transection of the medial collateral ligament and resection of the medial meniscus. In this mouse model of OA, Runx2 expression in osteoarthritic cartilage parallels collagen-10 expression but arises earlier than Mmp13. After induction of post-traumatic knee OA by the same surgical procedure, $Runx2^{+/-}$ mice displayed decreased cartilage destruction and osteophyte formation, along with reduced expression of collagen-10 and MMP13, as compared with wild-type mice (Kamekura et al., 2006). Human OA cartilage exhibits increased Runx2 expression when compared to control cartilage. Runx2 co-localizes with MMP13 in chondrocyte clusters of OA cartilage. Runx2 overexpression in cultured chondrocytes increases MMP 13 expression (Wang et al., 2004).

These findings suggest that Runx2 regulates chondrocyte differentiation both in the developmental and adult stages. Runx2 may stimulate the progression of OA by promoting articular chondrocyte hypertrophy (indicated by expression of Collagen-10) and expression of MMP13 in articular cartilage (**Figure 1**).

3.2.3 Nfat1

Nfat1 (NFAT1) is a member of the Nuclear Factor of Activated T-cells (NFAT) transcription factor family originally identified as a regulator of the expression of cytokine genes during the immune response (Hodge et al., 1996; Xanthoudakis et al., 1996). Recent studies have shown that Nfat1 plays an important role in maintaining the permanent cartilage phenotype in adult mice. Nfat1 knockout ($Nfat1^{-/-}$) mice exhibited normal skeletal development, but displayed most of the features of human OA in load-bearing joints in adults (Wang et al., 2009; Rodova et al., 2011). $Nfat1^{-/-}$ articular cartilage shows overexpression of multiple specific proinflammatory cytokines (**Figure 2A-B**) and matrix-degrading proteinases (**Figure 3A**) at the initiation stage of OA (2-4 months of age). These initial changes are followed by articular chondrocyte clustering, formation of chondro-osteophytes, progressive articular surface destruction, formation of subchondral bone cysts, and exposure of thickened subchondral bone (Wang et al., 2009), all of which resemble human OA (Pritzker et al., 2006). The expression of mRNA for cartilage structural proteins (e.g., collagen-2, -9, and -11) was down-regulated but mRNA for collagen-10 was up-regulated at 2-4 months of age (**Figure 3B**). However, both collagen-2 and collagen-10 were up-regulated to varying degrees at 6 and 12 months, suggesting that early dysfunction of articular chondrocytes triggers repair activity within the degenerating cartilage (Rodova et al., 2011). These new findings revealed a previously unrecognized role of Nfat1 in maintaining the physiological function of differentiated adult articular chondrocytes by regulating the expression of specific matrix-degrading proteinases and proinflammatory cytokines.

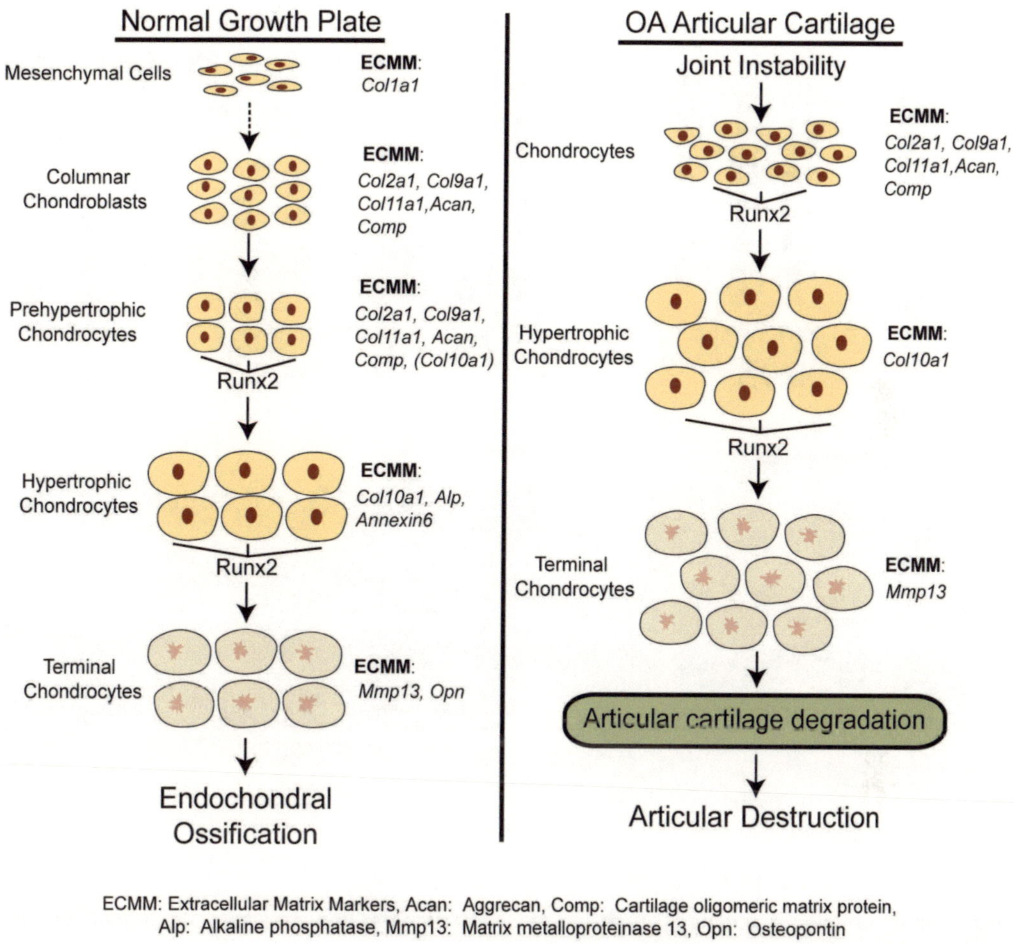

Fig. 1. A diagram shows Runx2 involvement in the chondrocyte differentiation pathways toward either physiological endochondral ossification in the growth plate or pathological chondrocyte hypertrophy in OA cartilage. Major morphological features and extracellular matrix markers for each step of chondrocyte differentiation are indicated.

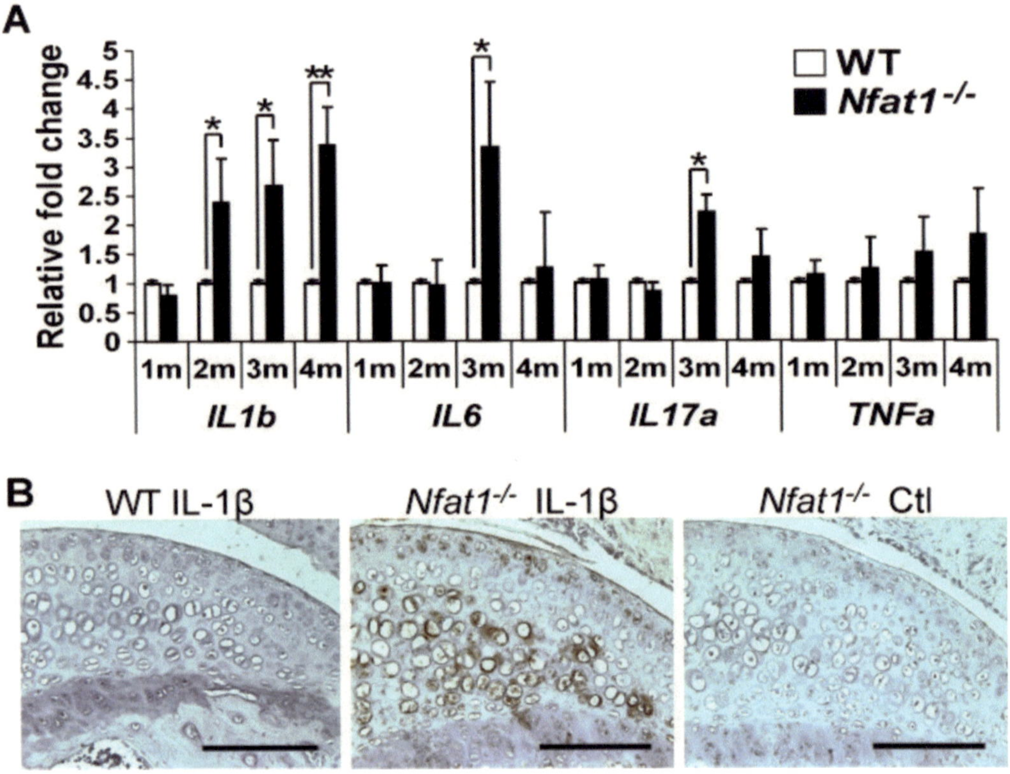

Fig. 2. Nfat1 deficiency causes dysfunction of adult articular chondrocytes with overexpression of specific proinflammatory cytokines. (**A**) Quantitative real-time PCR (qPCR) analyses indicate temporal changes in expression levels of various genes of proinflammatory cytokines in *Nfat1-/-* articular cartilage at 1-4 months (1-4m) of age. The expression level of each WT group has been normalized to "one". n = 3 pooled RNA samples, each prepared from the articular cartilage of 6-8 femoral heads. * $P < 0.05$; ** $P < 0.01$. (**B**) Immunohisto- chemical analyses using a polyclonal antibody against IL-1β (Santa Cruz) show substantially more intense expression of IL-1β (brown areas) in femoral head articular cartilage of 3-month-old *Nfat1-/-* mice compared to age-matched WT mice. *Nfat1-/-* Ctl represents a negative control using both IL-1β antibody and IL-1β blocking peptide (Santa Cruz) to validate the specificity of the immune reaction. Scale bar = 200 μm. Modified from the published figure (Wang, et al. J Pathol 2009; 219:163-72) with permission from the publisher.

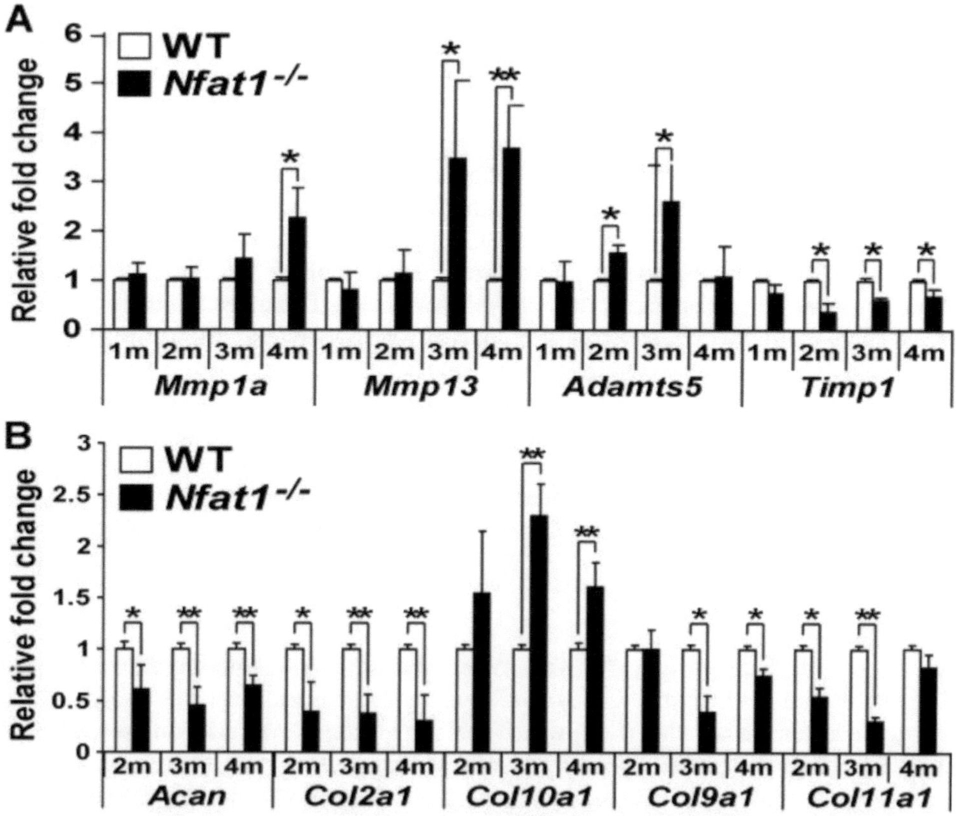

Fig. 3. Loss of Nfat1 leads to abnormal catabolic and anabolic activities of articular chondrocytes. (**A**) qPCR analyses demonstrate up-regulated expression of *Mmp1a, Mmp13, and Adamts5* and reduced expression of *Timp1* (tissue inhibitor of metalloproteinase-1) in femoral head articular cartilage of *Nfat1*-/- mice compared to age-matched WT mice at 1-4 months (1-4m) of age. (**B**) qPCR analyses indicate temporal changes in expression levels of various chondrocyte marker genes in *Nfat1*-/- articular cartilage at 2-4 months (2-4m) of age. The expression level of each WT group has been normalized to "one". n = 3 pooled RNA samples; * $P < 0.05$; ** $P < 0.01$. Modified from the published figure (Wang, et al. J Pathol 2009; 219:163-72) with permission from the publisher.

Thickening of subchondral bone is one of the characteristics of human OA. However, the precise biological mechanisms underlying the subchondral bone changes remain unclear. *Nfat1*-/- mouse joints display chondrocyte hypertrophy in the deep-calcified zones of articular cartilage, a feature of human OA cartilage. *Nfat1* -/- mesenchymal cells derived from subchondral bone marrow cavities differentiate into chondrocytes which subsequently underwent hypertrophy and endochondral ossification, leading to thickening of both subchondral plate and subchondral trabecular bone (Wang et al., 2009). These findings suggest that Nfat1 may prevent chondrocyte hypertrophy in adult articular cartilage and endochondral ossification in subchondral bone, thereby maintaining the integrity of cartilage-bone structure of synovial joints.

3.2.4 c-Maf

Transcription factor c-Maf, a member of the basic leucine zipper (bZIP) superfamily, is required for normal chondrocyte differentiation during endochondral bone formation. C-Maf is expressed in hypertrophic chondrocytes during fetal development. There is an initial decrease in the number of mature hypertrophic chondrocytes in *c-Maf*-null mouse tibiae, with decreased expression domains of collagen-10 and osteopontin (Opn), markers of hypertrophic and terminal hypertrophic chondrocytes, respectively. However, terminal chondrocytes, which express Opn and MMP13, appear later and persist for a longer period of time in *c-Maf* $^{-/-}$ fetuses than in control littermates, resulting in expanded chondrocyte maturation zones and a delay in endochondral ossification. These results suggest that c-Maf may facilitate both the initiation of terminal differentiation and the completion of the chondrocyte differentiation program (MacLean et al., 2003).

A recent study demonstrated transcriptional activation of human MMP13 gene expression by c-Maf in osteoarthritic chondrocytes. C-Maf enhances MMP13 promoter activity and RNAi-mediated knockdown of c-Maf leads to a reduced expression of MMP13. Chromatin immunoprecipitation assays reveal that c-Maf binds to the MMP13 gene promoter, suggesting that MMP13 is a potential target of c-Maf in human articular chondrocytes (Li et al., 2010).

3.2.5 β-catenin

In the canonical Wnt signaling pathway, Wnts bind the transmembrane Frizzled receptor (FRZ) family and co-receptors LRP5/6. FRZ receptor activation recruits the cytoplasmic bridging molecule Dishevelled (Dsh) which inhibits glycogen synthase kinase-3β (GSK-3β). This interaction prevents GSK-3β from phosphorylating β-catenin to avoid degradation of β-catenin, thereby allowing β-catenin to accumulate in the cytoplasm and translocate to the nucleus as a co-transcriptional activator with lymphoid enhancing factor 1/T cell-specific transcription factor (LEF/TCF) at specific DNA binding sites to activate downstream genes (Zou et al., 2006; Deng et al., 2008). Thus, β-catenin is a key mediator of the canonical Wnt signaling. Non-canonical Wnt signaling pathway, which does not involve β-catenin (Logan & Nusse, 2004), is probably best studied in *Drosophila* and its function is not covered in this chapter.

The canonical Wnt signaling pathway is known to induce chondrocyte maturation and endochondral ossification during skeletal development. This signaling pathway stimulates the commitment of mesenchymal stem cells to the preosteoblast and mature osteoblast phenotype, and blocks chondrogenic differentiation (Zou et al., 2006). Activation of the canonical Wnt signaling cascade during development in the limb bud and growth plate chondrocytes stimulates chondrocyte hypertrophy, calcification, and expression of MMPs and vascular endothelial growth factor (VEGF) (Tamamura et al., 2005; Day et al., 2005; Kawaguchi, 2009). Wnt-14 overexpression in chick limb mesenchymal tissue cultures causes a severe inhibition of chondrogenesis. Wnt-14 is necessary for joint formation since it might maintain the mesenchymal nature of the interzone by preventing chondrogenesis. In addition to Wnt-14, the interzone expresses Wnt-4, Wnt-16, and β-catenin. Conditional ablation of β-catenin in chondrocytes leads to the absence of joints. Ectopic expression of activated β-catenin or Wnt-14 in chondrocytes leads to ectopic expression of joint markers (Tamamura et al., 2005; Hartmann & Tabin, 2001; Guo et al., 2004).

The canonical Wnt signaling is also important in susceptibility to OA. Recent studies revealed that Wnt/β-catenin is involved in chondrocyte maturation and endochondral ossification in adult chondrocytes. The inhibition of Dickkopf-1 (Dkk1), a negative regulator of the Wnt signal, has been reported to allow conversion of a mouse model of rheumatoid arthritis to OA, due to increased endochondral ossification (Diarra et al., 2007). The conditional activation of β-catenin in articular chondrocytes of adult mice caused OA-like cartilage degradation and osteophyte formation. These pathological changes were associated with accelerated chondrocyte maturation and Mmp expression (Zhu et al., 2009). Interestingly, the same group also reported that selective suppression of β-catenin signaling in articular chondrocytes also caused OA-like cartilage degradation in Col2a1-ICAT (inhibitor of β-catenin and T-cell factor) transgenic mice, and this was mediated by enhancement of apoptosis of the chondrocytes (Zhu et al., 2008). These results suggest that both excessive and insufficient β-catenin levels may impair the homeostasis of articular chondrocytes.

Transcription factors and transcriptional co-activators that may be responsible for the maintenance of the physiological function of adult articular chondrocytes and development of OA are presented in **Figure 4**.

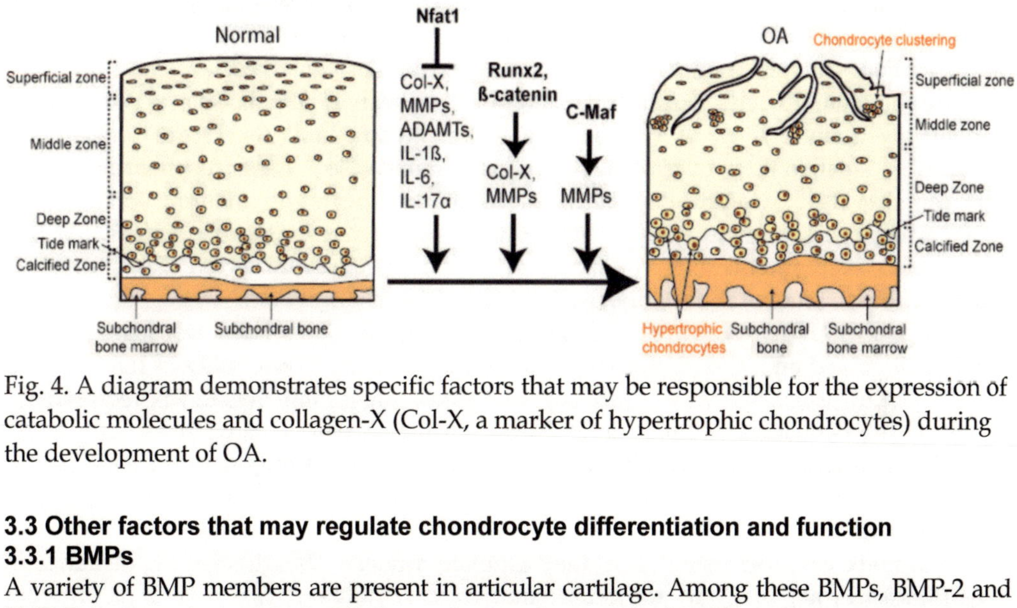

Fig. 4. A diagram demonstrates specific factors that may be responsible for the expression of catabolic molecules and collagen-X (Col-X, a marker of hypertrophic chondrocytes) during the development of OA.

3.3 Other factors that may regulate chondrocyte differentiation and function

3.3.1 BMPs

A variety of BMP members are present in articular cartilage. Among these BMPs, BMP-2 and BMP-7 (osteogenic protein-1, OP-1) are the two best studied BMPs with regard to cartilage homeostasis and OA. Both BMP-2 and BMP-7 have been shown to be capable of maintaining the chondrocyte phenotype. Inhibition of BMP-7 causes a reduction of aggrecan gene expression in chondrocytes. It has been reported that BMP-7 expression is decreased up to 9-fold in degenerated cartilage. In contrast to BMP-7, BMP-2 expression appears to increase with cartilage damage. In a study of BMPs in OA, BMP-2 is the only BMP member that demonstrates an increase in OA cartilage compared to cartilage from normal joints (Chubinskaya et al., 2007; Chubinskaya et al., 2000; Fukui et al., 2003; Sailor et al., 1996; Soder et al., 2005).

Multiple polymorphisms of the GDF-5 (BMP-14) gene have been found to produce an increased Odds Ratio of OA development, but the one that appears to have the most robust correlation is the rs143383 SNP in the 5′-UTR of GDF5. Miyamoto et al. reported a strong association between the rs143383 SNP of GDF5 and hip and knee OA in multiple Asian populations, with Odds Ratios ranging from 1.30-1.79 (Miyamoto et al., 2007). This association was confirmed in a large-scale meta-analysis; however, the magnitude of effect was less than previously reported (Evangelou et al., 2009). Interestingly, Egli *et al.* found that GDF5 expression imbalance was not limited to articular cartilage, but found in multiple joint tissues analyzed (synovium, fat pad, meniscus, ligaments) (Egli et al., 2009).

3.3.2 Insulin-like growth factor-1 (IGF-1)

IGF-1 is expressed in normal articular cartilage and is generally thought to be an important growth factor for maintenance of articular chondrocyte phenotype and articular cartilage repair (Fortier et al., 2002; Fortier et al., 2011). Chronic IGF-1 deficiency causes an increased severity of OA-like articular cartilage lesions in rat knee joints (Ekenstedt et al., 2006). Human OA cartilage responds to IGF-1 treatment by increasing proteoglycan synthesis; however, catabolism in OA cartilage is insensitive to IGF-1 treatment (Morales, 2008).

3.3.3 Indian hedgehog (Ihh)

Ihh is a member of the hedgehog proteins, and is essential for skeletal development. Ihh coordinates chondrocyte proliferation, chondrocyte differentiation, and osteoblast differentiation. Ihh is synthesized by prehypertrophic chondrocytes and by early hypertrophic chondrocytes during endochondral ossification. Ihh knockout (Ihh$^{-/-}$) mice demonstrate abnormalities of chondrocyte differentiation and bone growth. Cartilage elements are small in Ihh$^{-/-}$ mice because of a marked decrease in chondrocyte proliferation. Ihh$^{-/-}$ chondrocytes leaving the pool of proliferating chondrocytes prematurely because
Ihh$^{-/-}$ cartilage fails to synthesize parathyroid hormone-related protein (PTHrP) that acts primarily to keep proliferating chondrocytes in the proliferative pool. PTHrP, which is expressed by perichondral cells and early proliferative chondrocytes, down-regulates the expression of Ihh. This negative feedback loop mainly regulates the rate of chondrocyte differentiation and endochondral ossification. A third striking abnormality of Ihh$^{-/-}$ mice is the absence of osteoblasts in the primary spongiosa, suggesting that Ihh is required for osteoblast differentiation in endochondral bone formation (Kronenberg, 2003; Karp et al., 2000). Ihh is a critical and possibly direct regulator of joint development. In *Ihh*$^{-/-}$ mouse embryos, cartilaginous digit anlagen remained fused without interzones or mature joints (Koyama et al., 2007).

A recent study revealed that PTHrP may regulate articular chondrocyte maintenance in mice (Macica et al., 2011). In addition, parathyroid hormone (PTH) 1-34, a parathyroid hormone analog sharing the PTH receptor 1 with PTHrP, may inhibit the terminal differentiation of human articular chondrocytes *in vitro* and suppresses the progression of OA in rats (Chang et al., 2009).

3.3.4 Fibroblast growth factors (FGFs)

Recent evidence suggests that the FGF family plays an essential role in the proliferation and differentiation process of chondrocytes. The impact of many of these factors is not fully understood, but multiple FGF and FGFR (FGF receptor) genes are expressed at every stage of endochondral ossification. Within the chondrocyte pathway, FGFR3 is found in proliferating chondrocytes, FGFR1 in prehypertrophic and hypertrophic chondrocytes, and

FGFR2 is expressed among the earliest condensing mesenchyme (Ornitz & Marie, 2002). FGFs markedly enhance Sox9 expression in the early stages of development, likely through the mitogen-activated protein kinase (MAPK) pathway (Murakami et al., 2000).
The regulatory effects of FGF on adult articular chondrocytes are controversial in literature. A recent study showed that FGF-2 is an intrinsic chondroprotective agent that suppresses ADMTS5 and delays cartilage degradation in murine OA (Chia et al., 2009). However, other studies suggested that FGF-2 and FGF-23 may be involved in the progression of OA by stimulating MMP-13 expression through Runx2 (Orfanidou et al., 2009; Wang et al., 2004).

4. Future perspectives on pharmacological therapy

Over the past two decades, clinical trials applying a proinflammatory cytokine or proteinase inhibitor as a candidate disease-modifying OA drug (DMOAD) have been unsuccessful due to insufficient efficacy and/or severe side effects. A large number of candidate DMOADs have been tested but none have been approved (Hellio Le Graverand-Gastineau, 2009; Kawaguchi, 2009); suggesting that inhibition of a single catabolic molecule may not be sufficient for the treatment of OA because multiple catabolic factors are involved in its pathogenesis. Since specific transcriptional signaling molecules (e.g. Nfat1, Runx2, c-Maf, β-catenin) may regulate the expression of multiple catabolic and/or anabolic factors in articular chondrocytes, these regulatory factors may play more important roles in the development of OA than a single catabolic proteinase/cytokine. These findings have opened new avenues toward the development of DMOADs, using a more upstream factor as a molecular target than has been studied heretofore. In addition, OA not only affects articular cartilage but also involves other joint tissues such as the subchondral bone, synovium, capsule, menisci, and ligaments. Pathological changes in these joint tissues may affect the biological and mechanical properties of articular cartilage. Therefore, other joint tissues should not be ignored when designing pharmacological therapies. Furthermore, insufficient recognition of pathological changes in mechanical influence on the pathogenesis of OA may also negatively affect the efficacy of DMOAD candidates (Brandt et al., 2008). These recent research advances in the pathogenesis and treatment of OA may lead to the development of novel and effective therapeutic strategies using more up-stream pharmacological targets such as transcriptional signaling molecules, combined with biomechanical correction of abnormal joint loading if necessary, for the prevention and treatment of human OA.

5. Conclusion

OA is the most common form of joint disease and the major cause of chronic disability in middle-aged and older populations. All current pharmacological therapies are aimed at symptomatic control and have limited impacts on impeding or reversing the progression of OA, largely because the biological mechanisms of OA pathogenesis remain unclear. Previous studies have shown that overexpression of matrix-degrading proteinases and proinflammatory cytokines in articular cartilage is associated with osteoarthritic cartilage degradation. However, clinical trials applying an inhibitor of a proteinase or proinflammatory cytokine have been unsuccessful. Since multiple catabolic factors and pathological chondrocyte hypertrophy are involved in the development of OA, it is important to identify which upstream factors regulate the expression of catabolic molecules and/or chondrocyte hypertrophy in adult articular cartilage. This chapter summarizes the recent advances in the molecular regulation, with a main focus on transcriptional regulation, of the function of adult articular chondrocytes and its implication in the pathogenesis and treatment of OA. Recent studies have revealed that biological and mechanical abnormalities may affect transcriptional activity of specific transcription factors in articular chondrocytes. Transcription factor Sox9 is critical for the formation of cartilage, including articular cartilage, but its role in maintenance of adult articular chondrocyte function remains to be elucidated. Transcription factor Nfat1 plays an important role in maintaining the physiological function of adult articular chondrocytes. Nfat1-deficient mice exhibit normal skeletal development but display most of the features of human OA in their adult stage, including chondrocyte hypertrophy with overexpression of specific matrix-degrading proteinases and proinflammatory cytokines in articular cartilage. Transcription factor Runx2 and β-catenin transcriptional signaling may also be involved in the pathogenesis of OA via regulating the expression of anabolic and catabolic molecules in articular chondrocytes. These novel findings may provide new insights into the pathogenesis and treatment of OA.

6. Acknowledgments

This work was supported in part by the United States National Institutes of Health (NIH) grants AR 052088 (to J. Wang) and AR 059088 (to J. Wang), the Mary Alice and Paul R. Harrington Distinguished Professorship Endowment (to J. Wang), and the University of Kansas Medical Center institutional funds. The authors would like to thank Jamie Crist, James Bernard, Brent Furomoto, and Clayton Theleman for their assistance in graphic design and editing.

7. References

Aigner, T., Gebhard, P. M., Schmid, E., Bau, B., Harley, V. & Poschl, E. (2003). SOX9 expression does not correlate with type II collagen expression in adult articular chondrocytes. *Matrix Biology*, 22, 363-72.

Akiyama, H., Chaboissier, M. C., Martin, J. F., Schedl, A. & de Crombrugghe, B. (2002). The transcription factor Sox9 has essential roles in successive steps of the chondrocyte differentiation pathway and is required for expression of Sox5 and Sox6. *Genes Dev.*, 16, 2813-28.

Amano, K., Hata, K., Sugita, A., Takigawa, Y., Ono, K., Wakabayashi, M., Kogo, M., Nishimura, R. & Yoneda, T. (2009). Sox9 family members negatively regulate maturation and calcification of chondrocytes through up-regulation of parathyroid hormone-related protein. *Mol Biol Cell*, 20, 4541-51.

Bi, W., Deng, J. M., Zhang, Z., Behringer, R. R. & de Crombrugghe, B. (1999). Sox9 is required for cartilage formation. *Nat. Genet.*, 22, 85-9.

Block, J. A. & Shakoor, N. (2009). The biomechanics of osteoarthritis: implications for therapy. *Curr. Rheumatol Rep*, 11, 15-22.

Borrelli, J., Jr., Silva, M. J., Zaegel, M. A., Franz, C. & Sandell, L. J. (2009). Single high-energy impact load causes posttraumatic OA in young rabbits via a decrease in cellular metabolism. *J. Orthop. Res.*, 27, 347-52.

Bos, S. D., Slagboom, P. E. & Meulenbelt, I. (2008). New insights into osteoarthritis: early developmental features of an ageing-related disease. *Curr Opin Rheumatol,* 20, 553-9.

Brandt, K. D., Dieppe, P. & Radin, E. L. (2008). Etiopathogenesis of osteoarthritis. *Rheum. Dis. Clin. North Am.,* 34, 531-59.

Brandt, K. D., Radin, E. L., Dieppe, P. A. & van de Putte, L. (2006). Yet more evidence that osteoarthritis is not a cartilage disease. *Ann Rheum Dis,* 65, 1261-4.

Brew, C. J., Clegg, P. D., Boot-Handford, R. P., Andrew, J. G. & Hardingham, T. (2010). Gene expression in human chondrocytes in late osteoarthritis is changed in both fibrillated and intact cartilage without evidence of generalised chondrocyte hypertrophy. *Ann. Rheum. Dis.,* 69, 234-40.

Brunet, L. J., McMahon, J. A., McMahon, A. P. & Harland, R. M. (1998). Noggin, cartilage morphogenesis, and joint formation in the mammalian skeleton. *Science,* 280, 1455-7.

Buckwalter, J. A., Einhorn, T. A., O'Keefe, R. J. & American Academy of Orthopaedic Surgeons. 2007. *Orthopaedic basic science : foundations of clinical practice.* Rosemont, IL: American Academy of Orthopaedic Surgeons.

Buckwalter, J. A., Saltzman, C. & Brown, T. (2004). The impact of osteoarthritis: implications for research. *Clinical Orthopaedics & Related Research,* S6-15.

Burrage, P., Mix, K. & Brinckerhoff, C. (2006). Matrix metalloproteinases: role in arthritis. *Front Biosci,* 11, 529-43.

Chang, J. K., Chang, L. H., Hung, S. H., Wu, S. C., Lee, H. Y., Lin, Y. S., Chen, C. H., Fu, Y. C., Wang, G. J. & Ho, M. L. (2009). Parathyroid hormone 1-34 inhibits terminal differentiation of human articular chondrocytes and osteoarthritis progression in rats. *Arthritis Rheum* 60, 3049-60.

Chia, S. L., Sawaji, Y., Burleigh, A., McLean, C., Inglis, J., Saklatvala, J. & Vincent, T. (2009). Fibroblast growth factor 2 is an intrinsic chondroprotective agent that suppresses ADAMTS-5 and delays cartilage degradation in murine osteoarthritis. *Arthritis Rheum,* 60, 2019-27.

Chubinskaya, S., Hurtig, M. & Rueger, D. C. (2007). OP-1/BMP-7 in cartilage repair. *Int Orthop,* 31, 773-81.

Chubinskaya, S., Merrihew, C., Cs-Szabo, G., Mollenhauer, J., McCartney, J., Rueger, D. C. & Kuettner, K. E. (2000). Human articular chondrocytes express osteogenic protein-1. *J Histochem Cytochem,* 48, 239-50.

Clouet, J., Vinatier, C., Merceron, C., Pot-vaucel, M., Maugars, Y., Weiss, P., Grimandi, G. & Guicheux, J. (2009). From osteoarthritis treatments to future regenerative therapies for cartilage. *Drug Discov Today,* 14, 913-25.

Coffman, J. A. (2003). Runx transcription factors and the developmental balance between cell proliferation and differentiation. *Cell Biol Int,* 27, 315-24.

Day, T. F., Guo, X., Garrett-Beal, L. & Yang, Y. (2005). Wnt/beta-catenin signaling in mesenchymal progenitors controls osteoblast and chondrocyte differentiation during vertebrate skeletogenesis. *Dev Cell,* 8, 739-50.

Deng, Z. L., Sharff, K. A., Tang, N., Song, W. X., Luo, J., Luo, X., Chen, J., Bennett, E., Reid, R., Manning, D., Xue, A., Montag, A. G., Luu, H. H., Haydon, R. C. & He, T. C. (2008). Regulation of osteogenic differentiation during skeletal development. *Front Biosci,* 13, 2001-21.

Diarra, D., Stolina, M., Polzer, K., Zwerina, J., Ominsky, M. S., Dwyer, D., Korb, A., Smolen, J., Hoffmann, M., Scheinecker, C., van der Heide, D., Landewe, R., Lacey, D.,

Richards, W. G. & Schett, G. (2007). Dickkopf-1 is a master regulator of joint remodeling. *Nat. Med.,* 13, 156-63.

Drewniak, E. I., Jay, G. D., Fleming, B. C. & Crisco, J. J. (2009). Comparison of two methods for calculating the frictional properties of articular cartilage using a simple pendulum and intact mouse knee joints. *J. Biomech.,* 42, 1996-9.

Ducy, P., Zhang, R., Geoffroy, V., Ridall, A. & Karsenty, G. (1997). Osf2/Cbfa1: a transcriptional activator of osteoblast differentiation. *Cell,* 89, 747-757.

Eames, B. F., Sharpe, P. T. & Helms, J. A. (2004). Hierarchy revealed in the specification of three skeletal fates by Sox9 and Runx2. *Dev. Biol.,* 274, 188-200.

Egli, R. J., Southam, L., Wilkins, J. M., Lorenzen, I., Pombo-Suarez, M., Gonzalez, A., Carr, A., Chapman, K. & Loughlin, J. (2009). Functional analysis of the osteoarthritis susceptibility-associated GDF5 regulatory polymorphism. *Arthritis Rheum,* 60, 2055-64.

Ekenstedt, K. J., Sonntag, W. E., Loeser, R. F., Lindgren, B. R. & Carlson, C. S. (2006). Effects of chronic growth hormone and insulin-like growth factor 1 deficiency on osteoarthritis severity in rat knee joints. *Arthritis Rheum,* 54, 3850-8.

Evangelou, E., Chapman, K., Meulenbelt, I., Karassa, F. B., Loughlin, J., Carr, A., Doherty, M., Doherty, S., Gomez-Reino, J. J., Gonzalez, A., Halldorsson, B. V., Hauksson, V. B., Hofman, A., Hart, D. J., Ikegawa, S., Ingvarsson, T., Jiang, Q., Jonsdottir, I., Jonsson, H., Kerkhof, H. J., Kloppenburg, M., Lane, N. E., Li, J., Lories, R. J., van Meurs, J. B., Nakki, A., Nevitt, M. C., Rodriguez-Lopez, J., Shi, D., Slagboom, P. E., Stefansson, K., Tsezou, A., Wallis, G. A., Watson, C. M., Spector, T. D., Uitterlinden, A. G., Valdes, A. M. & Ioannidis, J. P. (2009). Large-scale analysis of association between GDF5 and FRZB variants and osteoarthritis of the hip, knee, and hand. *Arthritis Rheum,* 60, 1710-21.

Fernandes, J. C., Martel-Pelletier, J. & Pelletier, J. P. (2002). The role of cytokines in osteoarthritis pathophysiology. *Biorheology,* 39, 237-46.

Fitzgerald, J. B., Jin, M., Dean, D., Wood, D. J., Zheng, M. H. & Grodzinsky, A. J. (2004). Mechanical compression of cartilage explants induces multiple time-dependent gene expression patterns and involves intracellular calcium and cyclic AMP. *J Biol Chem,* 279, 19502-11.

Fortier, L. A., Barker, J. U., Strauss, E. J., McCarrel, T. M. & Cole, B. J. (2011). The Role of Growth Factors in Cartilage Repair. *Clin Orthop Relat Res,* 2011/03/16 (Epub ahead of print].

Fortier, L. A., Mohammed, H. O., Lust, G. & Nixon, A. J. (2002). Insulin-like growth factor-I enhances cell-based repair of articular cartilage. *J. Bone Joint Surg. Br.* , 84 276-88.

Francis-West, P. H., Abdelfattah, A., Chen, P., Allen, C., Parish, J., Ladher, R., Allen, S., MacPherson, S., Luyten, F. P. & Archer, C. W. (1999). Mechanisms of GDF-5 action during skeletal development. *Development,* 126, 1305-15.

Fukui, N., Ikeda, Y., Ohnuki, T., Tanaka, N., Hikita, A., Mitomi, H., Mori, T., Juji, T., Katsuragawa, Y., Yamamoto, S., Sawabe, M., Yamane, S., Suzuki, R., Sandell, L. J. & Ochi, T. (2008). Regional differences in chondrocyte metabolism in osteoarthritis: a detailed analysis by laser capture microdissection. *Arthritis Rheum,* 58, 154-63.

Fukui, N., Zhu, Y., Maloney, W. J., Clohisy, J. & Sandell, L. J. (2003). Stimulation of BMP-2 expression by pro-inflammatory cytokines IL-1 and TNF-alpha in normal and osteoarthritic chondrocytes. *J Bone Joint Surg Am,* 85-A Suppl 3, 59-66.

Glasson, S. S., Askew, R., Sheppard, B., Carito, B., Blanchet, T., Ma, H. L., Flannery, C. R., Peluso, D., Kanki, K., Yang, Z., Majumdar, M. K. & Morris, E. A. (2005). Deletion of active ADAMTS5 prevents cartilage degradation in a murine model of osteoarthritis. *Nature,* 434, 644-8.

Goldring, M. B. (2001). Anticytokine therapy for osteoarthritis. *Expert Opinion on Biological Therapy,* 1, 817-29.

Goldring, M. B. & Goldring, S. R. (2007). Osteoarthritis. *J Cell Physiol,* 213, 626-34.

Goldring, M. B. & Marcu, K. B. (2009). Cartilage homeostasis in health and rheumatic diseases. *Arthritis Res Ther,* 11, 224.

Goldring, M. B., Otero, M., Tsuchimochi, K., Ijiri, K. & Li, Y. (2008). Defining the roles of inflammatory and anabolic cytokines in cartilage metabolism. *Ann Rheum Dis,* 67 Suppl 3, iii75-82.

Goldring, M. B., Tsuchimochi, K. & Ijiri, K. (2006). The control of chondrogenesis. *J Cell Biochem,* 97, 33-44.

Guo, X., Day, T. F., Jiang, X., Garrett-Beal, L., Topol, L. & Yang, Y. (2004). Wnt/beta-catenin signaling is sufficient and necessary for synovial joint formation. *Genes Dev,* 18, 2404-17.

Hall, B. K. & Miyake, T. (2000). All for one and one for all: condensations and the initiation of skeletal development. *Bioessays,* 22, 138-47.

Hartmann, C. & Tabin, C. J. (2001). Wnt-14 plays a pivotal role in inducing synovial joint formation in the developing appendicular skeleton. *Cell,* 104, 341-51.

Haudenschild, D. R., Nguyen, B., Chen, J., D'Lima, D. D. & Lotz, M. K. (2008). Rho kinase-dependent CCL20 induced by dynamic compression of human chondrocytes. *Arthritis Rheum.,* 58, 2735-42.

Hellio Le Graverand-Gastineau, M. P. (2009). OA clinical trials: current targets and trials for OA. Choosing molecular targets: what have we learned and where we are headed? *Osteoarthritis Cartilage,* 17, 1393-401.

Hermansson, M., Sawaji, Y., Bolton, M., Alexander, S., Wallace, A., Begum, S., Wait, R. & Saklatvala, J. (2004). Proteomic analysis of articular cartilage shows increased type II collagen synthesis in osteoarthritis and expression of inhibin betaA (activin A), a regulatory molecule for chondrocytes. *J Biol Chem,* 279, 43514-21.

Hess, J., Porte, D., Munz, C. & Angel, P. (2001). AP-1 and Cbfa/runt physically interact and regulate parathyroid hormone-dependent MMP13 expression in osteoblasts through a new osteoblast-specific element 2/AP-1 composite element. *J. Biol. Chem.,* 276, 20029-38.

Hodge, M., Ranger, A., Charles de la Brousse, F., Hoey, T., Grusby, M. & Glimcher, L. (1996). Hyperproliferation and dysregulation of IL-4 expression in NF-ATp-deficient mice. *Immunity,* 4, 397-405.

Hogan, B. L. (1996). Bone morphogenetic proteins: multifunctional regulators of vertebrate development. *Genes Dev.,* 10, 1580-94.

Ijiri, K., Zerbini, L. F., Peng, H., Correa, R. G., Lu, B., Walsh, N., Zhao, Y., Taniguchi, N., Huang, X. L., Otu, H., Wang, H., Wang, J. F., Komiya, S., Ducy, P., Rahman, M. U., Flavell, R. A., Gravallese, E. M., Oettgen, P., Libermann, T. A. & Goldring, M. B. (2005). A novel role for GADD45beta as a mediator of MMP-13 gene expression during chondrocyte terminal differentiation. *J Biol Chem,* 280, 38544-55.

Ijiri, K., Zerbini, L. F., Peng, H., Otu, H. H., Tsuchimochi, K., Otero, M., Dragomir, C., Walsh, N., Bierbaum, B. E., Mattingly, D., van Flandern, G., Komiya, S., Aigner, T., Libermann, T. A. & Goldring, M. B. (2008). Differential expression of GADD45beta in normal and osteoarthritic cartilage: potential role in homeostasis of articular chondrocytes. *Arthritis Rheum,* 58, 2075-87.

Ikeda, T., Kamekura, S., Mabuchi, A., Kou, I., Seki, S., Takato, T., Nakamura, K., Kawaguchi, H., Ikegawa, S. & Chung, U. I. (2004). The combination of SOX5, SOX6, and SOX9 (the SOX trio) provides signals sufficient for induction of permanent cartilage. *Arthritis Rheum,* 50, 3561-73.

Inada, M., Yasui, T., Nomura, S., Miyake, S., Deguchi, K., Himeno, M., Sato, M., Yamagiwa, H., Kimura, T., Yasui, N., Ochi, T., Endo, N., Kitamura, Y., Kishimoto, T. & Komori, T. (1999). Maturational disturbance of chondrocytes in Cbfa1-deficient mice. *Dev Dyn,* 214, 279-90.

Iwamoto, M., Higuchi, Y., Koyama, E., Enomoto-Iwamoto, M., Kurisu, K., Yeh, H., Abrams, W. R., Rosenbloom, J. & Pacifici, M. (2000). Transcription factor ERG variants and functional diversification of chondrocytes during limb long bone development. *J. Cell Biol.,* 150, 27-40.

Iwamoto, M., Tamamura, Y., Koyama, E., Komori, T., Takeshita, N., Williams, J. A., Nakamura, T., Enomoto-Iwamoto, M. & Pacifici, M. (2007). Transcription factor ERG and joint and articular cartilage formation during mouse limb and spine skeletogenesis. *Dev. Biol.,* 305, 40-51.

June, R. K. & Fyhrie, D. P. (2008). Molecular NMR T2 values can predict cartilage stress-relaxation parameters. *Biochem. Biophys. Res. Commun.,* 377, 57-61.

Kamekura, S., Kawasaki, Y., Hoshi, K., Shimoaka, T., Chikuda, H., Maruyama, Z., Komori, T., Sato, S., Takeda, S., Karsenty, G., Nakamura, K., Chung, U. I. & Kawaguchi, H. (2006). Contribution of runt-related transcription factor 2 to the pathogenesis of osteoarthritis in mice after induction of knee joint instability. *Arthritis Rheum.,* 54, 2462-70.

Karp, S. J., Schipani, E., St-Jacques, B., Hunzelman, J., Kronenberg, H. & McMahon, A. P. (2000). Indian hedgehog coordinates endochondral bone growth and morphogenesis via parathyroid hormone related-protein-dependent and -independent pathways. *Development,* 127, 543-8.

Karsenty, G. (2005). An aggrecanase and osteoarthritis. *New England Journal of Medicine,* 353, 522-3.

Kawaguchi, H. (2009). Regulation of osteoarthritis development by Wnt-beta-catenin signaling through the endochondral ossification process. *J. Bone Miner. Res.,* 24, 8-11.

Kim, H. A. & Blanco, F. J. (2007). Cell death and apoptosis in osteoarthritic cartilage. *Curr Drug Targets,* 8, 333-45.

Kolettas, E., Muir, H. I., Barrett, J. C. & Hardingham, T. E. (2001). Chondrocyte phenotype and cell survival are regulated by culture conditions and by specific cytokines through the expression of Sox-9 transcription factor. *Rheumatology (Oxford),* 40, 1146-56.

Komori, H., Ichikawa, S., Hirabayashi, Y. & Ito, M. (1999). Regulation of intracellular ceramide content in B16 melanoma cells. Biological implications of ceramide glycosylation. *J Biol Chem,* 274, 8981-7.

Komori, T., Yagi, H., Nomura, S., Yamaguchi, A., Sasaki, K., Deguchi, K., Shimizu, Y., Bronson, R., Gao, Y., Inada, M., Sato, M., Okamoto, R., Kitamura, Y., Yoshiki, S. & Kishimoto, T. (1997). Targeted disruption of Cbfa1 results in a complete lack of bone formation owing to maturational arrest of osteoblasts. *Cell,* 89, 755-64.

Koyama, E., Ochiai, T., Rountree, R. B., Kingsley, D. M., Enomoto-Iwamoto, M., Iwamoto, M. & Pacifici, M. (2007). Synovial joint formation during mouse limb skeletogenesis: roles of Indian hedgehog signaling. *Ann. N Y Acad. Sci.,* 1116, 100-12.

Koyama, E., Shibukawa, Y., Nagayama, M., Sugito, H., Young, B., Yuasa, T., Okabe, T., Ochiai, T., Kamiya, N., Rountree, R. B., Kingsley, D. M., Iwamoto, M., Enomoto-Iwamoto, M. & Pacifici, M. (2008). A distinct cohort of progenitor cells participates in synovial joint and articular cartilage formation during mouse limb skeletogenesis. *Dev. Biol.,* 316, 62-73.

Kronenberg, H. M. (2003). Developmental regulation of the growth plate. *Nature,* 423, 332-6.

Kurz, B., Lemke, A. K., Fay, J., Pufe, T., Grodzinsky, A. J. & Schunke, M. (2005). Pathomechanisms of cartilage destruction by mechanical injury. *Ann Anat,* 187, 473-85.

Kypriotou, M., Fossard-Demoor, M., Chadjichristos, C., Ghayor, C., de Crombrugghe, B., Pujol, J. P. & Galera, P. (2003). SOX9 exerts a bifunctional effect on type II collagen gene (COL2A1) expression in chondrocytes depending on the differentiation state. *DNA Cell. Biol.,* 22, 119-29.

Lane, L. B., Villacin, A. & Bullough, P. G. (1977). The vascularity and remodelling of subchondrial bone and calcified cartilage in adult human femoral and humeral heads. An age- and stress-related phenomenon. *J Bone Joint Surg Br,* 59, 272-8.

Lefebvre, V., Li, P. & de Crombrugghe, B. (1998). A new long form of Sox5 (L-Sox5), Sox6 and Sox9 are coexpressed in chondrogenesis and cooperatively activate the type II collagen gene. *EMBO J,* 17, 5718-33.

Leung, K. K., Ng, L. J., Ho, K. K., Tam, P. P. & Cheah, K. S. (1998). Different cis-regulatory DNA elements mediate developmental stage- and tissue-specific expression of the human COL2A1 gene in transgenic mice. *J Cell Biol,* 141, 1291-300.

Li, T., Xiao, J., Wu, Z., Qiu, G. & Ding, Y. (2010). Transcriptional activation of human MMP-13 gene expression by c-Maf in osteoarthritic chondrocyte. *Connect Tissue Res,* 51, 48-54.

Loeser, R. F. & Shakoor, N. (2003). Aging or osteoarthritis: which is the problem? *Rheum Dis Clin North Am,* 29, 653-73.

Logan, C. Y. & Nusse, R. (2004). The Wnt signaling pathway in development and disease. *Annu. Rev. Cell Dev. Biol.,* 20, 781-810.

Lotz, M. (1999). The role of nitric oxide in articular cartilage damage. *Rheum. Dis. Clin. North Am.,* 25, 269-82.

Lotz, M. K. & Kraus, V. B. (2010). New developments in osteoarthritis. Posttraumatic osteoarthritis: pathogenesis and pharmacological treatment options. *Arthritis Res Ther,* 12, 211.

Macias, D., Ganan, Y., Sampath, T. K., Piedra, M. E., Ros, M. A. & Hurle, J. M. (1997). Role of BMP-2 and OP-1 (BMP-7) in programmed cell death and skeletogenesis during chick limb development. *Development,* 124, 1109-17.

Macica, C., Liang, G., Nasiri, A. & Broadus, A. E. (2011). Genetic evidence that parathyroid hormone-related protein regulates articular chondrocyte maintenance. *Arthritis Rheum,* 2011 Jun 23. doi: 10.1002/art.30515. [Epub ahead of print].

MacLean, H. E., Kim, J. I., Glimcher, M. J., Wang, J., Kronenberg, H. M. & Glimcher, L. H. (2003). Absence of transcription factor c-maf causes abnormal terminal differentiation of hypertrophic chondrocytes during endochondral bone development. *Dev. Biol.,* 262, 51-63.

Masuya, H., Nishida, K., Furuichi, T., Toki, H., Nishimura, G., Kawabata, H., Yokoyama, H., Yoshida, A., Tominaga, S., Nagano, J., Shimizu, A., Wakana, S., Gondo, Y., Noda,

T., Shiroishi, T. & Ikegawa, S. (2007). A novel dominant-negative mutation in Gdf5 generated by ENU mutagenesis impairs joint formation and causes osteoarthritis in mice. *Hum Mol Genet,* 16, 2366-75.

Mitrovic, D. (1978). Development of the diarthrodial joints in the rat embryo. *Am. J. Anat.,* 151, 475-85.

Miyamoto, Y., Mabuchi, A., Shi, D., Kubo, T., Takatori, Y., Saito, S., Fujioka, M., Sudo, A., Uchida, A., Yamamoto, S., Ozaki, K., Takigawa, M., Tanaka, T., Nakamura, Y., Jiang, Q. & Ikegawa, S. (2007). A functional polymorphism in the 5' UTR of GDF5 is associated with susceptibility to osteoarthritis. *Nat Genet,* 39, 529-33.

Mobasheri, A., Richardson, S., Mobasheri, R., Shakibaei, M. & Hoyland, J. A. (2005). Hypoxia inducible factor-1 and facilitative glucose transporters GLUT1 and GLUT3: putative molecular components of the oxygen and glucose sensing apparatus in articular chondrocytes. *Histol Histopathol,* 20, 1327-38.

Morales, T. I. (2008). The quantitative and functional relation between insulin-like growth factor-I (IGF) and IGF-binding proteins during human osteoarthritis. *J Orthop Res,* 26, 465-74.

Murakami, S., Kan, M., McKeehan, W. L. & de Crombrugghe, B. (2000). Up-regulation of the chondrogenic Sox9 gene by fibroblast growth factors is mediated by the mitogen-activated protein kinase pathway. *Proc Natl Acad Sci U S A,* 97, 1113-8.

Orfanidou, T., Iliopoulos, D., Malizos, K. N. & Tsezou, A. (2009). Involvement of SOX-9 and FGF-23 in RUNX-2 regulation in osteoarthritic chondrocytes. *J Cell Mol Med,* 13, 3186-94.

Ornitz, D. M. & Marie, P. J. (2002). FGF signaling pathways in endochondral and intramembranous bone development and human genetic disease. *Genes Dev,* 16, 1446-65.

Otto, F., Thornell, A. P., Crompton, T., Denzel, A., Gilmour, K. C., Rosewell, I. R., Stamp, G. W., Beddington, R. S., Mundlos, S., Olsen, B. R., Selby, P. B. & Owen, M. J. (1997). Cbfa1, a candidate gene for cleidocranial dysplasia syndrome, is essential for osteoblast differentiation and bone development. *Cell* 89, 765-71.

Pacifici, M., Koyama, E. & Iwamoto, M. (2005). Mechanisms of synovial joint and articular cartilage formation: recent advances, but many lingering mysteries. *Birth Defects Research Part C, Embryo Today: Reviews,* 75, 237-48.

Pelletier, J. P., Jovanovic, D. V., Lascau-Coman, V., Fernandes, J. C., Manning, P. T., Connor, J. R., Currie, M. G. & Martel-Pelletier, J. (2000). Selective inhibition of inducible nitric oxide synthase reduces progression of experimental osteoarthritis in vivo: possible link with the reduction in chondrocyte apoptosis and caspase 3 level. *Arthritis & Rheumatism,* 43, 1290-9.

Pfander, D., Swoboda, B. & Kirsch, T. (2001). Expression of early and late differentiation markers (proliferating cell nuclear antigen, syndecan-3, annexin VI, and alkaline phosphatase) by human osteoarthritic chondrocytes. *Am. J. Pathol.,* 159, 1777-83.

Piscoya, J., Fermor, B., Kraus, V., Stabler, T. & Guilak, F. (2005). The influence of mechanical compression on the induction of osteoarthritis-related biomarkers in articular cartilage explants. *Osteoarthritis Cartilage,* 13, 1092-1099.

Pritzker, K. P., Gay, S., Jimenez, S. A., Ostergaard, K., Pelletier, J. P., Revell, P. A., Salter, D. & van den Berg, W. B. (2006). Osteoarthritis cartilage histopathology: grading and staging. *Osteoarthritis Cartilage,* 14, 13-29.

Pullig, O., Weseloh, G., Gauer, S. & Swoboda, B. (2000a). Osteopontin is expressed by adult human osteoarthritic chondrocytes: protein and mRNA analysis of normal and osteoarthritic cartilage. *Matrix Biol.*, 19, 245-55.

Pullig, O., Weseloh, G., Ronneberger, D., Kakonen, S. & Swoboda, B. (2000b). Chondrocyte differentiation in human osteoarthritis: expression of osteocalcin in normal and osteoarthritic cartilage and bone. *Calcif. Tissue Int.*, 67, 230-40.

Rodova, M., Lu, Q., Li, Y., Woodbury, B. G., Crist, J. D., Gardner, B. M., Yost, J. G., Zhong, X. B., Anderson, H. C. & Wang, J. (2011). Nfat1 regulates adult articular chondrocyte function through its age-dependent expression mediated by epigenetic histone methylation. *J Bone Miner Res*, 26, 1974-1986.

Ross, M. H. & Pawlina, W. 2006. Cartilage. In *Histology, 5th Edition,* eds. M. H. Ross & W. Pawlina, pp 182-201. Philadelphia: Lippincott Williams & Wilkins.

Rothschild, B. M. & Panza, R. K. (2007). Lack of bone stiffness/strength contribution to osteoarthritis--evidence for primary role of cartilage damage. *Rheumatology (Oxford)*, 46, 246-9.

Sailor, L. Z., Hewick, R. M. & Morris, E. A. (1996). Recombinant human bone morphogenetic protein-2 maintains the articular chondrocyte phenotype in long-term culture. *J Orthop Res*, 14, 937-45.

Saito, T., Ikeda, T., Nakamura, K., Chung, U. I. & Kawaguchi, H. (2007). S100A1 and S100B, transcriptional targets of SOX trio, inhibit terminal differentiation of chondrocytes. *EMBO Rep*, 8, 504-9.

Sampath, T. K., Coughlin, J. E., Wheststone, R. M., Banach, D., Corbett, C., Ridge, R. J., Ozkaynak, E., Oppermann, H. & Rueger, D. C. (1990). Bovine osteogenic protein is composed of dimers of OP-1 and BMP-2A, two members of the transforming growth factor b superfamily. *J. Biol. Chem.*, 265, 13198-13205.

Sandell, L. J. & Aigner, T. (2001). Articular cartilage and changes in arthritis. An introduction: cell biology of osteoarthritis. *Arthritis Res*, 3, 107-13.

Segal, N. A., Anderson, D. D., Iyer, K. S., Baker, J., Torner, J. C., Lynch, J. A., Felson, D. T., Lewis, C. E. & Brown, T. D. (2009). Baseline articular contact stress levels predict incident symptomatic knee osteoarthritis development in the MOST cohort. *J. Orthop. Res.*, 27, 1562-8.

Smits, P., Li, P., Mandel, J., Zhang, Z., Deng, J. M., Behringer, R. R., de Crombrugghe, B. & Lefebvre, V. (2001). The transcription factors L-Sox5 and Sox6 are essential for cartilage formation. *Dev. Cell* 1, 277-90.

Soder, S., Hakimiyan, A., Rueger, D. C., Kuettner, K. E., Aigner, T. & Chubinskaya, S. (2005). Antisense inhibition of osteogenic protein 1 disturbs human articular cartilage integrity. *Arthritis Rheum*, 52, 468-78.

Stanton, H., Rogerson, F. M., East, C. J., Golub, S. B., Lawlor, K. E., Meeker, C. T., Little, C. B., Last, K., Farmer, P. J., Campbell, I. K., Fourie, A. M. & Fosang, A. J. (2005). ADAMTS5 is the major aggrecanase in mouse cartilage in vivo and in vitro. *Nature*, 434, 648-52.

Storm, E. E. & Kingsley, D. M. (1999). GDF5 coordinates bone and joint formation during digit development. *Dev Biol*, 209, 11-27.

Takeda, S., Bonnamy, J., Owen, M. J., Ducy, M. & Karsenty, G. (2001). Continuous expression of Cbfa1 in nonhypertrophic chondrocytes uncovers its ability to induce hypertrophic chondrocyte differentiation and partially rescues Cbfa1-deficient mice. *Genes Dev.*, 15, 467-81.

Tamamura, Y., Otani, T., Kanatani, N., Koyama, E., Kitagaki, J., Komori, T., Yamada, Y., Costantini, F., Wakisaka, S., Pacifici, M., Iwamoto, M. & Enomoto-Iwamoto, M. (2005). Developmental regulation of Wnt/beta-catenin signals is required for growth plate assembly, cartilage integrity, and endochondral ossification. *J Biol Chem*, 280, 19185-95.

Tsumaki, N., Nakase, T., Miyaji, T., Kakiuchi, M., Kimura, T., Ochi, T. & Yoshikawa, H. (2002). Bone morphogenetic protein signals are required for cartilage formation and differently regulate joint development during skeletogenesis. *J. Bone Miner. Res.*, 17, 898-906.

van der Meulen, M. C. & Huiskes, R. (2002). Why mechanobiology? A survey article. *J. Biomech.*, 35, 401-14.

Verzijl, N., DeGroot, J., Ben, Z. C., Brau-Benjamin, O., Maroudas, A., Bank, R. A., Mizrahi, J., Schalkwijk, C. G., Thorpe, S. R., Baynes, J. W., Bijlsma, J. W., Lafeber, F. P. & TeKoppele, J. M. (2002). Crosslinking by advanced glycation end products increases the stiffness of the collagen network in human articular cartilage: a possible mechanism through which age is a risk factor for osteoarthritis. *Arthritis Rheum*, 46, 114-23.

von der Mark, K., Kirsch, T., Nerlich, A., Kuss, A., Weseloh, G., Gluckert, K. & Stoss, H. (1992). Type X collagen synthesis in human osteoarthritic cartilage. Indication of chondrocyte hypertrophy. *Arthritis Rheum.*, 35, 806-11.

Wang, J., Gardner, B. M., Lu, Q., Rodova, M., Woodbury, B. G., Yost, J. G., Roby, K. F., Pinson, D. M., Tawfik, O. & Anderson, H. C. (2009). Transcription factor NFAT1 deficiency causes osteoarthritis through dysfunction of adult articular chondrocytes. *J. Pathol.*, 219, 163-72.

Wang, X., Manner, P. A., Horner, A., Shum, L., Tuan, R. S. & Nuckolls, G. H. (2004). Regulation of MMP-13 expression by RUNX2 and FGF2 in osteoarthritic cartilage. *Osteoarthritis Cartilage*, 12, 963-73.

Wilkins, R. J., Browning, J. A. & Ellory, J. C. (2000). Surviving in a matrix: membrane transport in articular chondrocytes. *J Membr Biol*, 177, 95-108.

Wozney, J. M., Rosen, V., Celeste, A. J., Mitsock, L. M., Whitters, M. J., Kritz, R. W., Hewick, R. M. & Wang, E. A. (1988). Novel regulators of bone formation: molecular clones and activities. *Science*, 242, 528-1534.

Xanthoudakis, S., Viola, J., Shaw, K., Luo, C., Wallace, J., Bozza, P., Luk, D., Curran, T. & Rao, A. (1996). An enhanced immune response in mice lacking the transcription factor NFAT1. *Science*, 272, 892-895.

Zehentner, B. K., Dony, C. & Burtscher, H. (1999). The transcription factor Sox9 is involved in BMP-2 signaling. *J Bone Miner Res*, 14, 1734-41.

Zhu, M., Chen, M., Zuscik, M., Wu, Q., Wang, Y. J., Rosier, R. N., O'Keefe, R. J. & Chen, D. (2008). Inhibition of beta-catenin signaling in articular chondrocytes results in articular cartilage destruction *Arthritis Rheum.*, 58, 2053-64.

Zhu, M., Tang, D., Wu, Q., Hao, S., Chen, M., Xie, C., Rosier, R. N., O'Keefe, R. J., Zuscik, M. & Chen, D. (2009). Activation of beta-catenin signaling in articular chondrocytes leads to osteoarthritis-like phenotype in adult beta-catenin conditional activation mice. *J. Bone Miner. Res.*, 24, 12-21.

Zou, H., Wieser, R., Massague, J. & Niswander, L. (1997). Distinct roles of type I bone morphogenetic protein receptors in the formation and differentiation of cartilage. *Genes Dev.*, 11, 2191-203.

Zou, L., Zou, X., Li, H., Mygind, T., Zeng, Y., Lu, N. & Bunger, C. (2006). Molecular mechanism of osteochondroprogenitor fate determination during bone formation. *Adv Exp Med Biol*, 585, 431-41.

22

TGF-β Action in the Cartilage in Health and Disease

Kenneth W. Finnson, Yoon Chi and Anie Philip
Division of Plastic Surgery, Department of Surgery, Montreal General Hospital, McGill University, Montreal, QC, Canada

1. Introduction

Transforming growth factor-β (TGF-β) is a pleiotropic cytokine that plays a critical role in the maintenance of healthy cartilage [1-4]. Aberrant TGF-β signaling has been implicated in a number of cartilage-related disorders including gout [5-6], lupus [7-8], rheumatoid arthritis [9] and osteoarthritis (OA) [1-3]. Although much progress has been made in understanding the molecular mechanism of TGF-β action in normal and OA cartilage, this knowledge has not translated into the development of a therapeutic strategy to slow or reverse the progression of the disease. In this chapter, we will highlight recent advances in understanding the role of TGF-β signaling in normal cartilage, the changes that occur in the TGF-β signaling pathway components in OA and the potential of targeting the TGF-β signaling pathway as a therapeutic strategy for the treatment of this disease.

2. TGF-β signaling

Members of the TGF-β superfamily, including TGF-βs, activins and bone morphogenetic proteins (BMPs), are critical for development and homeostasis [10-12]. They regulate diverse cellular processes including proliferation, differentiation and migration as well as extracellular matrix (ECM) production [11-14]. The three mammalian TGF-β isoforms (TGF-β1, -β2, -β3) share significant sequence (approximately 75% identity) and structural similarity [15-19]. However, the phenotypes of TGF-β isoform knockout mice do not overlap [20] and the isoforms exhibit distinct spatial and temporal expression in developing/regenerating tissues and in pathologic responses [21], suggesting distinct functions *in vivo*.

TGF-β is synthesized as a homo-dimeric pro-protein (pro-TGF-β) and is processed in the trans-Golgi network by furin-like enzymes. Cleavage by furin results in the formation of a mature TGF-β dimer along with its pro-peptide, known as latency associated peptide (LAP). TGF-β remains non-covalently associated with LAP and is in an inactive state. In most cases, this small latent complex associates with the latent TGF-β binding protein (LTBP) which forms a disulphide bond with LAP, giving rise to a large latent complex. Once secreted, the large latent complex becomes attached to the ECM by covalent cross-linking of LTBP with ECM proteins which is catalyzed by a transglutaminase [22-25].

TGF-β activation involves its dissociation from the latent complex which is necessary for TGF-β binding to its receptors and for mediating its biological effects [25]. Latent TGF-β can be activated by physical processes including acidification, alkalization and heat denaturation, and biological processes involving proteolysis or protein-protein interactions [22, 24-26]. Many serine proteases such as plasmin and thrombin, and several matrix metalloproteinases (MMPs) such as MMP-2, -9, -13 and -14 have been implicated in TGF-β activation [24]. In addition, thrombospondin-1 (TSP-1) has been shown to bind LAP directly and is thought to cause a conformational change in LAP that leads to activation of latent TGF-β [27]. Although the precise mechanisms of TGF-β activation *in vivo* in different tissues remain to be determined, it is likely to be a critical step for regulating TGF-β bioavailability [22, 24-26].

TGF-β signals through a pair of transmembrane serine/threonine kinases known as the type I (TβRI, also known as activin receptor-like kinase-5 or ALK5) and type II (TβRII) TGF-β receptors [10-12]. TGF-β binds TβRII, a constitutively active kinase, which then phosphorylates and activates TβRI/ALK5 [28-29]. Activated ALK5 phosphorylates intracellular Smad2 and Smad3 proteins, which then bind to Smad4 and accumulate in the nucleus where they interact with various co-activators, co-repressors and transcription factors to regulate gene expression [30-31]. TGF-β has also been shown to activate another TGF-β type I receptor known as ALK1 which phosphorylates Smad-1, -5 and -8 [32-34]. In addition, TGF-β activates several non-Smad pathways including mitogen-activated protein (MAP) kinase pathways (ERK, JNK and p38), Rho-like GTPase pathways and phosphatidylinositol-3-kinase (PI3K)/Akt pathways [35-36].

3. Regulation of TGF-β signaling

Intracellular regulation of TGF-β signaling involves the interplay of many cytoplasmic proteins including FKBP12, TRIP-1, STRAP, TRAP-1, SARA, HSP90 [37] and nuclear proteins such as TGIF, c-Ski, SnoN and Evi-1 [31]. The inhibitory Smads or I-Smads, which include Smad6 and Smad7, play critical roles in negative feedback regulation of TGF-β/BMP signaling by forming stable complexes with the activated type I receptors thereby blocking Smad phosphorylation [38-39]. Smad6 and Smad7 also act as adaptor proteins that recruit E3 ubiquitin ligases such as Smurf1 and Smurf2 to the TGF-β type I receptors and induce their ubiquitination and proteosomal degradation [40].

Extracellular control of TGF-β signaling is orchestrated by many factors including those that regulate activation of latent TGF-β as described in Section 2. In addition, several ECM components such as decorin and biglycan bind TGF-β and regulate its bioavailability [41]. Other extracellular molecules such as lipoproteins have been shown to sequester TGF-β ligand into an inactive pool [42]. TGF-β co-receptors such as endoglin, betaglycan and CD109 are emerging as important factors that regulate many aspects of TGF-β signaling in health and disease.

Endoglin (CD105) is a single-pass transmembrane homo-dimeric glycoprotein that is expressed mainly in endothelial cells. It binds TGF-β1 and TGF-β3 with high affinity in the presence of TβRII but does not bind the TGF-β2 isoform [43]. Endoglin has been shown to (i) alter TβRII and TβRI (ALK1 and ALK5) phosphorylation status, (ii) promote TGF-β/ALK1 signaling, (iii) suppress TGF-β/ALK5/Smad2/3 signaling and (iv) antagonize TGF-β-induced MAP kinase signaling through a β-arrestin-2-dependent mechanism [44-45].

Betaglycan, also known as TGF-β type III receptor, is a homologue of endoglin and is a more ubiquitously expressed transmembrane glycoprotein. It binds all three TGF-β isoforms (TGF-β1, -β2, -β3) with high affinity and enhances their binding to the signaling receptors, especially that of the TGF-β2 isoform [43, 46-47]. Betaglycan has been shown to direct clathrin-mediated endocytosis of TβRII and ALK5 [48], and enhance TGF-β signaling via Smad and MAP kinase pathways [49-51]. Conversely, betaglycan has also been reported to promote β-arrestin2-dependent TGF-β receptor internalization and down-regulation of TGF-β signaling [52].

CD109 is a glycosyl phosphatidylinostol (GPI)-anchored protein and a member of the α2-macroglobulin/complement family. It is found on activated T-cells and platelets, endothelial cells and many human cancer cell lines [53-56]. We have recently identified CD109 as a TGF-β co-receptor which binds TGF-β1 with high affinity, forms a heteromeric complex with the TGF-β signaling receptors and inhibits Smad2/3 signaling in different cell types [57-58]. Recent results indicate that CD109 inhibits TGF-β signaling by promoting TGF-β receptor internalization and degradation in a Smad7/Smurf2-dependent manner [57, 59]. Taken together, these studies demonstrate that the TGF-β co-receptors endoglin, betaglycan and CD109 play critical roles in regulating TGF-β signaling.

4. TGF-β and cartilage

Articular cartilage is an avascular tissue that receives its nutrients from synovial fluid, a thin layer of fluid surrounding the cartilage. The only cell type found in cartilage is the chondrocyte which are embedded in an extensive ECM made of mainly collagens and proteoglycans [60]. Type II collagen is the main collagen found in articular cartilage and is important for providing tensile strength [61-62]. Aggrecan is the main proteoglycan of articular cartilage and provides structural support by retaining water in the matrix [63]. Articular cartilage is commonly divided into four distinct zones, namely the superficial zone, middle zone, deep zone and calcified cartilage [60]. The zones differ in collagen organization, proteoglycan content and chondrocyte morphologies [60].

TGF-β plays a number of roles in the development, growth and maintenance of articular cartilage. During cartilage development, TGF-β stimulates chondrogenic condensation [64-65], chondroprogenitor cell proliferation and chondrocyte differentiation [66-67]. TGF-β also inhibits terminal differentiation or "hypertrophy" of chondrocytes thereby blocking endochondral bone formation [68-69] and allowing formation of articular cartilage at the end of the long bones [70]. The maintenance of mature articular cartilage is dependent on the action of TGF-β which not only stimulates production of ECM proteins such as type II collagen and aggrecan, but also blocks degradation of ECM proteins by increasing production of protease inhibitors such as tissue inhibitor of metalloproteases (TIMPs) [69, 71]. TGF-β also counteracts the catabolic effects of interleukin (IL)-1 and tumor necrosis factor (TNF)-α on cartilage[69, 71].

The potent anabolic effects of TGF-β on articular cartilage *in vivo* in animal models are well known. TGF-β injected into the periosteum of rat or mouse femur induces chondrocyte differentiation and cartilage formation [72-73]. Local administration of TGF-β into murine knee joints stimulated articular cartilage repair [74] and healing of full-thickness cartilage defects [75-76]. Conversely, blocking endogenous TGF-β using a soluble form of TβRII impaired articular cartilage repair in a murine model of experimental OA [77]. In addition, expression of a dominant negative TβRII in cartilage resulted in an OA-like phenotype in the mouse [78]. Furthermore, Smad3 knockout mice develop degenerative joint disease resembling human OA [70]. In addition, decreased TGF-β expression and Smad2 phosphorylation are associated with a reduced protective effect during OA progression [79]. Evidence for a causal relationship between TGF-β and OA in the human is further supported by the identification of asporin (a proteoglycan that sequesters TGF-β in the ECM and inhibits TGF-β function) as an OA susceptibility gene [80-83]. However, TGF-β also has been shown to have undesirable effects on cartilage. A number of studies have reported that TGF-β treatment of normal murine joints is associated with osteophyte outgrowth, inflammation and synovial fibroplasia [84-86]. Thus, normal cartilage function may dependent on a narrow range of bioactive TGF-β levels, and concentrations above or below this level may lead to alterations in TGF-β signaling, resulting in abnormal cartilage function.

5. Altered expression and function of TGF-β pathway components in osteoarthritis

OA is a chronic degenerative joint disease characterized by articular cartilage degradation, subchondral bone alterations and synovial inflammation [87-88]. The cause of OA is unknown but risk factors include aging, obesity, abnormal mechanical loading and anatomical abnormalities [89]. Subchondral bone alterations contribute to the initiation and/or progression of OA by producing catabolic factors that degrade the overlying cartilage [90]. Synovial inflammation is thought to be induced by cartilage matrix degradation products that are phagocytosed by macrophages of the synovial lining. The macrophages, in turn, secrete pro-inflammatory mediators into the synovial fluid that diffuse into the cartilage, thereby creating a vicious circle of synovial inflammation and cartilage degradation [90]. The current chapter focuses on the role of TGF-β signaling in articular cartilage homeostasis and its deregulation in OA.

5.1 TGF-β ligands and their activation

Several studies suggest that TGF-β isoform (TGF-β1, -β2, -β3) levels are down-regulated in OA cartilage. For example, TGF-β1 protein levels were shown to be decreased in human OA cartilage [91-92] and TGF-β3 levels were shown to be reduced in both spontaneous (STR/Ort) and collagenase-induced mouse models of OA [79]. In addition, TGF-β1 and TGF-β2 levels were moderately decreased in rabbit OA cartilage [93]. In constrast, a number of studies have demonstrated that TGF-β isoform expression is up-regulated in OA cartilage. TGF-β1, -β2 and -β3 levels were found to be increased in human OA [94-96] and TGF-β1 and -β3 levels were elevated in a papain-induced mouse model of OA [77]. Furthermore, TGF-β2 was increased in a surgically-induced model of early OA in rats [97]. One possible explanation for these discrepancies is that TGF-β isoform expression may vary during the course of OA. For instance, TGF-β levels might increase in the early stages of OA to counteract the catabolic effects of inflammatory cytokines such as IL-1β or TNF-α [98-99]. However, with the progressive loss of TGF-β receptor expression (see Section 5.2), chondrocytes may eventually lose their responsiveness to TGF-β, leading to a decrease in TGF-β levels due to the loss of TGF-β auto-induction [100]. Future studies using age-, race- and gender- matched normal and OA human articular cartilage and a better characterization of TGF-β isoform expression in the different animal models during OA progression will be needed to resolve this issue.

Although TGF-β isoform levels are altered in OA, it is not known whether these changes represent active TGF-β levels. Moreover, accumulating evidence suggests that components of the large latent complex may be disrupted in OA. For example, both LTBP-1 and LTBP-2 were shown to be increased in human OA cartilage [97, 101-102] and in experimental models of OA [97, 101]. Although LTBP-1 [103-104] and LTBP-2 [105] knockout mice do not display an OA phenotype suggesting that these proteins may not contribute to the OA process, LTBP-3 knockout mice develop an OA phenotype and display features resembling those of mice with impaired TGF-β signaling [106-107]. These results suggest that LTBP-3 might have a protective effect against OA progression. It is also possible that studies using LTBP-1 and LTBP-2 knockout mice in an experimental OA setting may reveal a role for these proteins in OA progression. Interestingly, the levels of TGF-β activators are also upregulated in human OA and in a variety of animal models of OA. Transglutaminase-2 (TG-2), the predominant transglutaminase subtype in hypertrophic chondrocytes, are higher in knee [108-109] and femoral [110] cartilage in human OA and in experimental OA models [97, 101, 111]. Whether the enhanced TG-2 expression in OA correlates with increased TGF-β activation or LTBP cross-linking to ECM remains to be determined. In addition, TSP-1 levels are increased in the cartilage in mild and moderate OA, but decreased in severe OA [112]. Intra-articular gene transfer of TSP-1 was shown to reduce disease progression in a collagen- or anterior cruciate ligament transection-induced OA in rats [113-114]. This is consistent with the notion that TSP-1 mediates latent TGF-β activation in OA cartilage and that the up-regulation of TSP-1 is an adaptive response in an attempt to increase cartilage repair.

5.2 TGF-β receptors

Increasing evidence indicates that TGF-β receptor expression levels are altered in OA. TβRII levels were shown to be decreased in human OA cartilage [92] and in a rabbit OA model [93]. In addition, TβRII mRNA expression was decreased in cultured human OA chondrocytes as compared to normal chondrocytes *in vitro* [115]. These results suggest that loss of TβRII during OA might represent an intrinsic defect of human OA chondrocytes. The notion that loss of TβRII might contribute to the initiation and/or progression of OA is supported by a study showing that a truncated, kinase-defective TβRII expressed in mouse skeletal tissue was associated terminal chondrocyte differentiation and the development of OA-like features [78]. A more recent study has shown that conditional expression of dominant negative TβRII inhibits cartilage formation in mice [116]. Thus, loss of TβRII expression and/or activity may not only promote an OA-like phenotype but may also contribute to OA progression by limiting the ability of cartilage to repair itself. Future studies using cartilage-specific knockout of TβRII may provide further insight into the role of this TGF-β receptor in OA pathogenesis.

Emerging evidence indicates that the expression of TGF-β type I receptors is also altered in OA. Our group has shown that in addition to the canonical TGF-β type I receptor ALK5, human chondrocytes also express ALK1 [34]. Both ALK5 and ALK1 are required for TGF-β-induced Smad1/5 phosphorylation whereas only ALK5 is essential for TGF-β-induced Smad3 phosphorylation in these cells [34]. We also demonstrated that ALK1 inhibits whereas ALK5 potentiates the expression of type II collagen and PAI-1 in chondrocytes, indicating that ALK1 and ALK5 elicit opposite efffects in chondrocytes [34]. More recent data suggest that both ALK5 and ALK1 levels are decreased in mouse models of OA, but that ALK1 expression decreases to a lesser extent than that of ALK5, suggesting that the ratio of ALK1/ALK5 increases during OA [117]. Interestingly, ALK1 has been identified as one of the genes upregulated in a mensical tear rat model of OA [101] whereas ALK5 levels were dramatically reduced in partial meniscectomy and post-surgery training rat model of OA [118]. These two latter studies are consistent with the notion that the ALK1/ALK5 ratio increases during OA. In human OA cartilage, ALK1 mRNA expression highly correlates with MMP-13 levels whereas ALK5 mRNA levels correlate with aggrecan and collagen type II levels [117]. Collectively, these data suggest that alterations in the expression of TGF-β signaling receptors (TβRII and ALK5/ALK1) play an important role in OA pathogenesis and that an increase in the TGF-β/ALK1 pathway activation relative to that of the TGF-β/ALK5 pathway activation is likely to be a critical event in the OA disease progression.

5.3 Smads

Since TGF-β receptor levels are altered in OA, it can be anticipated that activities of downstream signaling mediators such as Smad2 and Smad3 are also altered. Indeed, Smad2 phosphorylation levels are reduced in cartilage during OA progression in both spontaneous- (STR/Ort) and collagenase-induced mouse models of OA [79] and in cartilage of old mice as compared to young mice [119]. Although Smad3 phosphorylation was not examined in these models, a recent study has reported decreased Smad3 phosphorylation levels in the Smurf-2 transgenic mice which spontaneously develop an OA-like phenotype [120]. Together, these studies suggest that OA is associated with reduced TGF-β/ALK5/Smad2/3 signaling.

The potential importance of Smad3 in OA is further underscored by the finding that Smad3 knockout mice develop a degenerative joint disease resembling human OA [70] and intervertebral disc degeneration [121]. Moreover, several genetic studies in humans suggest that mutations in the Smad3 gene may be an important factor in OA. A missense mutation in the Smad3 gene was found in a patient with knee OA and was associated with elevated serum MMP-2 and MMP-9 levels [122]. A single nucleotide polymorphism (SNP) mapping to the Smad3 intron 1 was shown to be involved in risk of both hip and knee OA in European populations [123]. Furthermore, several mutations in the Smad3 gene were found in individuals that presented early-onset OA [124]. Although the functional significance of these mutations in Smad3 remains to be determined, these studies suggest that alteration in Smad3 function may play a role in the pathogenesis of OA.

A shift in the balance of signaling from Smad2/3 towards Smad1/5 is thought to play an important role in OA pathogenesis. TGF-β signals through both of these pathways in human chondrocytes with the Smad1/5 pathway opposing the Smad2/3 pathway [34]. This is consistent with the findings in endothelial cells [32-33], skin fibroblasts [125] and in chondrocyte terminal differentiation [126]. Although Smad-1, -5 and -8 expression levels and subcellular localization in human OA cartilage did not differ significantly from that of normal cartilage, two Smad1 gene splice variants of unknown significance were reduced in OA cartilage [127]. When the reported decrease in ALK5 expression and Smad2/3 signaling (see above) in OA cartilage is taken into account, it is possible to envision that a shift in TGF-β signaling away from the ALK5/Smad2/3 pathway and towards the ALK1/Smad1/5/8 pathway may occur, contributing to OA progression. However, whether such a shift is an adaptive response without a causal relationship to OA progression cannot be ruled out at this time.

As mentioned above, Smad7/Smurf2-mediated TGF-β receptor degradation is an important mechanism for the termination of TGF-β signaling [38-39]. Although Smad7 expression levels in human OA cartilage did not significantly differ from that of normal cartilage [128] it did show an age-related increased expression in murine cartilage [119] suggesting that age might be an important factor to consider when comparing Smad7 expression levels in OA versus normal cartilage. In addition, Smurf2 is increased in human OA cartilage as compared to normal cartilage [129] and Smurf2-transgenic mice spontaneously develop an OA-like phenotype [129]. Because Smad7 and Smurf-2 work in concert to promote TGF-β receptor degradation, these data suggest that increased Smad7/Smurf2 action resulting in decreased TGF-β receptor levels might be involved in OA pathogenesis.

5.4 MAP kinases

In addition to the Smad pathway, TGF-β also activates several non-Smad pathways including MAPK kinase (ERK, p38, JNK) pathways, Rho-like GTPase signaling pathways and PI3K/Akt pathways [35-36]. TGF-β-activated kinase-1 (TAK1), a MAP3 kinase activated by TGF-β and other pathways, plays a critical role in cartilage development and function [130]. TGF-β signaling via TAK-1 stimulates type II collagen synthesis in chondrocytes in a Smad3-independent manner [131]. On the other hand, activation of MAPK kinase activity by cytokines such as IL-1β or TNF-α decreases Smad3/4 DNA binding and ECM production in chondrocytes [132]. In addition, activating transcription factor (ATF)-2 works synergistically with Smad3 to mediate TGF-βs inhibition of chondrocyte maturation [133]. These studies suggest extensive cross-talk between Smad and non-Smad pathways in chondrocytes which should be taken into account when considering the role of aberrant TGF-β signaling in OA.

5.5 TGF-β co-receptors

TGF-β co-receptors such as endoglin, betaglycan and CD109 have emerged as important regulators of TGF-β signaling and responses with critical roles in diseases such as cancer and organ fibrosis [43, 47, 54, 58, 134-136]. This section focuses on the available information on these TGF-β co-receptors in cartilage health and disease.

Endoglin (CD105): We have previously shown that endoglin is detected in human articular cartilage *in vivo* and in primary human articular chondrocytes *in vitro* [137]. We have also demonstrated that endoglin enhances TGF-β-induced Smad1/5 signaling and suppresses Smad2/3 signaling and ECM production in human chondrocytes [138]. Importantly, we found that endoglin protein levels are increased in human OA cartilage as compared to normal cartilage [138]. These results are in agreement with the microarray data showing that endoglin mRNA levels are increased in human OA cartilage [102] and in a rat model of OA [97]. Interestingly, elevated circulating and synovial fluid endoglin are associated with primary knee OA severity, suggesting that endoglin may be a useful biomarker for determining disease severity and/or play a causative role in OA pathogenesis [139].

Betaglycan: Our group has shown that betaglycan is expressed in human chondrocytes and that it forms a complex with the signaling receptors and endoglin in a ligand- and TβRII-independent manner [137]. Betaglycan levels in damaged versus intact human OA cartilage were similar [140] although normal cartilage was not analyzed in this study. Furthermore, betaglycan levels did not change in a rat model of OA [97]. However, betaglycan expression was shown to be increased in adult human articular cartilage in response to mechanical injury [141]. These results suggest that elevated betaglycan expression might be important in secondary OA when joint trauma is involved. Interestingly, betaglycan expression was shown to be increased in mesenchymal stem cells from the femur channel [142] and in trabecular bone from the iliac crest [143] of OA patients. These studies suggest that altered betaglycan expression or function in bone might play a role in OA pathogenesis.

CD109: Information available on CD109 expression or function in cartilage is limited. CD109 was detected in conditioned media of human articular chondrocytes in monolayer culture [144-145] and in that of bovine cartilage explants treated with IL-1β or TNF-α [146]. These studies suggest that CD109 is released from the chondrocyte cell surface which is in agreement with our previous studies on skin cells [58, 147]. We have detected CD109 protein in conditioned media and cell lysates of human OA and normal human articular chondrocytes cultured in monolayer (Finnson and Philip, unpublished data). Recently, CD109 was detected in peripheral circulation and synovial fluid as a component of CD146-positive lymphocytes in patients with various musculoskeletal diseases [148]. The precise mechanisms by which TGF-β co-receptors may contribute to deregulation of TGF-β action in OA remain to be determined.

6. Targeting the TGF-β pathway for osteoarthritis therapy

Several components of the TGF-β signaling pathway display altered expression in human OA cartilage and in experimental models of OA. Genetic manipulation of some of the TGF-β pathway components in mice leads to OA-like phenotypes or to delayed OA progression in experimental OA models. These findings suggest that targeting specific components of the TGF-β pathway may represent a suitable therapeutic strategy for the treatment of OA. Many groups have studied the effect of exogenous TGF-β to promote cartilage repair and/or prevent cartilage degradation. Early studies showed that intra-articular injection of recombinant TGF-β1 into murine joints conferred protection against IL-induced articular cartilage destruction [149-150] although this effect was not observed in older mice [150-151]. Subsequently, exogenous delivery of TGF-β1 was shown to restore depleted proteoglycans in arthritic murine joints [74] and to stimulate proteoglycan synthesis and content in normal murine joints [152]. In addition, TGF-β injected into the osteoarthritic temporomandibular joint of rabbits was shown to have a protective effect on articular cartilage degradation [153]. Although these studies support the notion that TGF-β promotes cartilage repair, its use has been hampered by undesirable side effects including inflammation, synovial hyperplasia and osteophyte formation [84-86, 152, 154]. In this regard, several studies suggest that adjuvant therapies might be used to circumvent the undesirable effects TGF-βs on the osteoarthritic joint. For example, TGF-β was shown to stimulate cartilage repair and the resulting synovial fibrosis could be blocked by Smad7 overexpression in the synovial lining [155]. Such findings suggest that strategies designed to take advantage of the beneficial effects of TGF-β on cartilage repair and simultaneously block its unwanted side effects will be a fruitful avenue for the development of this molecule for OA therapy.

Another important factor to consider when developing a TGF-β-based strategy for OA therapy is that TGF-β may have differential effects on the chondrocyte itself, depending on the cellular context. We have shown that TGF-β signaling in chondrocytes occurs through two different TGF-β type I receptors, ALK5 and ALK1, with ALK1/Smad1/5 pathway opposing ALK5/Smad2/3 signaling and ECM production in human chondrocytes [34]. These data suggest that ALK1 signaling might interfere with the chondroprotective effects of TGF-β. Furthermore, others have shown that ALK1 expression is highly correlated with MMP-13 expression in human OA cartilage and that ALK1 stimulates MMP13 expression in chondrocytes [117]. Thus, a better approach for OA therapy might involve treatment with TGF-β while simultaneously blocking ALK1 activity in chondrocytes. Alternatively, targeting molecules that tip the balance of signaling away from ALK1 and towards ALK5 in OA chondrocytes might also prove to be beneficial. However, there are others who argue that the critical transition from a non-reparative to a reparative cell phenotype involves switching from ALK5-mediated fibrogenic signaling to ALK1-mediated chondrogenic signaling [156]. Therefore, further research on understanding the role of ALK5 and ALK1 signaling pathways in regulating chondrocyte phenotype is needed.

Targeting TGF-β co-receptors for the treatment of human diseases is an attractive concept. Endoglin, betaglycan and CD109 exist both as membrane-anchored and soluble forms due to enzymatic shedding of their ectodomains [134-135, 157-158] and soluble forms of these proteins have been shown to bind and neutralize TGF-β [58, 159, 160, 2001 #587]. One way that these soluble proteins might be used in combination with TGF-β for OA therapy would be to restrict TGF-β expression to the OA chondrocytes. For example, one can use an adenoviral vector containing a type II collagen-specific promoter to drive TGF-β expression in the cartilage while blocking the adverse side effects (synovial fibrosis) of exogenous TGF-β in the joint by co-administration of a soluble co-receptor protein into the synovial fluid. The soluble co-receptor because of its higher molecular weight would not readily diffuse into the cartilage from the synovial fluid [161-162] to block TGF-β action in chondrocytes but would sequester any TGF-β that diffuses from the cartilage into the synovial fluid. Alternatively, TGF-β co-receptor expression in chondrocytes might be targeted directly to promote cartilage repair. Our results indicate that endoglin inhibits TGF-β-induced ALK5-Smad2/3 signaling and ECM production and enhances TGF-β-induced ALK1-Smad1/5 signaling in human chondrocytes [138]. These findings suggest that reducing endoglin expression in OA chondrocytes might promote cartilage repair.

7. Concluding remarks

TGF-β is a critical regulator of articular cartilage development, maintenance and repair. Studies to date indicate that several extracellular, cell surface and intracellular components of the TGF-β pathway display altered expression or activity in OA suggesting that they might represent potential targets for therapeutic treatment of this disease. TGF-β has been shown to promote cartilage repair and its therapeutic use might be improved by "compartmentalized" inhibition of TGF-β activity in synovial tissues to halt or reverse synovial fibrosis and osteophyte formation. Targeting TGF-β co-receptors such as endoglin, betaglycan and CD109 represent new opportunities to explore aberrant TGF-β signaling in OA and to discover new strategies for manipulating the TGF-β pathway for OA therapy.

8. List of abbreviations

ALK, activin receptor-like kinase; ATF, activating transcription factor; ECM, extracellular matrix; ERK, extracellular signal-regulated kinase; Evi-1, ecotropic virus integration site 1 protein homologue; FKBP, FK506 binding protein; GPI, glycosyl phosphatidylinositol; HSP, heat shock protein; IL, interleukin; JNK, c-jun N-terminal kinase/stress-activated protein kinase; kDa, kilodalton; LAP, latency associated peptide; LTBP, latent TGF-β binding protein; MMP, matrix metalloproteinase; OA, osteoarthritis; PI3K, phosphatidylinositol 3-kinase; SARA, Smad anchor for receptor activation; Ski, Sloan Kettering Institute proto-oncogene; Sno, ski-related novel protein; SNP, single nucleotide polymorphism; Smurf, Smad ubiquitin regulatory factor; STRAP, serine-threonine kinase receptor-associated protein; TAK, TGF-β activated kinase; TG, transglutaminase; TGF-β, transforming growth factor-beta; TGIF, TGF-β-induced factor; TIMP, tissue inhibitor of metalloproteinase; TSP, thrombospondin; TNF, tumor necrosis factor; TRAP, TGF-β receptor-associated protein; TRIP, TGF-β receptor-interacting protein.

9. References

[1] van der Kraan PM, Goumans MJ, Blaney Davidson E, Ten Dijke P. Age-dependent alteration of TGF-β signalling in osteoarthritis. Cell Tissue Res 2011.

[2] van den Berg WB. Pathomechanisms of OA: 2010 in review. Osteoarthritis Cartilage 2011; 19: 338-341.

[3] Finnson K, Chi Y, Bou-Gharios G, Leask A, Philip A. TGF-β signaling in cartilage homeostasis and osteoarthritis. Front Biosci 2011; S4: 261-268.

[4] Song B, Estrada KD, Lyons KM. Smad signaling in skeletal development and regeneration. Cytokine Growth Factor Rev 2009; 20: 379-388.

[5] Chang SJ, Chen CJ, Tsai FC, Lai HM, Tsai PC, Tsai MH, et al. Associations between gout tophus and polymorphisms 869T/C and -509C/T in transforming growth factor β1 gene. Rheumatology (Oxford) 2008; 47: 617-621.

[6] Dalbeth N, Pool B, Gamble GD, Smith T, Callon KE, McQueen FM, et al. Cellular characterization of the gouty tophus: a quantitative analysis. Arthritis Rheum 2010; 62: 1549-1556.

[7] Kriegel MA, Li MO, Sanjabi S, Wan YY, Flavell RA. Transforming growth factor-β: recent advances on its role in immune tolerance. Curr Rheumatol Rep 2006; 8: 138-144.

[8] Kim EY, Moudgil KD. Regulation of autoimmune inflammation by pro-inflammatory cytokines. Immunol Lett 2008; 120: 1-5.

[9] Pohlers D, Brenmoehl J, Loffler I, Muller CK, Leipner C, Schultze-Mosgau S, et al. TGF-β and fibrosis in different organs - molecular pathway imprints. Biochim Biophys Acta 2009; 1792: 746-756.

[10] Heldin CH, Moustakas A. Role of Smads in TGFβ signaling. Cell Tissue Res 2011; DOI: 10.1007/s00441-011-1190-x.

[11] Wu MY, Hill CS. TGF-β superfamily signaling in embryonic development and homeostasis. Dev Cell 2009; 16: 329-343.

[12] Wharton K, Derynck R. TGF-β family signaling: novel insights in development and disease. Development 2009; 136: 3691-3697.

[13] Moustakas A, Heldin CH. The regulation of TGFβ signal transduction. Development 2009; 136: 3699-3714.

[14] Heldin C, Landstrom M, Moustakas A. Mechanism of TGF-β signaling to growth arrest, apoptosis, and epithelial-mesenchymal transition. Current Opinion in Cell Biology 2009; 21: 166-176.

[15] Schlunegger MP, Grutter MG. An unusual feature revealed by the crystal structure at 2.2 A resolution of human transforming growth factor-β2. Nature 1992; 358: 430-434.

[16] Mittl PR, Priestle JP, Cox DA, McMaster G, Cerletti N, Grutter MG. The crystal structure of TGF-β3 and comparison to TGF-β2: implications for receptor binding. Protein Sci 1996; 5: 1261-1271.

[17] Hinck AP, Archer SJ, Qian SW, Roberts AB, Sporn MB, Weatherbee JA, et al. Transforming growth factor β1: three-dimensional structure in solution and comparison with the X-ray structure of transforming growth factor β2. Biochemistry 1996; 35: 8517-8534.

[18] Daopin S, Piez KA, Ogawa Y, Davies DR. Crystal structure of transforming growth factor-β2: an unusual fold for the superfamily. Science 1992; 257: 369-373.

[19] Radaev S, Zou Z, Huang T, Lafer EM, Hinck AP, Sun PD. Ternary complex of TGF-β1 reveals isoform-specific ligand recognition and receptor recruitment in the superfamily. J Biol Chem 2010; 285: 14806-14814.

[20] Bottinger EP, Letterio JJ, Roberts AB. Biology of TGF-β in knockout and transgenic mouse models. Kidney Int 1997; 51: 1355-1360.

[21] Roberts AB, Sporn MB. Differential expression of the TGF-β isoforms in embryogenesis suggests specific roles in developing and adult tissues. Mol Reprod Dev 1992; 32: 91-98.

[22] Ramirez F, Rifkin DB. Extracellular microfibrils: contextual platforms for TGFβ and BMP signaling. Curr Opin Cell Biol 2009; 21: 612-622.

[23] Hynes RO. The extracellular matrix: not just pretty fibrils. Science 2009; 326: 1216-1219.

[24] Jenkins G. The role of proteases in transforming growth factor-β activation. Int J Biochem Cell Biol 2008; 40: 1068-1078.

[25] Annes JP, Munger JS, Rifkin DB. Making sense of latent TGF β activation. Journal of Cell Science 2003; 116: 217-224.

[26] Wipff PJ, Hinz B. Integrins and the activation of latent transforming growth factor β1 - An intimate relationship. Eur J Cell Biol 2008; 87: 601-615.

[27] Murphy-Ullrich JE, Poczatek M. Activation of latent TGF-β by thrombospondin-1: mechanisms and physiology. Cytokine Growth Factor Rev 2000; 11: 59-69.

[28] Massague J, Gomis RR. The logic of TGF-β signaling. FEBS Lett 2006; 580: 2811-2820.

[29] Shi Y, Massague J. Mechanisms of TGF-β signaling from cell membrane to the nucleus. Cell 2003; 113: 685-700.

[30] Schmierer B, Hill CS. TGFβ-Smad signal transduction: molecular specificity and functional flexibility. Nat Rev Mol Cell Biol 2007; 8: 970-982.

[31] Ross S, Hill CS. How the Smads regulate transcription. Int J Biochem Cell Biol 2008; 40: 383-408.

[32] Goumans M, Valdimarsdottir G, Itoh S, Rosendahl A, Sideras P, ten Dijke P. Balancing the activation state of the endothelium via two distinct TGF-β type I receptors. Embo J 2002; 21: 1743-1753.

[33] Goumans MJ, Valdimarsdottir G, Itoh S, Lebrin F, Larsson J, Mummery C, et al. Activin receptor-like kinase (ALK)1 is an antagonistic mediator of lateral TGF-β/ALK5 signaling. Mol Cell 2003; 12: 817-828.

[34] Finnson KW, Parker WL, ten Dijke P, Thorikay M, Philip A. ALK1 opposes ALK5/Smad3 signaling and expression of extracellular matrix components in human chondrocytes. J Bone Miner Res 2008; 23: 896-906.

[35] Mu Y, Gudey SK, Landstrom M. Non-Smad signaling pathways. Cell Tissue Res 2011; DOI: 10.1007/s00441-011-1201-y.

[36] Zhang YE. Non-Smad pathways in TGF-β signaling. Cell Res 2008; 19: 128-139.

[37] Wrighton KH, Lin X, Feng XH. Phospho-control of TGF-β superfamily signaling. Cell Res 2009; 19: 8-20.

[38] Yan X, Chen YG. Smad7: not only a regulator, but also a cross-talk mediator of TGF-β signalling. Biochem J 2011; 434: 1-10.

[39] Briones-Orta MA, Tecalco-Cruz AC, Sosa-Garrocho M, Caligaris C, Macias-Silva M. Inhibitory Smad7: Emerging Roles in Health and Disease. Curr Mol Pharmacol 2011; 4: 141-153.

[40] Inoue Y, Imamura T. Regulation of TGF-β family signaling by E3 ubiquitin ligases. Cancer Sci 2008.

[41] Macri L, Silverstein D, Clark RA. Growth factor binding to the pericellular matrix and its importance in tissue engineering. Adv Drug Deliv Rev 2007; 59: 1366-1381.

[42] Grainger DJ, Byrne CD, Witchell CM, Metcalfe JC. Transforming growth factor β is sequestered into an inactive pool by lipoproteins. J Lipid Res 1997; 38: 2344-2352.

[43] Bernabeu C, Lopez-Novoa JM, Quintanilla M. The emerging role of TGF-β superfamily co-receptors in cancer. Biochim Biophys Acta 2009; 1792: 954-973.

[44] Pardali E, ten Dijke P. Transforming growth factor-β signaling and tumor angiogenesis. Front Biosci 2009; 14: 4848-4861.

[45] ten Dijke P, Goumans MJ, Pardali E. Endoglin in angiogenesis and vascular diseases. Angiogenesis 2008; 11: 79-89.

[46] Bilandzic M, Stenvers KL. Betaglycan: A multifunctional accessory. Mol Cell Endocrinol 2011; 339: 180-189.

[47] Gatza CE, Oh SY, Blobe GC. Roles for the type III TGF-β receptor in human cancer. Cell Signal 2010; 22: 1163-1174.

[48] McLean S, Di Guglielmo GM. TβRIII directs clathrin-mediated endocytosis of TGFβ type I and II receptors. Biochem J 2010; 429: 137-145

[49] Finger EC, Lee NY, You HJ, Blobe GC. Endocytosis of the type III TGF-β receptor through the clathrin-independent/lipid raft pathway regulates TGF-β signaling and receptor downregulation. J Biol Chem 2008; 283: 34808-34818.

[50] Santander C, Brandan E. Betaglycan induces TGF-β signaling in a ligand-independent manner, through activation of the p38 pathway. Cell Signal 2006; 18: 1482-1491.

[51] You HJ, Bruinsma MW, How T, Ostrander JH, Blobe GC. The type III TGF-β receptor signals through both Smad3 and the p38 MAP kinase pathways to contribute to inhibition of cell proliferation. Carcinogenesis 2007; 28: 2491-2500.

[52] Chen W, Kirkbride KC, How T, Nelson CD, Mo J, Frederick JP, et al. β-arrestin 2 mediates endocytosis of type III TGF-β receptor and down-regulation of its signaling. Science 2003; 301: 1394-1397.

[53] Solomon KR, Sharma P, Chan M, Morrison PT, Finberg RW. CD109 represents a novel branch of the α2-macroglobulin/complement gene family. Gene 2004; 327: 171-183.
[54] Hashimoto M, Ichihara M, Watanabe T, Kawai K, Koshikawa K, Yuasa N, et al. Expression of CD109 in human cancer. Oncogene 2004; 23: 3716-3720.
[55] Schuh AC, Watkins NA, Nguyen Q, Harmer NJ, Lin M, Prosper JYA, et al. A tyrosine703serine polymorphism of CD109 defines the Gov platelet alloantigens. Blood 2002; 99: 1692-1698.
[56] Lin M, Sutherland DR, Horsfall W, Totty N, Yeo E, Nayar R, et al. Cell surface antigen CD109 is a novel member of the alpha 2 macroglobulin/C3, C4, C5 family of thioester-containing proteins. Blood 2002; 99: 1683-1691.
[57] Bizet AA, Liu K, Tran-Khanh N, Saksena A, Vorstenbosch J, Finnson KW, Buschmann MD, Philip A. The TGF-β co-receptor, CD109, promotes internalization and degradation of TGF-β receptors. Biochim Biophys Acta 2011; 1813: 742-753.
[58] Finnson KW, Tam BY, Liu K, Marcoux A, Lepage P, Roy S, et al. Identification of CD109 as part of the TGF-β receptor system in human keratinocytes. FASEB J 2006; 20: 1525-1527.
[59] Bizet AA, Tran-Khanh N, Saksena A, Liu K, Buschmann MD, Philip A. CD109-mediated degradation of the TGF-β receptors and inhibition of TGF-β responses involve regulation of Smad7 and Smurf2 localization and function. Journal of Cellular Biochemistry 2011; doi: 10.1002/jcb.23349
[60] Bhosale AM, Richardson JB. Articular cartilage: structure, injuries and review of management. Br Med Bull 2008; 87: 77-95.
[61] Eyre DR. Collagens and cartilage matrix homeostasis. Clin Orthop Relat Res 2004: S118-122.
[62] Eyre DR, Weis MA, Wu JJ. Articular cartilage collagen: an irreplaceable framework? Eur Cell Mater 2006; 12: 57-63.
[63] Heinegard D. Proteoglycans and more--from molecules to biology. Int J Exp Pathol 2009; 90: 575-586.
[64] Goldring MB, Tsuchimochi K, Ijiri K. The control of chondrogenesis. J Cell Biochem 2006; 97: 33-44.
[65] Onyekwelu I, Goldring MB, Hidaka C. Chondrogenesis, joint formation, and articular cartilage regeneration. J Cell Biochem 2009; 107: 383-392.
[66] Kawakami Y, Rodriguez-Leon J, Izpisua Belmonte JC. The role of TGF-βs and Sox9 during limb chondrogenesis. Curr Opin Cell Biol 2006; 18: 723-729.
[67] Quintana L, zur Nieden NI, Semino CE. Morphogenetic and regulatory mechanisms during developmental chondrogenesis: new paradigms for cartilage tissue engineering. Tissue Eng Part B Rev 2009; 15: 29-41.
[68] van der Kraan PM, Blaney Davidson EN, van den Berg WB. A role for age-related changes in TGF-β signaling in aberrant chondrocyte differentiation and osteoarthritis. Arthritis Res Ther 2010; 12: 201.
[69] van der Kraan PM, Blaney Davidson EN, Blom A, van den Berg WB. TGF-β signaling in chondrocyte terminal differentiation and osteoarthritis: modulation and integration of signaling pathways through receptor-Smads. Osteoarthritis Cartilage 2009; 17: 1539-1545.

[70] Yang X, Chen L, Xu X, Li C, Huang C, Deng C-X. TGF-β/Smad3 signals repress chondrocyte hypertrophic differentiation and are required for maintaining articular cartilage. J. Cell Biol. 2001; 153: 35-46.
[71] Blaney Davidson E, van der Kraan P, van den Berg W. TGF-β and osteoarthritis. Osteoarthritis Cartilage 2007; 15: 597-604.
[72] Chimal-Monroy J, Diaz de Leon L. Differential effects of transforming growth factors β1, β2, β3 and β5 on chondrogenesis in mouse limb bud mesenchymal cells. Int J Dev Biol 1997; 41: 91-102.
[73] Joyce ME, Roberts AB, Sporn MB, Bolander ME. Transforming growth factor-β and the initiation of chondrogenesis and osteogenesis in the rat femur. J Cell Biol 1990; 110: 2195-2207.
[74] Glansbeek HL, van Beuningen HM, Vitters EL, van der Kraan PM, van den Berg WB. Stimulation of articular cartilage repair in established arthritis by local administration of transforming growth factor-β into murine knee joints. Lab Invest 1998; 78: 133-142.
[75] Hunziker EB. Growth-factor-induced healing of partial-thickness defects in adult articular cartilage. Osteoarthritis Cartilage 2001; 9: 22-32.
[76] Hunziker EB, Rosenberg LC. Repair of partial-thickness defects in articular cartilage: cell recruitment from the synovial membrane. J Bone Joint Surg Am 1996; 78: 721-733.
[77] Scharstuhl A, Glansbeek HL, van Beuningen HM, Vitters EL, van der Kraan PM, van den Berg WB. Inhibition of endogenous TGF-β during experimental osteoarthritis prevents osteophyte formation and impairs cartilage repair. J Immunol 2002; 169: 507-514.
[78] Serra R, Johnson M, Filvaroff EH, LaBorde J, Sheehan DM, Derynck R, et al. Expression of a truncated, kinase-defective TGF-β type II receptor in mouse skeletal tissue promotes terminal chondrocyte differentiation and osteoarthritis. J. Cell Biol. 1997; 139: 541-552.
[79] Blaney Davidson EN, Vitters EL, van der Kraan PM, van den Berg WB. Expression of transforming growth factor-β (TGFβ) and the TGFβ signalling molecule Smad-2P in spontaneous and instability-induced osteoarthritis: role in cartilage degradation, chondrogenesis and osteophyte formation. Ann Rheum Dis 2006; 65: 1414-1421.
[80] Loughlin J. The genetic epidemiology of human primary osteoarthritis: current status. Expert Rev Mol Med 2005; 7: 1-12.
[81] Ikegawa S. New gene associations in osteoarthritis: what do they provide, and where are we going? Curr Opin Rheumatol 2007; 19: 429-434.
[82] Ikegawa S. Expression, regulation and function of asporin, a susceptibility gene in common bone and joint diseases. Curr Med Chem 2008; 15: 724-728.
[83] Dai J, Ikegawa S. Recent advances in association studies of osteoarthritis susceptibility genes. J Hum Genet 2010; 55: 77-80.
[84] van Beuningen HM, van der Kraan PM, Arntz OJ, van den Berg WB. Transforming growth factor-β1 stimulates articular chondrocyte proteoglycan synthesis and induces osteophyte formation in the murine knee joint. Lab Invest 1994; 71: 279-290.
[85] van Beuningen HM, Glansbeek HL, van der Kraan PM, van den Berg WB. Osteoarthritis-like changes in the murine knee joint resulting from intra-articular transforming growth factor-β injections. Osteoarthritis Cartilage 2000; 8: 25-33.

[86] Bakker AC, van de Loo FA, van Beuningen HM, Sime P, van Lent PL, van der Kraan PM, et al. Overexpression of active TGF-β1 in the murine knee joint: evidence for synovial-layer-dependent chondro-osteophyte formation. Osteoarthritis Cartilage 2001; 9: 128-136.

[87] Alcaraz MJ, Megias J, Garcia-Arnandis I, Clerigues V, Guillen MI. New molecular targets for the treatment of osteoarthritis. Biochem Pharmacol 2010; 80: 13-21.

[88] Goldring MB, Goldring SR. Articular cartilage and subchondral bone in the pathogenesis of osteoarthritis. Ann N Y Acad Sci 2010; 1192: 230-237.

[89] Zhang Y, Jordan JM. Epidemiology of Osteoarthritis. Clin Geriatr Med 2010; 26: 355-369.

[90] Martel-Pelletier J, Pelletier JP. Is osteoarthritis a disease involving only cartilage or other articular tissues? Eklem Hastalik Cerrahisi 2010; 21: 2-14.

[91] Wu J, Liu W, Bemis A, Wang E, Qiu Y, Morris EA, et al. Comparative proteomic characterization of articular cartilage tissue from normal donors and patients with osteoarthritis. Arthritis Rheum 2007; 56: 3675-3684.

[92] Verdier MP, Seite S, Guntzer K, Pujol JP, Boumediene K. Immunohistochemical analysis of transforming growth factor β isoforms and their receptors in human cartilage from normal and osteoarthritic femoral heads. Rheumatol Int 2005; 25: 118-124.

[93] Boumediene K, Conrozier T, Mathieu P, Richard M, Marcelli C, Vignon E, et al. Decrease of cartilage transforming growth factor-β receptor II expression in the rabbit experimental osteoarthritis-potential role in cartilage breakdown. Osteoarthritis Cartilage 1998; 6: 146-149.

[94] Xiao J, Li T, Wu Z, Shi Z, Chen J, Lam SK, et al. REST corepressor (CoREST) repression induces phenotypic gene regulation in advanced osteoarthritic chondrocytes. J Orthop Res 2010; 28: 1569-1575.

[95] Pombo-Suarez M, Castano-Oreja MT, Calaza M, Gomez-Reino JJ, Gonzalez A. Differential up-regulation of the three TGF-β isoforms in human osteoarthritic cartilage. Ann Rheum Dis 2009; 68: 568-571.

[96] Nakajima M, Kizawa H, Saitoh M, Kou I, Miyazono K, Ikegawa S. Mechanisms for asporin function and regulation in articular cartilage. J. Biol. Chem. 2007; 282: 32185-32192.

[97] Appleton CT, Pitelka V, Henry J, Beier F. Global analyses of gene expression in early experimental osteoarthritis. Arthritis Rheum 2007; 56: 1854-1868.

[98] Malemud CJ. Anticytokine therapy for osteoarthritis: evidence to date. Drugs Aging 2010; 27: 95-115.

[99] Pujol JP, Chadjichristos C, Legendre F, Bauge C, Beauchef G, Andriamanalijaona R, et al. Interleukin-1 and transforming growth factor-β1 as crucial factors in osteoarthritic cartilage metabolism. Connect Tissue Res 2008; 49: 293-297.

[100] Kim SJ, Angel P, Lafyatis R, Hattori K, Kim KY, Sporn MB, et al. Autoinduction of transforming growth factor β1 is mediated by the AP-1 complex. Mol Cell Biol 1990; 10: 1492-1497.

[101] Wei T, Kulkarni NH, Zeng QQ, Helvering LM, Lin X, Lawrence F, et al. Analysis of early changes in the articular cartilage transcriptisome in the rat meniscal tear model of osteoarthritis: pathway comparisons with the rat anterior cruciate transection model and with human osteoarthritic cartilage. Osteoarthritis Cartilage 2010; 18: 992-1000.

[102] Aigner T, Fundel K, Saas J, Gebhard PM, Haag J, Weiss T, et al. Large-scale gene expression profiling reveals major pathogenetic pathways of cartilage degeneration in osteoarthritis. Arthritis Rheum 2006; 54: 3533-3544.

[103] Todorovic V, Frendewey D, Gutstein DE, Chen Y, Freyer L, Finnegan E, et al. Long form of latent TGF-beta binding protein 1 (Ltbp1L) is essential for cardiac outflow tract septation and remodeling. Development 2007; 134: 3723-3732.

[104] Drews F, Knobel S, Moser M, Muhlack KG, Mohren S, Stoll C, et al. Disruption of the latent transforming growth factor-β binding protein-1 gene causes alteration in facial structure and influences TGF-β bioavailability. Biochim Biophys Acta 2008; 1783: 34-48.

[105] Shipley JM, Mecham RP, Maus E, Bonadio J, Rosenbloom J, McCarthy RT, et al. Developmental expression of latent transforming growth factor beta binding protein 2 and its requirement early in mouse development. Mol Cell Biol 2000; 20: 4879-4887.

[106] Dabovic B, Chen Y, Colarossi C, Obata H, Zambuto L, Perle MA, et al. Bone abnormalities in latent TGF-β binding protein (LTBP)-3-null mice indicate a role for LTBP-3 in modulating TGF-β bioavailability. J Cell Biol 2002; 156: 227-232.

[107] Dabovic B, Chen Y, Colarossi C, Zambuto L, Obata H, Rifkin DB. Bone defects in latent TGF-β binding protein (LTBP)-3 null mice; a role for LTBP in TGF-β presentation. J Endocrinol 2002; 175: 129-141.

[108] Johnson K, Hashimoto S, Lotz M, Pritzker K, Terkeltaub R. Interleukin-1 induces pro-mineralizing activity of cartilage tissue transglutaminase and factor XIIIa. Am J Pathol 2001; 159: 149-163.

[109] Heinkel D, Gohr CM, Uzuki M, Rosenthal AK. Transglutaminase contributes to CPPD crystal formation in osteoarthritis. Front Biosci 2004; 9: 3257-3261.

[110] Orlandi A, Oliva F, Taurisano G, Candi E, Di Lascio A, Melino G, et al. Transglutaminase-2 differently regulates cartilage destruction and osteophyte formation in a surgical model of osteoarthritis. Amino Acids 2009; 36: 755-763.

[111] Huebner JL, Johnson KA, Kraus VB, Terkeltaub RA. Transglutaminase 2 is a marker of chondrocyte hypertrophy and osteoarthritis severity in the Hartley guinea pig model of knee OA. Osteoarthritis Cartilage 2009; 17: 1056-1064.

[112] Pfander D, Cramer T, Deuerling D, Weseloh G, Swoboda B. Expression of thrombospondin-1 and its receptor CD36 in human osteoarthritic cartilage. Ann Rheum Dis 2000; 59: 448-454.

[113] Jou IM, Shiau AL, Chen SY, Wang CR, Shieh DB, Tsai CS, et al. Thrombospondin 1 as an effective gene therapeutic strategy in collagen-induced arthritis. Arthritis Rheum 2005; 52: 339-344.

[114] Hsieh JL, Shen PC, Shiau AL, Jou IM, Lee CH, Wang CR, et al. Intra-articular gene transfer of thrombospondin-1 suppresses the disease progression of experimental osteoarthritis. J Orthop Res 2010; 28: 1300-1306.

[115] Dehne T, Karlsson C, Ringe J, Sittinger M, Lindahl A. Chondrogenic differentiation potential of osteoarthritic chondrocytes and their possible use in matrix-associated autologous chondrocyte transplantation. Arthritis Res Ther 2009; 11: R133.

[116] Hiramatsu K, Iwai T, Yoshikawa H, Tsumaki N. Expression of dominant negative TGF-β receptors inhibits cartilage formation in conditional transgenic mice. J Bone Miner Metab 2011.

[117] Blaney Davidson EN, Remst DF, Vitters EL, van Beuningen HM, Blom AB, Goumans MJ, et al. Increase in ALK1/ALK5 ratio as a cause for elevated MMP-13 expression in osteoarthritis in humans and mice. J Immunol 2009; 182: 7937-7945.

[118] Gomez-Camarillo MA, Kouri JB. Ontogeny of rat chondrocyte proliferation: studies in embryo, adult and osteoarthritic (OA) cartilage. Cell Res 2005; 15: 99-104.

[119] Blaney Davidson EN, Scharstuhl A, Vitters EL, van der Kraan PM, van den Berg WB. Reduced transforming growth factor-β signaling in cartilage of old mice: role in impaired repair capacity. Arthritis Res Ther 2005; 7: R1338-1347.

[120] Wu Q, Huang JH, Sampson ER, Kim KO, Zuscik MJ, O'Keefe RJ, et al. Smurf2 induces degradation of GSK-3β and upregulates β-catenin in chondrocytes: a potential mechanism for Smurf2-induced degeneration of articular cartilage. Exp Cell Res 2009; 315: 2386-2398.

[121] Li CG, Liang QQ, Zhou Q, Menga E, Cui XJ, Shu B, et al. A continuous observation of the degenerative process in the intervertebral disc of Smad3 gene knock-out mice. Spine (Phila Pa 1976) 2009; 34: 1363-1369.

[122] Yao JY, Wang Y, An J, Mao CM, Hou N, Lv YX, et al. Mutation analysis of the Smad3 gene in human osteoarthritis. Eur J Hum Genet 2003; 11: 714-717.

[123] Valdes AM, Spector TD, Tamm A, Kisand K, Doherty SA, Dennison EM, et al. Genetic variation in the Smad3 gene is associated with hip and knee osteoarthritis. Arthritis Rheum 2010; 62: 2347-2352.

[124] van de Laar IM, Oldenburg RA, Pals G, Roos-Hesselink JW, de Graaf BM, Verhagen JM, et al. Mutations in SMAD3 cause a syndromic form of aortic aneurysms and dissections with early-onset osteoarthritis. Nat Genet 2011; 43: 121-126.

[125] Pannu J, Nakerakanti S, Smith E, Dijke Pt, Trojanowska M. Transforming growth factor-β receptor type I dependent fibrogenic gene program is mediated via activation of Smad1 and ERK1/2 pathways. J. Biol. Chem. 2007; 282: 10405–10413.

[126] Valcourt U, Gouttenoire J, Moustakas A, Herbage D, Mallein-Gerin F. Functions of transforming growth factor-β family type I receptors and Smad proteins in the hypertrophic maturation and osteoblastic differentiation of chondrocytes. J Biol Chem 2002; 277: 33545-33558.

[127] Bau B, Haag J, Schmid E, Kaiser M, Gebhard PM, Aigner T. Bone morphogenetic protein-mediating receptor-associated Smads as well as common Smad are expressed in human articular chondrocytes but not up-regulated or down-regulated in osteoarthritic cartilage. J Bone Miner Res 2002; 17: 2141-2150.

[128] Kaiser M, Haag J, Soder S, Bau B, Aigner T. Bone morphogenetic protein and transforming growth factor beta inhibitory Smads 6 and 7 are expressed in human adult normal and osteoarthritic cartilage in vivo and are differentially regulated in vitro by interleukin-1β. Arthritis Rheum 2004; 50: 3535-3540.

[129] Wu Q, Kim KO, Sampson ER, Chen D, Awad H, O'Brien T, et al. Induction of an osteoarthritis-like phenotype and degradation of phosphorylated Smad3 by Smurf2 in transgenic mice. Arthritis Rheum 2008; 58: 3132-3144.

[130] Gunnell LM, Jonason JH, Loiselle AE, Kohn A, Schwarz EM, Hilton MJ, et al. TAK1 regulates cartilage and joint development via the MAPK and BMP signaling pathways. J Bone Miner Res 2010; 25: 1784-1797.

[131] Qiao B, Padilla SR, Benya PD. TGF-β activated kinase 1 (TAK1) mimics and mediates TGF-β-induced stimulation of type II collagen synthesis in chondrocytes

independent of Col2a1 transcription and Smad3 signaling. J. Biol. Chem. 2005; 280: 17562-17571.

[132] Roman-Blas JA, Stokes DG, Jimenez SA. Modulation of TGF-β signaling by proinflammatory cytokines in articular chondrocytes. Osteoarthritis Cartilage 2007; 15: 1367-1377.

[133] Ionescu AM, Schwarz EM, Zuscik MJ, Drissi H, Puzas JE, Rosier RN, et al. ATF-2 cooperates with Smad3 to mediate TGF-β effects on chondrocyte maturation. Exp Cell Res 2003; 288: 198-207.

[134] Hagiwara S, Murakumo Y, Mii S, Shigetomi T, Yamamoto N, Furue H, et al. Processing of CD109 by furin and its role in the regulation of TGF-β signaling. Oncogene 2010; 29: 2181-2191.

[135] Hockla A, Radisky DC, Radisky ES. Mesotrypsin promotes malignant growth of breast cancer cells through shedding of CD109. Breast Cancer Res Treat 2009; 124: 27-38.

[136] Leask A. Targeting the TGFβ, endothelin-1 and CCN2 axis to combat fibrosis in scleroderma. Cell Signal 2008; 20: 1409-1414.

[137] Parker WL, Goldring MB, Philip A. Endoglin is expressed on human chondrocytes and forms a heteromeric complex with betaglycan in a ligand and type II TGFβ receptor independent manner. J Bone Miner Res 2003; 18: 289-302.

[138] Finnson KW, Parker WL, Chi Y, Hoemann C, Goldring MB, Antoniou J, et al. Endoglin differentially regulates TGF-β-induced Smad2/3 and Smad1/5 signalling and its expression correlates with extracellular matrix production and cellular differentiation state in human chondrocytes. Osteoarthritis Cartilage 2010; 18: 1518-1527.

[139] Honsawek S, Tanavalee A, Yuktanandana P. Elevated circulating and synovial fluid endoglin are associated with primary knee osteoarthritis severity. Arch Med Res 2009; 40: 590-594.

[140] Tsuritani K, Takeda J, Sakagami J, Ishii A, Eriksson T, Hara T, et al. Cytokine receptor-like factor 1 is highly expressed in damaged human knee osteoarthritic cartilage and involved in osteoarthritis downstream of TGF-β. Calcif Tissue Int 2010; 86: 47-57.

[141] Dell'accio F, De Bari C, Eltawil NM, Vanhummelen P, Pitzalis C. Identification of the molecular response of articular cartilage to injury, by microarray screening: Wnt-16 expression and signaling after injury and in osteoarthritis. Arthritis Rheum 2008; 58: 1410-1421.

[142] Rollin R, Alvarez-Lafuente R, Marco F, Garcia-Asenjo JA, Jover JA, Rodriguez L, et al. Abnormal transforming growth factor-β expression in mesenchymal stem cells from patients with osteoarthritis. J Rheumatol 2008; 35: 904-906.

[143] Sanchez-Sabate E, Alvarez L, Gil-Garay E, Munuera L, Vilaboa N. Identification of differentially expressed genes in trabecular bone from the iliac crest of osteoarthritic patients. Osteoarthritis Cartilage 2009; 17: 1106-1114.

[144] Polacek M, Bruun JA, Elvenes J, Figenschau Y, Martinez I. The secretory profiles of cultured human articular chondrocytes and mesenchymal stem cells: implications for autologous cell transplantation strategies. Cell Transplant 2011; 20:1381-93.

[145] Polacek M, Bruun JA, Johansen O, Martinez I. Differences in the secretome of cartilage explants and cultured chondrocytes unveiled by SILAC technology. J Orthop Res 2010; 28: 1040-1049.

[146] Stevens AL, Wishnok JS, Chai DH, Grodzinsky AJ, Tannenbaum SR. A sodium dodecyl sulfate-polyacrylamide gel electrophoresis-liquid chromatography tandem mass spectrometry analysis of bovine cartilage tissue response to mechanical compression injury and the inflammatory cytokines tumor necrosis factor-α and interleukin-1β. Arthritis Rheum 2008; 58: 489-500.

[147] Tam B, Larouche D, Germain L, Hooper N, Philip A. Characterization of a 150 kDa accessory receptor for TGF-β1 on keratinocytes: direct evidence for a GPI anchor and ligand binding of the released form. Journal of Cellular Biochemistry 2001; 83: 494-507.

[148] Dagur PK, Tatlici G, Gourley M, Samsel L, Raghavachari N, Liu P, et al. CD146+ T lymphocytes are increased in both the peripheral circulation and in the synovial effusions of patients with various musculoskeletal diseases and display pro-inflammatory gene profiles. Cytometry B Clin Cytom 2010; 78B: 88-95.

[149] van Beuningen HM, van der Kraan PM, Arntz OJ, van den Berg WB. Protection from interleukin 1 induced destruction of articular cartilage by transforming growth factor β: studies in anatomically intact cartilage in vitro and in vivo. Ann Rheum Dis 1993; 52: 185-191.

[150] van Beuningen HM, van der Kraan PM, Arntz OJ, van den Berg WB. In vivo protection against interleukin-1-induced articular cartilage damage by transforming growth factor-β1: age-related differences. Ann Rheum Dis 1994; 53: 593-600.

[151] Scharstuhl A, van Beuningen HM, Vitters EL, van der Kraan PM, van den Berg WB. Loss of transforming growth factor counteraction on interleukin 1 mediated effects in cartilage of old mice. Ann Rheum Dis 2002; 61: 1095-1098.

[152] van Beuningen HM, Glansbeek HL, van der Kraan PM, van den Berg WB. Differential effects of local application of BMP-2 or TGF-β1 on both articular cartilage composition and osteophyte formation. Osteoarthritis Cartilage 1998; 6: 306-317.

[153] Man C, Zhu S, Zhang B, Hu J. Protection of articular cartilage from degeneration by injection of transforming growth factor-β in temporomandibular joint osteoarthritis. Oral Surg Oral Med Oral Pathol Oral Radiol Endod 2009; 108: 335-340.

[154] Blaney Davidson E, Vitters E, van Beuningen HM, van de Loo F, van den Berg W, van der Kraan P. Resemblance of osteophytes in experimental osteoarthritis to transforming growth factorβ-induced osteophytes: limited role of bone morphogenetic protein in early osteoarthritic osteophyte formation. Arthritis Rheum 2007; 56: 4065-4073.

[155] Blaney Davidson EN, Vitters EL, van den Berg WB, van der Kraan PM. TGFβ-induced cartilage repair is maintained but fibrosis is blocked in the presence of Smad7. Arthritis Res Ther 2006; 8: R65.

[156] Plaas A, Velasco J, Gorski DJ, Li J, Cole A, Christopherson K, et al. The relationship between fibrogenic TGFβ1 signaling in the joint and cartilage degradation in post-injury osteoarthritis. Osteoarthritis Cartilage 2011.

[157] Velasco-Loyden G, Arribas J, Lopez-Casillas F. The shedding of betaglycan is regulated by pervanadate and mediated by membrane type matrix metalloprotease-1. J Biol Chem 2004; 279: 7721-7733.

[158] Hawinkels LJ, Kuiper P, Wiercinska E, Verspaget HW, Liu Z, Pardali E, et al. Matrix metalloproteinase-14 (MT1-MMP)-mediated endoglin shedding inhibits tumor angiogenesis. Cancer Res 2010; 70: 4141-4150.

[159] Vilchis-Landeros MM, Montiel JL, Mendoza V, Mendoza-Hernandez G, Lopez-Casillas F. Recombinant soluble betaglycan is a potent and isoform-selective transforming growth factor-β neutralizing agent. Biochem J 2001; 355: 215-222.

[160] Venkatesha S, Toporsian M, Lam C, Hanai J, Mammoto T, Kim YM, et al. Soluble endoglin contributes to the pathogenesis of preeclampsia. Nat Med 2006; 12: 642-649.

[161] Urech DM, Feige U, Ewert S, Schlosser V, Ottiger M, Polzer K, et al. Anti-inflammatory and cartilage-protecting effects of an intra-articularly injected anti-TNF{alpha} single-chain Fv antibody (ESBA105) designed for local therapeutic use. Ann Rheum Dis 2010; 69: 443-449.

[162] van Lent PL, van den Berg WB, Schalkwijk J, van de Putte LB, van den Bersselaar L. The impact of protein size and charge on its retention in articular cartilage. J Rheumatol 1987; 14: 798-805.

Part 6

Cellular Aspects of Osteoarthritis

23

How Important are Innate Immunity Cells in Osteoarthritis Pathology

Petya Dimitrova and Nina Ivanovska
Department of Immunology, Institute of Microbiology
Bulgaria

1. Introduction

Osteoarthritis (OA) is a chronic degenerative bone disorder leading to cartilage loss, frequently associated with the aging process. It is widely spread in society and often causes disability. Joint swelling which attends OA is due to osteophyte formation or to synovial fluid accumulation. Pathologically, focal damage of cartilage in load-bearing areas are observed together with the formation of new bone at the joint margins, as well as with changes in subchondral bone, and synovitis. Current diagnosis of OA is based on the clinical history and on the radiographical data which occur late at the disease and are very irreversible. Ideally, we wish to detect osteoarthritis at an early stage by following the changes in expression of particular molecular markers, assuming that these markers are sufficiently sensitive, specific, and quantitative for the disease. OA is no longer considered an exclusively degenerative joint disorder because it is related to changes in the synovial membrane as a result of more or less exerted inflammation (Hedbom & Hauselmann, 2002). Trauma or some mechanical problem might be the primary reason for OA initiation. The initiation and progression of OA is sometimes associated with synovial inflammation and the production of proinflammatory and destructive mediators from the synovium causing the invasion of chondrocytes into the cartilage. In early OA the influx of mononuclear cells is enhanced simultaneously with overexpression of inflammatory molecules compared with late OA (Benito et al., 2005). A fundamental question is which cell populations in OA contribute to and maintain synovial inflammation and cartilage destruction.

2. Neutrophils as the main participants in the development of OA

2.1 Phenotype of OA neutrophils

Neutrophils are an essential part of the innate immune system, triggering the initial inflammatory response and the development of host defense mechanisms. During inflammation they leave the circulation and enter the tissues in which they are under the influence of various local factors such as cytokines, endogenous growth factors, microbial products etc. In a result, neutrophils adopt effector functions of great importance for initiation and maintaining of many chronic inflammatory diseases (Duan et al., 2001; Edwards & Hallett, 1997; Mitsuyama et al., 1994).

Neutrophils develop from progenitor cells in bone marrow. They have short lifespans of several hours and then die via apoptosis. Constitutive apoptosis of neutrophils is regulated by two transcription factors: hypoxia-inducible factor 1 (HIF1) and forkhead box O3A. When certain stimuli such as granulocyte-macrophage colony-stimulating factor (GM-CSF), TNF-α, IL-8 and IFN-γ are provided, the lifespan of blood neutrophils is significantly prolonged (Brach et al., 1992; Kilpatrick et al., 2006). Increased neutrophil survival is related with an enhanced expression of anti-apoptotic genes (Marshall et al., 2007) and by death-inducing receptors belonging to the tumor necrosis factor (TNF)/nerve growth factor (NGF) receptor super-family, such as Fas, TNF-related apoptosis-inducing ligand (TNFSF10) receptors, TNFRSF9 (CD137), and the type I TNF receptor (Simon et al., 2003).

It has been shown that RA synovial fluid counteracts neutrophil apoptosis and leads to prolonged survival (Ottonello et al., 2002). Such inhibited apoptosis is characteristic for the earliest phase of RA in contrast to other early arthritides (Raza et al., 2006), suggesting that the suppression of apoptosis in RA patients at high risk is a possible therapeutic approach. RA neutrophils are also functionally different from healthy neutrophils as it has been demonstrated by up-regulated expression of complement receptors CR1, CR3 and CR4 (Felzmann et al., 1991). They show an increased chemotaxis to synovium (Pronai et al., 1991) promoted by TNF-α, IL-17, IL-20 and IL-24 (Kragstrup et al., 2008; Shen et al., 2005). Reports about apoptosis of neutrophils in OA are few and controversial. Bell et al. showed that synovial fluid from OA patients contains factors inhibiting neutrophil survival (Bell et al., 1995). There is also a hypothesis that pyrophosphate dihydrate (CPPD) and basic calcium phosphate (BCP) crystals present in the OA joint fluid and tissue can activate Ca2+ signal in neutrophils thereby prolonging their survival and reducing their apoptosis (Rosenthal, 2011). Chakravarti et al. isolated a subset of blood neutrophils which represents 8–17% of the total neutrophil population and persists beyond 72 h after an exposure to GM-CSF, TNF-α and IL-4. These neutrophils secrete IL-1, IL-1Ra and IL-8, and interact strongly with resident stromal cells (Chakravarti et al., 2009). The phenotype of "long-lived" neutrophils also differs from that of the circulating neutrophils. Although they express the common neutrophil cell surface markers CD32, CD18 and CD11b, they acquire new surface markers, such as HLA-DR and the co-stimulation molecule CD80 (Cross et al., 2003).

Neutrophils participate actively in joint inflammation as proven by their depletion in an experimental model of arthritis (Santos et al., 1997). They affect chemotaxis of macrophages and dendritic cells by cleaving prochemerin to chemerin. Neutrophils produce TNF-α and other cytokines like IL-1, IL-6 that drive the differentiation and activation of dendritic cells and macrophages. The destructive potential of neutrophils is related with their ability to release reactive oxygen species and granules with myeloperoxidase, defensins and MMP-8, MMP-9, MMP-25. MMPs are secreted in response to IL-8 and through ERK1/2 and Src-family kinase pathways (Chakrabarti & Patel, 2005).

2.2 RANKL expression on OA neutrophils

The uncoordinated bone remodeling events in OA results from the impaired balance between bone resorption mediated by mature osteoclasts and bone formation mediated by osteoblasts. The receptor activator of nuclear factor-κB ligand (RANKL) and its receptor RANK are actively involved in osteoclast formation (Yasuda et al., 1998). Immature osteoblasts express RANKL which binds to RANK on osteoclasts, initiating the recruitment of osteoclast precursors in bone marrow and promoting their differentiation.

Intracellularly, RANK interacts with TNF receptor-associated factor 6 (TRAF6), which unlocks signaling through NF-κB, p38 kinase, and c-Jun N-terminal kinase (Teitelbaum, 2000). OPG is released by osteoblasts and stromal cells and is expressed by macrophages in synovial lining layer. Bone resorption is controlled by the balance between RANKL, RANK and osteoprotegerin (Crotti et al., 2002). The inhibition of RANKL in serum transfer model (Ji et al., 2002), in TNF-α-induced model (Keffer et al., 1991) and in autoimmune type II collagen-induced arthritis (Kamijo et al., 2006) resulted in amelioration of bone destruction.

Recently, Poubelle and co-workers reported that RA neutrophils express RANKL and are activated through RANK/RANKL interaction (Poubelle et al., 2007). Despite the studies in RA, there are no investigations showing the involvement of RANKL positive neutrophils in the pathogenesis of OA. A little is known about the expression of RANKL in active or inactive stages of OA. We have conducted a study on RANKL expression by neutrophils in OA patients and in mouse models. OA patients have been divided into two groups depending on the presence of active inflammatory process. The first group, with active OA had swelling, local hyperthermia of one or more joints and high erythrocyte sedimentation rate (ESR). The second group with inactive OA lacked above mentioned painful swelling and local hyperthermia. A number of healthy controls have also been included (Table 1).

	healthy controls	active OA	inactive OA
No. of subjects (women/men)	10 (4/6)	12 (5/7)	14 (6/8)
Duration (years)	not assessed	4.5 ± 1.2	2.5 ± 1.2
ESR (mm/h)	<20	24.8 ± 6.2	14.0 ± 3.6
RF	not assessed	<20	<20
CRP	<0.01	58.9 ± 30.4	<0.01

CRP - C reactive protein; ESR-erythrocyte sedimentation rate; OA-osteoarthritis; RF-rheumatoid factor; Data are expressed as mean ± standard error of the mean

Table 1. Basic characteristics of healthy donors and OA patients

The intensification of OA symptoms at established phase of the disease can be due to calcium-containing crystals. The basic calcium phosphate (BCP) and hydroxyapatite (HA) crystals are often found in joint fluid and tissues of OA patients. The reason for their accumulation is not clear but their contribution to the aggravation of inflammation is obvious (Mebarek et al., 2011; Rosenthal et al., 2011). The elevated ESR might reflect their action on innate immunity cells, inducing inflammatory signals and amplification of already generated. Moreover, the increase of BCP concentration correlates with the severity of the disease (Yavorskyy et al., 2008). To provoke an inhibition of crystal deposition or their degradation represents a novel and tempting approach for application in chronic phase which can limit joint damage.

In our study low percentage of RANKL positive blood neutrophils was detected in healthy donors (0.8 ± 0.4%). After their *in vitro* stimulation with TLR2 agonist, zymosan, they responded with an increased RANKL expression (8.22 ± 0.07%). Significantly higher percentage of RANKL positive blood neutrophils were observed in patients with active OA (14.75 ± 5.07 %; p<0.001 vs healthy) and inactive OA (9.77 ± 2.16%; p<0.01 vs healthy) but only inactive group responded to zymosan stimulation (Fig. 1).

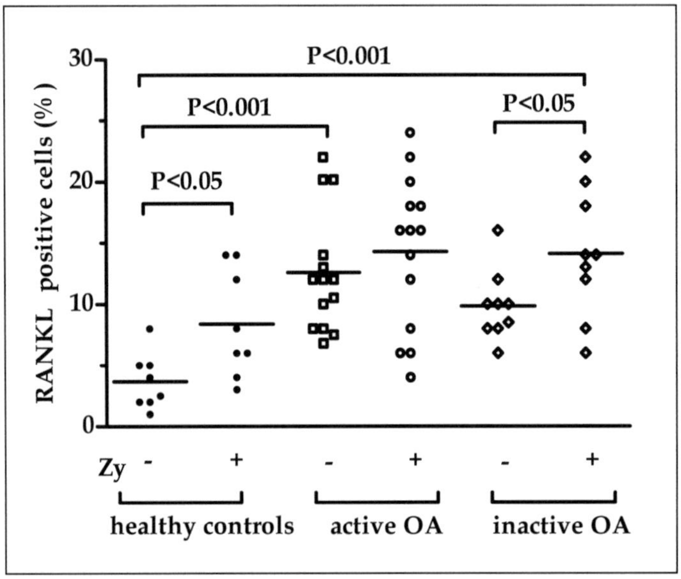

Fig. 1. RANKL expression on neutrophils isolated from healthy controls and patients with active and inactive osteoarthritis (OA). Cells (1x10⁶/ml) were incubated (37⁰C, 2 h) in the absence or presence of 10 µg/ml of zymosan (Zy). After washing neutrophils were stained with rat antibody against human RANKL and isotype control, followed by secondary FITC-conjugated anti-rat antibody. Data represent percentage of RANKL positive cells with the median value in the group (see lines in each group).

Experimental osteoarthritis was induced according to a method described by Blom et al. (Blom, et al. 2007). Mice received two intra-articular injections of collagenase (2 times x1U collagenase) at day 0 and 2. Arthritis onset occurs within 7 days. ZIA was induced by intra-articular injection of 180 µg (10 µl) of zymosan. In both models BALB/c mice 10-12 week old with weight 20-22 g were used. Whole-blood samples were collected in heparin and neutrophils were isolated by dextran sedimentation followed by gradient centrifugation, resuspended at 1x10⁶/ml and stimulated for 2 h with zymosan (10 µg/ml). After washing neutrophils were stained with rat antibody against mouse RANKL and isotype control, followed by secondary FITC-conjugated anti-rat antibody. Data from one representative experiment shows the mean fluorescence intensity and the percentage of RANKL positive cells.

Further, we have investigated RANKL expression on neutrophils in two mouse models: collagenase-induced osteoarthritis and zymosan-induced arthritis. We found low frequencies of RANKL positive neutrophils in blood of CIOA mice and a weak response to *in vitro* zymosan stimulation (Fig. 2). Blood neutrophis from ZIA mice expressed RANKL and responded to TLR2 engagement with increased RANKL expression (Fig. 2).

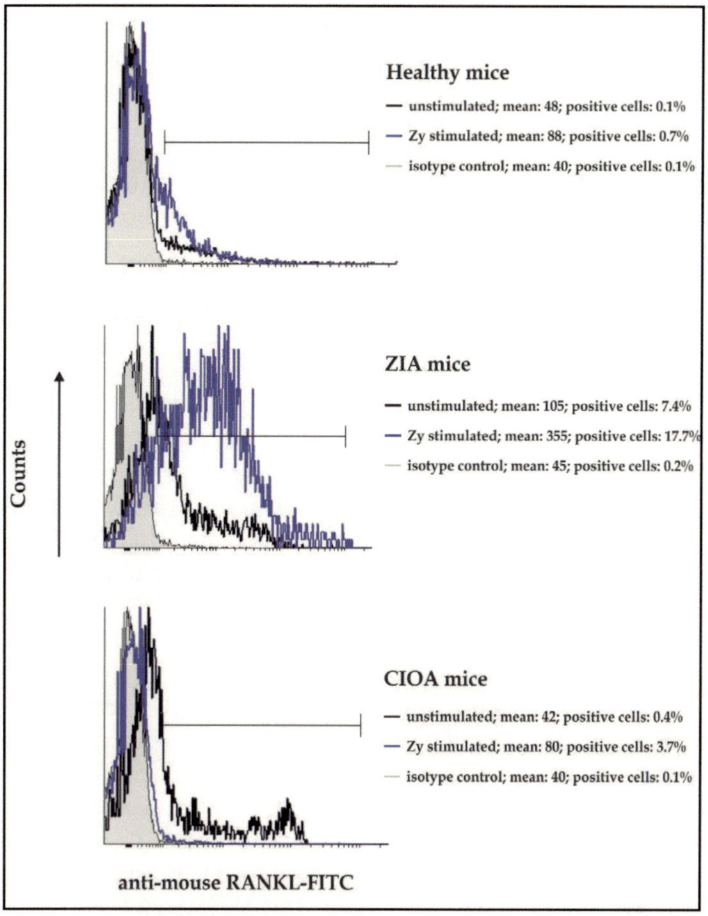

Fig. 2. RANKL expression by blood neutrophils isolated from mice with zymosan-induced arthritis (ZIA) and collagenase-induced osteoarthritis (CIOA) at day 30 of disease.

2.3 MRP8/MRP14 as a potential OA marker related to neutrophil recruitment

The rate of neutrophil and macrophage infiltration at the site of inflammation is associated with myeloid-related proteins (MRP)-8 and -14, belonging to S-100 family of calcium binding proteins. MRP8 and MRP14 are secreted by human monocytes after activation of protein kinase C (PKC) (Rammes et al., 1997). In inflammation they are expressed by infiltrating neutrophils, keratinocytes and monocytes in contrast to resting-tissue macrophages and lymphocytes (Frosch et al., 2000; Kerkhoff et al., 1998). Increased expression of these molecules has been established in various inflammatory disorders including RA (Youssef et al., 1999), psoriasis (Kunz et al., 1992), inflammatory bowel disease (Rugtveit et al., 1994), PsA (Kane et al., 2003). MRP8/MRP14 expression is very low in normal tissues and in RA patients in clinical remission, but high in patients with active disease (Brun et al., 1994). Similar levels of MRP8/MRP14 are found in synovial fluid from patients with psoriatic arthritis, RA and spondyloarthritis without a correlation with disease duration and clinical expression of arthritis activity (Bhardwaj et al., 1992). The proteins enriched more the synovial fluid than the blood circulation as a result of infiltration and activation of neutrophils and macrophages in the joints of RA patients. Very scarce data are available about MRP proteins in OA. It is supposed that the contact of phagocytes with activated endothelium leads to release of MRP8/MRP14, which induces the switch from selectin-mediated reversible adhesion to integrin-dependent tight contact (Frosch et al., 2000).

However, MRP8/MRP14 levels might be reliable prognostic marker for disease activity and for the effectiveness of immunosuppressive therapy. Methotrexate (MTX) treatment resulted in reduced MRP8/MRP14 serum levels (Kane et al., 2003; Ryckman et al., 2003). It is considered that in acute inflammation MRP8/14 and MRP14 are well represented, while MRP8 is associated with chronic inflammatory conditions (Roth et al., 2003). In our study we have included OA patients with or without an active inflammatory process in one or more joints (Toncheva et al., 2009). We observed high MRP8 plasma level in 30% of the patients with active OA (number of patients =37) and in 8% of the patients with inactive OA (number of patients =19). In healthy donors MRP8 level was very low (number of donors =31). Although our data suggest that the severity of OA might correlate with MRP8 plasma level it will be important to continue such investigations in larger groups of patients. The diagnostic value and advantage of MRPs over other disease markers is that they are released immediately upon activation of the particular cell population.

2.4 TLR2 expression by OA neutrophils

The progression of arthritic processes might be supported by the recognition of microbial or host-derived ligands found in arthritic joints. It has been shown that TLR2 and TLR4, but not TLR9, play distinct roles in disease pathogenesis (Abdollahi-Roodsaz et al., 2008). Knockout (IL1rn-/-) mice spontaneously develop T cell-mediated arthritis dependent on TLR activation since germ-free mice fail to develop arthritis. Activation of TLRs on macrophages and dendritic cells leads to the production of proinflammatory cytokines, including TNF-α and IL-1β. The role of the innate immune system in RA and in experimental models of RA has been the object of recent investigations. An increased expression of TLR2 and TLR4 on peripheral blood monocytes and in the synovial tissues from patients with RA has been observed (De Rycke et al., 2005; Iwahashi et al., 2004). Limited data exist on the quantitative TLR2 and TLR4 expression by synovial macrophages, but it is known that their expression was increased in RA compared with osteoarthritis or normal synovial tissue (Radstake et al., 2004). TLRs through NF-κB activation provoke the production of innate immunity mediators, like IL-1, IL-6, IL-8, and TNF-α (Takeuchi et al., 2000; Wang et al., 2001). Consequently, these molecules up-regulate TLR expression, e.g. TNF-α stimulates TLR2 gene expression in contrast to TLR4 (Matsuguchi et al., 2000). The stimulation of cultured RA synovial cells with IL-1β and TNF-α leads to an increase of TLR2 mRNA expression but such increase of TLR4 and TLR9 expression is not detected in the absence or in the presence of stimuli (Seibl et al., 2003). These results are not specific for RA, because cells derived from joints of patients with OA responded similarly to TNF-α stimulation.

Neutrophils express all known human TLRs except TLR3 (Hayashi et al., 2003). TNF-α and IL-6 production in neutrophils can be triggered upon the engagement of TLR2, TLR4, TLR9. In neutrophils the ligation of TLRs results in activation of MAPK and NF-kB but not always involves the adaptor protein MyD88. In respect to TLR4, recently it has been reported that

LPS can induce different response in adherent and in suspended neutrophils. In adherent cells TLR4 ligation triggers Jun activation and the release of the chemokine monocyte chemoattractant protein-1, an activated protein-1-dependent gene product that is important for monocyte recruitment. Adherent neutrophils interact with matrix proteins through sheded CD43. CD43 (leukosialin) is a heavily sialylated molecule that is cleaved by neutrophil elastase near the plasma membrane. In blood CD43 binds albumin that protects it from the elastase action. In inflammatory conditions neutrophils secrete elastase enhancing the spread and rolling of neutrophils. In RA the destruction of cartilage and bone might be associated with the activation of synovial cells through TLR2. The ligands of TLR2 include lipopetides and peptidoglycan (Aliprantis et al., 1999; Schwandner et al., 1999), and zymosan acting in collaboration with TLR6 and CD14 (Ozinsky et al., 2000). While TLR4 is weakly represented on the surface of human neutrophils, TLR2 and CD14 are well expressed (Kurt-Jones et al., 2002).

To investigate the involvement of TLR2 in OA we followed its constitutive and Zy-induced expression in blood neutrophils. Data in Fig. 3 show that the percentage of TLR2 positive neutrophils from OA patients was approximately 4 fold higher compared to healthy donors. Zymosan stimulation resulted in 2 fold enhancement of TLR2 expression on neutrophils from all groups.

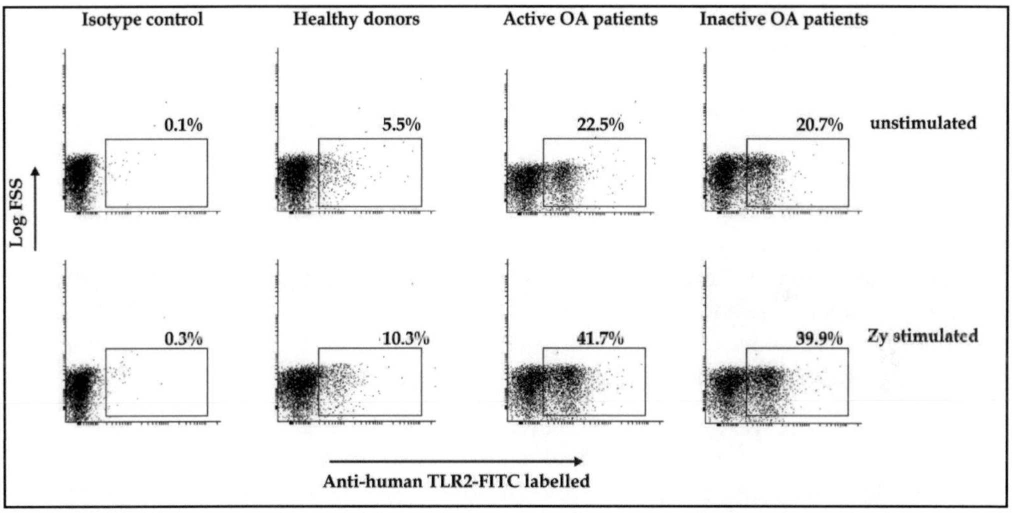

Fig. 3. TLR2 positive neutrophils from healthy donors and patients with active and inactive osteoarthritis (OA). Cells ($1x10^6$/ml) were incubated (37^0C, 2 h) in the absence or presence of 10 µg/ml of zymosan (Zy). Cells were collected, washed and stained with rat antibodies against human TLR2 (3 µg/ml), followed by secondary FITC-conjugated anti-rat antibody.

Neutrophils isolated from healthy and OA donors were *in vitro* simulated with zymosan and the secretion of TNF-α was determined. Neutrophils from patients with active OA spontaneously release the cytokine in contrast to healthy and inactive OA groups. Zymosan significantly enhanced TNF-α secretion of healthy donors and inactive OA (Fig. 4A). The spontaneous release of TNF-α was higher in ZIA and CIOA groups compared to healthy group. Neutrophils from arthritic mice did not respond significantly to zymosan stimulation, while healthy group showed increased TNF-α production (Figure 4B).

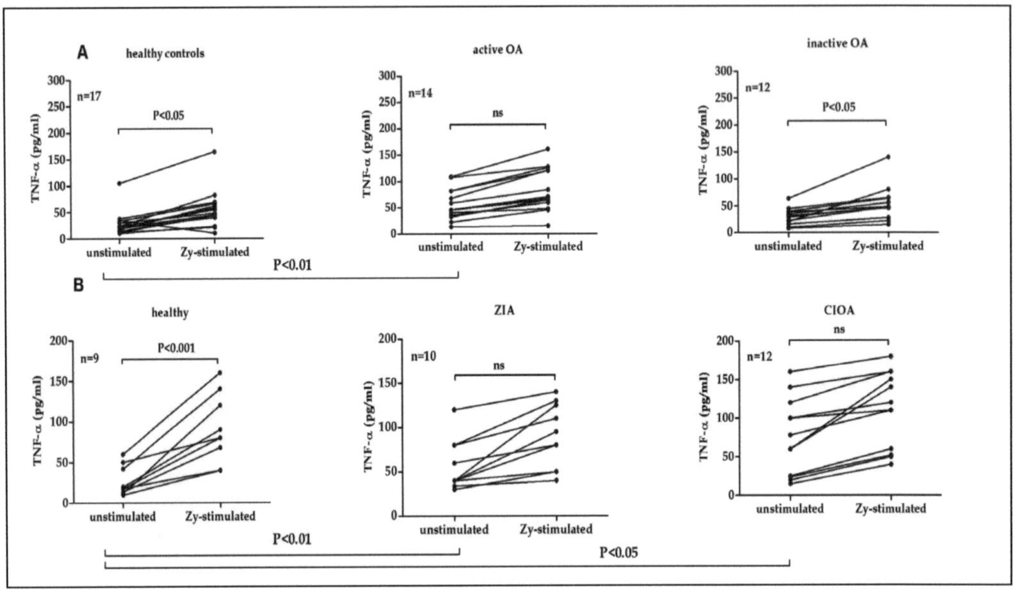

Fig. 4. Spontaneous and zymosan-induced TNF-α production by blood neutrophils. (A) Cells isolated from healthy donors and patients with active and inactive osteoarthritis ($1x10^6$/ml) were incubated (37^0C, 24 h) in the absence or presence of 10 μg/ml of zymosan. (B) Cells isolated from healthy mice and mice with zymosan-induced arthritis (ZIA,) and collagenase-induced osteoarthritis (CIOA) at day 30 of arthritis ($1x10^6$/ml) were incubated (37^0C, 24 h) in the absence or presence of 10 μg/ml of zymosan. TNF-α concentration in the supernatants was determines by ELISA.

The up-regulation of TLR2 corresponds either to a response to an exposure to microbial compounds or is secondary to the inflammatory milieu present in the rheumatoid joints. TNF-α is a key mediator in inflammatory joint diseases. We observed the activation state of neutrophils at least in active OA, which was witnessed by their spontaneous *ex vivo* TNF-α release. Our previous results showed that TLR4 ligand LPS is able to trigger *in vitro* TNF-α release by neutrophils from patients with inactive OA (Toncheva et al., 2009). Zymosan also enhanced TNF-α production of neutrophils from inactive OA patients. Probably in active OA, being in activated state cells has reached a threshold after which they become unresponsive. The results from ZIA and CIOA point on such possibility if we accept that ZIA is relevant to more severe inflammatory condition than CIOA. In synovial explant cultures it has been proved that a monoclonal antibody against TLR2 can inhibit the spontaneous release of TNF-α, IFN-γ, IL-1β and IL-8. Such data are a good base for future investigations on the use of TLR2 antagonists by clinicians, because the effect of anti-TLR2 antibodies is comparable with that of the TNF inhibitor adalimumab (Nic An Ultaigh et al., 2011).

2.5 Activation of monocytes and macrophages during OA

Monocytes and macrophages play an important role in various inflammatory conditions, depending on their stage of activation (Burmester et al., 1997; Tak et al., 1997). Monocytes are subdivided into two different populations with distinct phenotype and functional activity. While classical monocytes are $CD14^{hi}CD16-$ in humans and GR1+ in mouse, non-classical monocytes are $CD14^{low}CD16+$ in man and GR1- in mouse. Classical monocytes highly express the CC-chemokine receptor 2 (CCR2), CD62 ligand (CD62L) (Tacke et al., 2007) and vascular cell adhesion molecule 1 (VCAM1 or CD106), and produce low levels of proinflammatory cytokines like TNF-α and IL-1. The latter mediators activate synovial endothelial cells and other leukocytes and initiate inflammatory process. Non-classical monocytes or "resident" monocytes express high level of CX_3C-chemokine receptor 1 (CX_3CR1) and are potent antigen-presenting cells. It has been shown that monocytes from arthritic patients with active disease have reduced HLA–DR expression and decreased capacity to stimulate T cells *in vitro* than healthy cells (Muller et al., 2009). Moreover, TNF-α inhibits HLA-DR synthesis in arthritic myeloid cells via the expression of class II transactivator (CIITA). In comparison to RA, OA patients showed lower density of HLA-DR expression on peripheral monocytes (Koller et al., 1999) suggesting their intrinsic functional abnormality to act as antigen-presenting cells.

An accumulation of macrophages is found in the synovium of patients with early OA (Benito et al., 2005). These resident tissue cells are CD68 positive. CD68+ macrophages in OA synovium were restricted to the lining layer while in RA patients they were found in the sublining layer and the areas around newly formed micro-vessels. In the study of Bloom et al. macrophages are depleted prior the development of early OA by injection of clodronate liposomes (Blom et al., 2004). The lack of macrophages reduced the size of osteophytes and lining thickness, and inhibits chondrocyte ossification and fibrosis. Macrophage depletion also down-regulates the expression of bone morphogenetic proteins, BMP2 and BMP4 in synovium (van Lent et al., 2004). Both molecules are important regulators of bone remodeling process and their inhibition has good therapeutic potential in OA as we have observed in a model of CIOA (Ivanovska & Dimitrova, 2011).

Under OA conditions, CD68+ macrophages in synovial lining layer are persistently activated via NF-κB, STAT and Pi3K signaling pathways. They are the source of inducible nitric oxide and of proinflammatory cytokines like TNF-α and IL-1β (Benito et al., 2005) driving inflammatory process in OA and causing synovitis and bone erosion. Apart of this role, macrophages can participate directly in cartilage degradation. They are capable to produce enzymes degrading extracellular matrix macromolecules like disintegrin-metalloproteinases with thrombospondin motifs and MMPs like MMP-2, MMP-3 and MMP-9 (Smeets et al., 2003). While MMP-2 activates the expression of other MMPs in chondrocytes, MMP-3 is directly involved in cartilage destruction. Serum level of MMP-3 is associated with joint space narrowing in OA patients (Lohmander et al., 2005). MMP-3–deficient mice show significantly decreased cartilage damage (Blom et al., 2007). In rabbit model of experimental arthritis MMP-3 is initially up-regulated in the synovium contributing to the appearance of cartilage lesions while MMP-3 derived from chondrocyte exacerbate cartilage loss at late phases of OA (Mehraban et al., 1998). Blom et al. showed that at early experimental OA synovial macrophages are responsible for the initial MMP-3 production (Blom et al., 2007). These data are based on the observation that MMP-3 expression in the synovium is strongly reduced in the absence of synovial macrophages.

Secreted by macrophages MMPs are proteases that cleave not only collagen in bone matrix but also can modify other molecules present in the OA synovium. For example MMP-9 cleaves chemokines CXCL1 and CXCL8 increasing their potency to attract neutrophils and to amplify inflammation and bone erosion (Van den Steen et al., 2000).

Synovial macrophages can secrete pro-inflammatory mediators that increase MMP expression by synovial cells or chondrocytes. Macrophages isolated from synovial lining layer of OA patients produce spontaneously IL-1β and TNF-α. In synovial cell co-cultures macrophages stimulate the synovial fibroblasts to produce MMPs and cytokines like IL-6 and IL-8 via a synergistic action of IL-1β and TNF-α (Bondeson et al., 2006). IL-1β synthesis in OA is independent of TNF-α and correlates with OA severity. The biological activity of IL-1β is regulated by the balance between the expression of the active receptor IL-1RI and the inactive or decoy receptor IL-1RII. While the IL-1RI is highly expressed the decoy receptor IL-1RII is little or missing in OA. This receptor imbalance in turn decreases the ability of IL-1RII to neutralize completely and eliminate active IL-1. IL-1 together with TNF-α promotes osteoclast differentiation and bone resoption. It has been shown that IL-1 alone can induce osteoclastogensis but only in osteoclast precursors over-expressing IL-1R1 (Kim et al., 2009). Several *in vitro* studies show that IL-1 inhibition by natural inhibitors such as IL-1 receptor antagonist or soluble receptors decreases MMP expression and cartilage destruction in OA (Jacques et al., 2006).

Macrophages can produce pro-inflammatory cytokine IL-18. The administration of IL-18 at the initial and late phase of arthritis accelerates the development of disease. Despite that IL-18 is detected at low amounts in OA synovium (Gracie et al., 1999) it can stimulate the expression of MMP-3, MMP-13, aggrecanase-2, TIMP-1 in chondrocytes promoting bone destructive process. Recently, it has been shown that IL-21 is a proinflammatory cytokine that increases CXCL8 production by monocyte-derived macrophages. The receptor for IL-21 was detected on monocytes, monocyte-derived macrophages and on synovial macrophages from RA patients (Jungel et al., 2004). IL-21R has limited expression in OA synovium but it is expressed in the areas with enhanced catabolic processes and might participate in destructive process.

Macrophages also release factors that are important for tissue repair and suppression of inflammatory response. Among these factors are vascular endothelial growth factor CD106 (Haywood et al., 2003), prostaglandin E2, IL-10 and TGF-β. TGF-β expression from macrophages can be triggered by lipoxin A4 produced by activated neutrophils. TGF-β inhibits T cell proliferation and inflammatory responses. The anti-inflammatory cytokine IL-10 regulates the synthesis of IL-4, and inhibits IFN-γ production in T cells and TNF-α and IL-1β production in macrophages. The important role of anti-inflammatory cytokines IL-10 and IL-4 in OA has been well described in studies on experimental OA where these cytokine are administrated. The combined treatment with low dosages of IL-4 and IL-10 has potent anti-inflammatory effects and markedly protected against OA cartilage destruction. Improved anti-inflammatory effect was achieved with IL-4/prednisolone treatment (Joosten et al., 1999).

The progression of OA might result in an inappropriate differentiation of resident tissue macrophages, and expression of functionally distinct phenotype (Mantovani et al., 2007; Xu et al., 2005). Macrophage functions are tightly regulated by reversible histone acetylation with acetylases (HAT enzymes) and deacetylation with deacetylases (HDAC enzymes) (Grabiec et al., 2010).

Resident macrophages in different tissues such as lung, liver and synovium express Z39Ig (CRIg) protein (Helmy et al., 2006). The Z39Ig is a receptor for complement fragments C3b and iC3b and is a type 1 transmembrane protein of the immunoglobulin superfamily member. Significant Z39Ig staining is detected in macrophage-enriched areas in the lining and sublining areas of RA synovium (Lee et al., 2006). In OA synovial tissue the number of cells expressing Z39Ig was lower and the positive staining was restricted to the lining-layer macrophages. A significant number of Z39Ig+CD11c+cells observed in some cases of OA and PsA points that Z39Ig+CD11c+cells deserve extended investigations to clarify their functional activity in OA (Tanaka et al., 2008).

It has been shown that prostaglandin E2 secreted by macrophages contributes to pain hypersensitivity by promoting sensory neurons hyperexcitability. Tissue-resident macrophages constitutively express receptor P2X4 and the stimulation via P2X4R triggers calcium influx and p38 MAPK phosphorylation and COX-dependent release of PGE2 (Ulmann et al., 2010). These data suggest that synovial lining macrophages might be important effectors that control pain relieve in OA patients.

Osteoclasts and monocytes are not only derived from a common myeloid progenitor but their activity might be influenced by common mediators (Ross, 2000). Activation of CD40 signaling in monocytes/macrophages results in up-regulation of nitric oxide generation (Tian et al., 1995), and induction of metalloproteinase production (Malik et al., 1996). Recently, it was found that except CD40L, the known activator of monocytes/macrophages, also OPGL can express such function (Andersson et al., 2002). Mice deficient in CD40L expression display a deficiency in T cell-dependent macrophage-mediated immune responses (Stout et al., 1996). The development of osteoclasts is strongly dependent on the interactions between two members of TNF superfamily, OPGL and its receptor RANK (Lacey et al., 1998; Yasuda et al., 1998). One of the pathways for triggering inflammatory processes by OPGL is through p38 MAPK and p42/44 ERK and inducing cytokine and chemokine secretion (Suttles et al., 1996). Results from in vivo application of RANK-Fc in a model of antibody-mediated arthritis showed that it blocked OPGL activity and ameliorated arthritis development (Seshasayee et al., 2004).

3. TLR9 expression in OA

Toll-like receptors are involved not only in pathogen recognition but they can participate in triggering the inflammatory and joint destructive process in arthritis or they can enhance the progression of already established synovitis. TLR-mediated inflammatory response may induce further tissue damage and can provoke a self-sustaining inflammatory loop responsible for chronic progression of arthritis processes. The expression of TLR9 in the joints was assessed in chronic phase (day 30) of ZIA and CIOA. In healthy mice no detectable expression of TLR9 was found in the synovium in contrast to CIOA and ZIA, where synovial lining was extensively stained (Fig. 5A).

We observed stronger TLR9 positive staining in the bone and bone marrow of ZIA than of CIOA, in comparison to healthy mice showing only single positive cells (Fig. 5B). Most intensive accumulation of TLR9 positive cells was established in ZIA mice, especially well exerted in the sites of osteophyte formation (Fig. 5C)

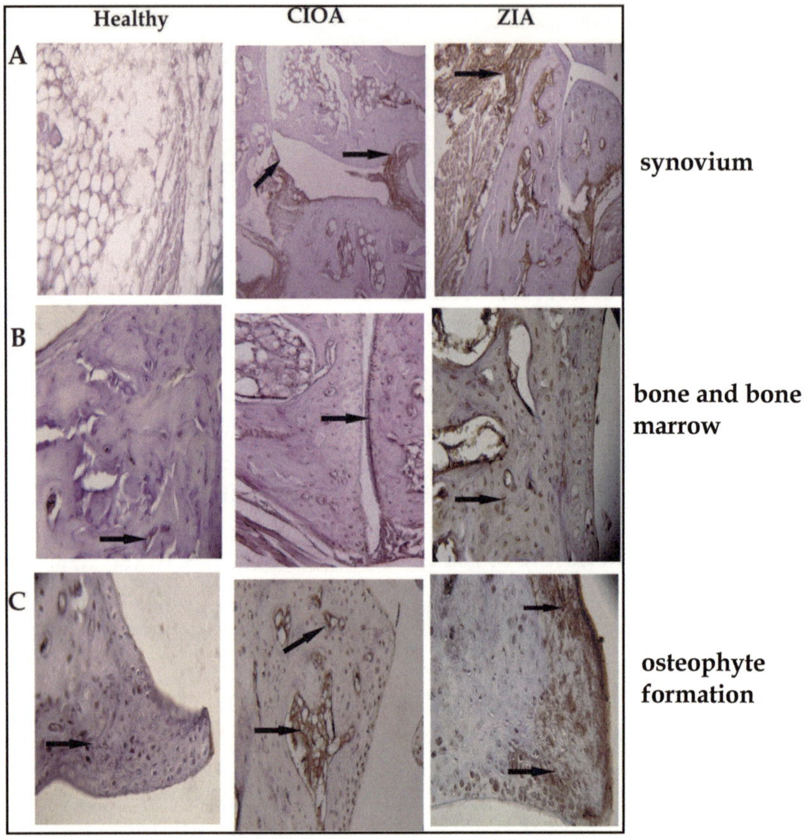

Fig. 5. Histological analyses of TLR9 expression in the joint. Dissected ankle joints were fixed in 10% paraformaldehyde/PBS, decalcified in 5% nitric acid for 1 week, dehydrated and embedded in paraffin. Sections (6 µm thickness) were blocked with 5% bovine serum albumin/PBS for 1 h and the endogenous peroxidase was blocked with 0.3% H_2O_2 in 60% methanol for 10 min. After washing, the sections were incubated for 40 min at room temperature with antibodes against mTLR9 (10 µg/ml). Isotype anti-mouse IgG was used as a background staining control. Then, the joint sections were incubated for 10 min with biotinylated anti-mouse IgGs and streptavidin-peroxidase was added for 10 min. The sections were washed and incubated with DAB solution kit (3',3'diaminobenzididne kit, Abcam) for 10 min and counterstained with Gill's hematoxylin. Arrows show positive TLR9 staining (magnification 40x).

The different TLR9 expression might be due to the difference in both models. Zymosan-induced arthritis is an example for proliferative arthritis, which is restricted to the joint injected with zymosan (Bernotiene et al., 2004). Using this model we found that histologically, joint sections showed cell infiltration into cartilage, capsule, osteoid and surrounding soft tissue and synovial hyperplasia without aggressive pannus formation. Proteoglycan depletion in cartilage, detected by loss of safranin O staining intensity, and changes in joint architecture were observed at late stage of arthritis. Interestingly, we observed the immunoreactivity for TNF-αR and C5aR in cartilage, along with C5aR positive inflammatory cells in the areas of bone and synovium. At the onset of ZIA, TNF-α plays a dominant role in inflammation. In the synovial extracts were found increased levels of IL-6 and C5a that can regulate the expression of C5aR on infiltrating neutrophils (Dimitrova et al., 2010; Dimitrova et al., 2011). CIA was provoked by intraarticular injections of collagenase, leading to acute ligament instability and prolonged inflammatory cartilage erosion over a period of six weeks. The model is relevant to human osteoarthritis pathology. In order to look for correlation between elevated TLR expression and the severity of arthritis we investigated the changes of TLR9 expression by macrophages from different origin in established ZIA. Data showed high presence of TLR9 positive cells in peritoneal exudates and PLNs in arthritic animals, while such elevation was not established for spleens (Fig. 6). These results deserve further experiments on the role of macrophages in the maintenance of inflammation in different organs. The elevation in lymph node population might be due to the fact that PLN is located most closely to the site of zymosan injection in inflamed joint.

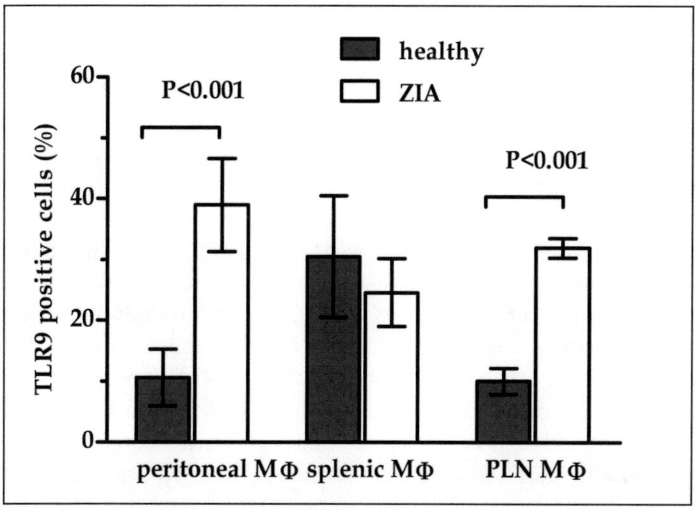

Fig. 6. TLR9 expression in macrophages isolated from different compartments at day 30 of ZIA. Differentiated macrophages isolated from peritoneal exudates (peritoneal Mϕ), spleens (splenic Mϕ) and popliteal lymph nodes (PLN Mϕ) of healthy and ZIA mice ($1x10^6$/ml) were stained with antibodies against mouse TLR9 (1 μg/ml), followed by secondary FITC-conjugated anti-mouse antibody and subjected to FACS analysis.

4. Natural killer cells

Natural killer cells are firstly described by their capacity to limit the growth of malignant cells and to eliminate virus-infected cells. They are innate immune effectors that produce immunoregulatory cytokines, such as interferon (IFN)-γ and granulocyte macrophage-colony-stimulating factor GM-CSF (Bancroft, 1993; Feng et al., 2006). Later, it became evident that NK cells can play a critical role in various autoimmune diseases, including rheumatoid arthritis by improving or exacerbating immune responses. They can play dual role in autoimmune diseases, either support or suppress pathogenic processes. In animal models it is established that NK cells are responsible for the induction and progression of K/BxN serum transfer model, being engaged through activation of their FcgIII receptors (Kim et al., 2006) and also being involved in the acceleration and exacerbation of CIA (Chu et al., 2007). The induction of CIA in NK-depleted mice reduces the severity of arthritis and almost completely prevents bone erosion (Soderstrom et al., 2010). In these experiments, also significantly reduced inflammation, pannus formation, and synovitis have been observed. NK cells are enriched within the joints of RA patients but how they contribute to disease pathology is currently not fully elucidated. In RA patients NK cells comprise 20 % of the synovial fluid cells at the early phase of disease (de Matos et al., 2007; Tak et al., 1994). These cells express CD56 and CD94/NKG2A phenotype, but failed to express CD16 similarly to peripheral RA NK cells.

Two distinct subsets of mature NK cells have been recognized, $CD56^{bright}$ and $CD56^{dim}$. $CD56^{bright}$ subset is the source of IFN-γ, TNF-β, IL-10, IL-13, and GM-CSF, whereas the $CD56^{dim}$ NK cell subset produces significantly less of these cytokines in vitro (Cooper et al., 2001). The $CD56^{bright}$ NK cells express a chemokine receptor pattern similar to that of monocytes including high-affinity receptors for IL-15 (Carson et al., 1994). This subset has been identified in the joints of patients with early synovitis in RA. Several studies have shown that IL-15 is a critical factor for the development of human and murine NK cells (Kennedy et al., 2000; Mrozek et al., 1996). This might be due to its stimulation of M-CSF and RANKL expression by NK cells. IL-15 alone did not change the ability of monocytes to enhance osteoclast formation, while this process was dramatically supported in the presence of both NK cells and IL-15, indicating that the effect of IL-15 is mediated through NK cells (Soderstrom et al., 2010).

NK cells may be implicated in the initiation, the maintenance or the progression of autoimmune diseases directly or through their interaction with dendritic cells, macrophages or T lymphocytes. Whether neutrophils are capable to regulate and influence the activity of NK cells is not well defined. Generally, data on neutrophils and NK cells concern RA and are focused mainly on cytokines. There are no available investigations in OA in regard to remodeling events and the participation of these cells in OA has been underestimated. The investigations of NK-cell functions in patients with OA will improve our capacity to monitor these cells as possible markers for disease activity and will provide new prospects for NK-cell–directed therapies.

5. Mast cells

Nearly two decades ago available data show that when compared with healthy individuals, patients with OA had elevated numbers of intact and degranulated mast cells in the synovium and synovial fluid of diseased joints. Histological studies confirmed significant numbers of mast cells in both RA and OA synovium (Dean et al., 1993; Kopicky-Burd et al., 1988). Moreover, the numbers of mast cells in OA are comparable with those in RA when clinically active arthritis is envisaged. Prednisone used as anti-rheumatic drug lowered synovial mast cell number (Bridges et al., 1991). Mast cells containing triptase (MCT) expanded in the SF of OA patients (Buckley et al., 1998), while cells containing triptase and chimase (MCTC) expand in RA but not in OA (Gotis-Graham et al., 1998). When mast cell numbers in RA and OA patients are compared without respect to mast cell distribution in the subsynovial layer or the stratum fibrosum, no statistical differences between the diseases could be observed (Fritz et al., 1984). Synovial fluid collected from patients with hand OA expressed elevated number of mast cells in correlation with high content of histamine and elevated levels of tryptase and NO (Renoux et al., 1996). Such data support the hypothesis that in OA the increase of mast cells may participate in the pathological process, at least they can contribute in concert with other inflammatory cells.

6. Adipokines as potential participants in OA

Although leptin has been discovered fifteen years ago, the investigations on adipokines as potential participants in arthritic diseases are now at its beginning. Innate immunity cells appeared to be a source of adipokines as well as an object of their action. Leptin realizes its action as a proinflammatory cytokine through modulation of monocytes, macrophages, neutrophils, basophils, eosinophils, natural killer and dendritic cells (Otero et al., 2005). It seems to play a role in auto immune diseases such as RA and OA, by expressing harmful as well protective action on joint structures in RA (Lago et al., 2007). Leptin has been detected in SF obtained from patients with OA, and it was strongly overexpressed in human OA cartilage and in osteophytes (Dumond et al., 2003). The administration of exogenous leptin in rats increases IGF1 and TGFβ1 production suggesting that high circulating leptin levels might protect cartilage from osteoarthritic erosion but it also can induce osteophyte formation. Although adiponectin was discovered almost at the same time as leptin, its role in obesity-related dis orders has now begun to be investigated. In joint disorders adiponectin might play proinflammatory role beimg involved in matrix degradation. The pathogenic role of adiponectin is largely unknown in concern to RA and OA. Recent data proved that in chronic RA patients adiponectin plasma levels are higher compared to healthy controls, but lower plasma levels than in OA (Laurberg et al., 2009). Another member of this group is resistin (FIZZ3) which is found in adipocytes, macrophages and other cell types. It has been determined in the plasma and the synovial fluid of RA patients. The injection of resistin into mice joints induces an arthritis-like condition, with typical leukocyte infiltration in the synovium and tissue hypertrophy (Bokarewa et al., 2005). There are not enough data to make firm conclusions about the exact role of adipokines in arthritic processes. Their physiological role in RA or OA and their use as disease markers deserve to be a subject of further studies.

7. Conclusions

In the hope of defining novel therapeutic targets in OA much attention has been paid on degenerative processes of cartilage and secondary bone damage. But in recent years, the synovium, and in particular the participation of synovial cells and their mediators are under intensive study. Macrophages, neutrophils and lymphocytes act together with resident fibroblasts in the destructive phases of arthritis through liberation of proinflammatory molecues. Activated macrophages produced chemoattractants such as chemoattractant protein 1, RANTES, MIP-2α and epithelial neutrophil activator (Choy & Panayi, 2001). Many studies have been devoted to investigating various signaling pathways involved in proinflammatory cytokine production from OA synovial macrophages. The promising results of anticytokine therapies in RA prompted that such approach might be used in OA (Bondeson, 2010). Major population of infiltrated cells in synovium are neutrophils. This is valid for the early phase of inflammation as well as for its maintenance. The injection of anti-neutrophil antibodies ameliorated the established disease in collagen-LPS-induced model and K/BxN model (Nandakumar et al., 2003; Tanaka et al., 2006). Instead of macrophage/monocyte or neutrophil depletion which can impair host resistance, neutralizing antibodies blocking their chemotaxis might be used. Promising results in animal models have been obtained with ant-MIP-1α antibodies (Kagari et al., 2003) and pertussis toxin blocking of signals from G protein-coupled receptors (GPCRs) (Becker et al., 1985; Painter et al., 1987; Spangrude et al., 1985).

There is a large unmet need for reliable biochemical markers that will predict the subset of patients who are at risk of the disease progression and will be used to find molecular targets in future therapies. Elevated RANKL levels in synovium and circulation, and particularly increased RANKL expression by neutrophils in OA, makes it a suitable candidate for disease prognosis.

The ability of known TLR agonists to activate neutrophil functions supports the notion that TLRs are an important pattern recognition receptors in the function of these cells. Consequently, while producing chemokines they trigger migration of other immune cells, such as more neutrophils, monocytes, macrophages, NK cells, and immature dendritic cells. These results prompt a possible correlation between the increase of TLR2 positive blood cells, including neutrophils and existing OA condition and strongly support the idea that OA inflammation might be influenced through TLR2. Also, elevated TLR9 expression is detected in the joints of arthritic mice. Whether TLRs involvement is similar for both inactive and active OA is a question to be resolved. TLR-dependent mechanisms may contribute to the activation of synovial cells, possibly leading to the destruction of cartilage and bone in the pathogenesis of RA and OA.

8. Acknowledgments

This work has been supported by the project BG051PO001/3.3-05-001 „Science and Business, financed by Operating Program "Development of human resources" to European Social Fund.

9. Abbreviations

CIOA – collagenase-induced osteoarthritis; ERK – extracellular signal-regulated kinase; FITC - fluorescein isothiocianate; GM-CSF - granulocyte-macrophage colony-stimulating factor; IFN-γ - interferon gamma; IL – interleukine; MAPK-mitogen-activated protein kinase; MIP-2 - macrophage inflammatory protein; MMP - matrix metalloproteinase; MRPs - myeloid-related proteins; NF-kB – nuclear factor-kappa B; NK cells – natural killer cells; OA – osteoarthritis; OPG - osteoprotegerin ; Pi3K - phosphatidylinositol 3-kinases; RA – rheumatoid arthritis; RANK – receptor activator of nuclear factor-kappa B; RANKL - receptor activator of nuclear factor-kappa B ligand; RANTES - Regulated upon Activation, Normal T-cell Expressed, and Secreted; STAT - Signal Transducer and Activator of Transcription; TGF-β – transforming growth factor beta; TIMP-1 - TIMP metallopeptidase inhibitor 1; TLR – Toll-like receptor; TNF - tumor necrosis factor; Z39Ig - Immunoglobulin superfamily protein Z39IG; ZIA – zymosan-induced arthritis

10. References

Abdollahi-Roodsaz, S., Joosten, L.A., Koenders, M.I., Devesa, I., Roelofs, M.F., et al. (2008). Stimulation of TLR2 and TLR4 differentially skews the balance of T cells in a mouse model of arthritis. *Journal of Clinical Investigation*, Vol.118, No1, pp. 205-216, ISSN 0021-9738

Aliprantis, A.O., Yang, R.B., Mark, M.R., Suggett, S., Devaux, B., et al. (1999). Cell activation and apoptosis by bacterial lipoproteins through toll-like receptor-2. *Science*, Vol.285, No5428, pp. 736-739.

Andersson, U., Erlandsson-Harris, H., Yang, H. & Tracey, K.J. (2002). HMGB1 as a DNA-binding cytokine. *Journal of Leukocyte Biology*, Vol.72, No6, pp. 1084-1091, ISSN 0741-5400

Bancroft, G.J. (1993). The role of natural killer cells in innate resistance to infection. *Current Opinion in Immunology*, Vol.5, No4, pp. 503-510, ISSN 0952-7915

Becker, E.L., Kermode, J.C., Naccache, P.H., Yassin, R., Marsh, M.L., et al. (1985). The inhibition of neutrophil granule enzyme secretion and chemotaxis by pertussis toxin. *Journal of Cell Biology*, Vol.100, No5, pp. 1641-1646, ISSN 0021-9525

Bell, A.L., Magill, M.K., McKane, R. & Irvine, A.E. (1995). Human blood and synovial fluid neutrophils cultured in vitro undergo programmed cell death which is promoted by the addition of synovial fluid. *Annals of the Rheumatic Diseases*, Vol.54, No11, pp. 910-915, ISSN 0003-4967

Benito, M.J., Veale, D.J., FitzGerald, O., van den Berg, W.B. & Bresnihan, B. (2005). Synovial tissue inflammation in early and late osteoarthritis. *Annals of the Rheumatic Diseases*, Vol.64, No9, pp. 1263-1267.

Bernotiene, E., Palmer, G., Talabot-Ayer, D., Szalay-Quinodoz, I., Aubert, M.L., et al. (2004). Delayed resolution of acute inflammation during zymosan-induced arthritis in leptin-deficient mice. *Arthritis Research and Therapy*, Vol.6, No3, pp. R256-263, ISSN 1478-6362

Bhardwaj, R.S., Zotz, C., Zwadlo-Klarwasser, G., Roth, J., Goebeler, M., et al. (1992). The calcium-binding proteins MRP8 and MRP14 form a membrane-associated heterodimer in a subset of monocytes/macrophages present in acute but absent in chronic inflammatory lesions. *European Journal of Immunology*, Vol.22, No7, pp. 1891-1897, ISSN 0014-2980

Blom, A.B., van Lent, P.L., Holthuysen, A.E., van der Kraan, P.M., Roth, J., et al. (2004). Synovial lining macrophages mediate osteophyte formation during experimental osteoarthritis. *Osteoarthritis and Cartilage*, Vol.12, No8, pp. 627-635, ISSN 1063-4584

Blom, A.B., van Lent, P.L., Libregts, S., Holthuysen, A.E., van der Kraan, P.M., et al. (2007). Crucial role of macrophages in matrix metalloproteinase-mediated cartilage destruction during experimental osteoarthritis: involvement of matrix metalloproteinase 3. *Arthritis and Rheumatism*, Vol.56, No1, pp. 147-157, ISSN 0004-3591

Bokarewa, M., Nagaev, I., Dahlberg, L., Smith, U. & Tarkowski, A. (2005). Resistin, an adipokine with potent proinflammatory properties. *Journal of Immunology*, Vol.174, No9, pp. 5789-95, SSN 0022-1767

Bondeson, J. (2010). Activated synovial macrophages as targets for osteoarthritis drug therapy. *Curr Drug Targets*, Vol.11, No5, pp. 576-585, ISSN 1873-5592

Bondeson, J., Wainwright, S.D., Lauder, S., Amos, N. & Hughes, C.E. (2006). The role of synovial macrophages and macrophage-produced cytokines in driving aggrecanases, matrix metalloproteinases, and other destructive and inflammatory responses in osteoarthritis. *Arthritis Research and Therapy*, Vol.8, No6, pp. R187, ISSN 1478-6362

Brach, M.A., deVos, S., Gruss, H.J. & Herrmann, F. (1992). Prolongation of survival of human polymorphonuclear neutrophils by granulocyte-macrophage colony-stimulating factor is caused by inhibition of programmed cell death. *Blood*, Vol.80, No11, pp. 2920-2924, ISSN 0006-4971

Bridges, A.J., Malone, D.G., Jicinsky, J., Chen, M., Ory, P., et al. (1991). Human synovial mast cell involvement in rheumatoid arthritis and osteoarthritis. Relationship to disease type, clinical activity, and antirheumatic therapy. *Arthritis and Rheumatism*, Vol.34, No9, pp. 1116-1124, ISSN 0004-3591

Brun, J.G., Jonsson, R. & Haga, H.J. (1994). Measurement of plasma calprotectin as an indicator of arthritis and disease activity in patients with inflammatory rheumatic diseases. *Journal of Rheumatology*, Vol.21, No4, pp. 733-738, ISSN 0315-162X

Buckley, M.G., Gallagher, P.J. & Walls, A.F. (1998). Mast cell subpopulations in the synovial tissue of patients with osteoarthritis: selective increase in numbers of tryptase-positive, chymase-negative mast cells. *Journal of Pathology*, Vol.186, No1, pp. 67-74, ISSN 0022-3417

Burmester, G.R., Stuhlmuller, B., Keyszer, G. & Kinne, R.W. (1997). Mononuclear phagocytes and rheumatoid synovitis. Mastermind or workhorse in arthritis? *Arthritis and Rheumatism*, Vol.40, No1, pp. 5-18, ISSN 0004-3591

Carson, W.E., Giri, J.G., Lindemann, M.J., Linett, M.L., Ahdieh, M., et al. (1994). Interleukin (IL) 15 is a novel cytokine that activates human natural killer cells via components of the IL-2 receptor. *Journal of Experimental Medicine*, Vol.180, No4, pp. 1395-1403, ISSN 0022-1007

Chakrabarti, S. & Patel, K.D. (2005). Regulation of matrix metalloproteinase-9 release from IL-8-stimulated human neutrophils. *Journal of Leukocyte Biology*, Vol.78, No1, pp. 279-288,

Chakravarti, A., Rusu, D., Flamand, N., Borgeat, P. & Poubelle, P.E. (2009). Reprogramming of a subpopulation of human blood neutrophils by prolonged exposure to cytokines. *Laboratory Investigation*, Vol.89, No10, pp. 1084-1099, ISSN 1530-0307

Choy, E.H. & Panayi, G.S. (2001). Cytokine pathways and joint inflammation in rheumatoid arthritis. *New England Journal of Medicine*, Vol.344, No12, pp. 907-916, ISSN 0028-4793

Chu, C.Q., Swart, D., Alcorn, D., Tocker, J. & Elkon, K.B. (2007). Interferon-gamma regulates susceptibility to collagen-induced arthritis through suppression of interleukin-17. *Arthritis and Rheumatism*, Vol.56, No4, pp. 1145-1151, ISS N0004-3591

Cooper, M.A., Fehniger, T.A., Turner, S.C., Chen, K.S., Ghaheri, B.A., et al. (2001). Human natural killer cells: a unique innate immunoregulatory role for the CD56(bright) subset. *Blood*, Vol.97, No10, pp. 3146-3151, ISSN 0006-4971

Cross, A., Bucknall, R.C., Cassatella, M.A., Edwards, S.W. & Moots, R.J. (2003). Synovial fluid neutrophils transcribe and express class II major histocompatibility complex molecules in rheumatoid arthritis. *Arthritis and Rheumatism*, Vol.48, No10, pp. 2796-2806.

Crotti, T.N., Smith, M.D., Weedon, H., Ahern, M.J., Findlay, D.M., et al. (2002). Receptor activator NF-kappaB ligand (RANKL) expression in synovial tissue from patients with rheumatoid arthritis, spondyloarthropathy, osteoarthritis, and from normal patients: semiquantitative and quantitative analysis. *Annals of the Rheumatic Diseases*, Vol.61, No12, pp. 1047-1054.

De Matos, C.T., Berg, L., Michaelsson, J., Fellander-Tsai, L., Karre, K., et al. (2007). Activating and inhibitory receptors on synovial fluid natural killer cells of arthritis patients: role of CD94/NKG2A in control of cytokine secretion. *Immunology*, Vol.122, No2, pp. 291-301.

De Rycke, L., Vandooren, B., Kruithof, E., De Keyser, F., Veys, E.M., et al. (2005). Tumor necrosis factor alpha blockade treatment down-modulates the increased systemic and local expression of Toll-like receptor 2 and Toll-like receptor 4 in spondylarthropathy. *Arthritis and Rheumatism*, Vol.52, No7, pp. 2146-2158, ISS N0004-3591

Dean, G., Hoyland, J.A., Denton, J., Donn, R.P. & Freemont, A.J. (1993). Mast cells in the synovium and synovial fluid in osteoarthritis. *British Journal of Rheumatology*, Vol.32, No8, pp. 671-675, ISSN 0263-7103

Dimitrova, P., Ivanovska, N., Schwaeble, W., Gyurkovska, V. & Stover, C. (2010). The role of properdin in murine zymosan-induced arthritis. *Molecular Immunology*, Vol.47, No7-8, pp. 1458-1466, ISSN0161-5890

Dimitrova, P., Toncheva, A., Gyurkovska, V. & Ivanovska, N. (2011). Involvement of soluble receptor activator of nuclear factor-kappaB ligand (sRANKL) in collagenase-induced murine osteoarthritis and human osteoarthritis. *Rheumatology International*, published online February 03 2011, DOI:10.1007/s00296-010-1723-8, ISSN0172-8172

Duan, H., Koga, T., Kohda, F., Hara, H., Urabe, K., et al. (2001). Interleukin-8-positive neutrophils in psoriasis. *Journal of Dermatological Science*, Vol.26, No2, pp. 119-124, ISSN0923-1811

Dumond, H., Presle, N., Terlain, B., Mainard, D., Loeuille, D. et al. (2003). Evidence for a key role of leptin in osteoarthritis. *Arthritis and Rheumatism*, Vol.48, No11, pp. 3118-29, ISSN0004-3591

Edwards, S.W. & Hallett, M.B. (1997). Seeing the wood for the trees: the forgotten role of neutrophils in rheumatoid arthritis. *Immunology Today*, Vol.18, No7, pp. 320-324, ISSN0167-5699

Felzmann, T., Gadd, S., Majdic, O., Maurer, D., Petera, P., et al. (1991). Analysis of function-associated receptor molecules on peripheral blood and synovial fluid granulocytes from patients with rheumatoid and reactive arthritis. *Journal of Clinical Immunology*, Vol.11, No4, pp. 205-212.

Feng, C.G., Kaviratne, M., Rothfuchs, A.G., Cheever, A., Hieny, S., et al. (2006). NK cell-derived IFN-gamma differentially regulates innate resistance and neutrophil response in T cell-deficient hosts infected with Mycobacterium tuberculosis. *Journal of Immunology*, Vol.177, No10, pp. 7086-7093, ISSN 0022-1767

Fritz, P., Muller, J., Reiser, H., Saal, J.G., Hadam, M., et al. (1984). Distribution of mast cells in human synovial tissue of patients with osteoarthritis and rheumatoid arthritis. *Zeitschrift fur Rheumatologie*, Vol.43, No6, pp. 294-298, ISSN 0340-1855

Frosch, M., Strey, A., Vogl, T., Wulffraat, N.M., Kuis, W., et al. (2000). Myeloid-related proteins 8 and 14 are specifically secreted during interaction of phagocytes and activated endothelium and are useful markers for monitoring disease activity in pauciarticular-onset juvenile rheumatoid arthritis. *Arthritis and Rheumatism*, Vol.43, No3, pp. 628-637, ISSN 0004-3591

Gotis-Graham, I., Smith, M.D., Parker, A. & McNeil, H.P. (1998). Synovial mast cell responses during clinical improvement in early rheumatoid arthritis. *Annals of the Rheumatic Diseases*, Vol.57, No11, pp. 664-671, ISSN 0003-4967

Grabiec, A.M., Krausz, S., de Jager, W., Burakowski, T., Groot, D., et al. (2010). Histone deacetylase inhibitors suppress inflammatory activation of rheumatoid arthritis patient synovial macrophages and tissue. *Journal of Immunology*, Vol.184, No5, pp. 2718-2728, ISSN 0022-1767

Gracie, J.A., Forsey, R.J., Chan, W.L., Gilmour, A., Leung, B.P., et al. (1999). A proinflammatory role for IL-18 in rheumatoid arthritis. *Journal of Clinical Investigation*, Vol.104, No10, pp. 1393-1401, ISSN 0021-9738

Hayashi, F., Means, T.K. & Luster, A.D. (2003). Toll-like receptors stimulate human neutrophil function. *Blood*, Vol.102, No7, pp. 2660-2669, ISSN 0006-4971

Haywood, L., McWilliams, D.F., Pearson, C.I., Gill, S.E., Ganesan, A., et al. (2003). Inflammation and angiogenesis in osteoarthritis. *Arthritis and Rheumatism*, Vol.48, No8, pp. 2173-2177, ISSN 0004-3591

Hedbom, E. & Hauselmann, H.J. (2002). Molecular aspects of pathogenesis in osteoarthritis: the role of inflammation. *Cellular and Molecular Life Sciences*, Vol.59, No1, pp. 45-53.

Helmy, K.Y., Katschke, K.J., Jr., Gorgani, N.N., Kljavin, N.M., Elliott, J.M., et al. (2006). CRIg: a macrophage complement receptor required for phagocytosis of circulating pathogens. *Cell*, Vol.124, No5, pp. 915-927, ISSN 0092-8674

Ivanovska, N. & Dimitrova, P. (2011). Bone resorption and remodeling in murine collagenase-induced osteoarthritis after administration of glucosamine. *Arthritis Research and Therapy*, Vol.13, No2, pp. R44, ISSN 1478-6354

Iwahashi, M., Yamamura, M., Aita, T., Okamoto, A., Ueno, A., et al. (2004). Expression of Toll-like receptor 2 on CD16+ blood monocytes and synovial tissue macrophages in rheumatoid arthritis. *Arthritis and Rheumatism*, Vol.50, No5, pp. 1457-1467, ISSN 0004-3591

Jacques, C., Gosset, M., Berenbaum, F. & Gabay, C. (2006). The role of IL-1 and IL-1Ra in joint inflammation and cartilage degradation. *Vitamins and Hormones*, Vol.74pp. 371-403, ISSN 0083-6729

Ji, H., Pettit, A., Ohmura, K., Ortiz-Lopez, A., Duchatelle, V., et al. (2002). Critical roles for interleukin 1 and tumor necrosis factor alpha in antibody-induced arthritis. *Journal of Experimental Medicine*, Vol.196, No1, pp. 77-85

Joosten, L.A., Lubberts, E., Helsen, M.M., Saxne, T., Coenen-de Roo, C.J., et al. (1999). Protection against cartilage and bone destruction by systemic interleukin-4 treatment in established murine type II collagen-induced arthritis. *Arthritis Research and Therapy*, Vol.1, No1, pp. 81-91, ISSN 1465-9905

Jungel, A., Distler, J.H., Kurowska-Stolarska, M., Seemayer, C.A., Seibl, R., et al. (2004). Expression of interleukin-21 receptor, but not interleukin-21, in synovial fibroblasts and synovial macrophages of patients with rheumatoid arthritis. *Arthritis and Rheumatism*, Vol.50, No5, pp. 1468-1476, ISSN 0004-3591

Kagari, T., Tanaka, D., Doi, H. & Shimozato, T. (2003). Essential role of Fc gamma receptors in anti-type II collagen antibody-induced arthritis. *Journal of Immunology*, Vol.170, No8, pp. 4318-4324, ISSN 0022-1767

Kamijo, S., Nakajima, A., Ikeda, K., Aoki, K., Ohya, K., et al. (2006). Amelioration of bone loss in collagen-induced arthritis by neutralizing anti-RANKL monoclonal antibody. *Biochemical and Biophysical Research Communications*, Vol.347, No1, pp. 124-132.

Kane, D., Roth, J., Frosch, M., Vogl, T., Bresnihan, B., et al. (2003). Increased perivascular synovial membrane expression of myeloid-related proteins in psoriatic arthritis. *Arthritis and Rheumatism*, Vol.48, No6, pp. 1676-1685, ISSN 0004-3591

Keffer, J., Probert, L., Cazlaris, H., Georgopoulos, S., Kaslaris, E., et al. (1991). Transgenic mice expressing human tumour necrosis factor: a predictive genetic model of arthritis. *EMBO Journal*, Vol.10, No13, pp. 4025-4031.

Kennedy, M.K., Glaccum, M., Brown, S.N., Butz, E.A., Viney, J.L., et al. (2000). Reversible defects in natural killer and memory CD8 T cell lineages in interleukin 15-deficient mice. *Journal of Experimental Medicine*, Vol.191, No5, pp. 771-780, ISSN 0022-1007

Kerkhoff, C., Klempt, M. & Sorg, C. (1998). Novel insights into structure and function of MRP8 (S100A8) and MRP14 (S100A9). *Biochimica et Biophysica Acta*, Vol.1448, No2, pp. 200-211, ISSN 0006-3002

Kilpatrick, L.E., Sun, S., Mackie, D., Baik, F., Li, H., et al. (2006). Regulation of TNF mediated antiapoptotic signaling in human neutrophils: role of delta-PKC and ERK1/2. *Journal of Leukocyte Biology*, Vol.80, No6, pp. 1512-1521, ISSN 0741-5400

Kim, H.Y., Kim, S. & Chung, D.H. (2006). FcgammaRIII engagement provides activating signals to NKT cells in antibody-induced joint inflammation. *Journal of Clinical Investigation*, Vol.116, No9, pp. 2484-2492, ISSN 0021-9738

Kim, J.H., Jin, H.M., Kim, K., Song, I., Youn, B.U., et al. (2009). The mechanism of osteoclast differentiation induced by IL-1. *Journal of Immunology*, Vol.183, No3, pp. 1862-1870, ISSN 1550-6606

Koller, M., Aringer, M., Kiener, H., Erlacher, L., Machold, K., et al. (1999). Expression of adhesion molecules on synovial fluid and peripheral blood monocytes in patients with inflammatory joint disease and osteoarthritis. *Annals of the Rheumatic Diseases*, Vol.58, No11, pp. 709-712, ISSN 0003-4967

Kopicky-Burd, J.A., Kagey-Sobotka, A., Peters, S.P., Dvorak, A.M., Lennox, D.W., et al. (1988). Characterization of human synovial mast cells. *Journal of Rheumatology*, Vol.15, No9, pp. 1326-1333, ISSN 0315-162X

Kragstrup, T.W., Otkjaer, K., Holm, C., Jorgensen, A., Hokland, M., et al. (2008). The expression of IL-20 and IL-24 and their shared receptors are increased in rheumatoid arthritis and spondyloarthropathy. *Cytokine*, Vol.41, No1, pp. 16-23.

Kunz, M., Roth, J., Sorg, C. & Kolde, G. (1992). Epidermal expression of the calcium binding surface antigen 27E10 in inflammatory skin diseases. *Archives of Dermatological Research*, Vol.284, No7, pp. 386-390, ISSN 0340-3696

Kurt-Jones, E.A., Mandell, L., Whitney, C., Padgett, A., Gosselin, K., et al. (2002). Role of toll-like receptor 2 (TLR2) in neutrophil activation: GM-CSF enhances TLR2 expression and TLR2-mediated interleukin 8 responses in neutrophils. *Blood*, Vol.100, No5, pp. 1860-1868.

Lacey, D.L., Timms, E., Tan, H.L., Kelley, M.J., Dunstan, C.R., et al. (1998). Osteoprotegerin ligand is a cytokine that regulates osteoclast differentiation and activation. *Cell*, Vol.93, No2, pp. 165-176, ISSN 0092-8674

Lago, F., Dieguez, C., Gomez-Reino, J., Gualillo, O. (2007). Adipokines as emerging mediators of immune response and inflammation. *Nature Clinical Practical Rheumatology*, Vol.3, No12, pp.716-24, ISSN 1745-8382

Laurberg, T.B., Frystyk, J., Ellingsen, T., Hansen, I.T., Jorgensen, A. (2009). Plasma adiponectin in patients with active, early, and chronic rheumatoid arthritis who are steroid- and disease-modifying antirheumatic drug-naive compared with patients with osteoarthritis and controls. *Journal of Rheumatology*, Vol.36, No9, pp.1885-1891, ISSN 0315-162X

Lee, M.Y., Kim, W.J., Kang, Y.J., Jung, Y.M., Kang, Y.M., et al. (2006). Z39Ig is expressed on macrophages and may mediate inflammatory reactions in arthritis and atherosclerosis. *Journal of Leukocyte Biology*, Vol.80, No4, pp. 922-928, ISSN 0741-5400

Lohmander, L.S., Brandt, K.D., Mazzuca, S.A., Katz, B.P., Larsson, S., et al. (2005). Use of the plasma stromelysin (matrix metalloproteinase 3) concentration to predict joint space narrowing in knee osteoarthritis. *Arthritis and Rheumatism*, Vol.52, No10, pp. 3160-3167, ISSN 0004-3591

Malik, N., Greenfield, B.W., Wahl, A.F. & Kiener, P.A. (1996). Activation of human monocytes through CD40 induces matrix metalloproteinases. *Journal of Immunology*, Vol.156, No10, pp. 3952-3960, ISSN 0022-1767

Mantovani, A., Sica, A. & Locati, M. (2007). New vistas on macrophage differentiation and activation. *European Journal of Immunology*, Vol.37, No1, pp. 14-16, ISSN 0014-2980

Marshall, J.C., Malam, Z. & Jia, S. (2007). Modulating neutrophil apoptosis. *Novartis Foundation Symposium*, Vol.280, pp. 53-66; discussion 67-72, 160-164, ISSN 1528-2511

Matsuguchi, T., Musikacharoen, T., Ogawa, T. & Yoshikai, Y. (2000). Gene expressions of Toll-like receptor 2, but not Toll-like receptor 4, is induced by LPS and inflammatory cytokines in mouse macrophages. *Journal of Immunology*, Vol.165, No10, pp. 5767-5772, ISSN 0022-1767

Mebarek, S., Hamade, E., Thouverey, C., Bandorowicz-Pikula, J., Pikula, S., et al. (2011). Ankylosing spondylitis, late osteoarthritis, vascular calcification, chondrocalcinosis and pseudo gout: toward a possible drug therapy. *Current Medicinal Chemistry*, Vol.18, No14, pp. 2196-2203, ISSN 0929-8673

Mehraban, F., Lark, M.W., Ahmed, F.N., Xu, F. & Moskowitz, R.W. (1998). Increased secretion and activity of matrix metalloproteinase-3 in synovial tissues and chondrocytes from experimental osteoarthritis. *Osteoarthritis and Cartilage*, Vol.6, No4, pp. 286-294, ISSN 1063-4584

Mitsuyama, K., Toyonaga, A., Sasaki, E., Watanabe, K., Tateishi, H., et al. (1994). IL-8 as an important chemoattractant for neutrophils in ulcerative colitis and Crohn's disease. *Clinical and Experimental Immunology*, Vol.96, No3, pp. 432-436, ISSN 0009-9104

Mrozek, E., Anderson, P. & Caligiuri, M.A. (1996). Role of interleukin-15 in the development of human CD56+ natural killer cells from CD34+ hematopoietic progenitor cells. *Blood*, Vol.87, No7, pp. 2632-2640, ISSN 0006-4971

Muller, I., Munder, M., Kropf, P. & Hansch, G.M. (2009). Polymorphonuclear neutrophils and T lymphocytes: strange bedfellows or brothers in arms? *Trends Immunol*, Vol.30, No11, pp. 522-530, ISSN 1471-4981

Nandakumar, K.S., Svensson, L. & Holmdahl, R. (2003). Collagen type II-specific monoclonal antibody-induced arthritis in mice: description of the disease and the influence of age, sex, and genes. *American Journal of Pathology*, Vol.163, No5, pp. 1827-1837, ISSN 0002-9440

Nic An Ultaigh, S., Saber, T.P., McCormick, J., Connolly, M., Dellacasagrande, J., et al. (2011). Blockade of Toll-like receptor 2 prevents spontaneous cytokine release from rheumatoid arthritis ex vivo synovial explant cultures. *Arthritis Research and Therapy*, Vol.13, No1, pp. R33, ISSN 1478-6354

Otero, M., Lago, R., Lago, F., Casanueva, F.F., Dieguez. C. et al. Leptin, from fat to inflammation: old questions and new insights. (2005). *FEBS Letters*, Vol.579, No2, pp.295-301, ISSN 0014-5793

Ottonello, L., Cutolo, M., Frumento, G., Arduino, N., Bertolotto, M., et al. (2002). Synovial fluid from patients with rheumatoid arthritis inhibits neutrophil apoptosis: role of adenosine and proinflammatory cytokines. *Rheumatology*, Vol.41, No11, pp. 1249-1260, ISSN 1462-0324

Ozinsky, A., Underhill, D.M., Fontenot, J.D., Hajjar, A.M., Smith, K.D., et al. (2000). The repertoire for pattern recognition of pathogens by the innate immune system is defined by cooperation between toll-like receptors. *Proceedings of the National Academy of Sciences of the United States of America*, Vol.97, No25, pp. 13766-13771.

Painter, R.G., Zahler-Bentz, K. & Dukes, R.E. (1987). Regulation of the affinity state of the N-formylated peptide receptor of neutrophils: role of guanine nucleotide-binding proteins and the cytoskeleton. *Journal of Cell Biology*, Vol.105, No6 Pt 2, pp. 2959-2971, ISSN 0021-9525

Poubelle, P.E., Chakravarti, A., Fernandes, M.J., Doiron, K. & Marceau, A.A. (2007). Differential expression of RANK, RANK-L, and osteoprotegerin by synovial fluid neutrophils from patients with rheumatoid arthritis and by healthy human blood neutrophils. *Arthritis Research and Therapy*, Vol.9, No2, pp. R25.

Pronai, L., Ichikawa, Y., Ichimori, K., Nakazawa, H. & Arimori, S. (1991). Association of enhanced superoxide generation by neutrophils with low superoxide scavenging activity of the peripheral blood, joint fluid, and their leukocyte components in rheumatoid arthritis: effects of slow-acting anti-rheumatic drugs and disease activity. *Clinical and Experimental Rheumatology*, Vol.9, No2, pp. 149-155.

Radstake, T.R., Roelofs, M.F., Jenniskens, Y.M., Oppers-Walgreen, B., van Riel, P.L., et al. (2004). Expression of toll-like receptors 2 and 4 in rheumatoid synovial tissue and regulation by proinflammatory cytokines interleukin-12 and interleukin-18 via interferon-gamma. *Arthritis and Rheumatism*, Vol.50, No12, pp. 3856-3865, ISSN 0004-3591

Rammes, A., Roth, J., Goebeler, M., Klempt, M., Hartmann, M., et al. (1997). Myeloid-related protein (MRP) 8 and MRP14, calcium-binding proteins of the S100 family, are secreted by activated monocytes via a novel, tubulin-dependent pathway. *Journal of Biological Chemistry*, Vol.272, No14, pp. 9496-9502, ISSN 0021-9258

Raza, K., Scheel-Toellner, D., Lee, C.Y., Pilling, D., Curnow, S.J., et al. (2006). Synovial fluid leukocyte apoptosis is inhibited in patients with very early rheumatoid arthritis. *Arthritis Res earch and Therapy*, Vol.8, No4, pp. R120, ISSN 1478-6362

Renoux, M., Hilliquin, P., Galoppin, L., Florentin, I. & Menkes, C.J. (1996). Release of mast cell mediators and nitrites into knee joint fluid in osteoarthritis--comparison with articular chondrocalcinosis and rheumatoid arthritis. *Osteoarthritis and Cartilage*, Vol.4, No3, pp. 175-179, ISSN 1063-4584

Rosenthal, A.K. (2011). Crystals, inflammation, and osteoarthritis. *Current Opinion in Rheumatology*, Vol.23, No2, pp. 170-173, ISSN 1040-8711

Ross, F.P. (2000). RANKing the importance of measles virus in Paget's disease. *Journal of Clinical Investigation*, Vol.105, No5, pp. 555-558, ISSN 0021-9738

Roth, J., Vogl, T., Sorg, C. & Sunderkotter, C. (2003). Phagocyte-specific S100 proteins: a novel group of proinflammatory molecules. *Trends Immunology*, Vol.24, No4, pp. 155-158, ISSN 1471-4906

Rugtveit, J., Brandtzaeg, P., Halstensen, T.S., Fausa, O. & Scott, H. (1994). Increased macrophage subset in inflammatory bowel disease: apparent recruitment from peripheral blood monocytes. *Gut*, Vol.35, No5, pp. 669-674, ISSN 0017-5749

Ryckman, C., Vandal, K., Rouleau, P., Talbot, M. & Tessier, P.A. (2003). Proinflammatory activities of S100: proteins S100A8, S100A9, and S100A8/A9 induce neutrophil chemotaxis and adhesion. *Journal of Immunology*, Vol.170, No6, pp. 3233-3242, ISSN 0022-1767

Santos, L.L., Morand, E.F., Hutchinson, P., Boyce, N.W. & Holdsworth, S.R. (1997). Anti-neutrophil monoclonal antibody therapy inhibits the development of adjuvant arthritis. *Clinical and Experimental Immunology*, Vol.107, No2, pp. 248-253.

Schwandner, R., Dziarski, R., Wesche, H., Rothe, M. & Kirschning, C.J. (1999). Peptidoglycan- and lipoteichoic acid-induced cell activation is mediated by toll-like receptor 2. *Journal of Biological Chemistry*, Vol.274, No25, pp. 17406-17409.

Seibl, R., Birchler, T., Loeliger, S., Hossle, J.P., Gay, R.E., et al. (2003). Expression and regulation of Toll-like receptor 2 in rheumatoid arthritis synovium. *American Journal of Pathology*, Vol.162, No4, pp. 1221-1227, ISSN 0002-9440

Seshasayee, D., Wang, H., Lee, W.P., Gribling, P., Ross, J., et al. (2004). A novel in vivo role for osteoprotegerin ligand in activation of monocyte effector function and inflammatory response. *Journal of Biological Chemistry*, Vol.279, No29, pp. 30202-30209, ISSN 0021-9258

Shen, F., Ruddy, M.J., Plamondon, P. & Gaffen, S.L. (2005). Cytokines link osteoblasts and inflammation: microarray analysis of interleukin-17- and TNF-alpha-induced genes in bone cells. *Journal of Leukocyte Biology*, Vol.77, No3, pp. 388-399.

Simon, T., Opelz, G., Weimer, R., Wiesel, M., Feustel, A., et al. (2003). The effect of ATG on cytokine and cytotoxic T-lymphocyte gene expression in renal allograft recipients during the early post-transplant period. *Clinical Transplantation*, Vol.17, No3, pp. 217-224, ISSN 0902-0063

Smeets, T.J., Barg, E.C., Kraan, M.C., Smith, M.D., Breedveld, F.C., et al. (2003). Analysis of the cell infiltrate and expression of proinflammatory cytokines and matrix metalloproteinases in arthroscopic synovial biopsies: comparison with synovial samples from patients with end stage, destructive rheumatoid arthritis. *Annals of the Rheumatic Diseases*, Vol.62, No7, pp. 635-638, ISSN 0003-4967

Soderstrom, K., Stein, E., Colmenero, P., Purath, U., Muller-Ladner, U., et al. (2010). Natural killer cells trigger osteoclastogenesis and bone destruction in arthritis. *Proceedings of the National Academy of Sciences of the United States of America*, Vol.107, No29, pp. 13028-13033, ISSN 0027-8424

Spangrude, G.J., Sacchi, F., Hill, H.R., Van Epps, D.E. & Daynes, R.A. (1985). Inhibition of lymphocyte and neutrophil chemotaxis by pertussis toxin. *Journal of Immunology*, Vol.135, No6, pp. 4135-4143, ISSN 0022-1767

Stout, R.D., Suttles, J., Xu, J., Grewal, I.S. & Flavell, R.A. (1996). Impaired T cell-mediated macrophage activation in CD40 ligand-deficient mice. *Journal of Immunology*, Vol.156, No1, pp. 8-11, ISSN 0022-1767

Suttles, J., Evans, M., Miller, R.W., Poe, J.C., Stout, R.D., et al. (1996). T cell rescue of monocytes from apoptosis: role of the CD40-CD40L interaction and requirement for CD40-mediated induction of protein tyrosine kinase activity. *Journal of Leukocyte Biology*, Vol.60, No5, pp. 651-657, ISSN 0741-5400

Tacke, F., Alvarez, D., Kaplan, T.J., Jakubzick, C., Spanbroek, R., et al. (2007). Monocyte subsets differentially employ CCR2, CCR5, and CX3CR1 to accumulate within atherosclerotic plaques. *Journal of Clinical Investigation*, Vol.117, No1, pp. 185-194, ISSN 0021-9738

Tak, P.P., Kummer, J.A., Hack, C.E., Daha, M.R., Smeets, T.J., et al. (1994). Granzyme-positive cytotoxic cells are specifically increased in early rheumatoid synovial tissue. *Arthritis and Rheumatism*, Vol.37, No12, pp. 1735-1743

Tak, P.P., Smeets, T.J., Daha, M.R., Kluin, P.M., Meijers, K.A., et al. (1997). Analysis of the synovial cell infiltrate in early rheumatoid synovial tissue in relation to local disease activity. *Arthritis and Rheumatism*, Vol.40, No2, pp. 217-225, ISSN 0004-3591

Takeuchi, O., Hoshino, K. & Akira, S. (2000). Cutting edge: TLR2-deficient and MyD88-deficient mice are highly susceptible to Staphylococcus aureus infection. *Journal of Immunology*, Vol.165, No10, pp. 5392-5396, ISSN 0022-1767

Tanaka, D., Kagari, T., Doi, H. & Shimozato, T. (2006). Essential role of neutrophils in anti-type II collagen antibody and lipopolysaccharide-induced arthritis. *Immunology*, Vol.119, No2, pp. 195-202, ISSN 0019-2805

Tanaka, M., Nagai, T., Tsuneyoshi, Y., Sunahara, N., Matsuda, T., et al. (2008). Expansion of a unique macrophage subset in rheumatoid arthritis synovial lining layer. *Clinical and Experimental Immunology*, Vol.154, No1, pp. 38-47, ISSN 0009-9104

Teitelbaum, S.L. (2000). Bone resorption by osteoclasts. *Science*, Vol.289, No5484, pp. 1504-1508.

Tian, L., Noelle, R.J. & Lawrence, D.A. (1995). Activated T cells enhance nitric oxide production by murine splenic macrophages through gp39 and LFA-1. *European Journal of Immunology*, Vol.25, No1, pp. 306-309, ISSN 0014-2980

Toncheva, A., Remichkova, M., Ikonomova, K., Dimitrova, P. & Ivanovska, N. (2009). Inflammatory response in patients with active and inactive osteoarthritis. *Rheumatology International*, Vol.29, No10, pp. 1197-1203.

Ulmann, L., Hirbec, H. & Rassendren, F. (2010). P2X4 receptors mediate PGE2 release by tissue-resident macrophages and initiate inflammatory pain. *EMBO Journal*, Vol.29, No14, pp. 2290-2300, ISSN 1460-2075

Van den Steen, P.E., Proost, P., Wuyts, A., Van Damme, J. & Opdenakker, G. (2000). Neutrophil gelatinase B potentiates interleukin-8 tenfold by aminoterminal processing, whereas it degrades CTAP-III, PF-4, and GRO-alpha and leaves RANTES and MCP-2 intact. *Blood*, Vol.96, No8, pp. 2673-2681, ISSN 0006-4971

van Lent, P.L., Blom, A.B., van der Kraan, P., Holthuysen, A.E., Vitters, E., et al. (2004). Crucial role of synovial lining macrophages in the promotion of transforming growth factor beta-mediated osteophyte formation. *Arthritis and Rheumatism*, Vol.50, No1, pp. 103-111, ISSN 0004-3591

Wang, J.E., Warris, A., Ellingsen, E.A., Jorgensen, P.F., Flo, T.H., et al. (2001). Involvement of CD14 and toll-like receptors in activation of human monocytes by Aspergillus fumigatus hyphae. *Infection and Immunity*, Vol.69, No4, pp. 2402-2406, ISSN 0019-9567

Xu, H., Manivannan, A., Dawson, R., Crane, I.J., Mack, M., et al. (2005). Differentiation to the CCR2+ inflammatory phenotype in vivo is a constitutive, time-limited property of blood monocytes and is independent of local inflammatory mediators. *Journal of Immunology*, Vol.175, No10, pp. 6915-6923, ISSN 0022-1767

Yasuda, H., Shima, N., Nakagawa, N., Yamaguchi, K., Kinosaki, M., et al. (1998). Osteoclast differentiation factor is a ligand for osteoprotegerin/osteoclastogenesis-inhibitory factor and is identical to TRANCE/RANKL. *Proceedings of the National Academy of Sciences of the United States of America*, Vol.95, No7, pp. 3597-3602.

Yavorskyy, A., Hernandez-Santana, A., McCarthy, G. & McMahon, G. (2008). Detection of calcium phosphate crystals in the joint fluid of patients with osteoarthritis - analytical approaches and challenges. *Analyst*, Vol.133, No3, pp. 302-318, ISSN 0003-2654

Youssef, P., Roth, J., Frosch, M., Costello, P., Fitzgerald, O., et al. (1999). Expression of myeloid related proteins (MRP) 8 and 14 and the MRP8/14 heterodimer in rheumatoid arthritis synovial membrane. *Journal of Rheumatology*, Vol.26, No12, pp. 2523-2528, ISSN 0315-162X

24

The Role of Synovial Macrophages and Macrophage-Produced Mediators in Driving Inflammatory and Destructive Responses in Osteoarthritis

Jan Bondeson[1], Shane Wainwright[2],
Clare Hughes[2] and Bruce Caterson[2]
[1]*Department of Rheumatology, Cardiff University, Heath Park, Cardiff,*
[2]*Connective Tissue Biology Laboratories, Cardiff School of Biosciences, Cardiff University, Museum Avenue, Cardiff, UK*

1. Introduction

Osteoarthritis (OA), one of the most common diseases among humans, is characterised pathologically by focal areas of damage on articular cartilage centred on load-bearing areas, associated with formation of new bone at the joint margins and changes in subchondral bone. Given the huge economic and personal burden of OA, and the fact that this disease is the major cause for the increasing demand for joint replacements, there is urgent need for disease modifying treatments to stop or at least slow the development and progression of OA.

But for this to be possible, we need further knowledge about the pathogenesis of disease initiation and progression in OA. The great success of targeted biologic therapy against rheumatoid arthritis (RA) in recent years has meant that much research has been devoted to investigating the pathophysiology of osteoarthritis (OA), in the hope of defining novel therapeutic targets. In contrast to RA, with its pannus and erosions, OA has long been thought of as a degenerative disease of cartilage, with secondary bony damage and osteophytes. In recent years, the importance of the synovium, and in particular the synovial macrophages, in OA, has been highlighted in both in vitro and in vivo studies. This article will give an overview of some important recent findings concerning the ability of macrophages to drive inflammatory and destructive disease mechanisms in OA, the role of their proinflammatory cytokines in doing so, and the potential for macrophages and macrophage-produced cytokines to be used as therapeutic targets for the development of disease-modifying anti-ostroarthritic drugs (DMOADs). There is also an abundance of potential downstream therapeutic targets in OA, including the matrix metalloproteinases, the aggrecanases, the inducible nitric oxide synthetase, and elements of the Wnt pathway.

2. Synovial macrophages and macrophage-produced mediators in driving inflammatory and destructive responses in osteoarthritis

2.1 Macrophage biology in RA and OA

In rheumatoid arthritis (RA), it is today accepted that both inflammatory and destructive features of the disease are driven through synovitis. The RA synovium has a plentiful infiltrate of activated macrophages, particularly at the cartilage-pannus junction (Kinne et al., 2007). These macrophages produce tumour necrosis factor α (TNFα), interleukin (IL)-1β and other proinflammatory cytokines. Since there is a 'cytokine cascade' with TNFα driving the other inflammatory mediators, this cytokine has become a key therapeutic target in RA, with several anti-TNFα biologic agents being used with considerable success (Feldmann & Maini, 2008). Although biologics with anti-B cell and anti-T cell co-stimulation properties have since been introduced, the anti-TNFα agents remain a mainstay of RA therapy. They have shown long-term sustained efficacy and safety, and are used all over the world with excellent results.

Clinically, RA and OA are usually easy to differentiate. X-rays of affected joints show erosions and periarticular osteoporosis in RA; in OA, they show reduction of joint space as a sign of cartilage degradation, and in later stages of the disease bony sclerosis and osteophytes. The joint pattern differs, with early RA affecting the proximal interphalangeal, metacarpophalangeal and metatarsophalangeal joints, and OA usually affecting the large joints, like the hips and knees, and also the distal (and sometimes proximal) interphalangeal joints. The typical RA patient has an elevated erythrocyte sedimentation rate, C-reactive protein and IL-6, the vast majority of OA patients do not. In RA patients, synovitis is a major feature of the disease, causing joint swelling and exudation, and driving cartilage degradation and the formation of pannus and erosive changes. In OA, there is much less joint swelling and exudation, and no pannus or erosions.

Many OA patients also have a variable degree of synovitis. Synovial inflammation is likely to contribute to disease progression in OA, as judged by the correlation between biological markers of inflammation and the progression of structural changes in OA (Clark et al., 1999; Sowers et al., 2002). Histologically, the OA synovium shows hyperplasia with an increased number of lining cells and a mixed inflammatory infiltrate mainly consisting of macrophages [Benito et al., 2005; Farahat et al., 1993]. Synovial biopsies from patients with early inflammatory OA may even resemble RA biopsies morphologically, although the percentage of macrophages is lower (1-3% as compared with 5-20%) and the percentages of T and B cells much lower [Bondeson et al., 1999a; Amos et al., 2006; Blom & van den Berg, 2007]. The synovial fluid of patients with active RA synovitis contains numerous polymorphonuclear leucocytes, something that is not the case in OA; another indicator that there is difference in pathophysiology between RA and OA synovitis.

In RA, it is today accepted that the synovitis is cytokine driven, through an disequilibrium between proinflammatory (TNFα, IL-1) and anti-inflammatory (IL-10, the IL-1 receptor antagonist, soluble TNF receptors). These proinflammatory cytokines are largely produced from a considerable infiltrate of synovial macrophages, which are particularly numerous and highly activated at the cartilage-pannus junction. Since macrophage-produced TNFα is the main mediator of disease, driving the other proinflammatory cytokines through a cytokine cascade, neutralisation of this one cytokine can reverse both synovitis and progression of joint damage (Brennan & McInnes, 2008).

Until recently, very little was known about the pathophysiology of synovitis in OA, or its role in promoting cartilage degradation, osteophytes and other features of the disease. The marked differences in cell percentages in the inflammatory infiltrate between RA and OA would speak in favour of differences also in the cytokine interdependence in these two diseases. For example, the great scarcity of T cells in the OA synovium would tend to rule them (and their cytokines) out as potential drivers of synovitis in this disease. Instead, it has been proposed that this OA synovitis is cytokine driven, possibly through macrophage-produced TNFα and/or IL-1β, although the levels of proinflammatory cytokines are lower than in RA. These cytokines can stimulate their own production and induce synovial cells and chondrocytes to produce IL-6, IL-8 and leukocyte inhibitory factor, as well as stimulate protease and prostaglandin production (Fernandes et al., 2002). The hypothesis that TNFα and IL-1 are key mediators of inflammation and articular cartilage destruction has raised the possibility of anti-cytokine therapy in OA, or the design of specific disease-modifying osteoarthritic drugs (Abramson & Yazici, 2006; Pelletier & Martel-Pelletier, 2005; Berenbaum, 2007; Qvist et al., 2008).

If it is accepted that synovial inflammation, and the production of proinflammatory and destructive mediators from the OA synovium, are of importance for the symptoms and progression of osteoarthritis, it is a key question which cell type in the OA synovium is responsible for maintaining synovial inflammation. In RA, where the macrophage is the main promoter of disease activity, macrophage-produced TNFα is a major therapeutic target. Much less is known about macrophage biology in OA, however, although histological studies have demonstrated that OA synovial macrophages exhibit an activated phenotype, and that they produce both proinflammatory cytokines and vascular endothelial growth factor (Benito et al., 2005; Haywood et al., 2003).

The spontaneous production of a variety of pro- and anti-inflammatory cytokines, including TNFα, IL-1β and IL-10, is one of the characteristics of synovial cell cultures derived from digested RA or OA synovium. In addition, the major MMPs and TIMPs are spontaneously produced by these cell cultures (Foxwell et al., 1998; Bondeson et al., 1999a; Amos et al., 2006). Less TNFα and IL-10 is produced from OA samples but the levels are still easily detectable by ELISA (Amos et al., 2006). It is possible to use effective adenoviral gene transfer in this model without causing apoptosis or disrupting intracellular signalling pathways. Using an adenovirus effectively transferring the inhibitory subunit IκBα, it was possible to selectively inhibit the transcription factor NFκB in synovial cocultures from RA or OA patients. Macrophage-produced TNFα and IL-1β was very strongly NFκB dependent in the RA synovium, but in OA synovium, adenoviral transfer of IκBα did not affect IL-1β production and had only a partial effect on TNFα. Effects on other cytokines were similar in RA and OA synovium, with IL-6 and IL-8 both being NFκB dependent, as well as the p75 soluble TNF receptor, whereas IL-10 and the IL-1 receptor antagonist were both NFκB independent. In addition, the matrix metalloproteinases (MMP) 1,3, and 13 were strongly NFκB dependent in both RA and OA, whereas their main inhibitor, tissue inhibitor of metalloproteinases (TIMP)-1 was not (Bondeson et al., 1999a; Amos et al., 2006).

The differential effect of NFκB downregulation on the spontaneous production of TNFα and IL-1β on RA and in OA would indicate that the regulation of at least one key intracellular pathway differs fundamentally between these diseases. It is known that both TNFα and IL-1β have functional NFκB elements on their promoters and that in various macrophage models, there are both NFκB dependent and NFκB independent ways of inducing TNFα and IL-1β (Bondeson et al., 1999b; Hayes et al., 1999). It would seem as if there are fundamental differences in the regulation of macrophage-produced TNFα and IL-1β between RA and OA, with cytokine levels being higher and NFκB playing a more important role in RA (Bondeson et al., 1999a; Amos et al., 2006; Brennan et al., 2002; Andreakos et al., 2003). The differential effect of NFκB downregulation on the spontaneous production of TNFα and IL-1β on RA and in OA would indicate that the regulation of at least one key intracellular pathway differs fundamentally between these diseases. There are not many other studies comparing RA and OA intracellular signalling, although a recent study demonstrated differences in the phosphorylation of the Pyk2 and Src kinases, belonging to the focal adhesion kinase family, between RA and OA (Shahrara et al., 2007).

2.2 Macrophages drive both inflammatory and destructive responses in the OA synovium

In cultures of osteoarthritis synovial cells, specific depletion of synovial macrophages could be achieved using incubation of the cells with anti-CD14-conjugated magnetic beads (Bondeson et al., 2006). These CD14+-depleted cultures of synovial cells no longer produced significant amounts of macrophage-derived cytokines like TNFα and IL-1β. Interestingly, there was also significant inhibition (40-70%) of several cytokines produced mainly by synovial fibroblasts, like IL-6 and IL-8, and also significant downregulation of MMP-1 and MMP-3 (Figure 1). This would indicate that OA synovial macrophages play an important role in activating fibroblasts in these densely plated cultures of synovial cells, and in perpetuating the production of proinflammatory cytokines and destructive enzymes (Bondeson et al., 2006). That the regulation is not tighter than observed is probably because the fibroblasts have an activated phenotype when put into culture, with considerable spontaneous production of cytokines and other mediators. It can be speculated that once the macrophages are removed, the synovial fibroblasts change their phenotype and downregulate their production of both proinflammatory cytokines and destructive MMPs.

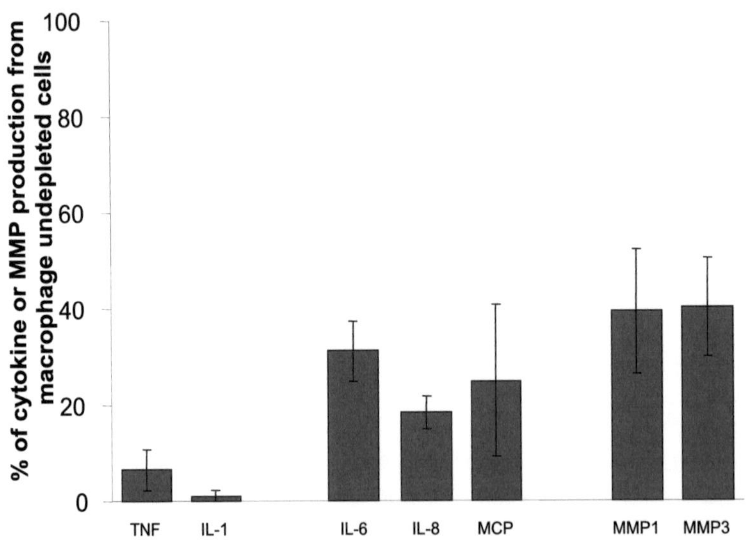

Fig. 1. OA cultures of synovial cells were either left intact or macrophage depleted. Cells were left to adhere for 24 h before the supernatants were removed for ELISA analysis of cytokines and MMPs, with data expressed as the percentage of cytokine/MMP production in the depleted culture as compared with the undepleted one, with the SEM given. Adapted from [23].

An important series of papers, using injections of liposome-encapsulated clodronate to induce depletion of synovial lining macrophages, has provided some intriguing new information about the role of macrophages in driving degenerative changes in a mouse model of experimental OA induced by injection of collagenase (Blom et al., 2004, 2007a). The collagenase injection causes weakening of ligaments leading to gradual onset of OA pathology within six weeks of induction, without any direct collagenase-induced cartilage damage being observed. If macrophage depletion had been achieved prior to the elicitation of experimental OA, there was potent reduction of both fibrosis and osteophyte formation (Blom et al., 2004, 2007a; van Lent et al, 2004). This would indicate that in this murine model of OA, synovial macrophages control the production of the growth factors that promote fibrosis and osteophyte formation, both key pathophysiological events in OA.

In this model of murine experimental OA, it was also possible to monitor the effect of macrophage depletion on the formation of the VDIPEN neoepitope that indicates MMP-induced cleavage of aggrecan (Blom et al., 2007). Between day 7 and day 14, however, VDIPEN expression more than doubled in non-depleted joints, whereas it remained unchanged in depleted ones. This would indicate that, in agreement with the data from human OA synovium discussed above, the production of MMPs in this murine model of OA is macrophage dependent. Analysis of samples of synovium and cartilage from the murine OA joints in this model demonstrated that MMP-2,3 and 9 were induced in both these tissues when murine OA was induced by collagenase. But whereas the MMP levels in the cartilage were unaffected by macrophage depletion, those in the synovium were inhibited, suggesting that removal of the macrophages would downregulate the production of MMPs from the synovial fibroblasts, and that the gradual decrease in the diffusion of these MMPs to the cartilage would prevent aggrecanolysis, as evidenced by the reduction in VDIPEN expression.

2.3 Macrophage-produced cytokines as therapeutic targets in OA

To investigate the mechanisms involved in this macrophage driven stimulation of inflammatory and degradative pathways in the OA synovium, specific neutralisation of the endogenous production of TNFα and/or IL-1β could be used in the cultures of OA synovial cell (Bondeson et al., 2006). OA synovial cell cultures were either left untreated, incubated with the p75 TNF soluble receptor Ig fusion protein etanercept (Enbrel), incubated with a neutralizing anti-IL-1β antibody, or incubated with a combination of Enbrel and anti-IL-1β. As could be expected, TNFα production was effectively neutralised by Enbrel treatment, and IL-1β by treatment with the neutralizing anti-IL-1β antibody (Figure 2). There was no effect of Enbrel on IL-1β production, nor did the neutralizing anti-IL-1β antibody affect the production of TNFα. This is in marked contrast to the situation in RA, where IL-1β is strongly TNFα dependent in these cultures of synovial cells (Brennan et al., 1989). This finding would seem to indicate yet another difference in macrophage cytokine biology between RA and OA: whereas TNFα is the 'boss cytokine' in the RA synovium, regulating the production of IL-1β, there is a redundancy between these two cytokines in the OA synovium, with neither TNFα nor IL-1β regulating the production of the other (Figure 2).

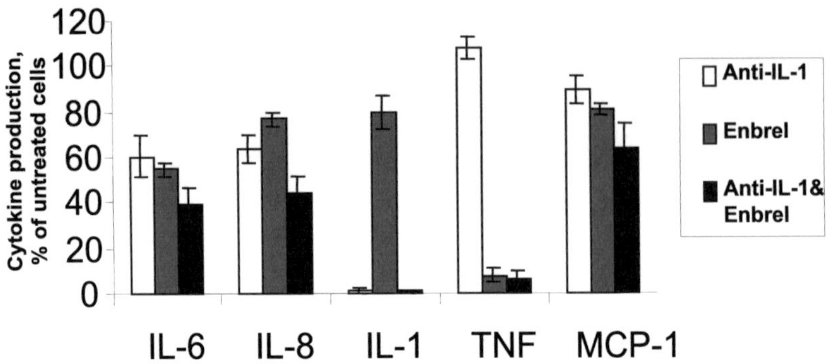

Fig. 2. Effect of neutralisation of TNFα and/or IL-1β on cytokine production in OA synovial cells. In these experiments, 2 x 10^6 cells per well were plated into 4 wells on a 24 well plate in 1 ml RPMI 1640 supplemented with 10% FCS. The cells in these 4 wells were either left untreated, incubated with the p75 TNF soluble receptor Ig fusion protein etanercept (Enbrel), incubated with a neutralizing anti-IL-1β antibody, or incubated with a combination of etanercept and anti-IL-1β. After incubation for 48 h the supernatants were removed for ELISA analysis of various cytokines. The data is expressed as percentage of the production of untreated cells, with the SEM given.

Both Enbrel and the neutralizing anti-IL-1β antibody inhibited IL-6 and IL-8, with 60% inhibition achieved when both IL-1β and TNFα were neutralized (Figure 2). The production of MCP-1 was not affected by the neutralizing anti-IL-1β antibody, but it was significantly decreased by Enbrel and by the combination of the two. It was also possible to study the effect of neutralizing IL-1β and/or TNFα on the mRNA expression and protein production of the major MMPs and aggrecanases, using RT-PCR and ELISA analysis in parallel (Bondeson et al., 2006, 2008). The results indicate that although neither Enbrel nor the neutralizing anti-IL-1β antibody had an impressive effect on the important collagenases MMP-1 and MMP-13, combination of the two led to significant inhibition both on the mRNA and protein levels (Figure 3). These findings indicate that in the OA synovium, the macrophages potently regulate the production of several important fibroblast-produced cytokines and MMPs, via a combined effect of IL-1β and TNFα.

There was no effect of either Enbrel or the neutralizing anti-IL-1β antibody on ADAMTS5 expression, nor was it at all affected by a combination of these treatments (Figure 3). Thus ADAMTS5 appears to be constitutive in OA synovial cells. In contrast, ADAMTS4 was significantly ($p<0.05$) inhibited by Enbrel, and more potently ($p<0.01$) inhibited by a combination of Enbrel and the neutralizing anti-IL-1β antibody (Figure 3). This would indicate that in the human OA synovium, the upregulation of ADAMTS4 is dependent on TNFα and IL-1 produced by the synovial macrophages, whereas ADAMTS5 is constitutive, and not changed by these cytokines (Bondeson et al., 2006, 2008).

After the success of targeted biological therapy in RA, there has been a good deal of interest in investigating anti-cytokine strategies also in OA (Malemud, 2004; Blom et al., 2007b). In RA, TNFα has become the major therapeutic target, whereas strategies targeting IL-1 have met with only moderate success. From the clinical data available, the same appears to be true for psoriasis, psoriatic arthritis, ankylosing spondylitis and juvenile chronic arthritis. In juvenile chronic arthritis, strategies directed against either TNFα or the IL-1 receptor antagonist have been successful (Burger et al., 2006; Kalliolas & Liossis, 2008). This may indicate that there are subtle differences in cytokine biology between these inflammatory arthritides, with IL-1 having a relatively more prominent role in juvenile chronic arthritis, and in adult Still's disease. Some of the potential small molecule disease-modifying anti-osteoarthritic drugs, like pralnacasan and diacerein, would appear to act at least in part as inhibitors of interleukin-1 (Rudolphi et al., 2003; Pavelka et al., 2007; Qvist et al., 2008).

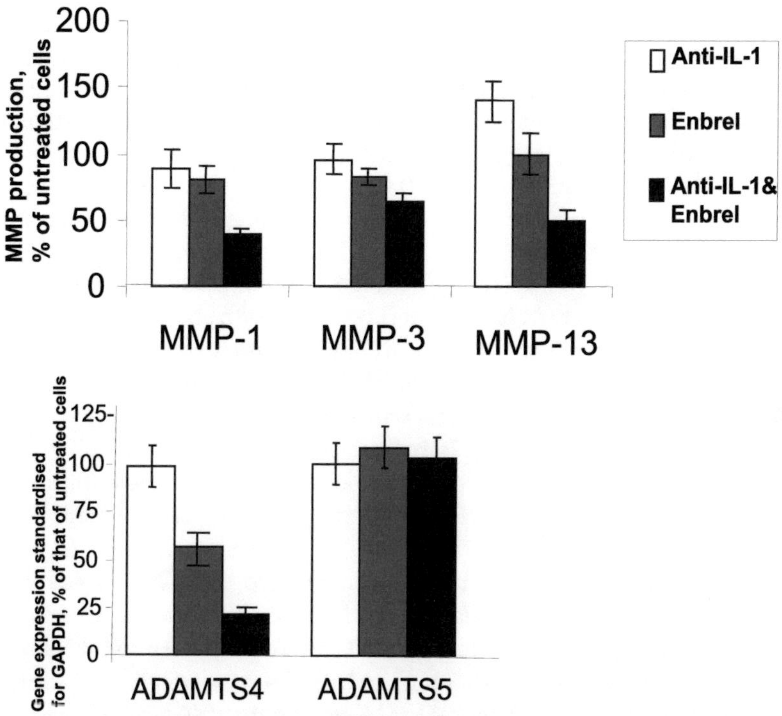

Fig. 3. Effect of neutralisation of TNFα and/or IL-1β on MMP production and ADAMTS gene expression in OA synovial cells. Experimental conditions were as in the Legend to Figure 2. After incubation for 48 h the supernatants were removed for ELISA analysis of MMPs. The cells were washed with PBS and the RNA extracted using Tri-reagent for RT-PCR analysis using oligonucleotide primers specific for ADAMTS4 and ADAMTS5. Analyis of GAPDH was used for comparison of gene expression, and in the right panel. ADAMTS4 and ADAMTS5 mRNA levels, expressed as percentage of the gene expression in untreated cells, as standardised for GAPDH, are given (n=4).

The experimental data described above would hint that unlike the situation in RA, there is redundancy between TNFα and IL-1 in the OA synovium. Both these cytokines appear to play important roles in driving the production of other proinflammatory cytokines, as well as MMPs and aggrecanases, however (Bondeson et al., 2006, 2010). In a patient with inflammatory knee OA, with synovitis visible on an MRI scan, an anti-TNF drug had marked benefit on pain and walking distance, as well as synovitis, synovial effusion and bone marrow oedema (Grunke & Schulze-Koops, 2006). In a pilot study involving 12 patients with inflammatory hand OA, the anti-TNFα antibody adalimumab had no significant effect (Magnano et al., 2007). Another pilot study involving 10 patients indicated that intra-articular injection of the anti-TNFα antibody infliximab caused significant symptomatic relief compared with placebo, although there was no significant difference in the radiological progression score after 12 months (Fioravanti et al., 2009). Interestingly, another study looked at the radiological progression of interphalangeal OA in a large cohort of RA patients treated with various disease-modifying drugs or with the anti-TNF antibody infliximab found that OA progression was significantly reduced in the patients receiving infliximab (Güler-Yüksel et al., 2008, 2010). An early study in 13 patients with knee OA indicated that intra-articular administration of the interleukin-1 receptor antagonist anakinra had some degree of analgesic effect (Chevalier et al., 2005; Goupille et al., 2007). Disappointingly, a later double-blind, placebo-controlled study could demonstrate no improvement in knee OA symptoms after intra-articular injection of anakinra, however (Chevalier et al., 2009). This may well be related to the short half-life of the drug, and the invention of an effective sustained-release system, or another alternative anti-IL-1 strategy that works intra-articularly, might still be worth trying (Martel-Pelletier & Pelletier, 2009).

There is a need for further clinical trials, with larger numbers of patients, to compare the effect of anti-cytokine strategies in large joint (knee/hip) with small joint (hand) OA, as well as correlating the results of targeted cytokine inhibition with the clinical amount of synovitis and macrophage infiltration. It would seem likely that inhibition of either TNFα or IL-1 would be much more efficacious in patients with significant inflammatory OA, as evidenced by joint exudation and active synovitis. In patients who already have significant irreversible bone and cartilage damage, the effect of these biologics would be less impressive. Since a combination of the anti-TNF biologic etanercept and the recombinant IL-1 receptor antagonist anakinra provided no added benefit and increased risk of infection and other side effects, such combination therapy is not recommended in RA (Genovese et al., 2004). In OA, however, such a combination could potentially be more attractive, due to the evidence that there is redundancy between TNFα and IL-1 in the OA synovium, if there is a way to solve the obvious safety concerns. As with all potential disease-modifying strategies in OA, a major obstacle for anti-cytokine therapy in OA will be the difficulty of recruiting patients with early inflammatory OA, before gross bone and cartilage loss is obvious on X-rays and clinical examination. In recent years, some exciting molecular imaging techniques, involving a tracer binding to the macrophage peripheral benzodiazepine receptor, or alternatively folate receptor β, have been invented (van der Laken et al., 2008; van der Heijden et al., 2009). Although hitherto published only for RA, there is no reason these methods could not be used also in OA, with the potential to identify a sub-group of patients with a higher degree of macrophage infiltration, or alternatively to correlate success with anti-cytokine approaches with the amount of macrophages detected.

2.4 Some potential downstream therapeutic targets in OA

Nitric oxide (NO) has been demonstrated to be a pathogenic mediator in OA. NO and its metabolites plays a role in the cyclooxygenase-2 activation leading to prostaglandin production, in activation of MMPs, in DNA damage, lipid peroxidation, chondrocyte apoptosis, and reduction of proteoglycan synthesis. NO production is regulated by the enzyme inducible NO synthetase (iNOS), which is in turn driven by proinflammatory cytokines and other pathologic stresses. In animal models of OA, the presence of iNOS and NO production was correlated with a higher rate of chondrocyte apoptosis and meniscal degeneration (Hashimoto et al., 1998; Hellio le Graverand et al., 2000). iNOS is overexpressed in human OA synovium and cartilage, and the levels of 3-nitrotyrosine and other NO metabolites is elevated in OA patients. Sustained high levels of NO leads to the formation of various harmful NO-derived metabolites, of which the radical peroxynitrite is an inducer of cytotoxicity and tissue damage.

Due to its many harmful effects on joint integrity, iNOS has long been of interest in both inflammatory and degenerative arthritis. It was defined as a potential therapeutic target in OA after a study in a murine model of joint instability-induced experimental OA showed that iNOS-deficient mice developed significantly less OA than wild-type animals, with about 50% reduction of both osteophytes and cartilage lesions (van den Berg et al., 1999). In a canine model of joint instability-induced experimental OA, treatment with a small-molecule iNOS inhibitor led to impressive inhibition of 3-nitrotyrosine formation, and significant (nearly 50%) reduction of OA lesions. A two-year Phase IIb/III clinical trial (Pfizer) is ongoing to evaluate the safety and efficacy of a selective iNOS inhibitor in the treatment of obese or overweight patients with knee OA (Hellio le Graverand-Gastineau, 2010).

An interesting and novel therapeutic target in OA is osteogenic protein-1 (OP-1), which exhibits potent anabolic activity in models of cartilage homeostasis and repair. This growth factor also has anti-catabolic actions, including MMP and aggrecanase inhibition (Badlani et al., 2008). It has been investigated in various animal models of OA with positive results: injected intra-articularly, it inhibited cartilage degeneration and the progression of OA (Sekiya et al., 2009). A Phase I clinical trial of intra-articular recombinant OP-1 (Stryker), assessing safety and effect on signs and symptoms, with dose escalation over 24 weeks, has been completed (Hellio le Graverand-Gastineau, 2010).

Another potential therapeutic target in OA is fibroblast growth factor (FGF)-18, which plays a role in chondrogenesis and osteogenesis during skeletal development and growth. In a rat model of meniscal tear-induced OA, bi-weekly intra-articular injections of recombinant FGF-18 induced a significant, dose-dependent reduction in cartilage degeneration, as well as an increased in chondrocyte size and subchondral bone remodelling (Moore et al., 2005). Intra-articular, recombinant FGF-18 (Merck Serono) has undergone a 12-month Phase II clinical trial in knee OA, and another Phase II study in acute cartilage injury is under way (Hellio le Graverand-Gastineau, 2010).

In recent years, the Wnt signalling pathways has been implicated in the pathophysiology of OA. The Wnts are a complex family of lipid modified, secreted glycoproteins that play a role in synovial joint formation, and are involved in the transcription of many proteins. Wnt signalling occurs through at least three pathways. Best known is the canonical Wnt pathway that induces β-catenin, but there is also a Wnt-Ca^{2+} pathway and a planar cell polarity pathway. It is canonical Wnt that is thought to play a role in OA, however. In this pathway, Wnt binds to the Frizzled receptor, and through several signalling steps this leads to accumulation of cytoplasmic β-catenin, which translocates to the nucleus and binds to TCF/LEF transcription factors, converting them from repressors to activators of the transcription of a great variety of genes, important MMPs, growth factors and chondrocyte hypertrophy markers among them (Blom et al., 2010). Whereas low levels of β-catenin are of importance to prevent chondrocyte apoptosis, intracellular accumulation of β-catenin appears to induce OA-like changes. In particular, increased levels of β-catenin are observed in areas of cartilage degeneration.

Recent data suggest a role for wnt-1 induced signalling protein 1 (WISP-1), a wnt-induced secreted protein, in the synovium during OA (Blom et al., 2009). During experimental OA wnt-signalling is not only occurring in the cartilage but also in the synovium, as was found by β-catenin staining. WISP-1, a gene in which a polymorphism was shown to be associated with spinal OA (Urano et al., 2007) was strongly upregulated in the synovium of two models for OA. Further investigation indicated that WISP-1 is a potent inducer of MMPs in macrophages, whereas the short term effect on chondrocytes is less pronounced. In addition, overexpression of WISP-1 specifically in the synovium induced MMP and aggrecanase mediated neoepitopes VDIPEN and NITEGE in the cartilage, indicating that WISP-1 expression in synovial cells leads to cartilage degradation. Interestingly, these effects were independent of IL-1, since WISP1 did not induce IL-1 production in macrophages, nor was cartilage damage decreased in IL-1 deficient mice after synovial WISP-1 overexpression. Blocking studies are needed in order to substantiate this role for WISP-1 in (experimental) OA.

The targeting of Wnt signalling in OA drug discovery is likely to be impaired by the lack of knowledge concerning the normal function of these signalling pathways. For example, the direct targeting of β-catenin is likely to be hazardous, considering its importance for normal chondrocyte physiology, and its role in carcinogenesis. Whereas intracellular accumulation of β-catenin is linked to the induction of OA-like pathology, conditional knockdown of β-catenin signalling is equally harmful, since it induces chondrocyte apoptosis (Blom et al., 2010). Importantly, there is an increasing amount of data concerning the change of expression of certain Wnt protein and their inhibitors in the OA synovium. For example, Wnt16 is strongly upregulated in the synovium in a model of experimental OA, and also as a result of cartilage injury. Although both WISP-1 and Wnt16 have promise, more knowledge of Wnt signalling in health and disease is needed before any member of this family of protein can be defined as a therapeutic target in OA.

2.5 Matrix metalloproteinases as potential therapeutic targets in OA

Matrix metalloproteinases (MMPs) are a family of zinc-dependent endopeptidases that are synthesized as inactive proenzymes and activated extracellularly through cleavage of their prodomains by other proteases. Since MMPs cleave many of the structural components of the extracellular matrix, they have long been known to play a part in both inflammatory and degenerative arthritis. Inhibition of their activity through various broad-spectrum MMP inhibitors was effective in both mouse and guinea-pig models of osteoarthritis, but in humans these nonspecific MMP inhibitors caused musculoskeletal side effects, with painful joint stiffening and adhesive capsulitis (Hutchinson et al., 1998). Since no specific MMP has been pointed out as being involved in this musculoskeletal syndrome, the lack of selectivity of these broad-spectrum MMP inhibitors has been blamed for this side effect.

Since there is evidence that MMP-13 may well be the dominant collagenase in OA cartilage, with higher activity against type II collagen than any of the others, this MMP has been a main target for drug discovery. In a mouse model, overexpression of MMP-13 via an inducible transgene caused an OA-like phenotype (Neuhold et al., 2001). Recently, a group of compounds with a high degree of potency against MMP-13, as well as selectivity against other MMPs, were presented as a novel class of MMP-13 inhibitors. In the rat medial meniscal tear model of OA, one of these compounds protected articular cartilage as effectively as a broad-spectrum MMP inhibitor (Baragi et al., 2009). Numerous MMP-13 inhibitors are in early phase clinical development as DMOADs.

In osteoarthritis, aggrecan degradation, caused by increased activity of proteolytic enzymes that degrade macromolecules in the cartilage extracellular matrix, is followed by irreversible collagen degradation. The degradation of aggrecan is mediated by various matrix proteinases, mainly the aggrecanases, multidomain metalloproteinases belonging to the ADAMTS family. There has been much interest in the possible role of these aggrecanases, mainly ADAMTS4 and ADAMTS5, as therapeutic targets in osteoarthritis. It has long been debated which of the ADAMTSs is the main aggrecanase in human OA. Due to observations of ADAMTS4 mRNA being inducible through interleukin (IL)-1 and other stimuli in human OA chondrocytes and synovial fibroblasts, this enzyme attracted a good deal of attention (Bondeson et al., 2008).

But in models of murine OA induced by antigen or surgical joint destabilisation, ADAMTS5 is the pathologically induced aggrecanase. ADAMTS4 deficient mice develop normally and develop surgically induced degenerative arthritis in a similar manner to wild-type mice, but deletion of ADAMTS5 protects mice from developing arthritis (Glasson et al., 2004, 2005; Stanton et al., 2005). These results suggest that at least in murine models of OA, ADAMTS5 is the major aggrecanase. The only caveat to this conclusion is that there is a discrepancy between human and murine cells with regard to the regulation of ADAMTS5: the murine, but not the human, ADAMTS5 gene responds to IL-1 stimulation. Furthermore, a study using a small interfering RNA approach could demonstrate that both ADAMTS4 and ADAMTS5 contribute to the aggrecanase activity in human cartilage explants (Song et al., 2007). The search for the primary aggrecanase in human OA is still ongoing (Bondeson et al., 2008; Tortorella & Malfait, 2008).

The available data on ADAMTS5 gene promoters would suggest that this enzyme is the antithesis of ADAMTS4, with regard to its regulation. ADAMTS5 activity is reduced by C-terminal processing, whereas ADAMTS4 activity is enhanced (Gendron et al., 2007; Fosang et al., 2008). Then, in human cartilage and synovium, ADAMTS5 is constitutive whereas ADAMTS4 is the inducible aggrecanase, responding to IL-1 and TNFα in an NFκB dependent manner (Bondeson et al., 2008). The contrast between murine and human chondrocyte studies indicates that the situation may well be profoundly different in mice, something that of course would affect the validity of OA animal studies using these animals.

Several pharmaceutical companies (Wyeth/Pfizer, Schering-Plough, Rottapharm SpA, Alantos Pharm, Japan Tobacco) have patented small-molecule inhibitors of ADAMTS4 and ADAMTS5, developed mainly as potential DMOADs. Some of these compounds are claimed to be specific, whereas others have effect against both enzymes, against other ADAMTS members, or even against MMPs (Wittwer et al., 2007; Tortorella et al., 2009). The Wyeth/Pfizer compound was recently used in a phase I clinical trial in osteoarthritis (Hellio le Graverand-Gastineau, 2010; Gilbert et al., 2011).

The main endogenous inhibitor of ADAMTS4 and ADAMTS5 is tissue inhibitor of metalloproteinases (TIMP)-3, with K_i values in the subnanomolar range (Kashiwagi et al., 2001). This inhibition may well be modulated by interactions between aggrecan and the C-terminal domain of ADAMTS4 (Wayne et al., 2007). Interestingly, reactive-site mutants of the N-terminal inhibitory domain of TIMP-3, also inhibit ADAMTS4 (Lim et al., 2010). TIMP-3 knockout mice spontaneously lose their articular cartilage (Sahebjam et al., 2007). There is a good deal of interest in recombinant full-length or N-terminal TIMP-3 as a potential DMOAD, to be delivered intra-articularly, although it is yet to enter clinical trials.

3. Conclusions

In a recent editorial about the development of biologic therapy in RA, its distinguished authors pointed out that two of the greatest impediment for drug discovery were preconceived ideas about disease mechanisms and vested interests among those responsible for investigating potential therapeutic targets (Maini & Feldmann, 2007). In the early 1990s, it was generally accepted that 'autoimmune' diseases like RA were T cell driven. The synovial T cells were driving both inflammatory and destructive pathways, it was presumed, and although immunosuppression with drugs like cyclosporine or azathioprine could ameliorate symptoms, the disease remained incurable. Although this concept was successively undermined by the demonstration of low levels of lymphokines in RA synovial tissue and exudates, and later by the failure of anti-CD4 therapy in RA, it was adhered to with a rigidity that today seems quite inexplicable. Another both unconstructive and nihilistic notion popular at this time was that there was redundancy between proinflammatory cytokines and other inflammatory mediators, meaning that the targeting of an individual cytokine would be pointless. The notion of TNFα as a therapeutic target was initially greeted with incredulity, leading to a significant delay in the clinical development of these strategies (Feldmann, 2009). An idea originating in Britain was overlooked by the biotech and pharmaceutical industry of that country, and later commercialized in the United States with remarkable success.

The discovery that the neutralization of a single cytokine could lead to lasting remission in RA, with regard to both inflammation and development of erosions, had several beneficial effects for medical research. Firstly, it inspired further research into the disease mechanisms of other forms of chronic inflammation, leading to the establishment of anti-TNFα biologic therapy also in inflammatory bowel disease, psoriatic arthritis, ankylosing spondylitis, juvenile chronic arthritis and psoriasis. Secondly, it blew aside the concept that RA was an incurable 'autoimmune' disease, and inspired intensive research into RA pathophysiology, with the aim to find other targets for directed biologic therapy. This research has been rewarded with considerable success, with effective anti-CD20 and anti-T cell costimulation biologics now being available for use in RA, and many other biologics on their way in clinical development. Thirdly, the successes for biologic therapy of RA opened the door for more energetic work to identify potential therapeutic targets also in other chronic diseases. Even OA, the 'ugly sister' of rheumatology, received considerable attention, since here was a disease with immense unmet need and no disease modifying strategies on the market.

It is of course important that the lessons learnt from the successful drug development for RA and other forms of inflammatory arthritis are implemented in the search for therapeutic targets in OA. First to go should be the counterproductive notion of OA as the incurable result of 'wear and tear'. Although mechanical trauma and strain definitely play a part in the pathogenesis of OA, it remains a multifactorial disease. Many sick and obese people never develop OA; some fit and healthy ones do. It would also be beneficial if the concept of OA an primarily a disease of cartilage was challenged. A more promising approach, conducive to the definition of potential therapeutic targets, would be to consider the pathophysiological contributions of both synovium and cartilage (Figure 4). Activated synovial macrophages stimulate synovial fibroblasts, leading to the production of proinflammatory cytokines and that will have the ability to activate chondrocytes into producing further degradative enzymes. Furthermore, the production of MMPs, and quite possible aggrecanases, from the synovium, would also have a pathophysiological potential.

Since OA is a heterogenous disease, with variable degree of synovitis and macrophage infiltration, this simplified diagram of inter-cell and inter-tissue signalling (Figure 4) is likely to differ between patients: some have a higher degree of macrophage activation, synovitis and joint exudation, whereas others have 'dry' OA.

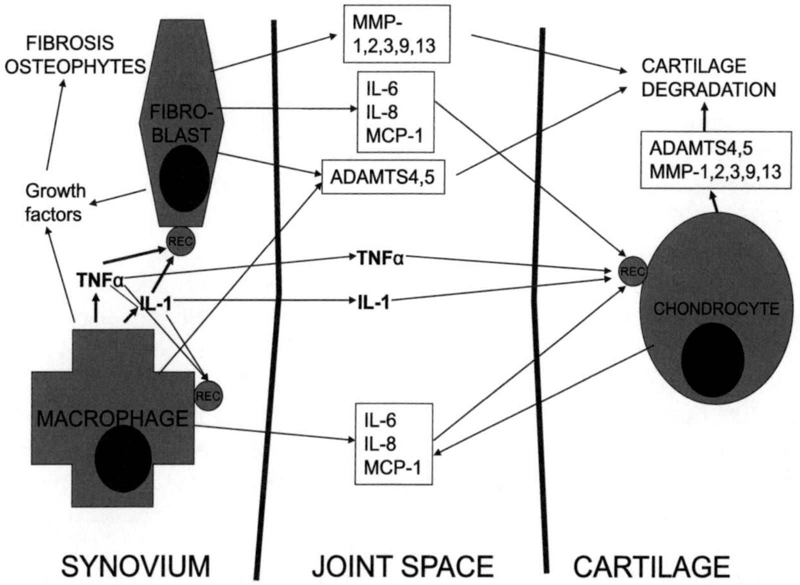

Fig. 4. A simplified view of the role of synovial macrophages in OA, in activating synovial fibroblasts and driving inflammatory and destructive responses. In this figure, 'REC' signifies all kinds of cell surface-related receptors. It remains unproven, although not unlikely, that ADAMTS4 and/or ADAMTS5 produced by synovial cells can be secreted into the synovial fluid, to influence cartilage degradation. Nor is it entirely clear that synovial macrophages produce ADAMTS4, although some preliminary data hints that this is possible.

Both in vitro and in vivo data point out the synovial macrophages and their main proinflammatory cytokines as potential therapeutic targets in OA. Macrophages drive the production of IL-6 and IL-8, the main MMPs (1,3,9,13) and ADAMTS4 from the synovial fibroblasts, and they are also crucial for the development of OA-related pathology, such as osteophyte formation and MMP-mediated cartilage breakdown (Bondeson et al., 2006, 2010; Blom et al., 2004, 2007). It should be remembered that the biology of OA synovitis is quite dissimilar from that in RA, with different cell composition, fewer macrophages, less synovial proliferation and synovial cell transformation, and no pannus or erosions. There are also differences in the regulation of key intracellular pathways between RA and OA macrophages (Amos et al., 2006) and important differences in cytokine biology (Bondeson et al., 2006), indicating that on the molecular as well as the clinical and histopathological levels, RA and OA are quite different diseases. The finding that there is redundancy between TNFα and IL-1 in the OA synovium, whereas TNFα drives IL-1 in RA, may well have some importance for the potential of anti-cytokine biologic treatment of OA. The concept of OA as a heterogenous disease would seem to be crucial for the application of anti-TNFα and/or anti-IL-1 strategies in this disease: in a patient with synovitis, exudation and bone marrow oedema, these strategies are likely to be more successful than in a patient with 'dry' OA secondary to obesity, or non-inflammatory OA of the distal interphalangeal joints. Had the clinical trials concerning anti-IL-1 and anti-TNFα strategies in OA selected patients with inflammatory knee OA verified by MRI, instead of patients with OA of the distal interphalangeal joints, the results may well have been different.

Disappointingly, there are currently no approved disease-modifying therapeutic strategies for OA. The three main impediments of drug development in OA have been the inadequacy of animal models of the disease, the difficulty in defining endpoints, finding validated biomarkers, and conducting worthwhile clinical trials in a disease that is so very slowly progressive, and the selection of patients for these clinical trials. Early OA is often asymptomatic, and the denudation of articular cartilage in advanced OA is likely to be an irreversible process. Many patients are likely to have some degree of denudation of cartilage, and exposure of subchondral bone, already at the time they exhibit radiographically obvious OA. Due to the slow progression of the disease, OA clinical trials need to take between one and three years, and use large numbers of patients. It would have been important to recruit patients with early disease, and a high risk of rapid progression, but the criteria currently used to define inclusion into clinical studies, and the lack of reliable predictors of disease progression, renders this very difficult. Furthermore, the commonly used measurement of OA progression, joint space narrowing on plain radiographs, is something of a blunt instrument, due to the slow progression of the disease.

The first criterium a DMOAD must fulfil is that its safety profile must be impeccable. Various drug companies and research organizations have performed clinical trials with existing drugs of proven safety, like the bisphosphonate drug Risedronate and the antibiotic Doxycycline but with unimpressive results. Nor has Diacerein, a compound with some degree of interleukin-1β inhibitory effect in vitro, or Licofelone, supposed to act as a combined cyclooxygenase and 5-lipoxygenase inhibitor, any obvious disease modifying potential in OA (see review by Hellio le Graverand-Gastineau, 2010). There is also a good deal of data concerning the widely available over-the-counter 'nutraceuticals' glucosamine and chondroitin sulphate. Although some early studies indicated that these substances at least had an analgesic effect, a recent meta-analysis found no evidence of them affecting neither joint pain, nor joint space narrowing, in OA (Wandel et al., 2010). Worryingly, there was also a discrepancy between industry sponsored and industry independent clinical trials, the latter indicating that the substances were close to worthless.

The situation appears to be that the existing drugs can provide little help to OA drug discovery: not only are they ineffective, but they provide no worthwhile clues as to future therapeutic targets in this disease. For some of them, their mechanisms are unknown, whereas others have been introduced from elements of serendipity rather than from understanding of the basic principles of OA pathophysiology. For OA drug discovery to move in the right direction, new ideas are required. Three compounds in phase III or phase IV development, namely calcitonin, vitamin D3 and avocado-soybean unsaponifiable; it would be an agreeable surprise if either of them has success as a DMOAD. Some more promising candidates are currently in phase II clinical trials. The Pfizer iNOS inhibitor benefits from quite solid preclinical data, and there is nothing to suggest it would be unsafe. Even a DMOAD leading to 20-30% slowing of the progression of OA would be in a strong market position, due to the absence of any competitor. Both OP-1 and FGF-18 are also in Phase II clinical trials. Albeit showing enormous future as a potential therapeutic target in OA, the canonical Wnt pathway is currently insufficiently understood, due to its complexity and its role in maintaining physiological function.

Non-selective MMP inhibitors are unlikely to have any future as potential DMOADs, but the selective MMP-13 inhibitors may well feature, although they do not appear to have progressed into clinical trials. Theoretically, the aggrecanase inhibitors have considerable promise as DMOADs. In mice, ADAMTS5 is clearly the dominant aggrecanase with regard to the development of OA in mice, but the dominant aggrecanase in human OA has not yet been identified. It is an important task for OA drug development that this is achieved, due to the need for an aggrecanase inhibitor used as a DMOAD to be as selective as possible. Another problem is that the normal function of ADAMTS4 and ADAMTS5 has not been elucidated. Both ADAMTS4 and ADAMTS5 knockout mice are fertile and phenotypically normal, speaking against these enzymes influencing the natural murine skeletal or joint development (Glasson et al., 2004, 2005). However, a recent study has indicated that ADAMTS5-deficient mice in fact had reduced apoptosis and decreased versican cleavage in the interdigital webs (McCulloch et al., 2010).

The search for a future DMOAD is reaching a critical time. There is a need for one of the abovementioned strategies to show definite promise in clinical trials, for the pharmaceutical industry to become convinced that the enormous effort and very considerable dollar costs to conduct preclinical and clinical OA research can be worth the effort. Some companies have already has OA projects, or even entire OA research departments, axed due to disappointing results in spite of vast financial spending. The window of opportunity for the search for therapeutic targets in OA, opened by the success of the anti-TNFs and other biologics for use in RA and other forms of inflammatory diseases, might be in danger of closing fast if some of the potential DMOADs in clinical development would join the long list of compounds used in 'failed' clinical studies in OA.

4. Acknowledgements

Address correspondence to Dr J. Bondeson at the Department of Rheumatology, Cardiff University, Heath Park, Cardiff CF14 4XN, UK; E-mail: BondesonJ@cf.ac.uk. This work has been supported by the Arthritis Research UK, grants no. W0596, 13172, 14570 and 18893.

5. Abbreviations

ADAMTS, A Disintegrin And Metalloproteinase with Transspondin Motives.
DMOAD, Disease-modifying anti-osteoarthritis drug
IL, Interleukin
MMP, Matrix metalloprotease.
NFκB, Nuclear factor κB.
OA, Osteoarthritis.
RA, Rheumatoid arthritis.
TIMP, Tissue inhibitor of metalloproteases.
TNF, Tumour necrosis factor.

6. References

Abramson, S.B. & Yazici, Y. (2006) Biologics in development for rheumatoid arthritis: relevance to osteoarthritis. *Advanced Drug Delivery Reviews* Vol. 58, No. 2 (May 2006), pp. 212-225. ISSN 0169-409X

Amos, N., Lauder, S., Evans, A., Feldmann, M. & Bondeson, J. (2006) Adenoviral gene transfer into osteoarthritis synovial cells using the endogenous inhibitor IκBα reveals that most, but not all, inhibitory and destructive mediators, are NFκB dependent. *Rheumatology* Vol. 45, No. 3 (March 2006), pp. 1201-1209. ISSN 1462-0324

Andreakos, E., Smith, C., Kiriakidis, S., Monaco, C., de Martin, R., Brennan, F.M., Paleolog, E., Feldmann, M. & Foxwell, B.M. (2003) Heterogenous requirement of IkappaB kinase 2 for inflammatory cytokine and matrix metalloproteinase production in rheumatoid arthritis: implications for therapy. *Arthritis and Rheumatism* Vol. 48, No. 7 (July 2003), pp. 1901-1912. ISSN 1529-0131

Badlani, N., Inoue, A., Healey, R., Coutts, R. & Amiel, D. (2008) The protective effect of OP-1 on articular cartilage in the development of osteoarthritis. *Osteoarthritis and Cartilage* Vol. 16, No. 5 (May 2008), 600-606. ISSN 1063-4584

Baragi, V.M., Becher, G., Bendele, A.M., Biesinger, R., Bluhm, H., Boer, J., Deng, H., Dodd, R., Essers, M., Feuerstein, T., Gallagher, B.M. Jr, Gege, C., Hochgürtel, M., Hofmann, M., Jaworski, A., Jin, L., Kiely, A., Korniski, B., Kroth, H., Nix, D., Nolte, B., Piecha, D., Powers, T.S., Richter, F., Schneider, M., Steeneck, C., Sucholeiki, I., Taveras, A., Timmermann, A., Van Veldhuizen, J., Weik, J., Wu, X. & Xia, B. (2009) A new class of potent matrix metalloproteinase 13 inhibitors for potential treatment of osteoarthritis: Evidence of histologic and clinical efficacy without musculoskeletal toxicity in rat models. *Arthritis and Rheumatism* Vol. 60, No. 7 (July 2009), pp. 2008-2018. ISSN 1529-0131

Benito, M.J., Veale, D.J., FitzGerald, O., van den Berg, W.B. & Bresnihan, B. (2005) Synovial tissue inflammation in early and late osteoarthritis. *Annals of the Rheumatic Diseases* Vol. 64, No. 9 (September 2005), pp. 1263-1267. ISSN 0003-4967

Berenbaum, F. (2007) The quest for the holy grail: a disease-modifying osteoarthritis drug. *Arthritis Research and Therapy* Vol. 9, No. 6 (December 2007), article no. 111. ISSN 1478-6354

Blom, A.B., van Lent, P.L.E.M., Holthuysen, A.E.M., van der Kraan, P.M., Roth, J., van Rooijen, N. & van den Berg WB. (2004) Synovial lining macrophages mediate osteophyte formation during experimental osteoarthritis. *Osteoarthritis and Cartilage* Vol. 12, No. 8 (August 2004), pp. 627-635. ISSN 1063-4584

Blom, A.B. & van den Berg, W.B. (2007) The synovium and its role in osteoarthritis. In: *Bone and Osteoarthritis,* F. Bronner & M.C. Farach-Carson (Eds.), Vol. 4, pp. 65-79, Springer Verlag, ISBN 9781846285134, Berlin, Germany.

Blom, A.B., van Lent, P.L., Libregts, S., Holthuysen, A.E., van der Kraan, P.M., van Rooijen, N. & van den Berg, W.B. (2007a) Crucial role of macrophages in matrix metalloproteinase-mediated cartilage destruction during experimental osteoarthritis. *Arthritis and Rheumatism* Vol. 56, No. 1 (January 2007), pp. 147-157. ISSN 1529-0131

Blom, A.B., van der Kraan, P.M. & van den Berg, W.B. (2007b) Cytokine targeting in osteoarthritis. *Current Drug Targets* Vol. 8, No. 2 (February 2007), pp. 283-292. ISSN 1389-4501

Blom, A.B., Brockbank, S.M., van Lent, P.L., van Beuningen, H.M., Geurts, J., Takahashi, N., van der Kraan, P.M., van de Loo, F.A., Schreurs, B.W., Clements, K., Newham, P. & van den Berg, W.B. (2009) Involvement of the Wnt signaling pathway in experimental and human osteoarthritis: prominent role of Wnt-induced signaling protein 1. *Arthritis and Rheumatism* Vol. 60, No. 2 (February 2009), pp. 501-512. ISSN 1529-0131

Blom, A.B., van Lent, P.L., van der Kraan, P.M. & van den Berg, W.B. (2010) To seek shelter from the WNT in osteoarthritis? WNT-signaling as a target for osteoarthritis therapy. *Current Drug Targets* Vol. 11, No. 5. (May 2010), pp. 620-629. ISSN 1389-4501

Bondeson, J., Foxwell, B.M.J., Brennan, F.M. & Feldmann, M. (1999a) Defining therapeutic targets by using adenovirus: blocking NF-κB inhibits both inflammatory and destructive mechanisms in rheumatoid synovium, but spares anti-inflammatory mediators. *Proceedings of the National Acadademy of Sciences of the USA* Vol. 96, No. 5 (May 1999), pp. 5668-5673. ISSN 0027-8424

Bondeson, J., Browne, K.A., Brennan, F.M., Foxwell, B.M.J. & Feldmann, M. (1999b) Selective regulation of cytokine induction by adenoviral gene transfer of IκBα into human macrophages: lipopolysaccharide-induced, but not zymosan-induced, proinflammatory cytokines are inhibited, but IL-10 is NFκB independent. *Journal of Immunology* Vol. 162, No. 5 (March 1999), pp. 2939-2945. ISSN 0022-1767

Bondeson, J., Wainwright, S.D., Lauder, S., Amos, N. & Hughes, C.E. (2006) The role of synovial macrophages and macrophage-produced cytokines in driving aggrecanases, matrix metalloproteinases and other destructive and inflammatory responses in osteoarthritis. *Arthritis Research and Therapy* Vol. 8, No. 6, (2006), article no. R187. ISSN 1478-6354

Bondeson, J., Wainwright, S., Hughes, C. & Caterson, B. (2008) The regulation of ADAMTS4 and ADAMTS5 aggrecanases in osteoarthritis: a review. *Clinical and Experimental Rheumatology* Vol. 26, No. 1 (February 2008), pp. 139-145. ISSN 1593-098X

Bondeson, J., Blom, A.B., Wainwright, S., Hughes, C., Caterson, B. & van den Berg, W.B. (2010) The role of synovial macrophages and macrophage-produced mediators in driving inflammatory and destructive responses in osteoarthritis. *Arthritis and Rheumatism* Vol. 62, No. 3 (March 2010), pp. 647-57. ISSN 1529-0131

Brennan, F.M., Chantry, D., Jackson, A., Maini, R. & Feldmann, M. (1989) Inhibitory effect of TNFa antibodies on synovial cell interleukin-1 production in rheumatoid arthritis. *Lancet* Vol. ii, No. 8657 (July 1989), pp. 244-247. ISSN 0140-6736

Brennan, F.M., Hayes, A.L., Ciesielski, C.J., Green, P., Foxwell, B.M.J. & Feldmann, M. (2002) Evidence that rheumatoid arthritis synovial T cells are similar to cytokine-activated T cells. *Arthritis and Rheumatism* Vol. 46, No. 1 (January 2002), pp. 31-41. ISSN 1529-0131

Brennan, F.M. & McInnes, I.B. (2008) Evidence that cytokines play a role in rheumatoid athritis. *Journal of Clinical Investigations* Vol. 118, No. 11 (November 2008), pp. 3537-3545. ISSN 0021-9738

Burger, D., Dayer, J.-M., Palmer, G. & Gabay, C. (2006) Is IL-1 a good therapeutic target in the treatment of arthritis? *Best Practice and Research: Clinical Rheumatology* Vol. 20, No. 5 (October 2006), pp. 879-896. ISSN 1521-6942

Chevalier, X., Girardeau, B., Conzorier, T., Marliere, J., Kiefer, P. & Goupille, P. (2005) Safety study of intraarticular injection of interleukin 1 receptor antagonist in patients with painful knee osteoarthritis: a multicenter study. *Journal of Rheumatology* Vol. 32, No. 7 (July 2005), pp. 1317-1323. ISSN 0315-162X

Chevalier, X., Goupille, P., Beaulieu, A.D., Burch, F.X., Bensen, W.G., Conrozier, T., Loeuille, D., Kivitz, A.J., Silver, D. & Appleton, B.E. (2009) Intraarticular injection of anakinra in osteoarthritis of the knee: a multicenter, double-blind, placebo-controlled study. *Arthritis Care and Research* Vol. 61, No. 3 (March 2009), 344-352. ISSN 0893-7524

Clark, A.G., Jordan, J.M., Vilim, V., Renner, J.B., Dragomir, A.D., Luta, G. & Kraus, V.B. (1999) Serum cartilage oligomeric protein reflects osteoarthritis presence and severity. *Arthritis and Rheumatism* Vol. 42, No. 11 (November 1999), pp. 2356-2364. ISSN 1529-0131

Farahat, M.N., Yanni, G., Poston, R. & Panayi, G.S. (1993) Cytokine expression in synovial membranes of patients with rheumatoid arthritis and osteoarthritis. *Annals of the Rheumatic Diseases* Vol. 52, No. 12 (December 1993), pp. 870-875. ISSN 0003-4967

Feldmann, M. & Maini, R.N. (2008) Role of cytokines in rheumatoid arthritis: an education in pathophysiology and therapeutics. *Immunological Reviews* Vol. 223 (June 2008), pp. 7-19. ISSN 1600-065X

Feldmann, M. (2009) Translating molecular insights in autoimmunity into effective therapy. Annual Review of Immunology Vol. 27 (2009), pp. 1-27. ISSN 0732-0582

Fernandes, J.C., Martel-Pelletier, J. & Pelletier, J.P. (2002) The role of cytokines in osteoarthritis pathophysiology. *Biorheology* Vol. 39, No. 1-2 (February 2002), pp. 237-246. ISSN 0006-355X

Fioravanti, A., Fabbroni, M., Cerase, A. & Galeazzi, M. (2009) Treatment of erosive osteoarthritis of the hands by intra-articular inflizimab injections: a pilot study. *Rheumatology International* Vol. 29, No. 8 (June 2009), pp. 961-965. ISSN 1437-160X

Fosang, A.J., Rogerson, F.M., East, C.J. & Stanton, H. (2008) ADAMTS-5: the story so far. *European Cells and Materials* Vol. 15 (February 2008), pp. 11-26. ISSN 1473-2262

Foxwell, B.M.J., Browne, K.A., Bondeson, J., Clarke, C.J., de Martin, R., Brennan, F.M. & Feldmann, M. (1998) Efficient adenoviral infection with IκBα reveals that macrophage TNFα production in rheumatoid arthritis is NF-κB dependent. *Proceedings of the National Academy of Sciences of the USA* Vol. 95, No. 14 (July 1998), pp. 8211-8215. ISSN 0027-8424

Gendron, C., Kashiwagi, M., Lim, N.H., Enghild, J.J., Thøgersen, I.B., Hughes, C., Caterson, B. & Nagase, H. (2007) Proteolytic activities of human ADAMTS-5. Comparative studies with ADAMTS-4. *Journal of Biological Chemistry* Vol. 282, No. 25 (June 2007), pp. 18294-18306. ISSN 0021-9258

Genovese, M.C., Cohen, S., Moreland, L., Lium, D., Robbins, S., Newmark, R. & Bekker, P. (2004) Combination therapy with etanercept and anakinra in the treatment of patients with rheumatoid arthritis who have been treated unsuccessfully with methotrexate. *Arthritis and Rheumatism* Vol. 50, No. 5 (May 2004), pp. 1412-1419. ISSN 1529-0131

Gilbert, A.M., Bikker, J.A. & O'Neil, S.V. (2011) Advances in the development of novel aggrecanase inhibitors. *Expert Opinion on Therapeutic Patents* Vol. 21, No. 1 (January 2011), pp. 1-12. ISSN 1354-3776.

Glasson, S.S., Askew, R., Sheppard, B., Carito, B.A., Blanchet, T., Ma, H.L., Flannery, C.R., Kanki, K., Wang, E., Peluso, D., Yang, Z., Majumdar, M.K. & Morris, E.A. (2004) Characterization of and osteoarthritis susceptibility in ADAMTS-4-knockout mice. *Arthritis and Rheumatism* Vol. 50, No. 8 (August 2004), pp. 2547-2558. ISSN 1529-0131

Glasson, S.S., Askew, R., Sheppard, B., Carito, B., Blanchet, T., Ma, H.L., Flannery, C.R., Peluso, D., Kanki, K., Yang, Z., Majumdar, M.K. & Morris, E.A. (2005) Deletion of active ADAMTS5 prevents cartilage degradation in a murine model of osteoarthritis. *Nature* Vol. 434, No. 7033 (March 2005), pp. 644-648. ISSN 0028-0836

Goupille, P., Mulleman, D. & Chevalier, X. (2007) Is interleukin-1 a good target for therapeutic intervention in intervertebral disc degeneration: lessons from the osteoarthritic experience. *Arthritis Research and Therapy* Vol. 9, No. 6 (2007), article no. 110. ISSN 1478-6354

Grunke, M. & Schulze-Koops, H. (2006) Successful treatment of inflammatory knee osteoarthritis with tumour necrosis factor blockade. *Annals of the Rheumatic Diseases* Vol. 65, No. 4 (April 2006), pp. 555-556. ISSN 0003-4967

Güler-Yüksel, M., Allaart, C.F., Watt, I., Goekoop-Ruiterman, Y.P., de Vries-Bouwstra, J.K., van Schaardenburg, D., van Krugten, M.V., Dijkmans, B.A., Huizinga, T,W,, Lems, W.F. & Kloppenburg, M. (2010) Treatment with the TNF-α inhibitor infliximab might reduce hand osteoarthritis in patients with rheumatoid arthritis. *Osteoarthritis and Cartilage* Vol. 18, No. 10 (October 2010), pp. 1256-1262. ISSN 1063-4584

Hashimoto, S., Takahashi, K., Amiel, D., Coutts, R.D. & Lotz, M. (1998) Chondrocyte apoptosis and nitric oxide production during experimentally induced osteoarthritis. *Arthritis and Rheumatism* Vol. 41, No. 7 (July 1998), pp. 1266-1274. ISSN 1529-0131

Hayes, A.L., Smith, C., Foxwell, B.M. & Brennan, F.M. (1999) CD45-induced tumor necrosis factor alpha production in monocytes is phosphatidylinositol 3-kinase-dependent and nuclear factor kappaB-independent. *Journal of Biological Chemistry* Vol. 274, No. 47 (November 1999), pp. 33455-33461. ISSN 0021-9258

Haywood, L., McWilliams, D.F., Pearson, C.I., Gill, S.E., Ganesan, A., Wilson, D. & Walsh, D.A. (2003) Inflammation and angiogenesis in osteoarthritis. *Arthritis and Rheumatism* Vol. 48, No. 8 (August 2003), pp. 173-177. ISSN 1529-0131

Hellio le Graverand, M.P., Vignon, E., Otterness, I.G. & Hart, D.A. (2000) Early changes in lapine menisci during osteoarthritis development Part II: Molecular alterations *Osteoarthritis and Cartilage* Vol. 9, No. 1 (January 2000), pp. 65-72. ISSN 1063-4584

Hellio Le Graverand-Gastineau, M.-P. (2010) Disease modifying osteoarthritis drugs: Facing development challenges and choosing molecular targets. *Current Drug Targets* Vol. 11, No. 5 (May 2010), pp. 528-535. ISSN 1389-4501

Hutchinson, J.W., Tierney, G.M., Parsons, S.L. & Davis, T.R. (1998) Dupuytren's disease and frozen shoulder induced by treatment with a matrix metalloproteinase inhibitor. *Journal of Bone and Joint Surgery (British volume)* Vol. 80, No. 5 (September 1998), pp. 907-908. ISSN 0301-620X

Kalliolias, G.D. & Liossis, S.N.C. (2008) The future of the IL-1 receptor antagonist anakinra: from rheumatoid arthritis to adult-onset Still's disease and systemic-onset juvenile idiopathic arthritis. *Expert Opinion on Investigational Drugs* Vol. 17, No. 3 (March 2008), pp. 349-359. ISSN 1354-3784

Kashiwagi, M., Tortorella, M., Nagase, H. & Brew, K. (2001) TIMP-3 is a potent inhibitor of aggrecanase 1 (ADAM-TS4) and aggrecanase 2 (ADAM-TS5) *Journal of Biological Chemistry* Vol. 276, No. 16 (April 2001), pp. 12501–12504. ISSN 0021-9258

Kinne, R.W., Stuhlmuller, B. & Burmester, G.-R. (2007) Cells of the synovium in rheumatoid arthritis: macrophages. *Arthritis Research and Therapy* Vol. 9, No. 6 (June 2007), article no. 224. ISSN 1478-6354

Lim, N.H., Kashiwagi, M., Visse, R., Jones, J., Enghild, J.J., Brew, K. & Nagase, H. (2010) Reactive-site mutants of N-TIMP-3 that selectively inhibit ADAMTS-4 and ADAMTS-5: biological and structural implications *Biochemical Journal* Vol. 431, No. 1 (October 2010), pp. 113–122. ISSN 0264-6021

McCulloch, D.R., Nelson, C.M., Dixon, L.J., Silver, D.L., Wylie, J.D., Lindner, V., Sasaki, T., Cooley, M.A., Argraves, W.S. & Apte, S.S. (2009) ADAMTS metalloproteases generate active versican fragments that regulate interdigital web regression. *Developmental Cell* Vol. 17, No. 5 (November 2009), pp. 687-698. ISSN 1534-5807

Magnano, M.D., Chakravarty, E.F., Broudy, C., Chung, L., Kelman, A., Hillygus, J. & Genovese, M.C. (2007) A pilot study of tumor necrosis factor inhibition in erosive/inflammatory osteoarthritis of the hands. *Journal of Rheumatology* Vol. 34, No. 6 (June 2007), pp. 1323-1327. ISSN 0315-162X

Martel-Peletier, J. & Pelletier, J.-P. (2009) Osteoarthritis: A single injection of anakinra for treating knee OA? *Nature Reviews Rheumatology* Vol. 5, No. 7 (July 2009), pp. 363-364. ISSN 1759-4790

Maini, R.N. & Feldmann, M. (2007) The pitfalls in the development of biologic therapy. *Nature Clinical Practice Rheumatology* Vol. 3 (2007), p. 1. ISSN 1745-8382

Malemud, C.J. (2004) Cytokines as therapeutic targets for osteoarthritis. *Biodrugs* Vol. 18, No. 1 (2004), pp. 23-35. ISSN 1173-8804

Moore, E.E., Bendele, A.M., Thompson, D.L., Littau, A., Waggie, K.S., Reardon, B., Ellsworth, J.L. (2005) Fibroblast growth factor-18 stimulates chondrogenesis and cartilage repair in a rat model of injury-induced osteoarthritis. *Osteoarthritis and Cartilage* Vol. 13, No. 7 (July 2005), pp. 623-631. ISSN 1063-4584

Neuhold, L.A., Killar, L., Zhao, W., Sung, M.L., Warner, L., Kulik, J., Turner, J., Wu, W., Billinghurst, C., Meijers, T., Poole, A.R., Babij, P. & DeGennaro, L.J. (2001) Postnatal expression in hyaline cartilage of constitutively active human collagenase-3 (MMP-13) induces osteoarthritis in mice. *Journal of Clinical Investigations* Vol. 107, No. 1 (January 2001), pp. 35-44. ISSN 0021-9738

Pavelka, K., Trc, T., Karpas, K., Vítek, P., Sedlácková, M., Vlasáková, V., Böhmová, J. & Rovenský, J. (2007) The efficacy and safety of diacerein in the treatment of painful osteoarthritis of the knee. *Arthritis and Rheumatism* Vol. 56, No. 12 (December 2007). pp. 4055-4064. ISSN 1529-0131

Pelletier, J.-P. & Martel-Pelletier, J. (2005) New trends in the treatment of osteoarthritis. *Seminars in Arthritis and Rheumatism* Vol. 34 (2005), pp. 13-14. ISSN 0049-0172

Qvist, P., Bay-Jensen, A.-C., Christiansen, C., Dam, B.E., Pastoreau, P. & Karsdal, M.A. (2008) The disease modifying osteoarthritis drug (DMOAD): Is it on the horizon? *Pharmacological Research* Vol. 58 (2008), pp. 1-7. ISSN 1043-6618

Rudolphi, K., Gerwin, N., Verzijl, N., van der Kraan, P. & van den Berg W. (2003) Pralnacasan, an inhibitor of interleukin-1 converting enzyme, reduces joint damage in two murine models of osteoarthritis. *Osteoarthritis and Cartilage* Vol. 11, No. 10 (October 2003). pp. 738-746. ISSN 1063-4584

Sahebjam, S., Khokha, R. & Mort, J.S. (2007) Increased collagen and aggrecan degradation with age in the joints of Timp3(-/-) mice. *Arthritis and Rheumatism* Vol. 56, No. 3 (March 2007), pp. 905-909. ISSN 1529-0131

Sekiya, I., Tang, T., Hayashi, M., Morito, T., Ju, Y.J., Mochizuki, T. & Muneta, T. (2009) Periodic knee injections of BMP-7 delay cartilage degeneration induced by excessive running in rats. *Journal of Orthopaedic Research* Vol. 27, No. 8 (August 2009), pp. 1088-1092. ISSN 0736-0266

Shahrara, S., Castro-Rueda, H.P., Haines, G.K. & Koch, A.E.. (2007) Differential expression of the FAK family kinases in rheumatoid arthritis and osteoarthritis synovial tissue. *Arthritis Research and Therapy* Vol. 9, No. 5 (2007), article no. R112. ISSN 1478-6354

Song, R.H., Tortorella, M.D., Malfait, A.M., Alston, J.T., Yang, Z., Arner, E.C. & Griggs, D.W. (2007) Aggrecan degradation in human articular cartilage explants is mediated by both ADAMTS-4 and ADAMTS-5. *Arthritis and Rheumatism* Vol. 56, No. 2 (February 2007), pp. 575-585. ISSN 1529-0131

Sowers, M., Jannausch, M., Stein, E., Jamadar, D., Hochberg, M. & Lachance, L. (2002) C-reactive protein as a biomarker of emergent osteoarthritis. *Osteoarthritis and Cartilage* vol. 10, No. 8 (August 2002), pp. 595-601. ISSN 1063-4584

Stanton, H., Rogerson, F.M., East, C.J., Golub, S.B., Lawlor, K.E., Meeker, C.T., Little, C.B., Last, K., Farmer, P.J., Campbell, I.K., Fourie, A.M. & Fosang, A.J. (2005) ADAMTS5 is the major aggrecanase in mouse cartilage in vivo and in vitro. *Nature* Vol. 434, No. 7033) (March 2005), pp. 648-652. ISSN 0028-0836

Tortorella, M.D. & Malfait, A.M. (2008) Will the real aggrecanase(s) step up: evaluating the criteria that define aggrecanase activity in osteoarthritis. *Current Pharmacological Biotechnology* Vol. 9, No. 1 (February 2008), pp. 16-23. ISSN 1389-2010

Tortorella, M.D., Tomasselli, A.G., Mathis, K.J., Schnute, M.E., Woodard, S.S., Munie, G., Williams, J.M., Caspers, N., Wittwer, A.J., Malfait, A.M. & Shieh, H.S. (2009) Structural and inhibition analysis reveals the mechanism of selectivity of a series of aggrecanase inhibitors. *Journal of Biological Chemistry* Vol. 284, No. 36 (September 2009), pp. 24185-24191. ISSN 0021-9258

Urano, T., Narusawa, K., Shiraki, M., Usui, T., Sasaki, N., Hosoi, T., Ouchi, Y., Nakamura, T. & Inoue, S. (2007) Association of a single nucleotide polymorphism in the WISP1 gene with spinal osteoarthritis in postmenopausal Japanese women. *Journal of Bone and Mineral Metabolism* Vol. 25, No. 4 (2007), pp. 253-258. ISSN 0884-0431

van den Berg, W.B., van de Loo, F., Joosten, L.A. & Arntz, O.J. (1999) Animal models of arthritis in NOS2-deficient mice. *Osteoarthritis and Cartilage* Vol. 7, No. 4 (July 1999), pp. 413-415. ISSN 1063-4584

van der Heijden, J.W., Oerlemans, R., Dijkmans, B.A., Qi, H., van der Laken, C.J., Lems, W.F., Jackman, A.L., Kraan, M.C., Tak, P.P., Ratnam, M. & Jansen, G. (2009) Folate receptor γ as a potential delivery route for novel folate antagonists to macrophages in the synovial tissue of rheumatoid arthritis patients. *Arthritis and Rheumatism* Vol. 60, No. 1 (January 2009), pp. 12-21. ISSN 1529-0131

van der Laken, C.J., Elzinga, E.H., Kropholler, M.A., Molthoff, C.F., van der Heijden, J,W,, Maruyama, K., Boellaard, R., Dijkmans, B.A., Lammertsma, A.A. & Voskuyl, A.E. (2008) Noninvasive imaging of macrophages in rheumatoid synovitis using ^{11}C-(R)-PK11195 and positron emission tomography. *Arthritis and Rheumatism* Vol. 58, No. 11 (November 2008), pp. 3350-3355. ISSN 1529-0131

Van Lent, P.L.E.M., Blom, A.B., van der Kraan, P., Holthuysen, A.E.M., Vitters, E., van Rooijen, N., Smeets, R.L., Nabbe, K.C. & van den Berg, W.B. (2004) Crucial role of synovial lining macrophages in the promotion of transforming growth factor beta-mediated osteophyte formation. *Arthritis and Rheumatism* Vol. 50, No. 1 (January 2004), pp. 103-111. ISSN 1529-0131

Wandel, S., Jüni, P., Tendal, B., Nüesch, E., Villiger, P.M., Welton, N.J., Reichenbach, S. & Trelle, S. (2010) Effects of glucosamine, chondroitin, or placebo in patients with osteoarthritis of hip or knee: network meta-analysis. *British Medical Journal* Vol. 341, (September 2010), c4675. ISSN 09598138

Wayne, G.J., Deng, S.J., Amour, A., Borman, S., Matico, R., Carter, H.L. & Murphy, G. (2007) TIMP-3 inhibition of ADAMTS-4 (Aggrecanase-1) is modulated by interactions between aggrecan and the C-terminal domain of ADAMTS-4. *Journal of Biological Chemistry* Vol. 282, No. 29 (July 2007), pp. 20991–20998. ISSN 0021-9258

Wittwer, A.J., Hills, R.L., Keith, R.H., Munie, G.E., Arner, E.C., Anglin, C.P., Malfait, A.M. & Tortorella, M.D. (2007) Substrate-dependent inhibition kinetics of an active site-directed inhibitor of ADAMTS-4 (Aggrecanase 1) *Biochemistry* Vol. 46, No. 21 (May 2007), pp. 6393–6401. ISSN 0001-527X

25

Cellular Physiology of Articular Cartilage in Health and Disease

Peter I. Milner, Robert J. Wilkins and John S. Gibson
University of Liverpool, University of Oxford & University of Cambridge
United Kingdom

1. Introduction

Articular chondrocytes live in an unusual and constantly changing physicochemical environment. Due to the structure of the extracellular matrix, adult cartilage is avascular, relatively hypoxic and acidic compared to other tissues (Wilkins et al., 2000). In this challenging environment the maintenance and regulation of extracellular matrix by chondrocytes is dependent on signals received through this milieu (Lai et al., 2002). In joint disease, such as osteoarthritis, the extracellular environment is altered and the cellular physiology of the chondrocyte will change to reflect this, leading to alterations in its key role of regulating matrix turnover and hence contributing to the pathophysiology of joint disease (Goldring 2006).

This chapter will discuss the challenges to the chondrocyte and how cellular physiology is affected in both health and disease. We will discuss how the structure of the matrix confers its biomechanical properties to cartilage and how this translates to physiological sensing by the cartilage during static and dynamic loading with particular emphasis on effects on membrane transporters and cell signalling pathways. We will also consider how other features of cartilage in the adult influence the chondrocyte, such as oxygen tension, osmolarity and pH. Finally we will consider the changes that occur in osteoarthritis and how these translate to alterations in cellular physiology and hence matrix integrity, the loss of the which is the key feature of osteoarthritis, and how these events may be new targets for treatment of this condition.

2. Structure of articular cartilage

Articular cartilage is a highly specialised tissue that provides a resilient, smooth, almost frictionless surface for joints to function efficiently and pain-free (Morris et al., 2002). In the adult, articular cartilage is avascular and predominately composed of extracellular matrix with a low density of resident cells, articular chondrocytes, which are responsible for the maintenance of the matrix in the healthy joint (Palmer & Bertone, 1994). Chondrocytes are embedded within a structurally organised matrix consisting of water, collagens, proteoglycans, glycosaminoglycans and non-collagenous proteins (Huber et al., 2000). The biochemical composition and structural alignment of these components within cartilage is responsible for the mechanical properties of this tissue and the cellular responses of the chondrocyte (Jeffery et al., 1991; Kuettner et al., 1991).

2.1 Articular chondrocytes and zonal organisation

Articular cartilage is organised to allow its main role to occur, that is, providing a smooth almost frictionless surface for pain-free mobility but also as a biomaterial that can also withstand compressive and shear forces. As well as the actual biochemical content of articular cartilage, the biomechanical properties rely on the structural organisation of the extracellular matrix and the cells embedded within them. The structure and organisation of articular cartilage not only varies with depth from the articular surface (divided into zones) but also the location within the joint (for example, weightbearing versus non-weightbearing surfaces).

Articular chondrocytes occupy 2-5% of the tissue volume and are sometimes considered relatively inactive metabolically due to an absence of a vascular supply but are responsible for maintaining the integrity of the extracellular matrix and can respond to mechanical stimuli, growth factors and cytokines. Articular cartilage has four distinct histological and biochemical zones (I-IV): superficial (tangential), intermediate (transitional), deep (radial) and calcified. The superficial zone is the thinnest along the articular surface and merges with the perichondrium at the articular margin. Type II collagen in the superficial zone is orientated tangentially to the articular surface to provide resistance to tensile forces. Proteoglycan composition in this zone acts as a non-selective barrier to diffusion of oxygen and water and a selective barrier to the diffusion of nutrients and hormones. This is largely due to the large amount of negatively charged anionic groups on the sulphated side chains on proteoglycans which allows smaller, non-ionic molecules through the matrix more readily than larger charged molecules. The pericellular matrix in the chondron (the chondrocyte and its pericellular microenvironment) consists of high levels of collagen type VI and aggregating proteoglycans and defines the physiochemical environment of the chondrocyte (Wang et al, 2008) and biochemical or mechanical signals perceived by the chondrocyte are therefore influenced by the structural and functional composition of the chondron (Guilak et al., 2006). Proteoglycans in the pericellular zone are thought to have a role in binding the chondrocyte to the matrix rather that the direct biomechanical role seen in the interterritorial matrix. Within the matrix surrounding the chondrocytes (territorial matrix) are thin type II and VI collagen fibrils, organised in a "basket-weave" formation and these fibrils extend out in a parallel arrangement to bind with larger type II collagen fibrils in the interterritorial matrix. In the intermediate zone the chondron structure is more typical. In this zone the collagen fibrils appears more widely spaced and their orientation is more random and there are increased amounts of proteoglycan compared to the superficial zone. In the deep zone the chondrocytes start to align themselves in columns perpendicularly to the joint surface along with thicker collagen fibrils. The collagen fibrils are orientated radially between these chondrocytic columns. The abundant proteoglycan within the interterritorial matrix with higher amounts of keratin sulphate side chains increases the permeability of the matrix in the deep zone and may be important in allowing diffusion of nutrients to the deeper layers of cartilage. Between the deep and calcified zones, there is a demarcation consisting of mineral associated with matrix vesicles within the interterritorial matrix and this is known as the tidemark.

2.2 The extracellular matrix

The extracellular matrix is a mechanically resilient structure comprising of collagens, proteoglycans and other non-collagenous proteins (Wilkins et al., 2000). Hydrated proteoglycans confer resistance to compression and are constrained by the collagen fibrillar meshwork (thought of as a "string-and-balloon" model). Proteoglycans, with highly sulphated glycosaminoglycan (GAG) side chains and fixed negative charges, attract free cations and osmotically obliged water, leading to a hydrated matrix of raised osmolarity and lowered pH. Avascularity of matrix means that movement of hormones, cytokines, nutrients and metabolites occurs over relatively large distances along steep gradients. The low partial pressures of oxygen denote that cells undergo predominately anaerobic glycolysis and must endure high concentrations of lactic acid. Added to these challenges, normal mechanical loading causes profound fluctuations in the physiochemical environment.

2.2.1 Collagen

There are a number of collagen types recognised in articular cartilage, but type II collagen is the primary collagen of articular cartilage, comprising 80-90% of the total collagen content (Becerra et al., 2010). Type II collagen acts primarily to provide tensile stiffness in cartilage (Kaab et al., 1998). Other collagens are formed due to different gene expression, translational splicing and post-translational modification and many have important regulatory and structural roles and may be associated with type II collagen (e.g. functional binding) or other components of the matrix (for example binding and interactions with proteoglycans and the chondrocyte).

Collagen fibrils extend out from the pericellular envelope into the territorial matrix (Morris et al., 2002). Further collagen fibrils extend out into the interterritorial matrix, intimately involved with proteoglycans. Numerous contacts are present between the plasma membrane, collagens and proteoglycans through the extracellular matrix. Pericellular matrix contains little or no fibrillar collagen but type VI collagen microfibrils that interact with hyaluronic acid (HA), small proteoglycans and cell surface molecules. Type IX collagen is found throughout cartilage matrix and type XI collagen is mainly localised to the territorial matrix interacting with type II collagen, adding to tensile strength. Type IX collagen appears to localise with type II collagen fibrils in particular regions and covalent cross-linking may alter size and stability and hence mechanical properties of the type II collagen fibrils.

2.2.2 Proteoglycans

Proteoglycans and glycosaminoglycans contribute compressive stiffness to articular cartilage (Hardingham & Forsang, 1992). There are a number of different types of these macromolecules present throughout cartilage and they can also function as regulatory proteins and binding sites for other matrix components. Aggrecan, one of the most common proteoglycans in cartilage, is a high molecular weight proteoglycan (1-2 x 10^6 kDa) that binds HA in the matrix. Proteoglycans and proteoglycan link proteins are present throughout the extracellular matrix including the pericellular matrix and have structural relationships with collagens. Proteoglycans act as a selective permeability barrier and the structure of the matrix will dampen kinetic responses as diffusion through the matrix is slow. As well as contributing important mechanical properties to cartilage, proteoglycans are also important modulators of cell signalling and function.

2.2.3 Glycosaminoglycans

Glycosaminoglycans contain highly negatively charged polyanionic sulphate groups. It is this, as well as the large molecular weight of the proteoglycan aggrecan, that attracts cations, such as Na^+ and thereby water into the cartilage matrix and thus increasing tissue osmotic pressure (Wilkins et al., 2000). The resistance of the collagen fibrillar network to expansion therefore provides cartilage with an ability to resist compressive forces. The main glycosaminoglycans identified in articular cartilage are chondroitin-4-sulphate, chondroitin-6-sulpate, keratin sulphate and hyaluronic acid (Morris et al., 2002).

In a typical aggrecan molecule there can be up to 100 chondroitin sulphate side chains attached to the core protein (via xyulose-serine bond), each with up to 1000 repeating disaccharide units. Keratan sulphate is a smaller polysaccharide and there are usually around 50 keratin sulphate side chains linked to the aggrecan core protein (via a galactose-*N*-acetyl-threonine or –serine bond). Hyaluronic acid ($1x10^4$ kDa) is also classified as a glycosaminoglycan although it lacks the sulphated groups on its D-glucosamine and D-glucuronic acid disaccharide chains. Each HA can bind up to 100 aggrecan proteins. Early release of HA of the cell during synthesis may be important in articular cartilage structure since the length of HA influences proteoglycan binding and may affect proteoglycan aggregation and function (Palmer & Bertone 1994).

2.2.4 Water and water flow in cartilage

Water makes up approximately 70% of cartilage weight. Negatively charged proteoglycans attract cations and water follows leading to swelling of proteoglycans, resisting tension and shear forces. Since the macromolecular composition of extracellular matrix of cartilage determines matrix hydration and tissue volume it therefore determines the space for molecular transport and offers compressive resistance (as water is essentially incompressible). The hydrodynamic processes controlling the water content include osmosis, filtration, swelling and diffusion.

Osmotic flow of water occurs up gradients of osmotic pressure and cartilage can be thought of as a gel consisting of cross-linked non-ideal macromolecules (i.e. yield parameters which vary nonlinearly with concentration, a feature of a number of biological systems). It is thought that within the proteoglycan network, an ensemble of segments interacting with each other may form "pores" through which the flow resistance for water is lowered (Comper 1996).

3. Cellular physiology of articular chondrocytes

The unusual biochemical structure of articular cartilage results in particular biomechanical properties that strongly influence the cellular physiology of the articular chondrocyte (Hall et al., 1996a). Due to the presence of fixed, highly negatively-charged polysulphated proteoglycans, there is an increase in cation (Na^+, K^+ and H^+) concentration in articular cartilage, compared to other tissues (e.g. plasma) leading to cartilage having raised osmolality ($350\text{-}450 mOsm.kg^{-1}$) compared to synovial fluid (around $300 mOsm.kg^{-1}$). Under load, the physical and ionic environment of cartilage alters. Dynamic load leads to increased hydrostatic pressure causing cartilage deformation/ membrane stretch and fluid flows (Urban, 1994). On removal of load the matrix regains its steady-state conformation. If loading continues, though, these dynamic components are followed by slower osmotic consequences. Under static loading conditions, fluid expression results in changes to the extracellular environment, raising fixed negative charge of glycosaminoglycans and hence increases osmotic pressure. These dynamic changes result in direct effects on articular chondrocyte function since not only does the extracellular environment change, intracellular cation concentrations fluctuate with load and altered membrane transport activities occur due to mechanical deformation of membranes and changes in pressure, osmolarity and pH. Additionally, this environment is altered in joint disease such as osteoarthritis since biochemical and biomechanical changes occur which will directly influence the chondrocyte.

3.1 Membrane transport in articular chondrocytes

Chondrocytes possess many of the membrane transport systems found in other cell types (Wilkins et al., 2000). Active membrane transport systems exchange cations whose intracellular concentrations fluctuate with load not only to maintain cellular homeostasis but these mechanisms can be linked to solute transport and intracellular signalling events and mechanotransduction events, important in the articular chondrocyte to maintain cartilage integrity through extracellular matrix synthesis.

3.1.1 Electrophysiology of articular chondrocytes

The resting membrane potential of articular chondrocytes is thought to be between -15mV and -44mV, maintained by Na^+/K^+ ATPase and is influenced by cyclical pressure (Clarke et al., 2010; Funabashi et al., 2010; Hall et al., 1996a). Potassium channels are integral membrane proteins, participating in cell membrane potential and belong to a large superfamily including voltage-activated potassium channels (K_v), Ca^{2+}-activated potassium channels (K_{Ca}) and inward rectifier potassium channels (Kir). Using whole cell-patch clamp techniques, a voltage-dependent, Ca^{2+}-independent K^+ current with rapid activation and very slow inactivation has been described in isolated canine articular chondrocytes (Wilson et al., 2004). ATP-sensitive K_{ATP} channels have also been demonstrated in articular cartilage (Mobasheri et al., 2007). K_{ATP} channels may couple metabolic events (i.e. intracellular ATP levels) to membrane electrical activity and potentially their activity may be may be important in low oxygen conditions since hypoxia is known to lead to activation of K_{ATP} channels in other systems (Miki & Seino, 2005). Additionally, electrophysiological responses of chondrocytes from osteoarthritic cartilage appears to differ from healthy cartilage (Sanchez & Lopez-Zapata 2010).

3.1.2 Volume regulation

The maintenance of cell volume in the face of alterations in the extracellular environment is an important cellular function (Hoffmann et al., 2009). Chondrocyte cell volume, as with other cell types, is determined by a pump-leak model where a double Donnan equilibrium exists between intracellular compartments and the matrix (Wilkins et al., 2000). Exclusion of Na^+ ions from the cell is maintained by Na^+-K^+ ATPase and cell volume is maintained by altered balance of leaks and pumps to hold cell water constant.

In articular chondrocytes, hypertonicity leads to regulatory volume increase (RVI) and raises intracellular potassium ($[K^+]_i$) via $Na^+/K^+/2Cl^-$ co-transporter (Hall et al., 1996b). Na^+/H^+ exchange (NHE), unlike in other cell systems in the body, does not appear to play a role in volume regulation in cartilage due to the lack of Cl^--HCO_3^- exchange activity which is required for RVI. During RVI, $[Na^+]_i$ is increased and the Na^+/K^+ pump is stimulated to keep $[K^+]_i$:$[Na^+]_i$ ratio optimal for protein and enzyme function. Removal of static load in cartilage results in cell swelling and the activation of regulatory volume decrease (RVD) processes. Cell swelling following hypotonic challenge leads to RVD in many cells via Cl^- -

dependent K^+ transporter, Ca^{2+}-activated K^+ (with associated Cl^- ions) channel or an "osmolyte" channel (e.g. taurine, sorbitol and myo-inositol) (Hoffmann et al., 2009). In chondrocytes, loss of osmolytes appears to occur via "osmolyte" channel and volume activated K^+ transport may also occur by this route (Hall & Bush 2001). Hypotonic challenge also leads to depolarisation via Na^+ influx through stretch activated cation channels (SACC) (Sanchez et al., 2003).

In cartilage, cells lysis is prevented by the ECM (akin to plant cells and cell wall) and thus avoiding the effects extremes of hyposmolarity (although static loading in normal joints only leads to fluid losses and decrease in cartilage hydration of only around 5% per day and these losses are restored when load is removed). However, in osteoarthritis (OA), proteoglycans are lost and reduced Na^+ and water content affects joint function. This increase in cartilage hydration under load is an early event in OA and could lead to changes in chondrocyte volume regulation (Bush & Hall 2005). Indeed the first changes in osteoarthritis are cell swelling suggesting the mechanisms for regulating cell volume are either lost or impaired.

3.1.3 Intracellular pH (pH_i) regulation

The acidic extracellular environment (pH 6.8) promotes inward leak of H^+ ions so chondrocytes are subjected to chronic acid loading. With low O_2 and anaerobic glycolysis as the primary source of metabolism resulting in lactate production, additional intracellular loading is also encountered. Articular chondrocytes have resting pH_i of around 7.1 and a relatively high intracellular buffering capacity of around 30mmol.l^{-1} (pH_i) (Wilkins & Hall 1992). Intracellular pH (pH_i) regulation in chondrocytes predominately occurs through the amiloride-sensitive sodium-dependent Na^+/H^+ exchanger (NHE). As discussed previously the extracellular matrix is rich in Na^+ but poor in anions and therefore it appears that anion-dependent pH regulation been sacrificed in favour of SO_4^- uptake; an essential precursor for proteoglycan synthesis.

Extracellular acidity is an important regulator of cartilage matrix metabolism and activity of degradative enzymes. Changes in extra-and intracellular pH both elicit a bi-modal response of matrix synthesis (Wilkins & Hall, 1995). Small changes in extracellular pH (pH_o) quickly and significantly (up to 50%) inhibit synthesis rates (particularly below pH 6.9). It is possible, in normal cartilage, that matrix acidification could provide a means of regulating proteoglycan synthesis by a negative feedback system such that increased proteoglycan content raises H^+, thereby inhibiting synthesis.

There are a number of NHE isoforms characterised but the main "housekeeping" form is NHE-1 (Pedersen & Cala, 2004). Static loading leads to hyperosmolarity and hyperosmosis results in increased acid efflux in chondrocytes through the activation of NHE (Yamazaki et al., 2000). Enhanced H^+ extrusion under conditions of loading may allow a defence versus cellular acidosis and a mechanism whereby effects of this loading can be transduced into changes in cartilage turnover. Hypotonic shock, however, leads to an increase in pH_i (alkalosis) via the opening of voltage-activated H^+ channels (VAHC) (Sanchez & Wilkins, 2003).

Serum leads to increased acid extrusion on response to intracellular acidosis. NHE3 is expressed following exposure to serum and cytokines (Tattersall et al., 2003), particularly IGF-1 (Tattersall et al., 2008). In contrast to NHE1, NHE3 is inhibited by hypertonicity and by PKA pathways but activated by hypotonicity. Exposure to serum factors occurring in osteoarthritic cartilage (damaged tissue more likely to be exposed to serum factors and IGF-1 is elevated in arthritic cartilage - van der Kraan & van den Berg, 2000) could therefore result in a differential response of NHE1 and 3 to hyperosmotic shock. Additionally this may have consequences for matrix synthesis which are dictated by pH. In addition to IGF-1, EGF has been shown to stimulate proton efflux by increasing activity of NHE involving PI3-kinase pathway (Lui et al., 2002).

Despite the chondrocyte already residing in an acidic extracellular matrix, further acidosis occurs in joint disease due to hypoxia and production of inflammatory cytokines altering blood flow. Since extracellular pH has a potent influence on cellular function (Das et al., 2010) any effect on the ability of the cell to regulate intracellular pH is likely to result in alteration in chondrocyte function, including matrix synthesis. Very low levels of oxygen, likely to be experienced in joint disease, reduce the activity of NHE resulting in intracellular acidosis in articular chondrocytes (Milner et al., 2006).

3.1.4 Intracellular calcium regulation

Intracellular calcium $[Ca^{2+}]_i$ in chondrocytes, as in many other cells has numerous physiological functions (Berridge et al., 1998). In articular chondrocytes, $[Ca^{2+}]_i$ is maintained at low levels (around 80nM) and Ca^{2+}-ATPase and Na^+-Ca^{2+} exchanger appear to be the dominant mediators of calcium homeostasis in these cells (Sanchez et al., 2003). The maintenance of calcium is a balance between Ca^{2+} extrusion, influx via membrane channels and Ca^{2+} release from intracellular stores, such as endoplasmic reticulum and mitochondria (Duchen, 2004; Sanchez et al., 2006).

Alterations in intracellular calcium can affect matrix synthesis (Wilkins et al., 2000) and calcium signaling has been implicated in mechanotransduction in articular chondrocytes (Guilak et al., 1999;). There are a number of studies showing that intracellular calcium in chondrocytes can be altered by hydrostatic pressure, osmotic stress and fluid flow (Kerrigan & Hall, 2008; Yellowley et al., 2002). Increased pressure and cell swelling induces a Gd^{3+}-sensitive $[Ca^{2+}]_i$ increase (Wilkins et al., 2003) and it has been shown that intracellular Ca^{2+} levels can also be modulated by pH (Sanchez and Wilkins, 2003).

3.1.5 Metabolite transport

Transport of metabolites across the plasma membrane has an important role in maintaining chondrocytic biosynthetic output and matrix integrity. The uptake of sulphate (SO_4^{2-}) is an important step in the synthesis of glycosaminoglycans and appears to occur in articular chondrocytes via a carrier-mediated mechanism that is Na^+-independent and sensitive to transmembrane H^+ gradient (stimulated by acidic extracellular pH) (Meredith et al., 2007). Probable candidates include SO_4^{2-} x Cl^- and SO_4^{2-} x OH^- exchanger (anion exchanger). Amino acid uptake occurs via Na^+-dependent (proline, glycine and glutamine) and independent (leucine) transporters (Wilkins et al., 2000).

Inorganic phosphate (P_i) uptake in chondrocytes appears to have both Na^+-dependent and –independent components and shows pH- sensitivity (Solomon et al., 2007). Transport of P_i across the cell membrane is an important component of the calcification process, particularly in the growth plate and the inappropriate formation of calcium-phosphate (hydroxyapatite) crystals in osteoarthritis could involve dysfunction of P_i-transporters.

Glucose provides energy source and is an essential precursor for glycosaminoglycan synthesis. GLUT transporters (e.g. IGF-1 modulated GLUT4) are mainly responsible for glucose uptake (Shikhman et al., 2004; Windhaber et al., 2003) whereas lactic acid transport appears via monocarboxylate family of transporters (MCT) including MCT1 ("housekeeper") and MCT4 (Meredith et al., 2002). MCT4 appears to be the main isoform in articular chondrocytes whose kinetics favour lactate export thereby allowing pyruvate conversion back to lactate to assist in NAD^+ regeneration and continued glycolysis.

4. Mechanotransduction in articular cartilage

The main functions of articular cartilage are concerned with load-bearing (Urban, 1994). During normal activity, pressures within cartilage may rise to 100-200 atmospheres (10-20 MPa) within milliseconds. The mechanical failure of extracellular matrix is a key event in the progression of degenerative joint disease since not only direct loss of function of the tissue occurs but detrimental effects on cellular activity and the potential repair process ensues. The ability of the chondrocyte to sense and respond appropriately to mechanical signals (mechanotransduction) is vital in maintaining cartilage integrity.

4.1 Mechano-electrochemical properties of cartilage and signal transduction

Physical environmental factors such as shear stress, fluid flow and electrical field alterations are known to be strong biologic factors in regulating cellular activities (Lai et al., 2002; Mow et al., 1999). During loading, a number of changes occur within cartilage, including increased hydrostatic pressure, cartilage/chondrocyte cell deformation, fluid flow and streaming potentials, changes in chondrocyte cell membrane and fluid loss resulting in changes to interstitial fluid osmolality/ionic content (Urban, 2000). Transducers of mechanotransduction in cells include activation of stretch activated channels allowing ingress of external Ca^{2+}, alteration of membrane transporter activity (eg Na^+/H^+ exchange) and activation of mechanosensitive ion channels and transporters such as transient receptor potential (TRP) channels and purinergic receptors. The ECM is directly linked to the cytoskeleton and nucleus of the cell via integrins. Integrins are central to many mechanotransduction pathways since they integrate a number of important intracellular signalling pathways, for example, focal adhesion kinase signaling via integrin-ECM (involving G-protein signaling) and other pathways (involving, for example MAPK and PI-3 kinases) (Loeser, 2002).

4.1.1 Streaming potential and diffusion potential

Streaming potentials and diffusion potentials can be used to describe the electrical forces generated during ionic species movement and these are thought to be important in mechanical signal transduction in cartilage. The potential induced by convection current (mechano-chemical force generated by cation and anion movement) in the presence of a pressure gradient gives the streaming potential of cartilage, whereas the potential induced by the diffusion in the presence concentration gradient is the diffusion potential and have been shown to be important modulators of chondrocyte metabolism (Kim et al., 1995).

4.1.2 Effects of mechanical load on chondrocyte function and matrix synthesis

Mechanical load is required to maintain cartilage integrity (Hasler et al., 1999). Matrix proteoglycan is lost from cartilage in immobilised joints and there is variation within a normal joint between unloaded and loaded regions. Regions subjected to load are often thicker and have higher proteoglycan content and therefore likely to be mechanically stronger. Dynamic or cyclic loading stimulates proteoglycan and protein synthesis whereas static loading is associated with decreased synthesis and in addition, load-induced solute movement can also influence rates at which growth factors or cytokines reach the cells and alter cellular metabolism.

When load is applied there is an increase in hydrostatic pressure, extracellular pH decreases and there is an increase in extracellular free cation concentration and osmolality. Alterations in the osmotic balance occurs as fluid is expressed to try to restore the hydrostatic equilibrium and this increases the concentrations of proteoglycans and hence cations, resulting in osmotic consequences. The changes in hydrostatic pressure and osmotic alteration lead to cellular deformation and change in volume resulting in changes in $[Na^+]_i$, $[K^+]_i$, pH_i and $[Ca^{2+}]_i$ due to altered transporter activity and therefore this can result in alterations in macromolecular synthesis.

During loading, cartilage from osteoarthritic joints will deform more than cartilage from non-diseased joints, since both the rate and amount of fluid loss are sensitive to proteoglycan concentrations. Therefore cartilage from degenerate joints will lose fluid faster than healthy cartilage and this is likely to alter the stimulus and hence the response of the chondrocyte in diseased tissue.

4.1.3 Hydrostatic pressure

During normal walking, articular cartilage cycles between a resting hydrostatic pressure of 0.2MPa and pressures of 4-5 MPa (2-50atm). It is known that pressures in the 5-50MPa range can alter cellular morphology, reduce exocytosis, dissociate cytoskeletal elements, reduce protein synthesis and inhibit membrane transport. The timing of the cycles is also important - application of cyclical pressures (>0.5Hz) have stimulatory effects on cartilage matrix synthesis. It also appears that isolated chondrocytes are more sensitive to pressure than *in situ* within the matrix and that the cytoskeleton and Golgi apparatus are involved in this response.

Physiological levels of hydrostatic pressure can affect membrane permeability to ions and amino acids and thus affect intracellular solute concentrations. Increase in hydrostatic pressure leads to increased rate of synthesis of matrix components and this may be exerted via alteration in intracellular pH. Browning et al., (1999) showed that application of 20-300atm to isolated cells led to NHE stimulation via phosphorylation-dependent processes. Additionally, hydrostatic pressure has been shown to inhibit membrane transport pathways (such as Na^+/K^+-pump, $Na^+/K^+/2Cl^-$ cotransporter) (Hall et al., 1999). Conformational alterations by cell deformation may be responsible for change in membrane transport activity as well as changes in their phosphorylation status. For example, pressure may uncouple ATP hydrolysis or alter lipid environment as to retard Na^+ binding or constrain conformational changes leading to altered activity of the Na^+/K^+ pump. Alteration in ion channel activity is therefore likely to be intimately linked to matrix synthesis.

4.1.4 Osmotic sensitivity of chondrocytes

Static loading leads to fluid expression and increased interstitial fluid osmolarity. The link between ECM hydration and chondrocyte metabolism appears to be via volume regulation. Cells respond to unequal tonicity by water movement across plasma membrane and this is usually rapid leading to cell volume changes within seconds. The osmometric behaviour of chondrocytes in situ and isolated from matrix appears to be similar although some differences in layers occur in situ (Bush & Hall, 2001). Superficial zone chondrocytes appear to swell more than middle or deeper zone cells and this may reflect less proteoglycan present in this zone. Additionally deeper zone chondrocytes may take longer to respond to water changes in cartilage so the response may depend on zone and local osmotic environment. Potentially, zone-specific alterations in physico-chemical signals may lead to differences in chondrocyte matrix biosynthesis.

Water can flux through membranes via aquaporins. Aquaporins (AQP) are water channel proteins that allow water to move in the direction of osmotic gradient and may also allow small solutes to pass, for example glycerol and urea. A role in cell volume regulation and mechanotransduction in chondrocytes has been proposed (Mobasheri et al., 2004). AQP1 and AQP3 are expressed in cartilage resulting in water permeability and may respond to environment changes since changes in aquaporin expression may be important in pathology.

Hyperosmotic stress induces a transient alteration in cellular volume and $[Ca^{2+}]_i$ (Erickson et al., 2001) but a latency appears to exist between minimum cell volume reached and peak Ca^{2+} levels. This may be explained by Na^+ entering the cell (possibly via voltage-gated sodium channels, VGSC, or epithelial sodium channels, ENaC), leading to depolarisation and subsequent increase in intracellular calcium levels. This then results in membrane hyperpolarisation and Ca^{2+} activated K^+ channels open causing K^+ efflux. Hypotonic shock also results in increased intracellular Ca^{2+} levels (Wilkins et al., 2003). Mechanosensitive Ca^{2+} channels appear to open in response to hypotonicity as well as calcium release from intracellular stores. Prolonged increase of intracellular calcium, however, is detrimental to the cell so mechanisms such as Na^+/Ca^{2+} exchanger are in operation to regulate this Ca^{2+} rise.

These stretch-activated ion channels may act as putative mechanical signal transducers since they lead to fluctuations in intracellular calcium levels that may affect gene expression. Potential mechanosensitive ion channels in chondrocytes could include VGSC, ENaC and N/L-type voltage gated calcium channels (VGCC). In epithelial cells, ENaC is linked to the actin cytoskeleton and integrin. In osteoarthritic cartilage, ENaC is absent and the lack of ENaC means that chondrocytes may have lost the ability to transduce mechanical signals effectively.

4.1.5 Integrins

Integrins play a key role in the interactions between the cell and the extracellular matrix including cell anchorage, growth, differentiation, migration and matrix synthesis and degradation (Loeser, 1993). Integrins are cell surface receptors that recognise and bind to an Arg-Gly-Asp sequence on ECM proteins and are heterodimeric (one α and one β subunit) transmembrane glycoproteins (Loeser, 2000). The importance of integrins, as well as being cell adhesion molecules, is that they may function as transmitters of information and be able to mediate intracellular responses to extracellular stimuli. The pericellular matrix and chondrocytes in the chondron contain collagen types II, VI and IV, aggrecan and fibronectin and integrins are known to interact with these proteins found in pericellular matrix. Immunoprecipitation and immunofluorescence experiments show co-localisation and association of integrin with ENaC and VGCC and therefore integrins may functionally activate ion transporters following deformation of the pericellular matrix.

Extracellular protein binding to the cell leads to receptor clustering and activates integrin. Integrins however, have no inherent kinase activity but will often complex with Shc, Crk, paxillin, vinculin, caveolin and/or FAK. Many of these proteins in the complex are activated by tyrosine phosphorylation which then leads to activation of other kinases such as Src, RhoA, Rac1, Ras, Raf1, Sos, Grb2, MEK kinase and member of the MAP kinase family (including ERK1/2, JNK and p38). This then leads to downstream signalling that regulate gene expression, for example MAP kinase, that lead to activation of transcription factors such as AP-1 and NF-κB.

The regulation of chondrocyte integrin function is important in the homeostasis of cartilage as well as in disease states in which interactions between chondrocytes and their ECM are altered. Factors that modulate chondrocyte ECM synthesis, such as IGF-1 and TGF-β, also appear to modulate integrin-mediated attachment of chondrocytes to ECM proteins (Loeser 1994, 1997). The effects of IGF-1 and TGF-β on chondrocyte integrin expression and function, however, in vivo may depend on the relative levels of each growth factor present and thereby providing a means for sophisticated control of cell-matrix interactions in cartilage. Growth factor receptor phosphorylation leads to increased integrin aggregation, possibly via MAP kinase activation. There appears to be co-localisation of IGF-1 receptor and β_1 integrin subunit in chondrocytes. Cross-talk exists between integrins and growth factors/cytokines and as well as integrin activity being affected by growth factors, growth factor activity itself is dependent on integrin binding. Therefore a two-way signalling process occurs with integrin occupying a central role in this system. Increased expression of IGF-1 has been noted in osteoarthritic cartilage and could act in an autocrine manner to increased $\alpha_1\beta_1$ possibly as part of a repair response mediating signals important for cell survival/proliferation.

Integrins have a central role in cell survival and inhibition of integrin function results in apoptosis (Loeser, 2002; Mobasheri et al., 2002). The Ras-MAPK pathway is important to chondrocyte survival and integrins are linked to Ras-MAPK pathway by downstream signaling factors including the docking protein Shc. Interruption of the Ras-MAPK pathway produces apoptosis (via increased expression of pro-apoptotic proteins or repression of anti-apoptotic proteins). Therefore disruption of the interactions between chondrocytes and the ECM (via integrins) may induce apoptotic cell death and may contribute to pathogenesis of osteoarthritis.

4.1.6 Purinergic signaling

The potential role of purinergic signalling in mechanotransduction in cartilage was postulated following the finding that compressive loading of bovine chondrocytes in chondrons or in agarose pellets leads to ATP release (Chowdhury & Knight, 2006). ATP is an important mediator involved in autocrine/paracrine signalling and it can be released following cell damage and as well as being directly involved in signalling via release.

Chondrocytes have been shown to express P2Y2 receptors (Millward-Sadler et al., 2004) and normal chondrocytes release ATP after mechanical stimulation involving calcium signaling. Recently, Varani et al., (2008) characterised the expression of $P2X_1$ and $P2X_3$ receptors in bovine chondrocytes. Unlike P2Y receptors that are G-protein coupled, P2X receptors are membrane ligand-gated ion channels that open in response to binding of extracellular ATP. Stimulation of purinergic pathways (via P2X receptors) may be important in the response to joint inflammation since ATP further stimulates NO and PGE_2 production in chondrocytes following IL-1β stimulation.

The link between P2 receptors and cell signalling may involve connexin hemichannel expression (Knight et al., 2009). Connexins are membrane proteins that form hemichannels and hemichannels are one of the potential ways of releasing ATP (as well as through anion channels and via exocytosis of ATP-filled vesicles). Cyclic loading leads to hemichannel opening and ATP release in chondrocyte constructs (Garcia & Knight, 2010). In human cartilage, connexion 43 has been found in cells in the superficial region. The presence of these potential mechanosensitive cells primarily in the superficial/middle zones may indicate different mechanotransduction pathways than deeper zone cells. Since hypoxia is known to regulate connexins 43 dephophosphorylation, translocation and proteosomal degradation in other cells the response to mechanical stimulation may be related to the oxygen environment of cartilage.

The primary cilium, a membrane-coated axoneme that projects from the cell surface into the extracellular microenvironment could also be involved in chondrocyte mechanotransduction. The function of primary cilium in chondrocytes has not established but in the study by Knight et al., (2009) approximately 50% of primary cilia had co-expression of connexin 43. It is postulated that deflection of the cilium may activate ATP release via hemichannels and once released, ATP may activate P2 receptors, triggering intracellular Ca^{2+} signalling cascades and mediate effects on proteoglycan and collagen synthesis and MMP expression and NO release.

In osteoarthritic chondrocytes, a reduction in purinergic signalling following mechanical stimulation has been reported. This could be due to desensitisation by ATP released into synovial fluid (increased ATP levels in synovial fluid are reported in OA patients) or by receptor down regulation (since reduction in receptor numbers has been described at the cell surface in OA chondrocytes). The changes in ATP-mediated signalling in OA cartilage is of importance since ATP is normally chondroprotective against proteoglycan loss.

4.1.7 Transient receptor potential (TRP) channels

Transient receptor potential (TRP) channels comprise a superfamily of more than 50 different ion channels with a preference of Ca^{2+}, playing a role in the transduction of several physical stimuli such as temperature, osmotic and mechanical stimuli. TRP channel opening induces membrane depolarisation while increasing cytosolic Ca^{2+} and/or Na^{+} concentrations. Most, but not all TRPC members act as store-operated Ca^{2+} channels whereas TRPV channels may be involved in a nonselective conductance of cations with a preference for Ca^{2+}. Since calcium entry through plasma membrane channels is recognised as a cellular signalling event per se, TPR channels provide an ideal candidate to link between mechanical stimuli and cellular response.

In human osteoarthritic chondrocytes, the majority of the investigated TRP genes are expressed (Gavenis et al., 2009) and a correlation appears between the degree of differentiation of chondrocytes and the expression of various members of the TRP family. Their role in cartilage health and disease is, as yet, unknown (Mobasheri &Barrett-Jolley, 2011).

5. Oxygen, mitochondria and reactive oxygen species in articular cartilage

Adult articular cartilage is avascular and hence long diffusion pathways exist for nutrients solutes and oxygen to cross. Synovial fluid has low oxygen tension (6-10%) and articular chondrocytes experience relatively low levels of oxygen, compared to other cell-types, with chondrocytes operating at oxygen tensions ranging from 6-10% at the articular surface to around 2% in the deep zones (Zhou et al., 2004). Despite this, articular chondrocytes not only survive but regulate extracellular matrix synthesis. Although energy production appears to be primarily via a glycolysis in this low oxygen environment, it is being recgonised that mitochondria might play an important role in the health and disease of the joint through their involvement in reactive oxygen species generation, calcium regulation and the intimate role in cell death/survival pathways in cartilage.

5.1 Cartilage oxygen tension and cell metabolism

The oxygen tension gradient in cartilage is determined by cell density and distribution, cartilage thickness, oxygen tension in synovial fluid, oxygen supply from subchondral surface and oxygen consumption rate per cell (Zhou et al., 2004). Articular chondrocytes have a characteristic morphology and metabolism depending on their position in cartilage and part of this may be due to the oxygen gradients that exist. Although the majority of diffusion of oxygen appears to come from the articular surface facing the synovial fluid, there is thought to be a component of diffusion from vessels in the subchondral bone plate and therefore extreme levels of hypoxia (i.e. 1% or less) may not exist *in situ* in cartilage (but could do in disease where subchondral bone plate thickening is a feature of osteoarthritis).
Despite these low oxygen conditions, articular chondrocytes do survive and are able to maintain their cartilage phenotype (Grimshaw & Mason, 2000; Pfander & Gelse, 2007). To survive low oxygen conditions cells possess highly conserved adaptive mechanisms. The most important component is mediated by transcriptional activation involving binding of the transcription factor hypoxia-inducible factor-1 (HIF-1). In cartilage, during physiological hypoxia, HIF-1α is expressed (Lin et al., 2004) and it appears to act as a survival factor since necrotic cartilage occurs in HIF-1 knock-out mice (Gelse et al., 2008).
Although articular chondrocytes reside in low oxygen levels, they are not unresponsive to hypoxia since changes in oxygen tension can have significant effects on matrix synthesis and cell growth. Indeed, matrix synthesis by articular chondrocytes may be optimal at lower tissue oxygen tensions, for example at 5% O_2, Sox9, type II collagen and aggrecan expression is higher than at 21% O_2 (Marty-Hartert et al., 2005). Oxygen diffusion and movement through cartilage may occur at differential rates in response to biochemical and loading differences in different regions and this could lead to local oxygen gradients within pockets of cartilage which could influence cell metabolism as well as differential gene expression.

5.1.1 Articular cartilage metabolism

Within the hypoxic environment of cartilage, articular chondrocytes predominately undergo glycolytic metabolism. Lactate is the major end-product of this process and this adds to the already acidic load experienced by these cells. ATP is generated by substrate level phosphorylation, whereas, apart from superficial layers where relatively higher oxygen levels can exist, oxidative phosphorylation appears to be a lesser component of ATP production.
Reduction of oxygen levels in other cells results in an increase in glucose usage and lactate production, thereby increasing ATP production - this is commonly known as the Pasteur effect. Articular chondrocytes, however, appear to display a negative Pasteur effect where

reductions in oxygen levels result in suppression of carbohydrate breakdown (Lee & Urban, 1997). This effect appears to be peculiar to articular cartilage since in fibrocartilaginous intervertebral disc, glucose uptake and lactate production increases under lowered oxygen levels.

5.1.2 Changes in oxygen tension in joint disease

Despite increased blood vessel formation in the synovial membrane and neoangiogenesis from the underlying bone into the deep zone of osteoarthritic cartilage, the hypoxic environment of cartilage appears more pronounced in osteoarthritis. Synovial fluid from osteoarthritic joints contains less oxygen than synovial fluids from healthy joints (Pflander & Gelse, 2007). Reductions in oxygen tension in joint disease could be due to increased oxygen usage by the synovial membrane, alterations in blood flow and gas exchange by fibrosis in the joint capsule and subchondral bone sclerosis (Svalastoga & Kiaet, 1989). Additionally, alterations in diffusion gradients caused by changes in matrix structure, altered biomechanical forces through the cartilage and alterations in oxygen consumption in inflammation (e.g. reactive oxygen species generation) contribute to the reduction in cartilage oxygen levels.

5.1.3 Hypoxia and HIF-1 in osteoarthritis

Chronic hypoxia in the osteoarthritic joint is associated with increased levels of HIF-1 in both synoviocytes and chondrocytes and related HIF-1 targeted genes, such as VEGF and iNOS. Additionally, HIF-1α accumulation can also be increased by other factors such as pro-inflammatory cytokines and changes in mechanical loading, as well as hypoxia (Pfander & Gelse, 2007). HIF-1α is important for anaerobic energy production and matrix synthesis by chondrocytes and appears to have a pivotal role for maintaining chondrocytic phenotype.

As well as the increased synthesis of matrix destructive enzymes, osteoarthritic chondrocytes show enhanced gene expression of type II collagen. This latter feature may be related to oxygen levels since increased accumulation of type II collagen induced by 1% oxygen is accompanied by stabilisation, nuclear translocation and increased activity of HIF-1α. The increase in posttranslational modification of type II collagen may contribute to the increased synthesis of collagen type II seen during osteoarthritis as an effort to restore extracellular matrix.

5.2 The role of mitochondria in articular chondrocytes

Mitochondria are extremely important cellular organelles traditionally seen as the source of cellular energy production (Duchen, 2004). Articular chondrocytes contain fewer mitochondria compared to other, more metabolically active cell types, and this difference may reflect the cellular environment (i.e. hypoxia) and reliance on glycolytic metabolism rather than oxidative phosphorylation for energy production. Despite this, mitochondrial physiology and function in the chondrocyte is still critical to cellular function and they are involved in many important aspects of cell physiology in both health and disease such as ROS generation, Ca^{2+} homeostasis and cell death and survival pathways. Indeed, mitochondrial dysfunction is a key component of a number of diseases, such as diabetes and cancer, and the role of the mitochondrion in osteoarthritis is now beginning to be more fully appreciated (Terkeltaub et al., 2002).

5.2.1 Mitochondria and the chemiosmotic principle of energy production

Mitochondria contain two membrane systems, an outer and inner mitochondrial membrane (Duchen, 2004). The inner mitochondrial membrane is folded into cristae and it is here that the membrane bound enzymes (a series of complexes) of the respiratory chain are located. The chemiosmotic principle of energy production involves the oxidation of cellular substrates to produce ATP. The reductants NADH and $FADH_2$, generated from the tricarboxylic acid (TCA) cycle, enter the mitochondrial electron transport chain. NADH is oxidised to NAD^+ at complex I and $FADH_2$ is oxidised to FAD^{2+} at complex II to provide electrons for ubisemiquinone at complex III. The electron chain complexes catalyse a series of redox reactions creating an electrochemical drive to transfer H^+ from the mitochondrial matrix into the intermembrane space across the inner mitochondrial membrane. This results in a large mitochondrial transmembrane potential of around-150 to -200mV and it is this membrane potential that provides the "protonmotive force" to cause H^+ influx through F_1-F_0 ATP synthase and drive the ATPase "backwards" thus phosphorylating ADP to release ATP. The respiratory rate is regulated by this proton gradient which in turn is dependent on substrate availability, inhibitors of respiration (for example anoxia) and any mechanism that results in the uncoupling of the enzyme complexes.

In articular chondrocytes, both mitochondrial density and activity appears to be lower than other cell types with mitochondrial density significantly reduced in the deep zones compared with the upper zones of articular cartilage, likely to reflect oxygen levels in these zones. There is also evidence that the cytochrome component of the electron transport chain in articular chondrocytes may be incomplete *in situ* and provides further evidence that ATP derived from mitochondrial oxidative phosphorylation is not a major component of energy production in cartilage. Interestingly though, following transfer of cells to a relatively "oxygen-rich" environment (for example during culturing of cartilage explants or isolated cells in ambient conditions), mitochondrial biogenesis occurs (Mignotte et al., 1991). This change within the chondrocyte appears to result in a switch to oxidative phosphorylation. It has to be noted, therefore, that these conditions may not represent *in vivo* conditions of the chondrocyte and interpretation of data on cartilage metabolism requires an appreciation of these potential changes.

5.2.2 Mitochondria and reactive oxygen/nitrogen species

The process of electron transfer along the electron transport chain in mitochondria is not completely efficient and electrons may be "lost" during the redox reactions, resulting in the transfer of electrons to oxygen and the generation of oxygen radicals (reactive oxygen species, ROS). These highly reactive species can result in cellular damage due to lipid peroxidation and DNA damage so efficient mechanisms in the mitochondrium (for example superoxide dismutase) and cytoplasm (for example catalase) exist to reduce the risk of this occurring. In mitochondria of articular chondrocytes, it seems that the main site of ROS generation is complex III (Milner et al., 2007).

As well as being a potential source of cellular damage if left unchecked, reactive oxygen species are now thought to be important mediators of cell signalling. A large number of intracellular signalling pathways are regulated by ROS including cytokine receptors, receptor tyrosine kinases, receptor serine/threonine kinases and p38 MAPK cascades. This can be through the redox status of component proteins. Oxidation and reduction of -SH groups on amino acids can result in conformational change and alteration in enzyme activity. ROS may also directly regulate activity of transcription factors through oxidative modifications of conserved cysteines. Redox-sensitive transcription factors include NF-kB, AP-1, sp-1, c-myb, p53 , egr-1, HIF-1α and c-fos (Lo & Cruz, 1995). DNA-binding by AP-1 is also regulated by post-translational modifications which are redox-sensitive and this is also seen with GTP-binding protein Ras.

Nitric oxide appears to have an important role in mitochondrial function (Duchen, 2004). Complex IV has a high affinity for NO and at low O_2 competes with oxygen to inhibit mitochondrial respiration and this may be of relevance in a low oxygen system. Mitochondria may also generate NO themselves and a specific NOS has been shown to be expressed by the mitochondrium. It appears that an intricate feedback mechanism involving NO, calcium, mitochondrial electron chain activity and ROS levels may exist in the mitochondrium that may be of particular importance in low-oxygen environments such as cartilage.

Cellular antioxidant mechanisms exist though, and it is seen as a balance between ROS production and removal that determine the difference between physiological and pathological ROS levels within the cell. As with ROS, the balance between physiological and pathological NO levels are also likely to be an important factor since high NO levels react with ROS resulting in peroxynitrite production and damage to the electron chain - a feature present in disease such as osteoarthritis.

5.2.3 Mitochondria and calcium uptake

Mitochondrial calcium handling is an important component of cellular calcium homeostasis since calcium "overload" is thought to be implicated in a number of pathological states including osteoarthritis. Mitochondrial calcium uptake is driven primarily by the electrochemical gradient established by the mitochondrial potential and the relatively low Ca^{2+} concentration (Duchen, 2004). When cytosolic calcium increases, calcium moves into the mitochondrial matrix. Intramitochondrial calcium concentration is kept low under "resting" conditions by the Na^{+}/Ca^{2+} exchanger that results in calcium efflux. Ca^{2+} appears to be taken up into the matrix through the IMM by a uniporter. Additionally, voltage-dependent anion channels (VDAC) permeant to calcium exist in the outer mitochondrial membrane and may affect inner mitochondrial membrane calcium uptake by acting as a fast filter. The VDAC also appears to form part of the mitochondrial membrane permeability pore in initiating apoptosis. Calcium microdomains can exist within cells and the proximity of mitochondria to endoplasmic reticulum calcium release sites may result in mitochondria experiencing relatively high local concentrations, promoting rapid calcium uptake to allow direct transfer of calcium between mitochondria and ER (Contreras et al., 2010). In addition, the proximity to the plasma membrane by mitochondria also could allow regulation of calcium influx and therefore mitochondrial positioning could be important regulators of signalling pathways involving calcium.

5.2.4 Mitochondria and cell death

Mitochondria are intimately involved in cell death pathways. In many cells a reduction in mitochondrially derived ATP leads to loss of maintenance of ion gradients and regulation of calcium and intracellular osmolarity causing cell swelling and death. Cell swelling is an early feature of osteoarthritis and mitochondrial dysfunction is likely to be a significant component of cell death in cartilage disease.

The opening of a large conductance pore (mPTP) occurs through a conformational change of several proteins of the mitochondrial membrane due to a number of conditions such as high $[Ca^{2+}]_m$, oxidative stress, ATP depletion, high inorganic phosphate (P_i) and mitochondrial depolarisation (Duchen 2004). This irreversible high conductance opening causes mitochondrial swelling, cytochrome c release, caspase activation and apoptotic cell death. Apoptotic cell death may be a normal feature of cartilage growth and development, particularly in the hypertrophic zone of the growth plate but factors resulting in abnormal activation are important causes of cellular death and subsequent loss of cartilage integrity in joint disease.

5.2.5 Mitochondria and osteoarthritis

Mitochondria are implicated in the pathogenesis of many diseases, including osteoarthritis and mitochondrial mediated diseases are often due to hypoxic cell stress or aging - relevant factors in joint disease. In diabetes mellitus, defects in the electron chain are described (especially Complexes I and IV) and in neuronal injury (ischaemia/reperfusion injury), mitochondrial injury leads to impaired intracellular Ca^{2+} buffering, increased ROS generation and promotion of apoptosis via release of cytochrome c. Additionally, ETC complex defects are present in Alzheimer's, Parkinson's and Huntingdon's disease and peroxynitrite-mediated nitration of tyrosines in Alzheimer's disease neurons are due to increased NO.

In osteoarthritis, mitochondrial content increases in number and size and mitochondrial swelling has been noted (Terkeltaub et al., 2002). Mitochondrial numbers increase at sites of crystal formation and matrix calcification is a feature of osteoarthritis. It appears that calcification is stimulated by NO/peroxynitrite and chondrocyte apoptosis and this is in turn is modulated by ATP metabolism. Mitochondrial energy reserve is required for matrix synthesis and crystal suppression and therefore altered mitochondrial energy metabolism may lead to crystal formation.

Mitochondrial dysfunction of the electron chain (particularly complexes II and III) has been described in osteoarthritic chondrocytes and this will alter the respiratory state and mitochondrial membrane potential of the mitochondrium (Maniero et al., 2003). A collapse of the mitochondrial membrane potential results in mitochondrial swelling, disruption of the outer mitochondrial membrane and release of pro-apoptotic factors such as cytochrome c, AIF and procaspases from the intermembrane space and hence cell death.

5.3 Oxidative stress and reactive oxygen/nitrogen species in joint disease

When ROS levels exceed the cellular defence mechanisms, cellular damage can occur. This is known as oxidative stress. Increased oxygen consumption by the synovium during inflammation and the exposure to inflammatory mediators can lead to increase in ROS and RNS generation to levels that can induce cellular damage. In the inflammed joint synoviocytes appear to be the key cell driving this response, as opposed to chondrocytes, although it is the effect on the chondrocyte that will lead to compromise in cartilage integrity and hence disease (Schneider et al., 2005). In synoviocytes there are a number of sources of ROS generation, as well as mitochondrial derived ROS including xanthine oxidoreductase and membrane-bound NADPH oxidase (Henroitin et al., 2003).

Oxidative stress results in protein, lipid membrane, DNA damage and therefore cell injury and death (Finkl 2003). Lipid peroxyl radical formation can result in lipid bond cross-linking and alteration in membrane properties as well as forming products, such as aldehydes and saturated hydrocarbons that are toxic to cells. Fragmentation of hyaluronic acid is reported following oxidative damage to the glycosidic bonds. Since hyaluronic acid is a key cartilage biomolecule both in structure and cell signalling, alterations to HA structure will lead to alterations in cytoskeletal polymerisation, for example and affect cell adhesive properties. Oxidative damage to other extracellular components and ROS-induced activation of matrix metalloproteinases can add to the degradative element of these molecules and additionally, the action of IL-1 on proteoglycan loss appears to be mediated by ROS and NO (Henroitin et al., 2003). The direct degradation of proteoglycans and collagen by ROS is due to upregulation of collagenases and other MMPs as well as decreased production of TIMPs. Additionally, NO is implicated in cartilage insensitivity to IGF-1 by inhibiting IGF-1 receptor autophosphorylation. Therefore the use of antioxidant therapy has justifiable support in joint disease.

6. Conclusion

Our knowledge of the cellular processes occurring in articular chondrocytes has grown immensely over recent years but it is the appreciation of the interaction and response of these cells to their unusual and challenging environment and how these change in diseases such as osteoarthritis that will open up new exciting opportunities for potential therapeutic modulation in joint disease. How the chondrocyte senses and adapts to the dynamic nature of the extracellular matrix in health and disease makes us realise the complexity of signals involved and the multiplicity of the component parts, such as, for example, the roles of cell volume regulation, intracellular pH homeostasis and mitochondrial function on cell function in cartilage. The challenge for the future then will be to tie all these elements together and be able to paint the big picture that reveals the many complex interactions occurring within the joint.

7. List of abbreviations

AQP	*Aquaporin*
ATP	*Adenosine triphosphate*
ECM	*Extracellular matrix*
ENaC	*Epithelial sodium channel*
ERK1/2	*Extracellular signal-regulated kinase 1/2*
ETC	*Electron chain transport*
$FADH_2$	*Flavin adenine dinucleotide H_2*
GAG	*Glycosaminoglycan*
GLUT	*Glucose transporter*
HA	*Hyaluronic acid*
HIF-1	*Hypoxia-inducible factor-1*
Hz	*Hertz*
kDa	*kiloDaltons*
IGF-1	*Insulin-like growth factor-1*
IL-1	*Interleukin-1*
IMM	*Inner mitochondrial membrane*

MAPK	*Mitogen-activated protein kinase*
MCT	*Monocarboxylate transporter*
MEK	*Mitogen-activated protein kinase kinase*
MMP	*Matrix metalloproteinase*
MPa	*Megapascals*
mPTP	*mitochondrial permeability transition pore*
NADH	*Nicotinamide adenine dinucleotide H*
NHE	*Na^+/H^+ exchange*
NO	*Nitric oxide*
OA	*Osteoarthritis*
OMM	*Outer mitochondrial membrane*
PGE_2	*Prostaglandin E_2*
PKA	*Protein kinase A*
TCA	*Tricarboxylic acid cycle*
TGF-β	*Transforming growth factor-β*
TRP	*Transient receptor potential*
VAHC	*Voltage-activated H^+ channel*
VDAC	*Voltage-dependent anion channel*
VGCC	*Voltage-gated calcium channel*
VGSC	*Voltage-gated sodium channel*

8. References

Becerra, J., Adrades, J.A., Guerado, E., Zamora-Navas, P., Lopez-Puertas, J.M. & Reddi, A.H. (2010). Articular cartilage: structure and regeneration. *Tissue Engineering Part B Review,* Vol.16, No.6, (December 2010), pp. 617-627

Berridge, M.J., Bootman, M.D. & Lipp, P. (1998). Calcium - a life and death signal. *Nature,* Vol.395, No. 6703 (October 1998), pp.645-648

Browning, J.A, Walker, R.E., Hall, A.C. & Wilkins, R.J. (1999). Modulation of Na^+ x H^+ exchange by hydrostatic pressure in isolated bovine articular chondrocytes. *Acta Physiologica Scandinavica,* Vol.166, No.1, (May 1999), pp. 39-45

Bush, P.G. & Hall, A.C. (2001). The osmotic sensitivity of isolated and in situ bovine articular chondrocytes. *Journal of Orthopaedic Research,* Vol.19, No.5, (September 2001), pp. 768-778

Bush, P.G. & Hall, A.C. (2005) Passive osmotic properties of in situ human articular chondrocytes within non-degenerate and degenerate cartilage. *Journal of Cellular Physiology,* Vol.204, No.1, (July 2005), pp.309-319

Chowdhury, T.T & Knight, M.M. (2006). Purinergic pathway suppresses the release of NO and stimulates proteoglycan synthesis in chondrocyte/agarose constructs to dynamic compression. *Journal of Cell Physiology,*Vol. 290, No.3, (December 2009), pp.845-853

Clarke, R.B., Hatano, N., Kondo, C., Belke, D.D., Brown, B.S., Kumar, S., Votta, B.J. & Giles W.R. (2010). Voltage-gated K+ currents in mouse articular chondrocytes regulate membrane potential. *Channels,* Vol.4, No.3, (May-June 2010), pp. 179-191

Comper, W.D. (1996). Water:Dynamic aspects, *In* Extracellular Matrix Volume 2 Molecular Components and Interactions, Comper W.D., pp.1-21. Harwood Academic Publishers, Amsterdam

Contreras, L., Drago, I., Zampese, E. and Pozzan, T. (2010). Mitochondria: the calcium connection. *Biochimica et Biophysica acta,* Vol.1797, No.6-7, (June-July 2010), pp.607-618

Das, R.H.J., van Osch, G.J., Kreukniet, M., Oostra, J., Weinans, H. & Jahr, H. (2010). Effects of individual control of pH and hypoxia in chondrocyte culture. *Journal of Orthopaedic Research,* Vol.28, No. 4, (April 2010), pp. 537-545

Duchen, M.R.(2004). Role of mitochondria in health and disease. *Diabetes,*Vol.53, Suppl.1, (February 2004), pp. S96-S102

Erickson, G.R., Alexopoulos, L.G. & Guilak, F. (2001). Hyper-osmotic stress induces volume change and calcium transients in chondrocytes. *Journal of Biomechanics,* Vol.34, No.12, (December 2001), pp. 1527-1535

Finkl, T. (2003). Oxidant signals and oxidative stress. *Current Opinion in Cell Biology,* Vol.15, No.2, (February 2003), pp.247-254

Funabashi, K., Fujii, M., Yamamura, H., Ohya, S. & Imaizumi, Y. (2010). Contribution of chloride channel conductance to the regulation of resting membrane potential in chondrocytes. *Journal of Pharmacological Science,* Vol.113, No.1, (April 2010), pp. 94-99

Garcia, M. & Knight, M. (2010). Cyclic Loading Opens Hemichannels to release ATP as part of a chondrocyte mechanotransduction pathway. *Journal of Orthopaedic Research,* Vol.28, No.4, (April 2010), pp. 510-515

Gavenis, K., Schumacher, C., Schneider, U., Eisfeld, J., Mollenhauer, J. and Schmidt-Rohlfing, B. (2009). Expression of ion channels of the TRP family in articular chondrocytes from osteoarthritic patients: changes between native and in vitro propagated chondrocytes. *Molecular Cellular Biochemistry,* Vol.321., No.1-2, (January 2009), pp.135-143

Gelse, K., Pfander, D., Obier, S., Knaup, K.X., Wiesener, M., Hennig, F.F. & Swoboda, B. (2008). Role of hypoxia-inducible factor 1 alpha in the integrity of articular cartilage in murine knee joints. *Arthritis Research Therapy,* Vol.10. No.5, (September 2008), pp. R111

Goldring, M.B. (2006). Update on the biology of the chondrocyte and new approaches to treating cartilage diseases. *Best Practice and Research Clinical Rheumatology,* Vol.20, No.5, (October 2006), pp. 1003-1010

Grimshaw, M.J. & Mason, R.M. (2000). Bovine articular chondrocyte function in vitro depends on oxygen tension. *Osteoarthritis Cartilage,* Vol.8, No.5. (September 2000), pp.386-392

Guilak, F., Zell, R.A., Erickson, G.R., Grande, D.A., Rubin, C.T., McLeod, K.J. and Donahue, H.J. (1999). Mechanically induced calcium waves in articular chondrocytes are inhibited by gadolinium and amiloride. *Journal of Orthopaedic Research,* Vol. 17, No.3, (May 1999), pp.421-429

Guilak, F., Alexopoulos, L.G., Upton, M.L., Youn, I. Choi, J.B., Cao, L., Setton, L.A. & Haider, M.A. (2006). The pericellular matrix as a transducer of biomechanical and biochemical signals in articular cartilage. *Annuals New York Academy of Science,* Vol. 1068, (April 2006), pp. 498-512

Hall, A.C., Horowitz, E.R. & Wilkins, R.J. (1996a). The cellular physiology of articular cartilage. *Experimental Physiology,* Vol.81, No.3, (May 1996), pp.535-545

Hall, A.C., Starks, I, Shoults, C.L. & Rashidbigi, S. (1996b). Pathways for K+ transport across the bovine articular chondrocyte membrane and their sensitivity to cell volume. *American Journal of Physiology,* Vol.270, No.5(Pt 1), (May 1996), pp. C1300-1310

Hall A.C. (1999). Differential effects of hydrostatic pressure on cation transport pathways of isolated articular chondrocytes. *Journal of Cellular Physiology,* Vol.178, No.2, (February 1999), pp. 197-204

Hall, A.C. & Bush, P.G. (2001). The role of a swelling-activated taurine transport pathway in the regulation of articular chondrocyte volume. *Pflugers Archive: European Journal of Physiology,* Vol.442, No.5, (August 2001), pp.771-781

Hardingham, T. & Fosang A.J. (1992) Proteoglycans: many forms and functions. *FASEB Journal.* 6, 861-870.

Hasler, E.M., Herzog, W., Wu, J.Z., Muller, W. & Wyss, U. (1999). Articular cartilage biomechanics: theorectical models, material properties, and biosynthetic response. *Critical Reveiw of Biomedical Engineering,* Vol.27, No.6, pp.415-488

Henroitin, Y.E., Bruckner, P. And Pujol, J.P. (2003). The role of reactive oxygen species in homeostasis and degradation of cartilage. *Osteoarthritis Cartilage,* Vol.11, No.10, (October 2003), pp.747-755

Hoffmann, E.K., Lambert, I.H. & Pedersen SF. (2009). Physiology of cell volume regulation invertebrates. *Physiological Reviews,* Vol.89, No.1, (January 1999), pp. 193-277

Huber, M., Trattnig, S. & Linter, F. (2000). Anatomy, biochemistry and physiology of articular cartilage. *Investigations in Radiology,* Vol.35, No.10, (October 2000), pp. 573-580

Jeffery, A.K., Blunn, G.W., Archer, C.W. & Bentley, G. (1991). Three-dimensional collagen architecture in bovine articular cartilage. *Journal of Bone and Joint Surgery,* Vol.73-B, No.5, (September 1991), pp. 795-801

Kaab, M.J., Ito, K., Clark, J.M., Notzi, H.P. (1998). Deformation of articular cartilage collagen structure under static and cyclic loading. *Journal of Orthopaedic Research,* Vol.16, No.6, (November 1998), pp.743-751

Kerrigan, M.J. & Hall, A.C. (2008). Control of chondrocyte regulatory volume decrease (RVD) by [Ca2+]i and cell shape. *Osteoarthritis and Cartilage,* Vol.16, No.3, (March 2008), pp.312-322

Kim, Y-J., Bonassar, L.J. and Grodzinsky, A.J. (1995). The role of cartilage streaming potential, fluid flow and pressure in the stimulation of chondrocyte biosynthesis during dynamic compression. *Journal of Biomechanics,* Vol.28, No.9, (September 1995), pp.1055-1066

Knight, M.M., McGlashan, S.R., Garcia, M., Jensen, C.G. & Poole, C.A. (2009) Articular chondrocytes express connexin 43 hemichannels and P2 receptors - a putative mechanoreceptor complex involving the primary cilium? *Journal of Anatomy,* Vol.214, No.2, (February 2009), pp.275-283

Kuettner, K.E., Aydelotte, M.B.& Thonar, E.J. (1991). Articular cartilage matrix and structure: a review. *Journal of Rheumatology Supplement,* Vol.27 (February 1991), pp. 46-48

Lai, W.M., Sun, D.D., Ateshian, G.A., Guo, X.E. & Mow, V.C. (2002). Electrical signals in cartilage. *Biorheology,* Vol.39, No.1-2, pp.39-45

Lee, R.B. and Urban J.P. (1997). Evidence for a negative Pasteur effect in articular cartilage. *Biochemical Journal,* Vol. 321, No.1, (January 1997), pp.95-102

Lo, Y.Y. and Cruz, T.F. (1995). Involvement of reactive oxygen species in cytokine and growth factor induction of c-fos expression in chondrocytes. *Journal of Biological Chemistry,* Vol.270., No.20., (May 1995), pp.11727-11730

Loeser, R.F. (1993). Integrin-mediated attachment of articular chondrocytes to extracellular matrix proteins. *Arthritis Rheumatism,* Vol. 36, No.8, (August 1993), pp. 1103-1110

Loeser, R.F. (1994). Modulation of integrin-mediated attachment of chondrocytes to ECM proteins by cations, retinoic acid and TGF-β. *Experimental Cellular Research,* Vol.211, No.1, (March 1994), pp. 17-23

Loeser, R.F. (1997). Growth factor Regulation of chondrocyte integrins. Differential effects of insulin-like growth factor 1 and transforming growth factor beta on alpha 1 beta 1 integrin expression and chondrocyte adhesion to type IV collagen. *Arthritis Rheumatism,* Vol.40, No.2, (February 1997), pp. 270-276

Loeser, R.F. (2000). Chondrocyte integrin expression and function. *Biorheology* Vol.37, No.1-2, pp.109-116

Loeser, R.F. (2002). Integrins and cell signalling in chondrocytes. *Biorheology,* Vol.39, No.1-2, pp. 119-124

Lin, C., McGough, R, Aswad, B, Block, J,A. & Terek, R. (2004) Hypoxia induces HIF-1alpha and VEGF expression in chondrocsarcoma cells and chondrocytes. *Journal of Orthopaedic Research,* Vol.22, No.6, (November 2004), pp. 1175-1181

Lui, K.E., Panchal, A.S, Santhanagopal, A, Dixon, S.J. & Bernier, S.M. (2002) Epidermal growth factor stimulates proton efflux from chondrocytic cells. *Journal of Cellular Physiology,* Vol.192, No.1, pp.102-112

Maneiro, E., Martin, M.A., de Andres, M.C., Lopez-Armada, M.J., Fernandez-Sueiro, J.L., del Hoyo, P., Galdo, F., Arenas, J. and Blanco, F.J. (2003). Mitochondrial respiratory activity is altered in osteoarthritic human articular chondrocytes. *Arthritis Rheumatism,* Vol.48, No.3, (March 2003), pp.700-708

Mathy-Hartert, M. Burton, S., Deby-Dupont, G. Devel, P., Reginster, J.Y. & Henroitin, Y. (2005). Influence of oxygen tension on nitric oxide and PGE2 synthesis by bovine chondrocytes. *Osteoarthritis Cartilage,* Vol.13, No. 1, (January 2005), pp.74-79

Meredith, D., Bell, P., McClure, B. & Wilkins, R.J. (2002). Functional and molecular characterisation of lactic acid transport in bovine articular chondrocytes. *Cellular Physiology and Biochemistry,* Vol.12, No.4, pp.227-234

Meredith, D., Gehl, K.A., Seymour, J., Ellory, J.C. & Wilkins, R.J. (2007). Characterisation of sulphate transporters in isolated bovine articular chondrocytes. *Journal of Orthopaedic Research,* Vol.25, No.9, (September 2007), pp. 1145-1153

Mignotte, F., Champagne, A.M., Froger-Gaillard, B., Benel, L., Gueride, M., Adolphe, M. and Mounolou, J.C. (1991). Mitochondrial biogenesis in rabbit chondrocytes transferred to culture. *Biology of the Cell,* Vol.71., No.1-2., pp.67-72

Miki, T. & Seino, S. (2005). Role of KATP channels as metabolic sensors in acute metabolic changes. *Journal of Molecular and Cellular Cardiology,* Vol.38, No.6., (June 2005), pp. 917-925

Milner, P.I., Fairfax, T.P., Browning, J.A., Wilkins, R.J. & Gibson, J.S. (2006). The effect of O2 on pH homeostasis in equine articular chondrocytes. *Arthritis Rheumatism,* Vol.54, No.11, (November 2006), pp.3523-3532

Milner, P.I., Wilkins, R.J. & Gibson, J.S. (2007). The role of mitochondrial reactive oxygen sepcies in pH regulation in articular chondrocytes. *Osteoarthritis Cartilage,* Vol.15, No.7, (July 2007), pp.735-742

Millward-Sadler S.J., Wright, M.O. Flatman, P.W. & Salter, D.M. (2004). ATP in the mechanotransduction pathway of normal human articular chondrocytes. *Biorheology,* Vol. 41, No.3-4, pp. 567-575

Mobasheri, A., Carter, S.D., Martin-Vasallo, P. & Shakibaei, M. (2002) Integrins and stretch activated ion channels; putative components of functional cell surface mechanoreceptors in articular chondrocytes . *Cell Biology International.* Vol.26, No. 1, pp. 1-18

Mobasheri, A., Trujillo, E., Bell, S., Carter, S.D., Clegg, P.D., Martin-Vasallo, P. & Marples, D. (2004) Aquaporin water channels AQP1 and AQP3 are expressed in equine articular chondrocytes. *The Veterinary Journal,* Vol.168, No. 2, (September 2004), pp.143-150

Mobasheri, A., Gent, T.C., Nash, A.I., Womack, M.D., Moskaluk, C.A. and Barrett-Jolley, R.B. (2007) Evidence for functional ATP-sensitive (K(ATP)) potassium channels in human and equine articular chondrocytes. *Osteoarthritis Cartilage,* Vol.15, No.1, (January 2007), pp.1-8

Mobasheri, A. & Barrett-Jolley, R.B. (2011) Transient receptor potential channels: emerging roles in health and disease. *The Veterinary Journal,* Vol. 187, No.2, (February 2011), pp. 145-146

Morris, N.P., Keene, D.R. & Horton, W.A. (2002) Morphology of Connective tissue: Cartilage, *In* Connective Tissue and Its Heritable Disorders, Royce, P.M. and Steinmann, B. pp. 41-66. Wiley-Liss Inc., New York

Mow, V.C., Holmes, M.H. & Lai,W.M. (1984). Fluid transport and mechanical properties of articular cartilage: a review. *Journal of Biomechanics,* Vol.17, No.5, pp.377-394

Palmer, J.L. & Bertone, A.L. (1994). Joint structure, biochemistry and biochemical disequilibrium in synovitis and equine joint disease. *Equine Veterinary Journal,* Vol.26, No.4, pp. 263-277

Pedersen, S.F. & Cala, P.M. (2004). Comparative biology of the ubiquitous Na+/H+ exchanger, NHE1: lessons from erthrocytes. *Journal of Experimental Zoology A Experimental Biology,* Vol.301, No.7, (July 2004), pp. 569-578

Pfander, D. and Glese, K. (2007). Hypoxia and osteoarthritis: how chondrocytes survive hypoxic environments. *Current Opinion in Rhuematology,* Vol.19., No.5., (September 2007), pp.457-462

Sanchez, J.C. and Wilkins, R.J. (2003). Effects of hypotonic shock on intracellular pH in bovine articular chondrocytes. *Comparative Biochemistry Physiology A Molecular Intregrated Physiology,* Vol.135, No.4, (August 2003), pp575-583.

Sanchez, J.C., Danks, T.A. & Wilkins, R.J. (2003). Mechanisms involved in the increase in intracellular calcium following hypotonic shock in bovine articular chondrocytes. *General Physiology Biophysics,* Vol.22, No.4, (December 2003), pp. 487-500

Sanchez, J.C. & Lopez-Zapata, D.F. (2010). Effects of osmostic challenges on membrane potential in human articular chondrocytes from healthy and osteoarthritic cartilage. *Biorheology,* Vol.47, No.5-6, pp. 321-331.

Shikhman, A.R., Brinson, D.C. & Lotz, M.K. (2004). Distinct pathways regulate facilitated glucose transport in human articular chondrocytes during anabolic and catabolic responses. *American Journal of Physiology Endocrinology and Metabolism,* Vol.286, No.6, (June 2004), pp.E980-E985

Solomon, D.H., Wilkins, R.J., Meredith, D. And Browning, J.A. (2007) Characterisation of inorganic phosphate transport in bovine articular chondrocytes. *Cellular Physiology and Biochemistry,* Vol.20, No.1-4, pp.99-108

Svalastoga, E. & Kiaet, T. (1989). Oxygen consumption, diffusing capacity and blood flow of the synovial membrane in osteoarthritic rabbit knee joints. *Acta Veterinaria Scandinavica,* Vol.30, No.2, pp. 121-125

Tattersall, A., Meredith, D., Furla, P., Shen, M. R., Ellory, C. & Wilkins, R.J. (2003). Molecular and functional identification of the NHE isoforms NHE1 and NHE3 in isolated bovine articular chondrocytes. *Cellular Physiology and Biochemistry* Vol. 13, No.4. pp. 215-222

Tattersall A.L. & Wilkins, R.J. (2008) Modulation of Na^{+}-H^{+} exchange isoforms NHE1 and NHE3 by insulin-like growth factor-1 in isolated bovine chondrocytes. *Journal of Orthopaedic Research.*, Vol.26, No.11, pp. 1428-1433

Terkeltaub, R., Johnson, K., Murphy, A. and Ghosh, S. (2002). Invited review: the mitochondrion in osteoarthritis. *Mitochondrion,* Vol.1, No.4, (February 2002), pp.301-319

Urban, J.P. (1994) The chondrocyte: a cell under pressure. *British Journal of Rhuematology,* Vol.33, pp. 901-908

Urban, J.P. (2000) Present perspectives on cartilage and chondrocyte mechanobiology/ *Biorheology,* Vol.37, No.1-2, pp.185-190

Van der Kraan, P.M. & van den Berg, W.B. (2000) Anabolic and destructive mediators in osteoarthritis *Current opinion in clinical nutrition and metabolic care,* Vol. 3, pp. 205-211

Varani, K., De Mattei, M., Vincenzi, F, Tosi, A., Gessi, S, Merghi, S, Pellati, A, Masieri, F., Ongaro, A.& Borea, P.A. (2008). Pharmacological characterisation of P2X1 and P2X3 purinergic receptors in bovine chondrocytes . *Osteoarthritis and Cartilage,* Vol.16, No. 11, (November 2008), pp 1421-1429

Wang, Q.G., El Haj, A.J. & Kuiper, N.J. (2008). Glycosaminoglycan in the pericellular matrix of chondrons and chondrocytes. *Journal of Anatomy,* Vol.213, No.3., (September 2008), pp.266-273

Wilkins, R.J. and Hall, A.C. (1992). Measurement of intracellular pH in isolated bovine articular chondrocytes. *Experimental Physiology* Vol.77, pp. 521-524

Wilkins, R.J. and Hall, A.C. (1995) Control of matrix synthesis in isolated bovine chondrocytesby extracellular and intracellular pH. *Journal of Cell Physiology,* Vol.164, No.3, (September 1995), pp.474-481

Wilkins, R.J., Browning, J.A. & Ellory, J.C. (2000). Surviving in a matrix: membrane transport in articular chondrocytes. *Journal Membrane Biology.* Vol.177, No.2 (September 2000), pp. 95-108

Wilkins, R.J., Fairfax, T.P. Davies, M.E., Muzamba, M.C. & Gibson, J.S. (2003). Homeostasis of intracellular Ca^{2+} in equine chondrocytes: response to hypotonic shock. *Equine Veterinary Journal,* Vol.35, No.5, (July 2003), pp. 439-443

Wilson. J.R., Duncan, N.A., Giles, W.R. and Clark, R.B. (2004) A voltage-dependent K+ current cotributes to membrane potential of acutely isolated canine articular chondrocytes. *Journal of Physiology,* Vol.557, No.1, pp93-104

Windhaber, R.A., Wilkins, R.J. & Meredith, D. (2003). Functional characterisation of gluocse transport in bovine articular chondrocytes. *Pflugers Archive: European Journal of Physiology,* Vol.446, No.5, (August 2003), pp. 572-577

Yamazaki, N., Browning, J.A. & Wilkins, R.J. (2000) Modulation of NHE by osmotic shock in isolated articular chondrocytes. *Acta Physiologica Scandinavica* Vol.169. No. 3, (July 2000), pp. 221-228

Yellowley, C.E., Hancox, J.C. & Donahue, H.J. (2002). Effects of cell swelling on intracellular calcium and membrane currents in bovine articular chondrocytes. *Journal of Cellular Biochemistry,* Vol.86, No.2, pp. 290-301

Zhou, S., Cui, Z. & Urban, J.P. (2004). Factors affecting the oxygen concentration gradient from the synovial surface of articular cartilage to the cartilge-bone interface: a modelling study. *Arthritis Rhuematism,* Vol.50, No.12, (December 2004), pp. 3915-3924